Paying the Hospital

William A. Glaser

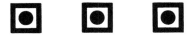

Paying the Hospital

*The Organization, Dynamics,
and Effects of
Differing Financial Arrangements*

Jossey-Bass Publishers

San Francisco   •   London   •   1987

PAYING THE HOSPITAL
The Organization, Dynamics, and Effects of Differing Financial Arrangements
by William A. Glaser

Library of Congress Cataloging-in-Publication Data

Glaser, William A.
  Paying the hospital.

  (A Joint publication in the Jossey-Bass health
series and the Jossey-Bass management series)
  Bibliography: p.
  Includes index.
  1. Hospitals—Finance.   2. Hospitals—Rates.
I. Title.   II. Series: Jossey-Bass health series.
III. Series: Jossey-Bass management series.
[DNLM: 1. Economics, Hospital.   2. Financial Manage-
ment.   3. Hospital Administration—economics.
WX 157 G658p]
RA971.3.G53   1987   362.1'1'0681   87-45421
ISBN 1-55542-048-6 (alk. paper)

Manufactured in the United States of America

The paper in this book meets the guidelines for
permanence and durability of the Committee on
Production Guidelines for Book Longevity of the
Council on Library Resources.

JACKET DESIGN BY WILLI BAUM

FIRST EDITION

Code 8727

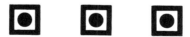

A joint publication in
The Jossey-Bass Health Series
and
The Jossey-Bass Management Series

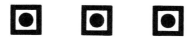

Contents

**Part Two: Methods for Financing Hospital Operations
and Capital Investment**

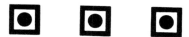

Preface

The entire fields of health economics and health financial policy hardly existed before 1974 and have exploded since. How to manage hospital finance and how to contain hospital costs—which account for between 3 and 5 percent of the gross national product (GNP) of every developed country—baffle every country's government policy makers, insurers, hospital associations, and scholars. Every country constantly tinkers with its methods of paying hospitals and searches for new techniques. And in every country there is considerable interest in learning whether another country has discovered a more effective method of managing and containing these costs.

Paying the Hospital analyzes in depth and compares the methods of paying hospitals across the principal developed countries—France, Germany, England, Holland, Switzerland, Canada, and the United States. It goes on to analyze the comparative effects of different payment methods—either within individual countries or across many countries—on administration, cost containment, and clinical performance. The volume is organized by topic, not country-by-country description, and offers information in the following sequence: methods of cost accounting, how budgets are screened and how rates are decided, units of payment, how capital is distributed for buildings and equipment, deciding wages of hospital employees and hospital doctors, the organization of medical staffs, the work of financial managers, effects of different methods on levels of costs, volume, types of services, quality of care, and so on.

Information given in this book has been gleaned from original field research (1979–1986) that involved my spending months in one country after another. Because of the importance of the subject, many books about hospital finance have been published within each country studied here. Each book, however, concerns that country alone, is written by a national of that country, and is intended as a basic textbook for courses in hospital finance or as a guide for hospital finance officers; none analyzes that country in the larger perspective of systems elsewhere. *Paying the Hospital* summarizes the highlights of studies of individual countries and includes the only information in the English language about hospital finance in France, Germany, Holland, and Switzerland.

Audience and Applications

The intended audiences for *Paying the Hospital* include policy makers, scholars, and practitioners in hospital administration, health care finance, health economics, and the politics of health care. The book is written for an international audience. Each chapter includes a summary of the advantages and disadvantages of particular arrangements, based on the experiences of different interest groups in various countries (especially the hospitals, payers, and general public); these advantages and disadvantages can also be looked at from the point of view of hospitals, payers, and government in all countries contemplating adoption of the same financial methods.

Everywhere there is constant tinkering with the hospital finance systems and requests for improvement. *Paying the Hospital* is designed to show how many different arrangements work in practice on a large scale, their successes and their defects. Before proposing new systems for their countries, policy makers can see from experiences described in this book their full setups, the presuppositions for their establishment, their weaknesses and their strengths.

The book should particularly interest Americans, who constantly debate the merits of their own hospital financing methods and who constantly look for something new. The research project began as one of my series of studies wherein I identify the principal public policy issues confronting the United States and then describe how the other developed countries try to solve them.

The volume will also interest the growing numbers of persons who teach courses in comparative health services. Most of the books available to them describe entire health care systems in general terms, but this one digs into a specific sector. It contains much about hospital services and payers in these countries and is not just about hospital finance.

Individual chapters may interest scholars outside the health field in rate regulation, capital investment, and labor relations. Hospitals now constitute a major sector in investment and employment in all developed countries, and *Paying the Hospital* provides such scholars a definitive summary of the variety of investment and wage-setting arrangements in health.

Overview of Contents

Paying the Hospital summarizes the principal forms of hospital finance among developed countries. It begins (Chapter One) with an overview of my approach to hospital finance, describing the importance and complexity of the topic and the research employed in studying it. Chapter Two summarizes the facts in the book by listing the forms of hospital organization and finance in all countries. In addition, it describes recent trends in hospital finance in the developed countries. Since every hospital's costs are the basis of the payment system, Chapter Three describes the structure of costs in the modern hospital and traces how the present situation evolved. It compares some variations among countries in the items of cost that can be included in the charges to patients and their third-party payers. The chapter also summarizes the types of forms used to report past costs, construct prospective budgets, and ask the third parties for specific payment. Chapter Four summarizes the units by which patients and third parties pay their bills. These include the widely used daily charge, itemized charges, the recently much-discussed case payments (or diagnosis-related groups), and the increasingly common global budgets. Chapter Five describes the insurance carriers, government programs, and other payers who provide the hospital's money.

The heart of the book is in Chapters Six through Nine. Chapters Six, Seven, and Eight describe methods of deciding reimbursement for operating costs. Chapter Six covers the organized negotiations between teams of insurance carriers and individual hospitals, but it also includes a few informal arrangements by individual carriers. Chapter Six also describes the unusual cases where hospitals control their own charges completely. Chapter Seven summarizes the methods wherein a neutral regulator—either government officials or an independent commission—investigates the hospital's prospective budget and sets its rates. Chapter Eight describes how some powerful payers—governments or (less often) coalitions of insurers—dictate the hospital's prospective budget and pay the budget in installments.

Chapter Nine shifts to the topic of capital investment. It summarizes the different forms of public grants for building and equipment and methods for planning them. Chapter Nine also summarizes the forms of self-financing, wherein the hospital decides its own capital priorities, borrows from special funds or from the general capital market, and then tries to retire the loan from its operating revenue.

Several chapters depict how certain principal determinants of hospital costs are themselves decided. The principal component of modern hospital costs is wages, and Chapter Ten summarizes the different forms of setting wages for nurses and other employees. The principal force determining the volume and type of work in the hospital is the medical staff, and Chapter Eleven describes how the doctors are organized, how they are paid, and problems of integrating them into modern hospital financial management. Chapter Twelve summarizes the forms of hospital ownership and management, and it examines the outcomes of whether the hospital cooperates with larger public policies or whether the hospital pursues its own goals.

Chapter Two is a summary of the facts of hospital finance, and Chapter Thirteen is a summary of results. The latter examines whether paying hospitals by one method or another makes any difference in levels of costs, in efficient treatment of patients, in appropriate access for patients, and in quality of care. The volume ends (Chapter Fourteen) with a summary of particularly salient strengths, weaknesses, policy dilemmas, and trends across all developed countries.

Each section about a payment arrangement contains generalizations about its main features and conclusions. But these cannot be fully appreciated without understanding the structure and practical operations of each arrangement. Publications about hospital finance are usually textbooks for managers, accountants, and regulators, explaining calculating methods. Because very little in any language describes how each country's arrangement works in practice, I have presented such information here. I include many details, so the reader can understand each arrangement fully.

The book goes considerably beyond merely comparing countries' current financing arrangements; it also explains *why* they differ. A full perspective is essential for the hospital administrators and politicians of any country who—submerged in their daily affairs—naturally tend to think their own arrangements normal and superior. In fact, every country's system results from a long and often conflict-ridden political give-and-take, not from a recent rational invention. Therefore, the book includes descriptions of the evolution of the current arrangements. In all countries, these changes continue today; what we call "the present situation" is merely a cross-section of a continuing history.

New York City   William A. Glaser
August 1987

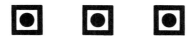

Acknowledgments

The research about hospital finance was supported by Grant No. 18P-97363/2, Health Care Financing Administration, U.S. Department of Health and Human Services. The findings do not necessarily reflect policies of HCFA. Work was also assisted by an earlier study of federal-provincial relations in health care finance, supported by Grant Number HS 02453 from the National Center for Health Services Research, OASH.

The field research was conducted while I was affiliated with the Center for the Social Sciences of Columbia University. In this—as in my previous work— the late Madeline Simonson made invaluable administrative contributions.

For their reading of my preliminary national monographs and other manuscripts, I am indebted to L. M. J. Groot, J. B. Stolte, and Kees Kleemans of the Netherlands; Pierre Gilliand, Danielle Bridel, Werner Frischknecht, and Jean-Paul Robert of Switzerland; John Perrin, Stuart Dimmock, and Robert Milne of Great Britain; Donald Stewart and A. Peter Ruderman of Canada; and the following Americans: George Silver, Odin W. Anderson, J. Michael Fitzmaurice, Eli Ginzberg, Dorothy P. Rice, Anders Richter, and Rosemary Stevens.

For expert typing of all manuscripts, I am grateful to Charlotte Fisher and Dorothy Mullen. As in all my peripatetic research, I was greatly helped by Richard Carlson and Teri Hilger of the Columbia Travel Service.

I am most indebted to the many administrators and scholars in Europe and North America who were so generous with their time and information. My principal informants are listed in Appendix B.

The epigraph by Roger Grégoire preceding the text is taken from "Pour une réforme hospitalière," in *Pour une politique de la santé* (Paris: Ministère de la Santé Publique et de la Sécurité Sociale, 1971), Vol. 3, p. 153. Quoted by permission of La Documentation Française. The translation into English is mine.

W.A.G.

For Gilberte

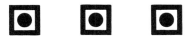

The Author

William A. Glaser is professor of health services administration and gerontological services administration at the New School for Social Research in New York. He received his B.A. degree (1948) from New York University in political science and his M.A. (1949) and Ph.D. (1952) degrees from Harvard University, also in political science.

His main research activities have been in cross-national comparative research about health services, government, and other topics. His books on comparative health care include *Paying the Doctor* (1970), *Social Settings and Medical Organization* (1970), and *Health Insurance Bargaining* (1978). From other cross-national research, he has written *The Brain Drain* (1978). From research about American government, he has written *Public Opinion and Congressional Elections* (1962) and *Pretrial Discovery and the Adversary System* (1968). In his many research projects, Glaser has prepared reports advising government agencies and private organizations.

From 1956 to 1982, Glaser was a senior research associate at Columbia University.

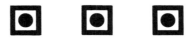

Paying the Hospital

Hospital payment for several years has been the target of criticisms and of proposals for recasting. To be sure, it has defects. But it is an illusion to expect from its transformation a better management and substantial savings. Without doubt a badly conceived payment system can encourage routine and even motivate certain expenditures. But the resources devoted to a public service ought in all circumstances cover its duties, and it should not happen that, while restraining the resources by modifying the methods of calculating them, the fulfillment of the duties themselves is substantially reduced.

Roger Grégoire
"Pour une réforme hospitalière"

1

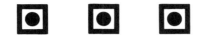

Introduction:
Studying Methods
of Hospital Finance

Hospitals were once charitable services; now they have become profitable industries. Once their users were the poor; now every hospital manager seeks the largest number of payers. Once the employees presumed that their rewards would come in Heaven; now they earn high incomes and have jobs rather than callings.

As evidence of their secularization, hospitals everywhere have become leading problems in economic policy. Total health expenditures now exceed 10 percent of gross national product (GNP) in several developed countries and approach that percentage in others. Hospitals account for about half of all health spending—more in some countries, less in others—and absorb between 3.5 and 6 percent of GNP.[1]

Once the public policy issue was how to improve the buildings, equipment, and staffs of hospitals; that is, how to spend more money on the capital and operations of hospitals, and how to find it. By the 1970s the problem was limits and balance. Finance officers of governments were the principal constituency for cost containment. In countries where expenditures for patient care was run through the general Treasury (as in Canada, Britain, and American Medicaid), government finance officers worried about the future bankruptcy of the accounts and the need to rescue them by Treasury subsidies; they also questioned whether stopgaps such as greater cost sharing by patients really reduced costs and were politically feasible. In countries where health and hospitals were paid by private carriers (as in Germany, Holland, and American Blue Cross and commercial insurance), government officials were responsible for setting or approving the premiums and payroll taxes, and they worried that too much of the national income was being redirected through this channel, that health providers were profiting without giving an adequate return, that health services were inefficient and wasteful, that the premiums and payroll taxes would destroy incentives to work and invest, and that the premiums and payroll taxes would become politically unacceptable. The executives of the carriers themselves worried that premiums and payroll taxes might soon be limited, causing them to go bankrupt, and that the steady rise of hospital costs was taking money better spent on other forms of care. (While health spending rises in all countries faster than consumer prices and GNP, hospital spending usually rises faster than other health spending. In other words, hospitals absorb a larger proportion of all money devoted to health.)[2]

By the 1970s the rise in all clinical-care expenditures—the greater share for inpatient hospital work—led to widespread misgivings by policy makers in clinical affairs and in public health, beyond fiscal concerns alone. They worried that technologically advanced hospitals might be overtreating patients, who might be better off with primary care; that many basic treatments and tests were being done unnecessarily in the more expensive hospital instead of in ambulatory facilities; and that too much effort and money went into treatment, not enough into prevention.

During the 1970s many conferences brought together health care leaders and economists from developed countries, ostensibly to present solutions to all these problems. But in their fleeting contacts, the participants merely presented separate descriptions of national methods and recited their woes. Mutual understanding in depth was scarce—largely because the participants were involved in the complex and demanding affairs of their own countries and therefore could not learn about others thoroughly enough to recognize and translate the lessons from abroad that applied to their own situations.

Purpose of This Book

This volume will analyze the principal methods of paying hospitals in developed countries. I will start with overviews of the hospital structures and third-party payment systems. Then I will summarize the construction of budgets, the units of payment, and the methods of collection. The book will convey the dynamics of each system—how the hospitals, payers, and public authorities interact to decide the hospital's allowable budget and to fix the unit of payment. It will summarize certain determinants of hospital costs, such as wages, investments, and levels of utilization. This volume is a companion to my two earlier books about the principal methods of paying doctors in the world.[3]

Much recent writing about health care finance compares aggregate outcomes and leaps to the conclusion that one system is better because the total national outcome is better. For example, if Country X has lower per capita costs than Country Y, and if the writer knows that the two countries have different payment systems, he may recommend Country X's system. Or, if Country Y has more modern facilities and no waiting lists, another writer with a different philosophy may recommend Country Y as a model. This book examines the mysterious "black boxes," how each system is constructed, how it operates, how it produces results—including many results unknown to distant foreign observers who focus on only a few macrostatistics. Generalizations about how to pay hospitals are premature unless one understands the complete dynamics, strengths, and difficulties of the alternatives.

This book provides an overview of methods of payment and their determinants, rather than an in-depth analysis of each individual country. It describes the organization and operation of programs in order to explain how the "black boxes" work, but it does not present full details. Included are some statistics—where they are available and reliable—in order to document statements about orders of magnitude and trends. But the book does not attempt extensive descriptions with full statistics. The notes at the back of the book refer readers to more extensive sources.

Identifying Effects. Ideally, an analysis of payment systems should compare the results, not merely the administration. One might ask whether one or another method of paying hospitals makes a difference in providing access to patients, motivating the best quality of care, stimulating efficiency, controlling costs, and encouraging innovation. Since a payment system for hospitals is usually standardized throughout a country, the effects can be identified only when entire countries are compared—preferably through comparisons of statistical rates among countries. Such comparisons require similar data among all the principal countries. At present, instead of collecting and reporting identical data about hospitals, each country does the opposite, generating only that information needed by its own administrative practices and policies. Therefore, complex comparisons about the effects of national payment systems cannot be made. However, the groundwork for standardized epidemiological, administrative, and financial statistics is now being negotiated among countries,[4] and comparisons might be possible in the future.

Data are reported in each country today. I will use them to make informed inferences about some variations in the operations and consequences of payment systems. However, these inferences must be made cautiously, since the data are imperfect in reliability as well as lacking in standardization.[5] One must understand the institutional systems and interpret statistical differences intelligently, disentangling real differences among the systems from the artifacts of current statistical reporting.[6]

One should search for the effects of different financial methods on the purpose of the entire exercise—that is, on the appropriateness and quality of care and on the recovery of patients. But the effects of hospital financial management on the performance of clinicians and on the experiences of patients are only now being identified in a few countries. Firm conclusions are not yet available in single countries, let alone possible in comparing their different national systems.

Recommending Solutions. In such a universally troubled field, a study ideally should find "the answers." The present book merely describes and analyzes the principal payment systems, to present reliable facts and a common understanding to persons whose roles and self-interest might make them adversaries in policy. My other publications from the research have attempted to make recommendations to policy makers in the United States. They have focused on the principal issues facing the United States, described how other developed countries and the Americans have dealt with these problems, and then offered lessons for the United States. I have not been financed by or associated with one client, but I have reported to all sides. My "lessons from abroad" have not been recommendations for any one scheme, but I have spelled out several options from foreign experience, and I have predicted possible outcomes from foreign precedents if a particular scheme were attempted in the United States. My proposals have been stimuli for thought rather than final blueprints.[7]

Research Methods

From 1979 through 1981, working alone, I collected information about the methods of paying hospitals in Switzerland, the Netherlands, France, Canada, England, and West Germany. (I list them in sequence followed.) I spent two or three months in each country learning the following information, where applicable to the financial system there. To learn about new developments, I returned to Holland, France, and Germany for several weeks during mid-1984 and for several months during 1986. In addition, I have kept in touch with American developments for many years.

- ☐ Overview.
  - General pattern of health and hospital services in the country.
  - General pattern of health insurance in the country.
- ☐ Accounting methods by hospitals. How they keep their books.
- ☐ Reporting by hospitals.
  - Financial reporting to the agency that decides the rates or that grants money to the hospital.
  - Financial, administrative, and clinical reports to the Ministry of Health or the Census Bureau.
- ☐ How the hospital develops its claim for higher rates or higher grants next year.
- ☐ How the paying agencies (such as the sickness funds or government Ministry) evaluate the hospital's claim and develop their own offer. How regulators and investigators work.
- ☐ Development of guidelines for use by the hospital, the regulator, or the grantor.
  - How guidelines (for example, personnel/bed ratios) are developed by parent organizations, such as Ministries of government, national associations of hospitals, and national associations of sickness funds.
  - How hospitals and sickness funds develop data systems in making their decisions. Principles of designing classes and peer group comparisons.
- ☐ How the components of the hospital's total costs are decided. Whether any of the following decisions are coordinated with the decision to set rates or grant budgets:
  - Wage rates and conditions of services of hospital workers. Labor negotiations. Any guidelines and restraints by higher authorities, such as wage policy by government.
  - Wage rates and conditions of service of hospital doctors. How their salaries are negotiated. How fee schedules are negotiated. The mix of salaries and fees in determining their work schedules and incomes.
  - Buildings and equipment.
    - Sources of investment money. Government funds, special public funds, private capital market.
    - How hospital develops its request.

       — Negotiations between the grantor or lender and the hospital. Whether future operating costs are considered.

       — Role of sickness funds in investment grants.

☐ What happens in the meetings between hospitals, on the one hand, and, on the other hand (depending on the country's system), rate regulators, negotiators from sickness funds, or grantors of government money.

☐ Appeals procedure.

☐ Billing and cash flow.

    • Collections from sickness funds.

    • Collections from patients if

       — Patient is not covered by any health insurance.

       — Patient is private.

☐ Variations in the payment system.

    • For-profit private hospitals compared with the nonprofits.

    • Teaching hospitals compared with the nonteaching.

    • Special payment rate different from the main ones.

    • Different administrative and decision-making arrangements in different parts of the country. For example, variations among provinces in federal systems.

☐ Statistics about the use and financing of hospitals.

☐ Perceptions of strong and weak points among persons in the country.

☐ Trouble spots in the politics, administration, and finance of hospital affairs.

In each country my field research has relied primarily on interviews with persons involved in hospital finance. The interviews have been qualitative in their flexible style of posing and answering questions, but a definite set of topics is covered in each instance, to elicit a systematic description of the respondent's work. Interviews lasted from one to three hours apiece.[8] My principal informants are listed in Appendix B.

In each country I interviewed the following persons about their work in the following topics (where applicable to the country):

☐ Ministry officials in national government.

    • Finance and Budget.

       — Social security taxes, subsidies to sickness funds, subsidies to hospitals.

       — Appropriations for the hospitals' operating costs.

    • Ministry that oversees the health insurance system.

    • Ministry that oversees the hospitals.

       — Guidelines for rate regulators.

       — Distribution of grants to hospitals for operating costs and investments.

       — Drafters of new laws and regulations about hospital finance.

    • Statisticians who gather and report data about hospitals.

☐ Headquarters of national and regional hospital associations.

    • Participants in any negotiations about new laws and regulations.

    • Participants in any negotiations about contracts and principles of payment.

- ☐   •   Experts in giving advice about finance to member hospitals.
- ☐   Headquarters of national and regional health insurance associations.
  - •   Participants in any negotiations about new laws and regulations.
  - •   Participants in any negotiations about contracts and principles of payment.
  - •   Experts in giving advice about hospital finance to member sickness funds.
- ☐   Directors and finance officers of several individual hospitals. Occasionally, a chief of service.
- ☐   Officials of some local sickness funds who:
  - •   Negotiate with hospitals over rates.
  - •   Testify before rate regulators.
  - •   Review the hospitals' bills and order payment.
- ☐   Officials of the rate regulation office.
- ☐   Local officials of the national or provincial government who distribute money to the hospital.
- ☐   Officials of the medical association who specialize in negotiating the pay rates for specialists.
- ☐   Officials of the trade unions who negotiate pay and working conditions of hospital workers.
- ☐   Scholars who have done research about hospital finance.

Besides field notes from interviews, in each country I collected recent publications and statistics about hospital finance. Many sources appear in the notes at the back of the book. The voluminous citations might make this book seem a review of the literature, but it is not. The text is based on my interviews, with additional details relegated to the source notes. In particular, my text contains few statistical tables, but the interested reader can find many in the sources.

In addition, I performed equivalent but less structured fieldwork in the United States. I conducted interviews and made site visits in many parts of the country at various times from 1978 through 1983.

Earlier Research

The present work is built on previous efforts. During 1961 and 1962, I traveled continuously in sixteen countries, to learn about the social structure of hospitals and the payment of physicians.[9] Revisiting the same countries for my cross-national research in subsequent years, and revisiting many of the same hospitals during the late 1970s, I have watched their evolution in organization and in finance. In addition, I conducted studies of medical and nursing education in American teaching hospitals.[10] Additional background for the current research came from my research about how national health insurance is administered and financed in Europe and North America.[11]

Exchange Rates

Because we are interested in the structure of payment systems rather than in the international equivalence of incomes and services, the text will deal entirely with local currencies. However, I present here a convenient summary of the figures for the principal countries I investigated. Since this was a period of great fluctuations in exchange rates, I include the numbers at the start and finish of my research:

Country	Currency	*Number of units of each European currency equaling one American $ in:*	
		1979	*mid-1985*
Canada	Dollar ($)	1.17	1.35
France	Franc (F)	4.25	8.70
Germany (Federal Republic)	Deutsche Mark (DM)	1.83	2.85
Great Britain	Pound (£)	0.47	0.72
Netherlands	Guilder (fl)	2.01	3.22
Switzerland	Franc (Fr S)	1.66	2.35

Abbreviations

Abbreviations and non-English words repeatedly used in the text are defined in the Glossary of Abbreviations, pp. 473–476.

2

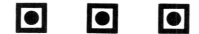

Characteristics
of Hospitals
and Finance Systems

A simple taxonomy of the world's hospital systems is difficult to find. Hardly anyone has attempted to write an overview, and authors get bogged down in detailed variations.[1] A very few books collect separate descriptions of hospitals in several countries.[2] A more manageable effort is to focus on a few themes and generalize about them across several countries,[3] but few researchers have attempted even this. This chapter will summarize the principal methods of organizing and paying hospitals in developed countries. Appendix A describes each individual country where I did extensive field research.

Ownership

Voluntary Associations, Churches, and Religious Orders. These associations and orders once owned nearly all hospitals in Europe and North America. They still own most of them. In a few countries (notably, France and Great Britain), however, government has taken them over. In a few Catholic countries, such as Italy and Spain, the churches and religious orders could no longer afford to maintain hospitals, and the responsibilities have been assumed by voluntary associations of laymen, as charitable good works.

Government. There is a growing trend toward local government ownership and management of hospitals—largely because government intervention has proved necessary to resolve health crises or to meet needs in areas unserviced by private groups. Government hospitals have the advantage of more money for investment than the voluntary associations have. As a result, most public hospitals today are owned and managed by local governments. Britain, with its National Health Service, is the only Western country where the hospitals are owned nearly exclusively by the national government. Before 1946 British hospitals were owned by voluntary associations and by local governments, but the bankruptcy of the financing system required greater government intervention. The medical profession pressed to take all hospitals out of the hands of local governments.[4]

If one or more waves of anticlericalism and expropriation of church property occur in a country, as they did in France and Italy, most of its hospitals fall into the hands of local governments (although Italy still has many church-owned establishments). A distinction should be made, however, between ownership and management. The national government of France assumed title to many church-owned hospitals during the 1790s; they later became public corporations affiliated with the *communes,* and now they are managed by intricate coalitions of representatives from both national and communal governments.[5]

In federal systems (such as Germany, Switzerland, parts of Canada, and in many cases the United States), provincial governments own the public universities and therefore the teaching hospitals. Provincial governments also often own the principal mental hospitals. Sweden's regional governments (the "counties") are responsible for the social services; therefore, Sweden is one of the few countries where regional governments own and manage all the acute hospitals.

Doctors. Until the late nineteenth century, the large hospitals owned by associations, churches, and governments were patronized by the poor. Richer persons were treated at home by their personal physicians. When surgery and obstetrics became more successful, doctors created small "private clinics" with a few beds apiece, extending their private offices. Throughout Europe and the United States during the late nineteenth and twentieth centuries, the private clinics became very common. They have steadily diminished in number as the nonprofit and public hospitals modernized, but such proprietary establishments owned by individual doctors can still be found in France, Germany, and the Mediterranean countries.[6]

The complexities and costs of modern acute care make unviable the small private clinics with only one doctor and a few dozen beds. Some partnerships of several doctors have created larger and better-provided private clinics in France, Switzerland, and the United States.

Business Firms Owned by Laymen. Nursing homes evolved out of rooming houses and old-age homes, and many are owned and managed by persons other than doctors. Physicians prefer acute care to the mix of social services and health maintenance involved in geriatric care. Laymen rarely own individual private clinics for acute care, since these clinics evolved out of physicians' office practices.

Some large corporations owned by laymen have created chains of acute hospitals, either by buying existing ones or by creating new ones in underprovided areas. They are active in only a few countries, most conspicuously the United States.[7] A nursing home chain and a private insurance company have created acute hospitals in England, to provide a private alternative to the National Health Service.

Combinations. Only in a few countries, such as Sweden, are all acute hospitals owned and managed uniformly. Even when government intervenes to take over and rationalize a patchwork—as in France in 1793–1795 and Britain in

1946–1948—additional new forms later spring up. Most developed countries today have a mixture of nonprofit and municipal acute hospitals, with the latter growing in budgets and utilization. Many countries have proprietary hospitals, usually still owned by doctors; but some (such as the Netherlands) do not. If the health insurance carriers refuse to pay private clinics (as in Holland), the clinics can no longer survive.

(Throughout this book the term "private hospitals" refers both to the nonprofit hospitals owned by associations or churches and to the for-profit hospitals owned by doctors or laymen. The term "public hospitals" refers to those owned by national, regional, or local governments. In some countries—such as Canada and West Germany—the word "private" is reserved for the for-profit hospitals, and "public" for the nonprofits. But I do not employ that usage here.)

The Entity

The traditional image of a "hospital" refers to a building with walls and a definite boundary. Its staff and patients are located within the walls. Outsiders are identified with other organizations. However, during the late twentieth century, the "hospital" in several countries is becoming less clear-cut.

Differentiated Services. As health care has become more elaborate, the services within one building have become more differentiated, and a set of buildings may be created with a division of labor. For example, as French public hospitals modernized in many *communes,* the new building became the acute hospital, while the old building became the home (the *hospice*) for elderly persons, who once shared space with the younger short-stay patients. Recently a triad has become common: an even more modern building houses the acute-care patients, while extended-care and *hospice* patients occupy older buildings. The same ownership and management apply to all three installations; patients are transferred back and forth as needed; and many services are shared. It is often difficult to compare the performance of hospitals both within and among countries; a complication is inclusion of some of these differentiated sets.

Another additional service is the outpatient department. In some countries, such as Britain, outpatient departments provide care that precedes and follows inpatient hospitalization. In others, such as Sweden and the United States, they are full-scale providers of routine ambulatory care. In a few countries, such as Germany, the acute hospitals still lack outpatient facilities. A flourishing outpatient department brings much revenue and work to the hospital and might even overshadow the inpatient work. Therefore, when studying a country's hospitals and analyzing its data, one must understand the magnitude and functions of outpatient services.

Multihospital Systems. When several hospitals have a common owner— such as a religious order in Germany, a nonprofit trust in Britain, or a business corporation in America—they can share common services. Examples are accounting, billing, purchasing, the pharmacy, laboratory work, and personnel management. Individual hospitals may seem to be simpler and more economical than free-standing establishments in this and other countries, because the common services appear only in the accounts of the headquarters. The efficiencies and financial advantages of such arrangements enable the for-profit companies to buy marginal free-standing organizations in the United States.

Multihospital arrangements can be negotiated among free-standing hospitals as well as created by a parent headquarters. Many cooperative agreements have recently been negotiated among hospitals in the same communities in the United States, to share laundries, pharmacies, laboratories, expensive diagnostic equipment, ambulances, and so on. America readily adopts such methods, because hospital management is not standardized and because each hospital constantly looks for methods to maximize revenue and minimize costs.[8]

Debundling. Organizational innovation in the United States has altered the free-standing autonomous organization, not only by widespread multihospital arrangements but also by fragmentation.[9] Departments that once were parts of the traditional hospital organization are often incorporated separately. They continue to do the hospital's work—plus some outside work—but as nominally autonomous entities. Examples are radiology, the laboratory, the emergency room, and anesthesiology. Separate incorporation has been designed to evade planning regulations and reimbursement controls. Whether these methods will spread within America and to other countries remains to be seen. Meanwhile, when generalizing about the American hospital sector and comparing hospitals, one has to include these nominally separate services.

Management

Governing Boards. In developed countries each individual hospital often is managed by a Governing Board. Its membership and powers are spelled out by the rules of the private association (if the owner is a nonprofit organization) or by the laws of the government. In publicly owned systems, the board may be a committee responsible to the legislature (as in Sweden) or a collection of locally influential politicians and citizens (as in France). In countries with national health services (such as Great Britain and the Soviet Union), the individual hospital is not autonomous and therefore lacks its own governing board. But in Britain monitoring and planning boards exist at higher tiers in the hierarchy, dealing with clusters of publicly owned facilities. In privately owned chains—as in European religious arrangements or in American private hospital corporations—boards exist at the top.

The individual hospital board monitors the managers and provides a link between the managers and the community. Sometimes it acts as representative of the community, ensuring that the managers are responsive. In many countries the board acts as the political arm of the managers, helping them find new investment funds and seeking exceptions to regulations and cost controls.

Directors. In every Western country, the hospital is directed not by a "medical director" but by a layman who has graduated from courses in health administration. The medical director survives in countries with many doctors and vertical bureaucracies (as in the Soviet Union), where the doctor rises in his career by moving into executive positions.

When hospitals were simple and stagnant organizations, the financial functions were modest and the finance officer was merely a clerk. As budgeting, accounting, and cost control have become important, the chief financial officer everywhere has risen in power, skills, and salary. This officer is particularly important in the United States, where raising revenue, fixing charges, and writing bond issues are crucial to the hospital's survival.

Medical Staffs

Doctors decide the utilization and level of costs of hospitals. How they are organized is fundamental to the structure and financing of the hospital more generally.

Extent of Staff Privileges. Urban areas in nearly all developed countries now have predominantly closed staffs. That is, only a specified group of doctors has admitting and treatment privileges in each hospital. This distinction has produced two classes within medicine: (1) the hospital specialists, who have a monopoly on teaching and on remunerative advanced care, and (2) the office doctors, who are confined to simpler care in ambulatory settings or in private clinics.

In rural areas and small towns, places without specialists, open staffing prevails, so that any qualified physician can admit and treat in the locality's hospitals. In its familiar spirit of open opportunity, the United States once permitted open staffing in many city hospitals as well. Recently, however, problems of quality control and administrative order have produced a compromise in the United States: many office doctors are screened and approved as "attending" or "courtesy physicians," but the hospital is led by an inner core of specialists. The result still makes American hospital organization more amorphous than any foreign one, and more office doctors are able to do specialized work.

Time Devoted to the Hospital. Once no senior doctors spent all their time inside the hospital. They saw a few patients, taught students, and managed their service for a few hours at a nominal salary but spent most of their time in private practice in offices and private clinics. The trend in every country has been toward full-time salaried practice for the seniors as well as for the juniors. Part-timers are still found in Europe among the office doctors who work in local hospitals in rural areas and small towns. Some medium-sized European hospitals lack the work load for a full-timer in certain specialties (such as orthopedics, ENT, and ophthalmology), and they sign local specialists to part-time contracts. The United States is the only country where the typical hospital doctor still spends most of his time outside, seeing only his own patients and a few others inside.

In recent decades in almost every country, the hospital system has stabilized its organization by persuading its senior doctors to stay on the grounds all the time. To do so, the government and sickness funds have had to agree to very high pay for these doctors and also to limited rights of private practice within the hospital. Junior doctors have always been full-time salaried.

Service Structure. The tradition in Europe has been hierarchical. A service is headed by one chief for life, such as a chief in surgery. Under this chief is a hierarchy of juniors. Another specialist may be affiliated, with a title that makes him sound like the chief's colleague and not a subordinate. This hierarchical structure has several drawbacks. The chief becomes too powerful, too rich, and too difficult to influence. His span of control is too wide, since he rules many beds and all subspecialties in the clinical area. Young doctors wait too long for promotion.

A departmental structure is being introduced into French hospitals during the 1980s. Senior doctors in many related subspecialties become colleagues in a department and elect a chairman for a fixed term.

Britain has an egalitarian medical staff. Within a service are several coequal specialists, each with a subordinate group of juniors and very clear jurisdiction, such as his own set of beds and patients.

Some countries have diffuse medical staff structures. The hospital on paper may have several services, with full-timers administering the clinical aspects but with many other doctors—full time or part time—affiliated. An example is the United States. Or the departmental structure itself is not clear. An example is the Netherlands.

Paying the Hospital Doctor. At one time senior doctors earned most of their income from fees, in private practice and under national health insurance. Senior hospital doctors got small salaries but earned most of their incomes from fees outside. Doctors in offices and in proprietary hospitals still earn fees, both from patients' health insurance and from their out-of-pockets. Other hospital doctors rely less on fees, although some full-time senior hospital staffs (for example, in the Netherlands and Canada) are still paid by fee-for-service. American attendings also are still paid by fee-for-service.

A trend has been toward full-time hospital affiliations in almost every country, and usually (not always) this has involved full-time salaries. The salaries are counted in the comprehensive daily charge or global budget collected by hospitals from sickness funds and governments; but fees usually mean that the doctor bills the sickness funds directly, without a role for the hospital. Often the salaried arrangements forbid private fee-earning practice (as in France and Sweden), but sometimes the specialist may also see private patients for fees (as in Germany).

Once many American radiologists and pathologists collected a proportion of the earnings of their departments from itemized billing. No other country has ever used this method. It has rapidly declined in the United States because Medicare has preferred paying all doctors by fee-for-service.

Sources of Revenue for the Hospital

National Health Insurance. NHI is the common method in Europe. Payroll taxes are levied on workers and employers and are paid into special sickness funds. Government helps pay the premiums of the elderly and the unemployed by subsidizing the carriers. The sickness funds (carriers) pay the hospitals and doctors.

Government Revenue. Government revenue commonly pays for construction and heavy equipment but is unusual for patient care. It is adopted only if national health insurance proved inadequate financially (Great Britain and Italy) or if NHI was never tried and private insurance was inadequate (Canada).

Private Insurance. The Netherlands is the only European country with a substantial number of persons not covered by NHI; nearly all these persons have private policies. The United States is the only developed country without NHI on a large scale; it has a mixture of different nonprofit and private policies. (The American mixture includes a kind of small-scale NHI for the aged and revenue-supported charity care for the poor.)

Cash Payments by Patients. Once common, cash payments by patients are now rare in all countries, except for extra benefits. Health insurance evolved to enable patients to pay; and the sickness funds then became third parties, paying hospitals directly. Cash payments for part or all of the fees are still common in the payment of doctors in a few countries, such as the United States and Belgium.

Charitable Donations. Donations once were common for investments and operating costs in all countries. They have now disappeared almost everywhere, except for some gifts of buildings and equipment for special programs. In the absence of general public financing and national health insurance, many American hospitals still depend on donations, even for shortfalls in their operating budgets.

Reinvestment of Profits. In the past, hospitals in many countries had endowments of land, buildings, vineyards, orchards, and the like. The fortunate ones could pay for much of their operations from rents and from sales of merchandise. Periods of inflation, depression, and wars have forced most to sell their valuable properties; or the yields did not keep up with the growing magnitude of hospital operations. Not many foreign hospitals still have profitable endowments, but a few do.

In all countries except the United States, hospitals cannot earn profits from the mainstream of national health insurance or from governmental payments. A few proprietary hospitals earn profits, but they have private clienteles. Rate regulators from government and negotiators from sickness funds abroad never allow profits; their calculations cover the hospital's costs and no more. The United States is the only country where the proprietaries can earn a profit and where the nonprofits can receive a return on capital under the principal health insurance and the principal public grants for operations.

How the Hospital's Revenue is Decided

Hospital Sets Its Own Charges. Once this was the rule, but it is unrealistic today, when every country has one or several organized payers and when governments intervene on behalf of the public interest to prevent waste, profiteering, and fraud. The United States is the only country where hospital managers come close to setting their own budgets and price schedules: in most American states, the managers face separate organized payers and are constrained over each arrangement, although they have discretion over certain prices and over the total mix.

Adversarial Bargaining. Bargaining between the individual hospital (backed up by the provincial or national hospital association) and all organized payers forming a team is the standard method for determining the contracts and fees of office doctors; bilateral negotiation in hospital finance, however, is unusual. It exists for all hospitals in West Germany and for the proprietary hospitals in France. In limited form, such bilateral negotiation sets the contracts and rates between America's Blue Cross and individual hospitals.

Screening Agency. An arrangement whereby a screening agency represents all the hospitals and all the sickness funds sometimes replaces bilateral negotiation between hospitals and sickness funds. The screening agency is both expert investigator and arbitrator. An example is the *Centraal Orgaan Tarieven Gezondheidszorg* (COTG) in the Netherlands, which also could function as a government regulatory commission under some circumstances. A few such joint commissions exist in French-speaking Switzerland, but with wider scope, since they involve the cantonal governments as well; a few American committees created either by the hospital association or by Blue Cross—for instance, in Michigan and Indiana—operate in a somewhat similar way.

Government Regulation of Hospital Budgets and Rates. In France and some American states, such as New York and New Jersey, a government agency regulates hospital budgets and rates. In other American states, such as Maryland and Washington, an independent commission—which is created by law and is part of government but is not directed by a line agency reporting to the chief executive—serves as the regulatory agency. This device is peculiar to the United States, with its suspicion of politicians and fear that line agencies can be captured by one side.

Government Pays Hospitals Their Operating Costs and Sets the Amounts. In Britain, Canada, and Italy, hospitals may initiate requests, or government may allocate its available money among hospitals without reviewing the hospital managers' requests first; in either case, the final word is determined by interaction between the Treasury and the Ministry of Health. In Switzerland the cantonal governments decide the shares of the hospital budgets coming from the sickness funds and their own public budgets.

Ubiquity of Change. In every country the payment of hospitals encounters recurrent difficulties in the form of cost overruns or deficits in services, or both. The method of paying hospitals is the object of frequent adjustment and periodic transformation. Each reform produces unexpected complications and further corrections. Several countries have changed their payment methods during the course of my research, and in the future many others will depart substantially from their current practices.

In contrast, each country tends to freeze its method of paying doctors. National health insurance and national health services usually adopt the traditional method, since the doctors, payers, and government cannot easily agree on a new one. Once a deal is struck, everyone lets sleeping dogs lie.

Unit of Payment

Global Budget. When government pays all or nearly all the hospital's revenue, as in Britain and Canada, payments usually are made in twelve or twenty-four installments to cover the entire amount allotted for operating costs during the coming year. A British hospital's budget is part of a hierarchy of budgets in the National Health Service. Each Canadian hospital is autonomous and gets its own global grant from its provincial government.

Daily Charge. A standard daily charge is averaged over the complete or nearly complete costs of caring for all patients. A hospital is paid for the number of days of each individual patient's hospitalization multiplied by the standard daily charge. This has been the most common way of paying for hospital care under third-party payment systems.

The daily charge can take various forms. It can be all-inclusive, including physicians' salaries. It can be averaged across all clinical services in the hospital. An example is West Germany's nonprofit and public hospitals.

The daily charge can be all-inclusive except for physicians' fees, which are paid by the sickness funds separately according to fee schedules. Examples are all hospitals in the Netherlands and most European private clinics.

The daily charge can be all-inclusive—including physicians' salaries—but with separate rates for the principal clinical services. An example is France before 1984.

Itemized Billing. Charge lists are used most extensively by nonprofit and for-profit hospitals in the United States. Even when the third party will pay the hospital a per diem, the hospital sends the patient an itemized bill for a basic daily charge, for many clinical services, and for many extra amenities. Itemized billing is never done completely in Europe, but substantial deviations from the all-inclusive daily charge occur. For example, Swiss hospital bills distinguish basic average daily charges for basic nursing and medical care and for housing and food. Some hospitals (particularly the European proprietaries) break certain clinical items out of the basic daily charges and bill for them separately, such as the use of the operating room, drugs, medical supplies, physiotherapy, and physicians' fees. In all European hospitals, patients also are billed separately for first-class or second-class rooms and for extra amenities.

Case Payments. A system of payment based on diagnosis—at first practiced experimentally for all payers in New Jersey and Maryland—is now widely used in the United States. In 1983 Medicare began paying by diagnosis-related groups for all its inpatients.

Recent Trends

The United States and Sweden had the first modern—and expensive—hospital systems. During the 1950s they built many new hospitals, installed much new equipment, and relied more on wage workers and less on unpaid labor (such as religious sisters and student nurses). Europe then used old buildings with multibedded wards; its nursing and domestic staffs were smaller, worked longer hours, and received little pay. During the 1960s and 1970s, European health administrators and sickness funds intentionally caught up with the United States and Sweden by modernizing or completely replacing hospital buildings, installing modern equipment and comforts, and adding many technicians to the wage bill. The nursing and domestic staffs became much more expensive in Europe: recruitment into religious nursing orders diminished, all employees got the same hours and wages as other nonhealth workers, and the new hospital workers unions obtained salaries for the work by the nursing students. Medical education was expanded, clinical experience in hospitals was required of all doctors, and the unions obtained normal salaries for the junior doctors. In order to catch up with the United States, nearly every country during the 1960s and 1970s had a higher annual increase in health and hospital spending than did the United States.[10]

The United States continued to grow in spending from its high base during the 1960s and 1970s. Numbers of hospital employees continued to rise. America's costs might have increased very substantially but for the fact that it reduced numbers of beds, even before the downturns began abroad. Other countries followed the American precedent of shorter stays, a smaller acute bed supply, greater service intensity, and a steadily increasing cost per patient-day.

Some policy makers recently have been unpleasantly surprised that health care costs in general and hospital costs in particular have been rising faster than the consumer price index and have been increasing in their share of GNP. But this has been true of every country nearly every year since each began its statistical time series about health care spending. During the nineteenth and earlier centuries, hospitals were simple, doctors earned low incomes, and daily costs were low. As the staffing and technology of hospitals modernized, hospital costs were bound to go up faster than other indicators in the economy.

But countries rise to a different degree. Britain's health care costs consistently increase more slowly than other countries'. Canada's costs in recent decades have increased no more than the general price level, a unique pattern. In the United States, health care costs usually increase more than prices generally, but not every year. Increases were about equal to or less than the general price rise during periods of general wage and price controls—for instance, during World War II and the Economic Stabilization Program of the Nixon administration.

The clinical problems facing hospitals in all developed countries changed while the Europeans were trying to modernize along the early American lines. Acute and extended care became distinct. While some acute care continued to involve the restoration of the temporarily ill and injured to health, new technology and treatment made possible the prolongation of life in varying levels of discomfort. Since it seemed possible to save patients who earlier were doomed, many acute hospitals became busy and expensive centers for technology and expert staffing. To control costs and free beds, efforts were made in all countries to shorten stays and (recently) to perform the simpler tests and treatments in outpatient services. The cost-control efforts came from sickness funds and governments; freeing beds for interesting new clinical challenges was often proposed from within the hospitals and medical staffs.

More numerous than ever were the infirm elderly who required nonacute care. Less advanced technically, the nonteaching European general hospital had long housed them on wards with acute cases. The European countries with the more ambitious building programs (such as France and the Netherlands) were able to create a division of function among acute, extended, and chronic care, either in separate buildings or in separate services in the same building complex. Because of the aging of their populations and the ability of modern medicine to keep people alive, many of the acute patients are elderly.

In the Anglo-Saxon countries (Britain, the United States, and Canada), private enterprises created nursing homes for the elderly, thereby freeing beds in acute hospitals. A persistent management problem has been their coordination with the acute hospitals. Problems exist in financing—adequacy of provision for the patient and honesty in institutional provision—since the financing system in these countries (health insurance in the United States and Treasury payments in Britain and Canada) are oriented toward acute care.

In contrast to the countries that developed extended-care hospitals and nursing homes with varying success, a few countries—for example, Germany— have not yet altered their tradition of mixing the infirm elderly into the acute services. Several statistical aberrations result. Length of stay and total patient-days in acute hospitals appear longer in Germany than elsewhere. The daily charge is averaged over budgets and patient-days that include extended-care as well as acute patients, and it seems lower than that of many other countries, even though total costs of the system are high.

One might think that level of expenditure is related to type of social and health system. As several researchers have noticed, the richer the country, the higher the proportion of GNP spent on health care.[11] But among developed countries not even this pattern holds true, and countries with dissimilar organizations have comparable levels of spending. For example, the biggest spenders are the citadel of medical capitalism (the United States), a decentralized government health service (Sweden), and two systems of national health insurance involving much bilateral bargaining (Germany and Holland). Among the lower spenders are a National Health Service (Great Britain) and three forms of national health insurance (Belgium, Japan, and Italy until recently). Levels of health spending depend on social priorities, political will, and the leverage of payers over providers. The purpose of this book is to explain how these forces operate.

3

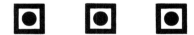

Tracking and Reporting Operating Costs

Payments to hospitals are designed to cover their costs, as calculated from written summaries of current and expected costs. Financial decisions are based on the expected trends in costs, utilization, and revenue. This chapter will examine the growth of hospital costs over time and will compare modern options in the inclusion of certain items in the total charged to payers. It will also discuss the evolution of hospital financial reports and the various options in their design today.

In this chapter, as in all later ones, I summarize the history of the topic in Europe and North America and describe current practices. An understanding of past practices and their development is essential if we are to understand why current national practices vary—why the "obvious" method in one society is hard for officials elsewhere to understand, let alone to emulate. Short-term historical change also demonstrates the difficulties besetting some methods and the reasons for innovation.

This book would seem diffuse without a guiding structure for each topic. Therefore, most chapters begin with the principal options for organizing those topics, the possible range of institutions among developed countries. For example, following are the principal options in the design and use of hospital financial reporting systems, to be illustrated in the rest of this chapter:

☐ Purposes of financial reports.
- Calculation of prices charged to patients and third parties. Unit prices times volume cover costs.
- Inventory of assets and accounts receivable, in order to prevent waste and fraud.
- Identify costs of departments within the hospitals. Identify weak and wasteful managements.
- Identify costs of processes within hospitals. Identify losing and profitable services.
- Strategic planning by hospital management. Identify the changes that will be profitable and unprofitable.

- • Inform higher decision makers about the social value of the hospital.
- ☐ Financial reports follow styles of others' reports.
  - • Government agencies.
  - • Business firms.
  - • Charities.
- ☐ Whether obligatory or not. If so, who requires them?
  - • Rate regulators.
  - • Government auditors.
  - • Regulators of the financial solvency of:
    - — Business firms.
    - — Nonprofit charities.
  - • Ministry of Finance.
  - • Hospital association.
  - • Accountants' association.
- ☐ Legal status of the report.
- ☐ Sanctions for omissions, errors, or falsification.
- ☐ Whether uniformity is required among all hospitals in:
  - • Their reports.
  - • Their internal accounts.
- ☐ Length, degree of detail, whether aggregate or departmentalized.
- ☐ Inclusion of certain items in the costs.
  - • Capital.
  - • Profits.
  - • Teaching and research.
  - • Others.

Early Cost Structures and Their Reports

When hospitals were primarily charitable homes for the poor, their cost structures were simple. They were self-supporting and had little need for cash. The nurses, many workers, and many doctors lived on the grounds, consuming the food and fuel grown on the estate and wearing the clothing made in the workshops of the hospital, archdiocese, or religious order. Wages were a combination of cash and fixed quantities of food and other commodities. (For example, the chief clerk of a denominational hospital in Würzburg in 1802 was paid 414 Gulden, 15 Kreuzer, and the following quantities in Mandelliter: 6 wheat, 18 corn, 2 oats, 2 peas, and 2 lentils. He received no wine or wood, but other employees did.[1])

The distinction between patients and employees was imprecise: the more able-bodied patients were expected to do some work. If they had no home or could not cope with the outside world, they stayed on, in return for room and board. If they did not work in the hospital, they might work in the workshops and farms. (I will describe the early wage structure further, at the beginning of Chapter Ten.)

Simple financial lists can be found in the archives of medieval hospitals. The largest and most expensive hospitals prepared them annually.[2] A particular administrator had the tasks of collecting income, calculating costs, writing the reports, and explaining them to the owners. These lists usually included the following items:

- *Inventory of the hospital's property.* The endowments were often substantial, including treasures kept in the hospital chapel or adjacent cathedral, farmlands, and buildings. Inventories were necessary to guard against thefts, register new donations, and record sales. The more prominent hospitals received gifts each year.
- *Revenue.* Lists were made of rentals of land and buildings, sales of materials from farms and workshops, and charitable donations of cash and materials. One important function of the lists was to record the rents and confirm that they were collected. Well-endowed hospitals had many tenants. Such lists of the holdings and transactions of estates were common among European churches, governments, and feudal orders for centuries.[3]
- *Costs.* These lists were primitive and could be compared with the revenue lists only in approximate totals. Until the early twentieth century, complete accounts, combining revenue and costs in a single budget, could not be made because not all expenditures (including wages) and not all income were completely monetized.

The expenditure lists of the pre-nineteenth-century hospitals had miscellaneous purposes. Many were really memoranda, confirming for everyone agreements to pay particular wages—often complicated lists of cash and commodities—to each worker. The memoranda prevented disputes and were the basis for continued payments to that jobholder or to his successor. The expenditure lists also permitted the owners, such as the religious order, to monitor the management in order to determine whether agreements with employees were reasonable, whether resources were being wasted, and whether payments were actually being made or whether resources were being diverted fraudulently.

Even though costs could not be compared precisely with revenue each year, the owners and managers sensed when serious deficits were occurring over time. For example, during wars and plagues, the hospital had more patients, revenue in kind and cash from the farms and workshops diminished, and charitable fund raising dwindled. Therefore, the managers had to struggle to reduce operating costs, even selling part of the endowment if deficits were protracted.[4]

Origins of Modern Cost Reports

Systematic reporting of the work and finances of hospitals requires government action. Many hospitals are then compelled to keep internal accounts and fill out forms in the same way. Government prescribes the categories according to new financial ideas. Government becomes involved in hospitals as either owner, regulator, payer, or creditor.

Health care finance was modernized first in France. As it is everywhere, the reporting was shaped by the country's policy priorities. The hospitals were nationalized during the 1790s, their management was turned over to the *communes*, and all local agencies were required to adopt new reporting forms and procedures. One goal was to eliminate the embezzlement of public funds and property—a common affliction of pre-Revolutionary France—so that the poor would benefit from the resources appropriated for them. Another goal was to implement national unity and efficient centralized management of public services. By means of a hierarchy of financial accounts, the public sector's expenditures and property could be aggregated at successively higher tiers; and inspectors from Paris could easily spot-check public finances at any degree of detail anywhere in the country. The basic ideas and the laws were created under Napoleon. The methodology of financial reporting evolved gradually during the nineteenth and twentieth centuries. (Meanwhile, France was also leading Europe in the modernization of commercial accounting.)

Standardization was essential. The reports and books of every public agency had to be kept in categories that could be readily understood by the elite corps of investigators based in Paris (the *Inspecteurs des Finances*), if a member arrived on a surprise visit. The papers of any public agency also had to be easily understood by the court that spot-checks all audits and issues judgments about inefficiency and wrongdoing (the *Cour des Comptes*).

Conventions for writing charts of accounts and assigning items of expenditure to categories developed in French accounting. The accounting methods of the *communes* are now expected to follow a nomenclature and assignment methods prescribed by decrees issued by the national government in 1947 and afterward. The reports from the *communes* are submitted to the representative of the Ministry of Finance in each prefecture (the *trésorier-payeur général*) and are ultimately forwarded to the Division of Public Accounting *(Direction de la Comptabilité Publique)* in the Ministry of Finance. The Division of Public Accounting also studies and updates the accounting methods and drafts changes in the decrees.[5]

By the 1950s the *communes* followed a strict chart of accounts, a prescribed list of account numbers, and assignment conventions. The hospitals followed the same rules as the other local government agencies. The nomenclature of the expenditures reports included, among others, the following broad categories (that is, a "categorical" and not a "functional" style):[6]

Personnel
Materials purchased
Construction work and furnishings
Transportation
Administration

Within each category were specific subparts. For example, under "Materials purchased," items such as food, consumable supplies, and pharmaceuticals were included. Under "Personnel," items such as wages and social security contributions were included.

When the hospital paid bills, each payment was counted in its special category. Auditors checked whether the totals could be reconstructed by valid invoices and by actual payments to the appropriate workers and suppliers.

The administrative procedure was designed to prevent fraud, not improve efficient performance. A pay order for each expenditure was made out by a hospital manager (the *ordonnateur*). It was double-checked and countersigned by a second financial officer (the *receveur*), who double-checked all pay orders for the communal government and sometimes was assigned full time to a very large

Table 3-1. A German Hospital's Cash Expenditure in 1851.

	Reichstaler
Food	571
Wages:	
Honorarium for the principal doctor	50
Lump sum for the community of deaconesses	23
Craftsmen	39
Service workers	66
Supplies:	
Medications	27
Surgical instruments	9
Wearing apparel	9
Bedding and linen	64
Household and kitchen utensils	25
Furniture	8
Writing materials	1
Printing and paper	8
Laundry supplies and wages	41
Light and heating	62
Postage	1
Total	1,004

Source: Adapted from Theodor Kogge, *Hundert Jahre Evangelisches Krankenhaus Düsseldorf* (Düsseldorf: privately printed, 1949), p. 36.

hospital. Auditors later checked all the hospital's expenditures for accuracy and honesty.

The nomenclature was designed to be very general, since it applied to all accounts of the *communes*. Figures for hospitals could be aggregated with the reports for other communal activities. The reports were useless for insight into the distinctive operations of hospitals, and they could not be used as guides to managers—both internal and external—searching for areas of inefficiency and waste. Hospitals could not be compared on performance. Examiners from Paris could use the reports only to detect fraud, not to monitor and improve services— that is, to determine whether a worker had received his paycheck, not whether his employment was necessary.

Modernization of Operating Costs

Table 3-1 shows the cash expenditures of a German denominational hospital in the mid-nineteenth century, just before the scientific revolution transformed all hospitals.[7] At this time more than half of the spending budget was devoted to food. The proportion devoted to wages was much lower, because staffing was still low, wages were low, employees got free meals, and many employees got free housing.

As the nineteenth century progressed, the work pace grew, more doctors and lay employees were added, individuals' wages rose, and larger proportions were paid in cash rather than food. More staff lived outside the hospital. By the late nineteenth century, hospitals' cash budgets were much higher, and wages were the largest single category. Not until the 1930s or 1940s were wages more than half the total budget, but now they are two-thirds or more in most countries.[8] Employees now are paid completely in cash, no longer in commodities.

Cost Reports to Obtain Reimbursement

By the late nineteenth century, as I will explain in Chapters Four and Five, nonprofit and public hospitals in Europe and North America no longer depended on mixtures of charitable fund raising by their owners and revenue from endowments. More affluent persons came as patients, health insurance originated, and hospitals began to charge self-paying and insured patients. For a long time, the charges were fixed by the arbitrary judgment of the managers and governing board, based on guesses about the probable costs of caring for the average patient. Gradually, each country's hospitals improved their reports about the annual operations, so that the managers could estimate the costs of care.

The daily charge—covering all costs except the doctor's fee—became the common billing unit in Europe and North America during the late nineteenth and twentieth centuries. Since the nonprofit and public hospitals were not supposed to pay profits, the daily charge should not exceed the patient's costs and the hospital tried to collect enough money so that it would not lose. The growing sickness funds were willing to pay daily charges provided they had evidence that the charges were justified by costs. During the twentieth century in every country, hospital cost reports were developed for reimbursement calculations. Reluctant to reveal more than was necessary and unwilling to perform extra paper work, hospitals usually resisted including in cost reports information not related to reimbursement.

Until the new requirements, all cost reports had been retrospective, summarizing expenditures during the previous year. The hospital manager was now expected to submit to the payer or rate regulator a prediction of its costs during the next year, making a case for the money it needed. The payer or rate regulator required every hospital to fill out a standard form. If the hospitals were paid under statutory health insurance, eventually government in each country made payment contingent on submission of the standard form by all.

The new forms for submission of prospective budgets were "categorical" in nomenclature; that is, there were separate lines for personnel, materials purchased, services purchased, and so on. In contrast to some earlier cost reports, these items were subcategorized in lines that specified the work of the hospital. For personnel, wages were usually subtotaled for doctors, nurses, domestics, technicians, and so on; the total for materials was usually subtotaled for food, medical supplies, pharmaceuticals, office supplies, and so on.

The lists at first were simple, without the functional categories and cost-finding rearrangements that have been introduced only recently. They were designed merely to explain the principal divisions of the hospital's total expected expenditure for the next year. The categories and the general format resembled whatever had been common before. In France the hospital prepared a prospective budget (the interim *budget primitif* and the updated *budget supplémentaire*) with the nomenclature of public-sector accounting, since it had earlier been applied to the hospitals' end-of-the-year cost reports. In other countries each hospital had produced its own budget and cost reports for internal purposes; the styles were crude and heterogeneous; and few hospitals employed skilled accountants conversant with the advanced methods used in business. Government regulators, the sickness funds, and the hospital association had to devise forms that all hospital managers could fill out; and the sickness funds could not press for forms more complex than their own auditors could quickly review in large numbers. Therefore, until recently the hospitals' prospective budgets devised for reimbursement decisions have been very simple.

Because the prospective budget was designed to justify a daily rate, it had to include the number of patient-days expected during the fiscal year. The total costs divided by total expected patient-days produced the all-inclusive daily rate, to be charged every patient and third party.

The prospective budget provided supporting evidence for the hospital's formal request for a new daily rate for the next fiscal year. Prepared by the chief executive officer and the chief financial officer, the prospective budget was then approved by the hospital's governing boards, signed by the chairman of the governing board, and forwarded to the regulatory agency (in countries with rate regulations) or to the other side (in countries with bilateral rate negotiation).

Hospital accounting and rate setting became intensely calendar-conscious. The prospective budget summarized all expected costs during a single calendar or fiscal year, and the rate was awarded for that period. Once the period began, the hospital's accountants had to record the payments and the receipts for that period, and accounting rules became common in each country to reconcile total accounts payable and accounts receivable for the period. These figures had to be distinguished from the accounts for each previous year, so that time series could be calculated. Accounting for current time periods became more precise, so that quarterly financial progress reports could be presented to owners, regulators, and governments.

(Calculating the daily charge from a prospective budget became the rule after reimbursement methods matured. Prospective budgets rather than retrospective cost reports became the base after it became evident that hospital costs rose every year. But at first in France, under the law of 1893 setting an official daily charge for the welfare patient, the calculation used average costs for the previous five years. The retrospective cost reports provided the data.)

Restraining Cost Increases

Controlling hospital costs became a public policy problem during the 1950s. Sickness funds were no longer willing to pay whatever the hospital wanted and then only grumble privately. Sickness funds questioned the hospitals' simple prospective budgets in rate negotiations, as in Germany; existing rate regulators were prepared to be more critical, as in France; and new regulatory agencies were created, as in the Netherlands. The sickness funds and the regulators pressed governments to mandate new forms for submitting prospective budgets, so that negotiators and regulators could judge whether the hospitals' financial claims were reasonably related to the expected work or were wasteful. At first, during the 1950s and 1960s, the negotiators and rate regulators did not question the hospitals' utilization but only the resources that the payers were expected to cover.

The key to cost control was thought to be restraint over selected inefficiencies within the hospitals; therefore, hospitals were expected to report their prospective budgets in ways that would disclose their internal operations. Costs then could be controlled in three ways:

- Selected lines within the hospital's prospective budget would be cut if they exceeded levels allowed by guidelines.
- The hospital's spending should not exceed that of comparable hospitals.
- The hospital's spending next year should not exceed its trends in recent years.

Hospitals resisted such scrutiny, and the political struggles between hospitals and payers produced reports of varying detail. Line-item prospective budgets were short in some countries (such as Germany) and much longer in others (such as France, Holland, and Switzerland). In some countries the categories of spending (such as all wages of nursing employees) were reported for the entire hospital; in others they were reported for individual departments.

In several countries the prospective budget forms asked for more than money. In particular, numbers of personnel of each type were listed. The forms began to ask about work performed, such as numbers of tests in radiology and in the laboratory.

Establishment of Guidelines. Without standards or guidelines, the individual lines in the hospital's prospective budget would be disputed endlessly. As I shall explain in Chapter Seven, on rate regulation, governments and headquarters of sickness funds announced guidelines. If a proposed level of expenditure or a proposed number of employees exceeded a ratio, it could be challenged. Usually the ratio related these items to the number of beds or the number of expected patient-days. The prospective budget included all the numbers for these calculations.

The reports merely provided accurate facts, not automatic outcomes. If the negotiators or regulators deemed a hospital's budget too high, the entire hospital association might challenge the guidelines as a bureaucratic threat to the quality of care; or the individual hospital might argue that the unique requirements of its patients justified an exception.

Peer Comparisons. Unable to disprove the hospital managers' claims about their unique merits, negotiators soon adopted the standard of average costs of all hospitals. The idea had originated in the payment of doctors in Germany and had become the foundation of utilization control in several other countries. If a doctor submitted far more bills for a procedure than other doctors did, he was probably writing false claims or was overproducing tasks, and he was not paid for all his bills.

Applying peer comparisons to hospitals was much more laborious. Every hospital had to fill out a prospective budget according to the same format. The sickness funds or the rate regulators had to employ staffs to read the entries into computers and had to maintain very large computing capabilities to read and process the data. Hospitals had to be clustered into peer groups that could withstand the hospital association's protests. Only during the 1970s did Europe have the computing power and staffs to generate and analyze such peer comparisons of lines in prospective budgets. Such peer group comparisons were then being produced by the headquarters of the rival sides in negotiations in Germany (the *Bundesverband der Ortskrankenkassen* and the *Deutsche Krankenhausgesellschaft*), by the rate regulation agency in Holland (*Stichting Centraal Orgaan Ziekenhuistarieven*, or COZ) and (in order to advise the individual hospitals) by the hospital associations in Holland and Switzerland. The regulators in France were beginning to generate computerized nationwide peer comparisons for the large hospitals by the time the country switched to other methods of paying hospitals. Within each district the French regulators made visual comparisons among their hospitals' prospective budgets; a district had neither the computing capability nor a sufficient number of cases for statistical identification of outliers.

Like a deviation from a guideline, a deviation from a peer group average provided only evidence for judgment. The managers could still argue that the hospital was different from others in that peer group: they might even argue that the regulators had misclassified it in the wrong peer group. Such a debate required comparing the hospital and its peer group over several years. Therefore, past end-of-the-year cost reports and past prospective budgets had to be computerized as well.

Comparisons to Previous Years. As hospital costs rose during the 1960s and 1970s, sickness funds and government financial officers complained that many hospitals were increasing staffing, wages, tests, and equipment beyond the growth justified by the clinical load. Some regulatory guidelines suggested that annual increases in the lines of prospective budgets should not exceed increases in utilization, the country's prices, the GNP, or other baselines.

To provide the facts, the prospective budget forms in most countries during the 1970s asked the hospital to report its operating costs and utilization in the previous one, two, or three years. The cost reports usually had to be certified by the hospital's external auditor. Therefore, the end-of-the-year cost reports and the prospective budgets were connected, followed the same nomenclature, and were pooled in the same data files maintained by the sickness funds (in rate negotiation systems) and by the regulatory agencies (in rate regulation systems). Comparing lines in the hospital's previous cost reports and next prospective budget became a common screening device by regulators during the 1970s.

Hospitals' Own Accounts. The reports were part of the hospitals' cases for higher rates. The hospitals could keep their internal books any other way, presumably in the manner most appropriate to internal management. However, accounting skills came late to hospitals. In most hospitals the internal books had been oriented to recording payments and were simpler than the reports mandated for reimbursement applications. During the 1960s hospitals throughout Europe became accustomed to maintaining all their accounts in these new forms. But by the 1980s these forms were becoming obviously inadequate for the internal assignment of costs and the evaluation of the efficiency of cost centers.

In some countries government intervention pressed the hospitals to keep their books to fit the prospective budget forms—that is, to maintain uniform recording as well as uniform reporting. For example, German laws on the payment of hospitals by sickness funds prescribed the forms (the *Selbstkosten-blätter*) that hospitals sent the funds for negotiation. The provincial government then had legal power to review and amend the agreement between the hospital and the sickness funds. If they could not agree, the provincial government conducted a full investigation—extending to the hospital's accounts, which were normally closed to all outsiders, including the sickness funds—and then decided what amounts were to be paid. Therefore, the laws and regulations about hospital payment have included requirements about how the hospital should keep its accounts.[9] Even though they could not see the hospital's accounts, the sickness funds therefore could presume that the *Selbstkostenblätter* were an honest summary.

An accounting system is a method of thinking about an organization. A uniform accounting system therefore influences hospital managers to adopt a common organizational structure, including the various centers of responsibility that report costs. Uniform accounting is often part of the organizational reforms pushed by hospital associations and governments.

Resistance to Uniform Reporting. To be guaranteed full coverage of their costs, hospitals in nearly every developed country have had to concede to payers and governments extensive disclosure of their financial operations and accept standard rules on costs chargeable to payers. Detailed uniform reporting is a price the hospitals pay, but hospitals in some countries have been able to limit what they tell their adversaries and also to limit the adversaries' ability to verify. In the Netherlands for example, hospital rate regulation at one time was handicapped because the rate regulators (COZ) and the sickness funds were unable to obtain complete information from the hospitals' cost reports and prospective budgets.

Businessmen in America's vast free economy have always resisted the nationwide uniform financial reports common in other developed countries. American business widely uses only certain "generally accepted accounting principles" and fills out forms limited to the purposes of certain national and local regulations. American hospitals have always resisted the mandating of uniform financial reports, since they can survive without a single comprehensive payment system and since the national government has never enacted a general hospital cost-containment law. At the most, Medicare requires all hospitals in the country to fill out reports about the costs of their Medicare business, and a few states with rate regulation require reports about all costs. Attempts to mandate universal financial reports, or even to pursuade hospitals to submit such reports voluntarily, have always floundered, since American hospitals collectively wish to preserve their privacy and market power.[10] Since individual American hospitals are competitors, they resist any openings that might eventually lead to standardization within their industry in accounting, organization, and services.

Improving Management

Reimbursement trends made reports more demanding. As the economic organization of hospitals improved, schools of health administration taught the modern financial management that had long been central to business and government. Hospital associations fostered more efficient methods, including modern accounting and cost finding. Hospital associations convinced individual hospital managements that such performance was essential for hospitals to get favorable rulings from regulators. Also, such capacities were essential for hospitals to perform efficiently when rate awards were disappointing and when cost pressures rose.

The hospital associations in several countries—particularly Switzerland, the Netherlands, the United States, and Canada—devised accounting methods and cost reports that could accomplish the same goals as a private business management's. Management would constantly know what was happening at lower units throughout the organization—an innovation in the traditionally diffuse hospital. Favorable and unfavorable trends in the parts could be spotted quickly. The costs of the hospital could be attributed to those work sites that generated them. Efficient and inefficient work sites could be identified.

At first, during the 1970s, the new methods were intended to improve management during a period of growing revenue. Income was still usually derived from all-inclusive daily rates calculated from the totals in steadily rising prospective budgets. During the 1980s, however, much tighter lids were imposed on revenue in all countries, and management was forced to become more economical. Costs no longer dictated revenue but must be set within available revenue. The new methods of internal financial monitoring and cost finding enabled hospital managers to locate and improve their less efficient subdivisions and to ensure that the flows of expenditure did not exceed the expected flows of revenue.

Cost-Center Accounting. During the twentieth century, large business firms became producers of distinct products, successful companies created product divisions, each division became responsible for its own performance, and headquarters judged them all by their net profits. Headquarters set general strategy, the management of each division had considerable discretion in the acquisition and use of resources, and headquarters used financial reports to monitor performance and evaluate outcomes.[11]

A hospital might also be considered a multiproduct firm. Several functions can be identified as centers generating costs, and all the hospital's costs can be attributed ultimately to one or another of these cost centers. Switzerland was one of the first countries to adopt modern accounting and reporting in all hospitals, including the redistribution of the costs of all departments among principal cost centers. The methodology has been developed and the data processed by the national hospital association (the *Vereinigung Schweizerische Krankenhäuser,* or VESKA). In a country with limited governmental power and small public bureaucracies, VESKA was created in 1930 to improve hospital operations and to collect statistics. The national government wanted to have comprehensive information; and each cantonal government wished to know about the situation within its own boundaries, since it owned several hospitals and subsidized most others.

A committee of VESKA members has drafted reporting forms, with the help of the VESKA secretariat. The draft forms have been circulated for comment by cantonal hospital associations and have been pretested by individual hospitals.

Major revisions—including the complex forms for cost-center accounting—are studied and approved by the standing committee of all cantonal health ministers.

The same reports are used for many purposes. Since the 1930s, aggregated statistics about hospital work and finance have been published annually by VESKA and by the national government. The cantonal governments examine the reports from individual hospitals when deciding the next year's daily charge and the cantonal subsidy. (All hospitals are forced to comply because the cantons' subsidies are conditioned on submission of the VESKA cost reports.) Many individual hospitals publish their responses to the questionnaires in their annual reports. Individual responses from several hospitals are compared with each other and with peer group averages at meetings of the national and cantonal hospital associations for discussions about improving management.

The first ten pages of the annual cost report include the usual lines in communications with payers and regulators—for example, numbers of personnel at each rank; numbers of hospital beds, admissions, and patient-days in the clinical departments; and total expenditure for each class of personnel, medical supplies, food, maintenance, and energy.

During the late 1970s, the basic forms were supplemented by cost-center accounting *(Kostenstellenrechnung)*. Three classes of cost center are identified in each hospital:

- Clinical services (surgery, medicine, pediatrics, obstetrics, psychiatry, and so on, depending on the hospital's service structure).
- Medical-technical central services used by the clinical departments (for instance, operating theaters, anesthesia, radiodiagnosis, laboratories, and physical therapy).
- Infrastructure services (building maintenance and operations, administration, laundry, central stores, kitchen, pharmacy, and so on).

The goal is to distribute all costs of the hospital among the clinical services, which are the ultimate responsibility centers. This is done in four steps:

- During the year, costs are posted in the ledgers for the clinical, medical-technical, and infrastructure services. They are totaled before the redistribution.
- The infrastructure service costs are attributed to the clinical and medical-technical services according to formulas: building operation costs according to the square meters occupied by each clinical and medical-technical service; laundry costs according to the kilograms sent there by each clinical and medical-technical service; central store costs according to the orders placed in thousands of francs; and so on.
- The new total of medical-technical service costs is attributed to the clinical services according to reported utilization during the year. Each medical-technical service has recorded use by each clinical service by a point system, a *Taxpunkttabelle* written by VESKA, itemizing the services within hospitals.
- Finally, the total costs of the hospital are distributed among the clinical services. Their resource consumption can be compared in cost per patient-day.

The method requires considerable internal recording of procedures (by such methods as the *Taxpunkttabelle*) and requires computer capabilities. Switzerland gradually phased in the method during the late 1970s and the 1980s. It was not used for reimbursement but only to improve management. Swiss hospitals continue to be paid by all-inclusive per diems, not differentiated by service.[12]

Cost-center accounting can be implemented in various ways and can be associated with a restructuring of the hospital. Such an effort might occur in France during the late 1980s if the medical staff structure is changed. For centuries the hospital has consisted of a few general services (such as medicine, surgery, or obstetrics), each headed by a chief. All other physicians in the subject area have been his subordinates. Under a long-discussed reform, several senior physicians in related subspecialties will form a department; for example, cardiologists, gastroenterologists, endocrinologists, oncologists, and others will form a department of internal medicine. One doctor will be elected to the rotating chairmanship, but the group will share power. Each department will be a "center of responsibility" *(centre de responsábilité).*

If the reform is implemented, French accounting methods and reporting forms will be rewritten completely. A hospital's total prospective budget will be the total of all departmental budgets. Even without the departmentalization reform, each hospital now receives global grants from the sickness funds in the form of monthly installments of the total. The hospital no longer receives daily charges. Under the reform the departments will not be paid individually, such as a fixed amount for each case; instead, each department will be required to perform its work within its share of the total budget. Any deficit for the hospital will be due to cost overruns in one or more of the departments, and the books will quickly reveal the problems.[13]

Revenue-Center Accounting. For several decades before the adoption of payment by global budgeting, the French hospital had separate all-inclusive daily charges for its principal clinical services. Instead of one for the average patient, it had one for the average surgical patient, one for the average medical patient, and so on. Small hospitals had two or three; large ones (such as teaching hospitals with many specialties) had over a dozen. In order to obtain the separate daily rates from the regulator, the French hospital's prospective budget included estimates of the costs of the different services. The methods of cost-center accounting were used to assign the costs of central services—the administration, the pharmacy, capital depreciation, and so on—to each of the services with separate daily rates. The methods were simple, and the calculations were done by hand rather than by computer.[14]

When Americans applied to hospitals the methods of cost finding and cost assignment that had flourished in American business and finance, the uses resembled those in the commercial marketplace. American nonprofit and for-profit hospitals set their own prices and could maximize their revenue, like any nonmedical business firm and unlike their counterparts in European health. One task for the American hospital was to set its charges to achieve maximum profits; another task was to determine when the marginal costs of producing work were excessive.

The cost centers in American hospital accounts were the ones that the hospital itemized when it billed patients: nursing and domestic services as a whole, the operating theater, the delivery room, intensive care, anesthesia, radiology, the laboratory, the pharmacy, physical therapy, and several others. The American hospital did not group all its costs under clinical services as the French hospital did; that is, it did not calculate the costs of surgery (including surgery's use of nursing, the operating theater, the laboratory, and so on), it did not calculate the all-inclusive costs of internal medicine, and therefore it did not make separate clinical services into cost centers in the accounts. Rather, the American hospital grouped all nursing and domestic services into one cost center related to one daily charge, it charged separately for the other technical services, and the other technical services became separate cost centers. The American hospital could not have made cost and revenue centers out of the separate clinical services, since it lacked medical chiefs of service interested in financial management. A principal task of the American hospital's chief financial officer has been to identify the most profitable revenue centers and set high charges that will bring in the most revenue. Management tries to persuade the lay administrators in these departments to increase utilization and limit costs.[15]

Calculating costs for each revenue center is not only traceable to the revenue-maximizing strategy of the American hospital management but is due also to the expenditure-minimizing strategy of American sickness funds. Except for temporary demonstration projects in a few American states, the United States has always lacked an all-payers system, wherein all third parties and patients pay the same charges and total hospital costs are averaged across everyone. American sickness funds insist that they will pay only for the costs of their subscribers, requiring the hospital to distinguish resource use for different types of patients. In particular, the elderly use more nursing and domestic care and fewer technical services (such as the operating theater, the delivery room, or radiodiagnosis) than younger patients. Before adopting payment by diagnosis-related groups (DRGs), Medicare for the elderly insisted that the costs of the technical services be included in Medicare bills only in the proportion of their use by the Medicare patients, and hospital cost analysis had to include certain estimating formulas.[16] Except in a few states with all-payers rate regulation, the different cost reimbursers (primarily Medicare, Medicaid, and Blue Cross) recognized *different* cost bases and required *different* stepdown calculations in the *same* hospital. Elaborate maneuvers ensued between American hospital finance officers and payers, wherein the finance officers tried to assign activities to revenue centers in ways to maximize total revenues from all payers.[17] Such ambiguity, discretion by hospital managers, unexpected cost increases, and disputes are avoided in rate regulation and public grants in other countries.

Cost finding by revenue center proves inadequate for understanding the internal dynamics of hospitals. Before the changes in cost accounting triggered by the adoption of DRGs during the 1980s, each American hospital defined its cost centers by its own charging customs, and hospitals could be compared only in their Medicare reports rather than in their total work. Therefore, general statistics about internal hospital costs—such as those developed in Switzerland— were not possible in the United States. Most of the American hospital's costs were grouped into one large uninformative category ("nursing administration") and into many small ancillary services (labor and delivery, radiology, inhalation therapy, and so on).[18]

Identifying the Cost of Each Clinical Procedure. A goal in business accounting is to identify the firm's cost of generating each product and service. Even if some are deliberately underpriced, management knows the profits and losses from different levels of output of each product and service. A variety of decisions can then be made about increasing or decreasing the output of each item, attacking high costs, changing methods of production, repricing, changing market strategy, and so on.

In the past the crude forms of costing and reporting in hospitals in every country prevented such precise cost assignment. Perhaps some simple and recurrent procedures in the hospital's industrial services can be costed plausibly; for example, the cost of each laboratory test, the cost of each X ray, and the cost of laundering can be estimated just as the costs of each output of a business firm are estimated. But many other procedures—such as a thoracic operation or a physiotherapy session—are not so standardized and vary in their resource use each time. The inputs throughout a hospital appear more heterogeneous than the inputs throughout an industrial factory, and clustering them to estimate the costs of an output is more difficult than cost assignment in a factory.

In every sector the cost of an individual output is a function of the cost assignment rules of that accounting scheme. That is certainly true in hospital accounting, which is not yet standardized. Therefore, different schemes can produce widely different estimates of the costs of a procedure, such as a thoracic operation.[19] Charge lists for procedures reflect the hospital's economic strategy and are only loosely related to the costs of the procedures.

Identifying the Cost of Each Clinical Case. No country, therefore, can describe hospital costs by procedure in any generally agreed manner. All costing in practice involves estimates and aggregation. Americans during the 1980s developed detailed methods of cost accounting, wherein the ultimate assignments are grouped by clinical case. The groundwork existed in America, since its itemized billing had long recorded resource consumption for each patient. Extensive clinical and financial information was recorded for each patient, and the two types of information could be linked. Computing was introduced into hospital records early. Americans criticized flat-rate and all-inclusive payment methods earlier than Europeans and favored itemization. Americans introduced into hospital finance ideas that business had developed about costing individual products. Americans also became interested in incentive reimbursement schemes, whereby hospitals would know that they could profit from efficient care of particular types of patients.

In all previous types of hospital accounts, the units of information were the many individual bills posted under accounts payable and totaled on the lines of the expenditure budget. The totals of each line or of entire sections of the expenditure budget have been the bases of decisions by managers, regulators, and payers. In contrast, the unit of data for costing by diagnosis-related groups is the discharge record of each patient. On the discharge form, several facts must be entered with high accuracy: primary and secondary diagnoses, length of stay, all procedures, all pharmaceuticals, and so on. The methodology of diagnosis-related costing is being developed during the 1980s in the United States and in several European countries. First, patients have been classified into clusters of diagnoses that use distinct levels of resources. The cost per diagnosis in each hospital and (on average) in all hospitals has been done by statistical estimation. However, each hospital has an incentive to identify the precise cost of each input in patient care in order to learn the exact cost of each course of treatment.[20]

In particular, the elusive concept of "cost of nursing care" must be operationalized. In several research projects in the United States, various patient classification systems—particularly DRGs—incorporate correlational methods of estimating the average component for time and skill of nursing care.[21] Several management consulting firms have gone further by offering bedside-based medical information systems that enable every nurse and employee to record every service rendered to each patient.

When and if these forms of detailed costing can be implemented throughout a country, many different aggregate cost reports can be generated, and they can be used for intelligent management decisions concerning the entire hospital, individual departments, and individual cases.

- *Entire hospital.* As at present, the hospital's total costs can be summarized. But with this method, unlike traditional methods, the hospital's costs can be related to its clinical case mix. Hospitals can be compared in total costs, not merely in relation to bed sizes or total patient-days; and one can also question whether differentials in costs are justified by case mixes. Cost reports become more meaningful to managers, payers, and planners. Understanding and reforming the hospital as a whole were objectives of the first research projects that developed diagnosis-related groups in the United States.
- *Department within the hospital.* Departments' expenditures also can be evaluated in the light of their case mixes. Managers can press the less efficient departments. Diagnosis-related groups might be used in this fashion in France during the late 1980s.
- *Case.* Average cost per case can be calculated across all hospitals in the country or among all hospitals in a region. Hospitals can be compared in their efficiency in treating the same case. A division of labor might develop, with the most efficient hospital taking more cases with that diagnosis. Hospitals and doctors generally might judge that certain clinical conditions are treated more wastefully than others and might economize. Or they might judge that certain clinical conditions are undertreated and should be priced higher. Diagnosis-related groups have been used in these ways in the United States during the 1980s.

Allowable Costs

As long as revenue was not intimately related to costs, there was no need to delineate the components of costs. But as more revenue was earned from the users of hospitals and as payers agreed to reimburse costs, the exact boundaries and amounts had to be defined. For purposes of calculating the accounts for reimbursement, each European country now designates a particular set of allowable costs in a precise and stable fashion. Most have legalistic political cultures and courts that implement rather than imaginatively reinterpret laws.

Several countries have uniform hospital accounting as well as uniform reporting. Several countries have all-payers systems of cost reimbursement and therefore need to fix definite boundaries. Most prefer to minimize wrangling; since dispute occurs over the monetary level of costs, governments can limit the level of contention by specifying which items will be included as allowable costs.

For several decades the European pattern was to settle on a definition of allowable costs, add some items through negotiation or legislation, and pay amounts that represented reasonable annual increases in costs. A new trend is to reverse the dependence of revenue on costs by making costs fit into revenue. Certain sums are made available, and the hospital is no longer told in the law or negotiations that the award can fully cover specific lines in the prospective budget; but the hospital is given discretion in use of its revenue. Few countries have abandoned cost reimbursement completely. Even in countries where payers—particularly governments—try to force hospitals to work within available revenue, hospitals can make a case for higher reimbursement this year or next by proving that operating costs and utilization are unavoidably higher.

Personnel. A perennial issue in hospital accounting is whether wages, capital, administration, and some other items should be attributed to the hospital organization or to the hospitals' owners. Until the nineteenth century, hospital revenue did not come from selling health care and housing; therefore, such items could not be considered "costs" of the hospital's "business," and these items were supplied by the owners. Many hospitals were owned by religious orders and churches, which recruited, supported, and managed the nurses and many other employees. Hospitals varied widely in their cost accounts, and personnel costs were listed quite variously.

During the late nineteenth and twentieth centuries, hospital revenue was tied to medical and housing services to patients, and revenue grew to cover all costs. Accounting conventions began to differentiate the hospital from other organizations run by their owners, such as municipal departments or a religious sisterhood. The entire wage bill is now included in hospital costs in every country, to be covered in full from the revenue from charges or operating grants. Since all hospitals are labor intensive, personnel now constitutes 60 to 80 percent of operating costs, depending on how many other items are included in that country's definition of hospital costs.

The trend has been to individualize salaries. During the nineteenth century and the first half of the twentieth century, many acute hospitals in Europe and North America still had groups of religious sisters as executives and ward nurses, often provided by religious associations that owned the hospital. As hospital affairs became rationalized and monetarized, the hospitals paid lump sums to the parent association for the sisters' services, in addition to room and board. Fewer sisters now serve in acute hospitals, and work has been done by laywomen on salary.

Partial payment in room and board has nearly disappeared. Employees are expected to pay rent for any housing and to pay for their meals in cafeterias. Their salaries have been increased accordingly. The housing and food costs in hospital accounts are supposed to be parts of patient care. Where a few employees still share in these, no serious financial complications result, since such hospitals are paid by all-inclusive daily charges or by global budgets, both of which pool the personnel, housing, and food costs.

The trend in the world is to mandate wage rates by nationwide collective bargaining. Laws mandate social security contributions by all employers, including hospitals. Hospital managers are bound by these rates. Their only discretion in the personnel budget is over the number of employees and over the mix of full-timers and part-timers.

If certain key workers are not paid by the hospital, the managers cannot control them and they may pursue their own goals, using the hospital for their own ends. Inclusion of the nursing and domestic staffs in hospital budgets has been part of the secularization of hospitals and the rising power (and responsibility) of their managements. A difference that continues today is the payment of the senior physicians: in some countries (such as France and Germany), they are becoming full-time salaried, and their incomes are parts of the hospital budgets; in other countries (such as the United States, the Netherlands, and Great Britain), they remain independent in payment and in behavior.

Capital. Whether certain items are included in the definition of a hospital's costs reflects that country's definition of the nature of a hospital and that country's strategy about how a hospital should be managed. An important variation today is whether the acquisition, renovation, and replacement of buildings and heavy equipment are defined as operating costs and are charged to patients and their payers.

For centuries the capital needs of hospitals were modest and were covered by owners and by charitable donors. Buildings and furniture were given by benefactors or were created in the workshops maintained by the owners. In many countries this practice continues today: a new building or expensive equipment is donated by a government capital fund or by private philanthropists. A trend is toward more reliance on government and less on private donations.

The idea of capital depreciation originated in industrial business accounting. The production process not only used up supplies but wore out the equipment. The firm had to replace the equipment, and it saved some of its revenue for that purpose. Funds for current maintenance and for replacement (that is, depreciation) were created from revenue and therefore were normal operating costs. If purchases of new equipment required borrowing, repayment of the interest was a cost, and the depreciation dedicated to amortizing the principal also was a cost.

In all countries the new hospital accounting of the nineteenth and twentieth centuries adopted the idea of depreciation for smaller equipment. Many such items were involved, they clearly wore out, donors could be enlisted only for glamorous items, and depreciation funds replaced the small items. Eventually it became obvious that medical technology was never merely replaced: the new item was more advanced and more expensive. Therefore, depreciation covered modernization, and hospital managers tried to increase the line in prospective budgets.

As long as buildings and heavy equipment were supplied by owners and by donors, hospitals were limited in their capacity to modernize, and managers and their medical staffs were dependent on outsiders. In several countries—as I will explain in Chapter Nine—rate regulators and payers preserved this approach. They accepted as allowable costs in prospective budgets only the interest costs for short-term cash management at the hospital's bank and only a low depreciation line sufficient to cover equipment with short expected lives. The large amounts of new capital needed by modern hospitals come from public capital grants, not from the operating costs paid by sickness funds and by other third parties.

The dynamics of hospital finance have differed where regulators and payers have allowed the hospitals to incur large debts for the purpose of modernizing buildings and buying heavy equipment, and to increase the lines for interest and depreciation substantially. Examples are the United States and the Netherlands. Hospital managers and senior doctors have developed their own strategies regardless of any public policy, the hospitals have constantly modernized, and hospital costs have risen steeply.

If cost reports are used only to understand the internal operations of the hospital and are not the base for reimbursement calculations, they can include items that are not covered by the payment unit. Therefore, they can include the use of capital, even when the capital is granted rather than paid for under the patient charges. In Switzerland, for example, the VESKA cost accounts were amended in 1985 to include the consumption of all capital, calculated annually by the straight-line method. Swiss cost reports are not converted directly into units of payment, as I will explain later: the cantonal governments cover some of the operating costs (not including amortization of larger capital) by subsidies; the sickness funds pay the rest of operating costs by per diems; and the cantonal governments pay for heavy capital by grants to the hospitals.

Profits. In prospective budgets covered by cost-based reimbursement in every country, except for the United States, profits are not recognized as costs chargeable to payers. The methods of calculating the payment of expected work in Europe and Canada have been designed to break even, with neither profits or losses.[22] Last year's profits are included as new revenue in the next year's prospective budget; all such extra revenue is deducted from total expected costs; and the balance of the costs is the basis for next year's rates, paid by the sickness funds or government. Last year's profits have resulted in an increase in the hospital's balance at its bank (that is, accounts receivable have exceeded accounts payable), and the hospital is expected to use them up next year by charging the payers less than the full operating costs.

By the same procedures, the nonprofit and public hospitals in Europe and Canada do not suffer losses. The hospital has incurred a short-term debt at its bank, since accounts payable have exceeded accounts receivable. Repayment of the debt is included among the costs in next year's prospective budget. Most forms provide such a line. Next year's rate covers the full budget, including the extra amount over basic operating costs, so the hospital's bank account comes back into balance.

Amendments to the German hospital finance law terminated this practice in 1985. The hospital may keep its end-of-the-year profits but also must adjust to its losses. Carry-overs into next year have been eliminated. Profits and losses last for no more than one year, since the hospital and the sickness funds negotiate a new daily charge based on a new prospective budget.

One result of the prevalent European and Canadian break-even practice has been to squeeze the profitability of proprietary hospitals. For-profit hospitals flourish in the United States in large part because profits were allowed them under the cost reimbursement rates of Medicare, Medicaid, and several Blue Cross Plans. Because the for-profits got this extra cash, the nonprofits argued that they needed a "return on equity" in order to guarantee a flow of capital; without it, they said, investors would place their capital in for-profit hospitals and in for-profit nonmedical opportunities.[23] Blue Cross Plans have usually agreed to a return on equity; at times Medicare and Medicaid appeased the nonprofit hospitals by adding a "plus factor," thereby giving them extra discretionary cash.

Costs Resembling a Business Firm's. In most countries the nonprofit hospital is still viewed as a humanitarian service, as a public utility. Items that a self-centered business firm might incur to fight its adversaries never arise in hospital management or—if they are proposed—are never allowed as costs by regulators and payers. If such items are accepted, the image of the hospital becomes fundamentally different.

Traditionally, European hospitals were paternalistic toward their employees. When workers became secularized and unionized, hospital managers recognized the unions, however unenthusiastically. Unions were recognized by government and the social services at high national levels. On the other hand, private business remained free to fight unions. In the United States alone, the managers of nonprofit and for-profit hospitals have emulated businessmen in labor relations as in many other respects. Unions have been weak in health, hospital managers have resolutely opposed recognizing them, and hospital managers have successfully fought strikes. Hospital managers—like business managers—have included the costs of contesting union recognition among the costs of their business, chargeable to all payers. The third parties—including all government programs, such as Medicare and Medicaid—have agreed that these are allowable costs.

One might suppose that subsidizing hospitals' litigation against payers and planners assists noncooperation, when it is cooperation that should be rewarded. Business firms include all their legal costs in their cost bases, but they are not guaranteed reimbursement. Outside of America hospitals are guaranteed their costs, and the preparation of appeals against adverse rate rulings is part of routine administrative costs; but the hospitals do not pursue expensive lawsuits. In the United States, however, hospitals were often in court against Medicare and Medicaid rulings during the period of cost reimbursement, and the hospitals were allowed to include these substantial amounts in their Medicare and Medicaid cost bases.

Teaching and Research. For many years hospitals in all countries have been used to teach student doctors and student nurses. At one time the students' presence was a financial windfall, since they donated labor for no or little pay. In many hospitals until shortly after World War II, most nursing care was given by students, so that the personnel budget remained low.

As money flowed into hospitals from sickness funds and governments during the 1960s, the junior doctors and student nurses obtained salaries. Education was no longer confined to listening to bedside lectures; instead, students were expected to test and treat. When they were modernized, the hospital buildings added classrooms, libraries, and research laboratories. Several of the senior nurses became specialists in classroom teaching and student evaluation. Sickness funds in all countries complained that they were obligated to pay only for the care of their subscribers, that someone else should pay the costs of teaching and research.

Allocating the costs of patient care and the costs of teaching and research is a universal problem with universally elusive solutions. In most of Europe, certain hospitals affiliated with medical schools are classified as teaching establishments. Often they are owned by the Ministries of Education of the national or provincial governments. The faculty members and many employees are full-time salaried employees of the Ministries, and much of the building-maintenance cost is borne by the Ministries.

Several countries have conducted research projects to identify the extra costs of patient care due to teaching and research. They compare teaching and nonteaching hospitals and then estimate the amount of extra testing and extra staffing in the teaching hospitals.[24] Some additional costs are inevitable, since the teaching hospitals get the more complex cases and longer stays within each diagnostic group, and they use the newest methods. No country has yet settled on such proportions, and the sickness funds are still expected to bear the full operating costs of care, beyond those charged to the Ministries of Education and the Ministries of Health. Switzerland is an exception; all cantonal Treasuries share support of all hospitals' operating costs with the sickness funds, and the cantons pay high shares of patient care in the academic medical centers. In France the sickness funds pay hospital operating costs in full, but government subsidizes the funds in order to reduce the burden from the teaching hospitals.

Perverse Incentives. Items included under a country's reimbursable costs and in the allowable prospective budget may later give rise to "perverse incentives"; that is, hospitals and payers may respond to the rules in unexpected and troublesome ways, and changes in the rules then are resisted by their beneficiaries. For example, interest from debt and depreciation of capital were separate allowable costs under American Medicare, Medicaid, and Blue Cross in the past; but repayment of the borrowed principal was not an allowable cost, since it was an acquisition of capital assets. The cost-reimbursing payers covered interest in full; therefore, the hospital had no incentive to bargain for lower debt charges or to postpone borrowing until interest rates dropped. Interest is a large proportion of repayments during the first year of the debt and a progressively small proportion later, when the bulk of the principal is repaid. Cost-reimbursing third parties paid large proportions of the hospital's debt during the first years of the repayment and steadily declining proportions later. Therefore, American hospitals had an incentive to acquire buildings and equipment by borrowing rather than by savings; they had an incentive to refinance old debt, even at less favorable interest rates, rather than retire it. The treatment of interest under the cost-reimbursement rules—along with the availability of tax-exempt bonds, to be described in Chapter Nine—led to much higher indebtedness by hospitals in the United States than in any other country.[25]

The treatment of interest costs illustrates how a single country's practices over a particular item can produce unexpected and controversial results. Some perverse incentives are widespread. For example, countries have always assumed that cost reimbursement should cover hospital staffs' numbers and salaries in full. They have assumed that health in general and hospitals in particular are labor intensive. Until governments and payers screened hospitals' prospective budgets more critically during the 1970s and 1980s, hospital employees steadily increased in numbers and in wages. Other industries in every country substituted capital for labor, but hospitals did not. New capital in hospitals was clinical and increased rather than reduced labor costs. Hospitals and the medical equipment industries made no effort to invent and install labor-saving equipment in the departments with the greatest scope—such as administration, catering, laundry, pharmacy, and housekeeping—since employment there too was fully covered by cost reimbursement and was included in the prospective budgets.[26] Not until countries moved toward strict revenue caps—such as global budgets and DRGs— were hospitals pressed to cut back on employment and to seek labor-saving technology.

Wider and Longer Perspectives

Hospital financial reports in every country have focused on the individual hospital alone. And they have had short time frames serving their limited purposes: calculating the reimbursement rates for next year, understanding the hospital's net financial condition this year, and identifying downturns or stability in immediate solvency. But hospital managers—in some countries more than others—are being oriented toward a wider scope and longer time perspective, and new forms of arranging and reporting financial information are being developed.

Larger Entities. The headquarters of multihospital systems—for example, the nonprofit Nuffield Nursing Homes Trust of the United Kingdom and the several for-profit chains in the United States—have their own objectives beyond those of individual hospitals, and they develop appropriate reporting methods. The accounts and reports of individual hospitals fit into the larger system. Some costs borne by other independent hospitals are carried by the headquarters of the multihospital systems. At a still wider level—the level of a country or a region as a whole—special reports are prepared for facilities planning. Other reports are prepared to estimate the total volume of hospital spending in the country's or the region's total health accounts.

Since this book concentrates on the mainstream of hospital financial management, it will not examine the reports and finances of wider societal levels, as in facilities planning and national health accounts. Other publications are devoted to those topics.

Longer Time Frames. Instead of assuming perpetual survival and stability, hospitals in some countries foresee possible financial bankruptcy, expansion, or transformation. Such projections are particularly salient for individual hospitals and multihospital systems in the volatile health economy of the United States. Methods are developed there to appraise alternative investments and programs and to estimate whether the new actions will enhance or handicap the financial position and social mission of the hospital or chain. Certain data are sought, and reports are designed for the decision makers.[27] Since hospital strategic financial planning is only beginning, since its methods are in flux, and since it is almost entirely American, I will not examine its reports and financial methods in this book.

4

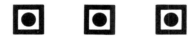

Units of Payment

After the hospital's operating costs are defined, the next issue is the owners' revenue strategy. Do they seek reimbursement that exceeds, equals, or fails to cover their total costs? At one time revenue from medical services was less than the total medical costs of the hospital. But, as I mentioned in the last chapter and will explain further in the next, payment for clinical care and the hospitals' housing has steadily increased, so that hospitals can recapture at least their full costs.

Although hospital owners everywhere might like extra cash, sickness funds and government payers refuse to give more money than the costs of care. Extra cash, they say, should stay with its owners—the insurance subscribers or the taxpayers. Any hospital earning its entire revenue from such sources earns its expected operating costs and no more.

Hospitals earn profits only if they provide care in a private market; that is, where the hospital is owned by doctors or by businessmen, and many or all of its patients are private self-payers who are billed charges set by the management. The United States is the only developed country where the principal payers (such as Blue Cross and Medicare) officially agree to a profit margin over the hospital's costs. In Europe the proprietary hospitals collect no profits above costs from the basic daily rates of sickness fund patients, but each earns extra cash by extra-billing for first-class rooms, second-class rooms, and extra amenities (such as meals). (In a few countries, such as Germany, the sickness funds try to force the hospitals to divulge this extra revenue in the prospective budget and then pay less than the full operating costs.) Many European proprietary hospitals—as in France and Switzerland—bill for individual services, such as diagnostic tests, and the charges exceed costs.[1]

The problem for the hospital is to cover its costs by collection from one or more payers, each paying by some formula. This chapter describes the units of payment; their sum total now equals the hospital's costs, more or less. Chapter Five will describe the payers.

The formulas for paying a particular hospital are set by some method of decisions. The hospital may set its own charges unilaterally, or adversarial bargaining may take place between the hospital and payers, or a screening agency may mediate between the hospital and the payers. Another possible method is rate regulation by a government agency. Finally, the payers may set their own payments unilaterally, through global budgets and direct grants. Chapters Six through Eight of this book will describe each of these methods of deciding the units of payment and their monetary value.

The following basic units of payment to hospitals are discussed in this chapter:

☐ *Global budget*—the entire amount for operating costs during the coming year. The usual method when government pays all or nearly all the hospital's revenue. Payments are made in twelve or twenty-four installments. Examples are Britain and Canada. In Britain the budgets are successively subdivided on each tier of the National Health Service; the hospital is one of several entities with parts of the total district budget. In Canada each hospital gets a distinct budget from the provincial Ministry of Health.

☐ *Daily charge.* A hospital is paid for the number of days of a patient's hospitalization multiplied by the standard daily charge averaged over all patients. In some form this unit of payment is nearly universal for basic ward care in countries with health insurance and direct payments by or on behalf of the patient. It has existed for nearly a century in most countries, even longer in a few.

   • All-inclusive, including physicians' salaries. Standard for all services in the hospital. Example is West Germany, except in its proprietary hospitals and its smaller hospitals.

   • All-inclusive except for physicians' fees, which are paid separately by sickness funds according to fee schedules negotiated with the medical association. Example is Medicare in the United States before 1983. Many European proprietary hospitals have this arrangement when they are paid under statutory health insurance, since the physicians are not salaried.

   • All-inclusive, including physicians' salaries, but with separate rates for the principal clinical services. This requires the hospital's finance office and the rate regulators to break the total prospective budget into cost centers. Example is France before 1984.

☐ *Itemized charges for services.* Some hospitals (particularly the proprietaries) break certain clinical items (such as use of the operating room, drugs, medical supplies, physiotherapy, and physicians' fees) out of the basic daily charges and bill for them separately. If a patient gets a first-class or second-class room and special amenities, these are billed separately in every country. In the United States, the hospital bill for each patient usually lists separately the basic daily charge, charges for many clinical services ("ancillary services"), and many extra amenities. (Usually the attending doctor sends a separate bill.) Such extensive itemization is unusual in Europe, even in proprietary hospitals. Where American Blue Cross Plans have large numbers of patients and use cost reimbursement, the ancillary use by all their members may be averaged. A per diem use of the ancillaries is then calculated and added to the basic daily charge to produce a more inclusive payment per patient-day; that is, the hospital sends an itemized bill for each patient but gets from Blue Cross an all-inclusive per diem.

☐ *Case payments.* Rates vary by diagnosis. An American idea, at first practiced experimentally only in New Jersey and Maryland. It became the method of paying under Medicare after 1983.

☐ *Prepaid subscription fees.* Subscribers (individuals and families) pay flat amounts to a hospital every week, month, or quarter. The hospital uses the money for its current operations. When the subscriber is ill, he can be hospitalized there, usually with low or no out-of-pockets. The method was one of the fund-raising techniques of British voluntary hospitals before the National Health Service. A few such "capitation" experiments were attempted in the United States during the 1980s.

Some hospitals are paid by combinations of different units, without a standardized nationwide pattern. Dutch hospitals until the mid-1980s collected per diems plus itemized charges. Swiss hospitals receive all-inclusive per diems from sickness funds, but the rates are not high enough to cover costs in full, and cantonal governments pay the rest in lump sums.

The following pages will summarize the incentives associated in theory with each payment method. Actual effects depend on how a method is administered and how it relates to many other conditions. Chapter Thirteen will summarize evidence about the effects of each unit of payment.

Global Budgets

The most recent method of paying hospitals, the "global budget" method, presumes a single source that can plan and pay. (Until recently nonprofit and even public hospitals pieced their revenue together from many sources.) Once established, it is the simplest method. Hospital and payer agree on the total expected budget (as described in Chapter Three). The payer then sends the money in installments, once a month or once every two weeks. Suppose that the Ministry of Health in the Canadian province of Ontario has agreed on a prospective budget of $25,000,000 for large urban Hospital A and $8,000,000 for small rural Hospital B. At approximately two-week intervals throughout the fiscal year (twenty-four times), the provincial paymaster transfers $1,040,000 to Hospital A and $330,000 to Hospital B. (A little is held back from the first payment and from each subsequent payment to cover end-of-the-year settlements.)

In some global budgeting systems, no deviations occur in the grantors' regular payments if the volume of work is higher or lower than predicted. In contrast, British Columbia allows small increases or decreases if actual work, measured by number of patient-days, is higher or lower than expected. All systems allow the grantor to reopen the commitment if the hospital greatly diminishes its work. One of the principal goals of payment by global budgeting is predictability, even if payment is not precisely calibrated to work. The revenue of hospitals paid by daily charges or by itemized charges always deviates somewhat from the predicted budget, because utilization was not predicted exactly and is not controlled by the payers or regulators.

The method's conformity to the budget is attractive to government finance officers, who usually must cope with chronic overruns from health. In theory, the method should make everyone in the hospital more cost-conscious, since the organization must perform all its work—even including higher utilization—within the prospective budget. The method should force the hospital to reorganize more efficiently, with closer cooperation between managers and doctors. However, the method might have some perverse incentives if the hospital is not monitored. For instance, to avoid overspending, the hospital might cut costs by underservicing.

At first hospital administrators welcome payment by prospective global budgeting. They think that they can economize and keep the savings, that they will get all the money they need, and that the grants of lump sums will give them complete freedom to manage. But they soon become disenchanted. Costs usually exceed predictions, and the hospital's executives constantly struggle with their staffs to keep within limits. Savings are rare and are not permanent, since the grantors give less money next year.

Administrative and financial statistics on health usually are generated from bills. Therefore, the drawback of simple payment methods is the loss of information. Countries with global budgeting systems usually learn very little about numbers and costs of medical procedures, the work of different clinical services in hospitals, and so on. They cannot compare the effects of global budgeting and other payment systems; they cannot make extensive financial comparisons of countries and their health service systems; and they cannot accumulate data about the costs of each case, defined by diagnosis or by any other principle. Therefore, they can never learn whether certain cases are more or less expensive, or whether one organization or treatment strategy is more or less expensive.

During the 1980s France is adopting global budgeting methods of payment in order to control expenditure; at the same time, it is improving the internal management of hospitals and, consequently, the reporting of information about procedures and costs in each hospital. Considerable effort in record keeping and computerization will be needed if the usual connection between simpler finance and less management information is to be reversed.

Daily Charge

The per diem has been the most common unit in paying the hospital. The names in several languages are:[2]

Words	*Countries*
charge per day, or per diem	Anglophone
prix de journée	Francophone
Pflegesatz	Germany, Switzerland, Austria
verpleegdagprijs	Netherlands
retta di degenza	Italy
sygedagstakst	Denmark

Hints of the modern daily charge appeared during the eighteenth and nineteenth centuries. Since the hospital basically provided housing and custodial care, the idea of itemized charging for specific services could not yet exist. The few payers were billed a certain amount each day for housing and food. The hospital was reimbursed by government agencies that pledged to support soldiers and foundling infants. As the population began to acquire cash, some hospitals billed other adult patients. In practice, collections fell short of charges because patients and their families lacked enough cash.[3] The hospital owners made up the bulk of the revenue budget from other sources. Not until the twentieth century did the sum total of all collected daily charges come close to full operating costs.

The simple daily charge resembled the earliest method of paying the doctor: a total payment for each home visit or for each office visit, covering all procedures. The apothecary sold individual medications and thus rendered itemized bills. As the scientific revolution in the nineteenth and twentieth centuries gave the physicians and surgeons more procedures, their fee schedules became more differentiated.[4]

When organized third parties agreed to pay for the care of certain hospitalized patients, perennial issues quickly arose: Should the payment be set by the payer or by the hospital? What should be the rationale for the payment? The first highly formalized arrangement was created in France. The armed forces lacked their own hospitals, and soldiers were placed in nearby local ones. But the soldiers were not local residents and taxpayers with rights to use the municipal hospital. Therefore, the national government agreed to pay but had to use an objective method for setting the rates. Laws of Parliament and regulations by the Department of War listed the services and amenities that should be provided soldiers, noncommissioned officers, junior commissioned officers, and senior commissioned officers. The department then estimated the costs per day in every French urban public hospital and set a *prix de journée* for each hospital and for each of the four military ranks. Payment was used as leverage for detailed regulation of the hospitals: each had to meet meticulous standards in order to care for the military.[5]

A second *prix de journée* arose during the late nineteenth century in France and was decided quite differently. One office in the *commune* government owned and managed the local hospital, another office provided social welfare to the indigents, and the social welfare office transferred some of its budget to the hospital office by daily charges when its beneficiaries were hospitalized. Eventually, the prefect—the local representative of the national Ministry of Interior—mediated between the two agencies of local government by setting a fair amount, thus initiating the rate regulation to be described in Chapter Seven.[6] For several decades different *prix de journée* were set by different procedures for different classes of patients, such as the military, the indigent, and victims of work accidents.[7] Eventually, standard daily charges—calculated by the prefect—were set for everyone.

When European and North American hospitals became more attractive to the middle classes during the middle and late nineteenth centuries, establishments created private and semiprivate wards. The patients usually were asked for all-inclusive daily charges, not including the fee of the principal doctor, who billed the patient separately. Unlike the early daily charges in the public wards, the hospital did not encounter widespread collection problems among the paying patients and did not have to settle for a sliding scale. The private daily charges were one of the many methods of fund raising and may have brought in profits over the costs of care. But the amount of profit—if any—was not clear, since the hospitals did not employ modern cost accounting until long afterward.[8]

Norway and Sweden by the 1880s were the first countries where every hospital patient was expected to pay something. Every patient was classified by income, and charges varied by class. Therefore, charges were based on ability to pay, not on the costs of services. The method could be used harmoniously only in countries where personal income was public knowledge.

Calculation. The daily charge was conceived when hospital work and hospital finance were simple. Its principal virtue continues to be the avoidance of administrative complexity. The hospital need not calculate the unique costs of each patient's care. The expected total budget for the forthcoming year is divided by the expected total number of patient-days. The daily charge is set by this arithmetic at the start of the year; all bills to patients and sick funds use it. The expected budget can be either the hospital's application or the last available cost report, trended for price changes. The expected patient-days can be either the hospital's prediction or the last available total, trended according to changes in the population, morbidity, or the hospital's mission. These premises require screening by a regulator, as I will report in Chapter Seven.

For example, a 580-bed West German urban hospital had gross operating costs of 45,717,628 DM in 1980. It had revenue other than payments from sickness funds, such as fees for private rooms; and health insurance daily charges would cover the remaining 41,242,551 DM. The hospital had 202,488 patient-days. The daily cost was 41,242,551 DM divided by 202,488 = 203.68 DM. The hospital had tried to get nearly this amount in the negotiations during the spring of 1980, but the sickness funds refused, since they believed that the hospital could find some additional revenue, such as raising the rental for the private practices of the senior doctors. The two sides had agreed on 197.25 DM as the *Pflegesatz* for 1980. The hospital predicted that its total net costs for 1981 would be about 46,192,000 DM. The two sides agreed that total patient-days should remain the same, and—after the usual haggling about probable costs and offsetting revenue from other sources—they also agreed on a daily charge of 221.30 DM for 1981. Sickness funds were then billed this amount for every patient day.

Deviation from the simple averaging results in complicated and inexact calculation, as French experience shows. Instead of a single daily charge for the entire hospital, France long had different ones for the principal clinical services, reflecting different costs. This procedure was possible when the technical level of medical care produced only a few general clinical services (surgery, internal medicine, pediatrics, and a few others); the rates were merely informed guesses. But after World War II, clinical services multiplied in number, the larger teaching hospitals had over a dozen daily rates apiece, and the rates were supposed to be calculated accurately from the prospective budget, necessitating elaborate cost-center accounting *(comptabilité analytique).*[9] This work was done before hospital accounting offices were thoroughly computerized; it was done without itemized information about exactly what procedures (such as clinical tests in the general departments) were done for which patients in which services.

For example, in Burgundy in 1980, the university hospital in Dijon had eighteen *prix de journée,* including:

	Francs per day
Medicine	752.80
Surgery	808.00
Obstetrics and gynecology	814.60
Psychiatry	567.20
Intensive care	4,940.00

A smaller urban hospital had six *prix de journée,* including:

	Francs per day
Medicine	339.20
Surgery, obstetrics, gynecology	534.20
Intensive care	2,223.00

A rural hospital's *prix de journée* were:

	Francs per day
Medicine	185.00
Extended care for elderly	154.80
Hospice for infirm elderly	115.80
Hospice for healthy elderly	66.30

Because of the increasing unwieldiness of this method, France abandoned the traditional system of daily charges in 1984 and tried to assign sickness funds fixed shares of each hospital's aggregate operating costs.

Unique or Collective Rates. The daily charge is supposed to cover costs, and therefore each hospital's charge is supposed to be individual. But administering an individualized payment system is very difficult: an impartial investigator must examine each hospital's accounts intelligently, and there must be enough investigators for all the hospitals. France has had to employ several financial analysts in every prefecture in the country to do little else.

When the information, staffing, and legal authority are lacking, short-cuts must be employed. One method is to classify hospitals in groups and to fix an average daily charge for every hospital in the group. The method resembles the fixing of a standard fee schedule for all doctors, the common method in medical pay.

Germany demonstrated the reasons for adopting group rates and the reasons for abandoning them in favor of individualization. German hospital operations before 1954 were simple, daily charges were low, accounting was primitive, and cost finding in the accounts was impossible. A series of price-control laws to revive the country after World War II included a regulation on rate setting. One permissible method was to group hospitals and fix a group-wide daily charge. This method seemed reasonable, since hospitals of similar type were not too dissimilar in costs and since neither the provincial governments nor the sickness funds had sufficient staffs and power to investigate each hospital thoroughly. Most provincial governments defined categories of hospitals according to their size and the complexity of clinical services. The sickness funds then agreed to pay a daily charge for all hospitals of the same class in the region, with individual rates for the very large and unique establishments.

As medical care became more complex and expensive, an aspiring hospital that wished to exceed the group average found itself underfunded by a rate set for others. The sickness funds saved money by pointing to the simpler hospitals in each category and agreeing to pay low charges appropriate to them. Aspiring hospitals pressed the provincial government to give them a higher group classification; but promoting them would lower the norm and average charge in the higher group. The only objective resolution seemed to be the individual costing and rate setting for each hospital.[10] The hospitals succeeded in replacing group rates by individual rates in the Hospital Finance Law of 1972 (*Kranken-hausfinanzierungsgesetz*, or KHG).

Billing. Once the daily charge is calculated—whether the simple one for the entire hospital or the distinct French one for each service—its simplicity saves effort in billing and collection. Since each patient's daily charge is the average for all patients, the hospital merely sends an aggregate bill to that patient's sickness fund: the number of patient-days that week (or other time period) for that patient and all other patients belonging to that sickness fund, multiplied by that hospital's daily rate. The sickness fund then makes a prompt payment into that hospital's account, without laborious and time-consuming scrutiny of each patient's claim form. The mail delivers a stream of aggregate bills and aggregate payments: each hospital sends to several sickness funds lists of their members' patient-days multiplied by that hospital's standard daily charge; each sickness fund sends to all hospitals prompt payment, calculated from its members' days in each hospital multiplied by each hospital's unique daily charge.

Modern computerization makes the work automatic. In the larger Dutch cities, the hospital clerks read into each of their computers the admissions that day, and the computers send notices to the patients' sickness funds to make sure the patients are covered. When patients are discharged, the clerks read that information in, and the computers send notices to the sickness funds. Subtracting date of entry from date of discharge shows length of stay for each patient. The sickness fund's own computer is programmed with the daily rates for all hospitals in the area, announced by the current Dutch regulatory rate commission (*Centraal Orgaan Tarieven Gezondheidszorg,* or COTG) once a year. The sickness fund's computer can multiply the month's total patient-days for its patients (those discharged or even those still hospitalized) by the hospital's daily rate, and the computer then instructs a transfer from the sickness fund's bank account to the hospital's bank account. Variations occur in different localities in Holland: some hospitals have their own computers, and others share them; some sickness funds have their own computers, and others share them; some hospitals bill the sickness funds, and some allow the funds to do the calculation. In a small and compact country such as Holland, all billing and payment might be centralized in a single installation in the future.

Daily charges are flexible enough to fit health insurance systems with many sickness funds as well as systems with a few big ones. For example, besides its regimes run by a few large funds, France has a regime for professionals and managers (*Caisse Nationale d'Assurance Maladie et Maternité des Travailleurs Non Salariés des Professions Non Agricoles,* or CANAM), where the actual financial administration is done by many smaller funds. The same daily charge of a hospital applies to all of them; rate setting protected their interests as well as the interests of the large funds. Having many third parties makes other methods of payment difficult: when France experimented with global budgeting during the 1980s, the many small payers had to be pooled.

Averaging. The daily charge presumes that each third party has a large volume of patient-days, that third parties have similar patient compositions, and that third parties cooperate. Some patients are more expensive than the average, and some are less expensive; but they average out for the hospital as a whole. They should also average out for each sickness fund. If one sickness fund argues that it should pay less because its members require less intensive care each day, the method becomes unworkable.

Inclusiveness. The daily charge began to cover room and board when clinical services were simple; gradually—by pooling all hospital costs in the calculations—it covered more services as they were added. Doctors' salaries are included in the pool, but fees-for-service are not included. Such a method could be a windfall for the hospital doctors, since they would be paid fees according to a fee schedule negotiated between the medical association and the sickness funds to cover the practice costs of office doctors as well as the honoraria for their personal incomes. The Dutch solution is three schedules: the honoraria for physicians, paid by the sickness funds to the hospital doctors on receipt of their bills; a list of costs to the hospital for each act performed by hospital doctors where the sickness funds will pay the honorarium part to the doctor directly (the *tarievenlijst*); and a daily rate for all other hospital costs. The hospital using "all-out" billing asks from the sickness fund for each patient the daily rate plus the items on the *tarievenlijst*.

In most countries the daily charge began with household costs and added clinical work, but this is not inevitable. The original political design of health insurance produced a different structure in Switzerland. Before the national law of 1911, Swiss health insurance was designed to pay for medical care; the patient was supposed to pay the hospital's household costs. The law of 1911 merely provided subsidies by the national government to approved health insurance carriers, to supplement subscribers' premiums, since employers were not compelled to give payroll taxes. This money has been used only for medical care, in the form of sickness funds' fees to the doctors and daily charges to the hospitals (the *Spitaltax*). The hospitals calculate and the cantonal government regulators approve the daily costs of room and board (the *Pensionszuschlag*). Therefore, the patient is liable for two daily charges. In practice, most cantons require the subscriber to be insured for both medical and household costs, and the subscriber pays a single premium for policies with both benefits. In cantons where an option remains, nearly all subscribers voluntarily buy policies covering the *Pensions-zuschlag;* and the sickness funds send both daily charges to the hospital on behalf of their subscribers.

Effects on Length of Stay. The most common criticism of the daily charge is its supposedly perverse incentive to prolong the length of stay. That is, its arithmetic discourages the reduction of stays and occupancy, and third parties pay for excessive days of hospitalization. The charge is an average of all the hospital's daily costs over all patient-days, but each patient's pattern differs. Usually a patient's tests and treatments are packed into the first days, and he convalesces at the end; therefore, his first days are more expensive than the average, his last days are less expensive, and the hospital can earn large profits by keeping the patient longer and billing the sickness funds at the full rate. This practice might occur particularly in a daily-rated system that lacks a rate regulator. Elsewhere, a rate regulator could spot hospitals with apparently excessive stays and penalize them by reducing rates, so that the hospital earns no more revenue than it would at the national average for stays.

Some have proposed a degressive daily rate, higher at the start and steadily lower later. It is most commonly proposed in Germany, where rates are settled by negotiations between sickness funds and hospitals but no regulator exists to penalize a hospital with excessive stays. The Germans seek a payment unit that will bring about greater efficiency through incentives.[11]

A degressive rate is easier to propose than to design. The present per diem is a simple accurate average reflective of costs: all costs are divided by all days. A lower rate for later parts of a stay would have to be offset by higher rates for the earlier stages; every day's typical costs would have to be calculated for each kind of case. The present per diem calculations were designed to avoid this impossible task.[12] A further problem is the ubiquity of perverse incentives: if the original method corrupts hospital managers, evil ingenuity can manipulate the reform as well. A degressive charge is an incentive to discharge helpless patients early. A few proposals for degressive payment aim at the physicians: they are said to lack incentives to speed up work; therefore, they should be paid lower proportions of the full rate if they perform procedures later during stays.[13] But I have encountered no serious degressive daily-rate designs for the *hospital's* costs.

Attempting to fine-tune the daily charge may be unproductive as well as technically impossible. Decisions by doctors and hospital managers in nonprofit hospitals may not be governed by such simple pecuniary incentives. Stays have been shortening in all countries, even those using the per diem, as I will report further in Chapter Thirteen. When variable per diems are substituted for flat per diems in experiments, length of stay does not change.[14]

Nevertheless, a few crude variations by length of stay are used in some countries, since medical costs are lower and since sickness funds press the acute hospital to refer the long-stay patient to the less expensive extended-care establishment. This method picks a day when the patient is reclassified as chronic long-stay rather than acute, and the daily rate suddenly drops. In contrast, a degressive rate gradually diminishes as stay lengthens. For example, in the Swiss canton of Zurich, the daily rate drops to 40 percent of the full rate after the thirtieth day; in the larger hospitals of Bern, the rate halves after the ninetieth day. France's per diem system—in effect until 1984—involved review and judgment. Each hospital had several daily rates. Larger hospitals had extended-care services as well as acute-care services, and the former had lower rates. Hospitals were supposed to transfer convalescent inpatients to the extended-care installations at the lower rates. When patients stayed over twenty days, the hospital was supposed to notify the sickness fund, whose control doctor (the *médecin conseil*) advised either continued acute hospitalization, continued nonacute (and therefore less expensive) hospitalization, or discharge. But this procedure was cumbersome to administer: papers reached the sickness funds late, and the control doctors were overloaded with this and other work.

Dutch experience further demonstrates the difficulty in eliminating all perverse incentives from the all-inclusive daily charge. Shortly after World War II, the Dutch government decided to combat wasted building space by discouraging the survival of less occupied hospitals. Beds with occupancy rates of less than 90 percent should not be built. A hospital would be paid a daily rate calculated to yield revenue sufficient to pay costs when its total number of patient-days equaled 90% × 365 × bed size. While hospitals could break even by shutting underused beds (the intent of the rule), more often they filled the beds at least 90 percent of the time. Additional patient-days from higher occupancy resulted in profits.

Around 1972 the new rate regulation commission, COZ, appointed an expert committee to devise new calculations.[15] The payment formula would no longer be used in futile attempts to pursue facilities-planning goals. After the committee reported, COZ scrapped the 90 percent break-even point. The denominator of the fraction was based on actual experience, not a theoretical goal: calculations used the actual number of patients last year or the expected number this year.

But the new method also had bugs. Under the new calculations, staffing and other costs kept pace with number of patient-days, since each item was a fixed part of each daily rate. If patient-days diminish, revenue declines, and staff should be reduced to cope with the lower level of work. The reasoning assumed that the need for staff and facilities depends on patient-days. This relationship flew in the face of the modern trend for greater service intensity; that is, stays are reduced, but the same amount of work is performed more rapidly or simultaneously by several persons. Patient-days, occupancy rate, and bed size were not confined to the denominator when the daily charge was calculated; they were also entered into the numerator. Holland had rate regulation wherein an examiner restrained the hospital's total costs by determining whether personnel and provision were appropriate. Staff and facilities were supposed to be related to "need"; bed size and patient-days were not good measures of "need," but no better measures could be substituted. The examiner scrutinized the hospital's prospective budget in the light of guidelines that related staff and facilities to numbers of patient-days, beds, and occupied beds. I will explain the methodology of these guidelines further in Chapter Seven.

Money still depended on patient-days, and the hospital was not motivated to reduce stays. If the number of occupied beds diminished, if it expected lower occupancy and fewer beds next year and the year after, it could plan an orderly reduction of its staff in accordance with COZ personnel/bed ratios. The problem was short-run deviations, and particularly the constant need to cover the present payroll. Reduction of stays below the budgetary expectations should be encouraged, but the hospital was committed to pay all its current employees, and the slightest decrease in patient-days below expectations created a deficit. To play safe, the hospital was motivated to exceed its planned occupancy slightly, instead of taking opportunities to reduce it further.

So that extra reductions in occupancy would not be penalized, the application of the guidelines for nursing personnel was cushioned during successive years when occupancy was diminishing. The problem arises during the retrospective balancing of accounts by the regulatory agency at the end of the year and the start of the next: without a cushion, if the hospital had a lower occupancy rate, it should have been paying fewer people under the guidelines; therefore, the COZ examiner would calculate a lower tariff. Since the hospital would have earned a "profit" under last year's cost report and actual tariff, it should repay the "profit" through additional deductions from the new year's reduced tariff. But such a hospital had hired and paid its nursing staff in good faith; it should not suffer from heeding the ministry's call to shorten stays and reduce costs.

The cushion took the form of retrospective calculations during periods when occupancy was declining: if the actual occupancy was less than the predicted rate, only half of the reduction was counted. The hospital got less money than it expected, but not to the full extent of the reduction. Presumably, the manager knew that his occupancy was declining below his budgetary expectations during the year and was making some adjustments in his staff. If the cushion provided no reductions in the hospital's allowable income during that period, the manager would have no incentive to reduce staff, he could keep "profits" resulting from reduced work, and the policy goal of lower spending would be defeated.

To illustrate the calculations, suppose a general hospital has 400 beds. Each 1 percent of occupancy represents 4 beds ($1\% \times 400 = 4$). If the COZ guideline allows 1 full-time-equivalent employee per 1.8 occupied beds, every 1 percent of occupancy in this hospital allows 2.22 employees (4 divided by 1.8 = 2.22). Suppose that the hospital expected to cut its occupancy from 90 percent to 85 percent during the year and actually cut it to 81 percent. Instead of a retrospective financial ceiling of 9 percent below the previous level of 90 percent occupancy, the COZ examiner imposes 7 percent: the 5 percent reduction in the year's cost report plus only half the difference between 85 percent and 81 percent; that is, $5\% + \frac{1}{2}(85\% - 81\%) = 7\%$, which represents a reduction of 15.4 jobs, since $7 \times 2.2 = 15.4$. Without the cushion, $5\% + (85\% - 81\%) = 9\%$; and $9 \times 2.2 =$ a retrospective reduction of 19.8 jobs. The economic manager knew in advance that his planned reduction of occupancy from 90 percent to 85 percent would necessitate a reduction of 11 jobs (that is, $5 \times 2.2 = 11$).

In the long run, the hospital was supposed to stabilize at its lower bed complement and its lower number of patient-days. The cushion was a delaying mechanism, not a nullification of the guidelines. After a few years' lag, the hospital's personnel level must fall within the guideline, without a cushion. In order to combat perverse effects and pursue these new aims, Holland had to introduce complex formulas and install a rate regulation system. But this did not succeed either, and major changes were made during the 1980s in the units of payment, the guidelines, and the method of regulation. I will describe these events in Chapter Seven.

Relation to Resource Use. The all-inclusive average daily rate sometimes is criticized because it does not represent anything. Economists are accustomed to individual prices for each product, reflecting the costs of production plus a markup. If each hospital day were priced according to its true costs, one could understand the hospital's output. The hospital would be equally rewarded for all its work and no longer experience the present mix of windfalls and shortfalls.[16]

Instead of scrapping the daily rate in favor of an itemized charge list, one might try to design a daily rate for each type of case. One such scheme has been designed in Germany and tested in a hospital. It requires far more internal information processing than German hospitals have needed under the traditional method. The German proposal has a two-part *Pflegesatz*. The basic nursing and housing cost per day is the same for every patient in the hospital. The patient is also charged per day the costs of treating his illness.[17] This procedure is an alternative to estimating the cost of each case and paying by admission, to be described later in this chapter. This cost-based *Pflegesatz* might still carry disincentives against early discharge, particularly for expensive cases. Payment by DRG is designed to encourage shorter stays.

Limited Information. Like the global budget, the daily charge has the drawback of gathering little information about utilization. The country lacks statistics about numbers and costs of medical procedures. One cannot make extensive comparisons among countries' health service systems or between the per diem and other methods of payment. Similarly, one cannot estimate the costs of treating cases under different payment systems.[18]

Information problems also arise for the hospital management itself. Enterprising managements can keep their own books, so that they can understand their internal affairs and can find costs. But this requires leadership by the hospital association and pressure by government, as in the example of Switzerland, described in Chapter Three. More often, hospitals in countries with per diem payment systems keep their accounts in highly aggregated fashion, without much internal cost-center accounting.

Itemized Charges for Services

Billing. Nonprofit and public hospitals in nearly all European countries have been paid by aggregated units, either the daily charge or the global budget. On the other hand, physicians and surgeons have long been small businessmen, charging for individual services. When doctors created private clinics, they continued to bill patients by itemized services. Distinctive inpatient procedures (extensive tests, surgery, anesthesia, and nursing care) were included in bills, along with other procedures that could be performed in ambulatory modes as well.

Sickness funds and government regulators fixed the flat rates for nonprofit and public hospitals in all countries; in a few countries, the for-profit hospitals were included as well. For example, German proprietary hospitals contracted with sickness funds have a *kleine Pflegesatz* covering all daily costs except the physician's fee. In most countries with private clinics (such as France), the all-inclusive daily rate does not apply to private clinics; the sickness funds and/or rate regulators review and approve the hospital's particular schedule of charges. In all countries (including Germany), a proprietary hospital without a contract with the sickness funds is free to send itemized bills to its patients. If such hospitals survive without sickness funds contracts, it is because of affluent clienteles.

Following are the items that French private clinics bill separately:

Each medical service, by each doctor. Laboratory tests and radiological examinations as well as treatments.

Use of special equipment (for instance, in the operating theater or the delivery room) whose operating costs and amortization are expensive.

Basic housing, nursing, administration, and food. Includes basic medical supplies, such as routine changes of bandages. This figure is often called the *prix de journée*, although its composition differs from the one used in public hospitals.

Special clinical supplies (such as drugs, blood, and prostheses).

Supplement for private room. Higher for one-bed than for two-bed rooms.

Extra services (such as telephone, television, flowers, special food).

The method used to set charges varies by country and by the individual hospital. The owner would like a free hand, but that is unusual today. If the private clinic has a contract with the official sickness funds governed by statutory health insurance, the entire charge schedule may be negotiated with the sickness funds or reviewed by the rate regulators. Even if the private clinic has no such contract and official restrictions, medical procedures charged to the physicians' payment accounts under statutory health insurance are paid according to the negotiated fee schedule. If treatment is done outside of statutory health insurance, the patient probably seeks reimbursement from private health insurance; those companies may have discussed the charge list with the private clinic, and the ordinary private clinic cannot charge too much. Glamorous establishments catering to the very rich are less inhibited. (I will examine the strategies of charge setting again at the beginning of Chapter Six.)

The methods of calculating global budgets and daily charges ensure that revenue equals costs. But the relation between charges and costs is more tenuous. Hospital accounting methods can produce only guesses about the fixed and variable costs of each procedure. Managers of these hospitals want only an approximation, since they usually aim to charge more and earn profits.

The all-inclusive daily charge is designed to incorporate all work that is routine in the hospital. As medical care has increased in complexity, more elaborate and more expensive procedures are included in the aggregate costs. But some very advanced and unusually expensive services are kept out and paid separately, at least until they become routine. For example, hospitals in Germany and in several other countries are paid individual fees for hemodialysis, open-heart surgery, transplants, and other unusual procedures. The planners and sickness funds screen hospitals' applications to install such special capabilities, confine them to a few sites, and monitor their utilization by separate billing.

Some European and Canadian hospitals have itemized price lists for charging inpatients not covered by national health insurance. But such a procedure is unusual; normally, the official per diem is charged. Price lists are used more often in the outpatient department for self-paying and privately insured patients.

The Netherlands demonstrates the difficulties in combining itemized charges and cost-based reimbursement. It is the only European country where a nonprofit or public hospital can elect to bill for tests and for many other services instead of pooling them under the all-inclusive daily charge. Each hospital until the mid-1980s could decide whether its tariff was "all-in" (an all-inclusive per diem) or "all-out" (a basic per diem plus many charges). But the hospital (in theory) could not earn profits, and therefore the selection of option was supposed to follow custom rather than financial gain.

The charges were not set for each hospital but followed a nationwide fee schedule (the *tarievenlijst*) written by the rate regulation agency (COZ). Exact calculation of the hospital's costs per service supposedly was not necessary. Therefore, the economist's hope that a price should reflect an interaction between production costs and market demand was not fulfilled. If the Dutch hospital lost money on an official fee, the rest of the costs were included in the cost base for the daily charge; if the hospital gained money on a fee, the profits were counted as hospital revenue and reduced the cost base used to calculate the daily charge. In Chapter Seven I will explain how the *tarievenlijst* was written.

The European method of cost-based all-inclusive daily charges was designed to be simple and easy to understand. The Dutch system proved complicated, difficult to understand, and possibly in violation of the nonprofit philosophy of reimbursement. Hospitals had many different "all-out" arrangements, the regulatory agency (COZ) could not monitor them, and no research was even done to count and classify them or to distinguish the costs attributed to the charges and to the daily rates. Since the COZ could not easily understand each hospital's application for daily rates and lacked access to the hospital's books, the revenue from charges may have been understated and the remaining costs of the hospital overstated.[19] The hospital had an incentive to increase the numbers of tests and treatments to earn extra revenue, and downward compensating corrections in the daily rate were not made by COZ for years, if at all. Increased revenue from charges could offset declining revenue from per diems as length of stay diminished. The confusion contributed to the unexpected increases in Dutch hospital costs, to be described in Chapter Thirteen. The difficulty in coping with this hybrid of daily rates and itemized charges was an important motive for substituting global budgeting in Holland during the 1980s. Total costs could then be predicted and enforced.

The United States is the only country where nonprofit and public hospitals collect charges that they themselves set.[20] The lists of charges developed long before World War II. Third-party payment of the hospital developed late in America, and until recently no third party had the large volume of claims conducive to averaging under flat rates; since each paying patient was billed individually, each person's liability had to be calculated exactly. Charge lists have become very extensive; they are matched by the hospital's computer to the itemized list of services for every patient, and the computer than generates an itemized bill for each patient. The charges usually exceed the hospital's costs— often substantially—particularly for diagnostic tests, the pharmacy, and amenities. Medicare and Medicaid by law refuse to pay such itemized bills unless the charges are below the hospital's costs for a particular patient, a virtually impossible event. Blue Cross also prefers average per diems covering the costs of its patients.

The patients expected to pay the itemized bills are those who pay from personal funds or who are then reimbursed by commercial insurance companies.

Usually these are upper-income people, but the total bills can be very high, and considerable complaint results. Lower-income self-payers leave bad debts; to make up for them, hospitals keep high the charges in bills for those who can pay. Most commercial insurance policies reimburse the patients in large part but not in full. Blue Cross in half the states is not able to negotiate all-inclusive per diems with hospitals, agrees to pay a large share of the posted charges, but usually tries to negotiate discounts with individual hospitals. The existence and size of the charges are the principal reasons why Americans have higher out-of-pocket payments for inpatient hospital care than the citizens of any other country, but there are no reliable estimates of the magnitude.[21] Each hospital has its own arrangement; hospitals are secretive about pricing, collections, and income.

Incentives. The usual assumptions about pricing and economic motivation apply to hospital charges. The hospital should be motivated to produce more of a particular service until marginal cost equals marginal revenue. Compared to a profit-maximizing business firm in an average market, the hospital is usually far more constrained in setting prices and in obtaining new capital to expand production. But it has considerable discretion in determining volume of a service if the price is attractive.

When postulating the incentives of "the hospital," one must quickly ask, "Whose incentives?" Hospital organizations vary among countries in the identity of their leaderships, the relations between managers and doctors, the authority of managers and doctors in deciding utilization, and the financial gains to the organization and to the individuals from ordering more services on the charge list. Charges can indeed be an incentive to much higher utilization and costs if the system creates an alliance of self-interest between managers and doctors. But hospital charges lack such effects if the doctors are unmoved.

A charge system in theory should persuade the hospital to organize its management and its resources more efficiently: unit costs should be kept low, so that high profits can be made on each service. However, total costs of the system may increase if revenue grows with larger volume of output, possible only from larger investments of labor and equipment.

A charge system may be an incentive to greater efficiency in calculating costs and in performing work, but not necessarily to greater accuracy in billing. Every procedure should be counted in the billing, but the system may invite exaggeration and fraud—revealed, for example, in occasional audits by American commercial insurers.[22] The third party cannot know the precise services consumed by each patient. Medical care and itemized bills are so complicated that patients cannot detect errors. The principal victims—the commercial insurance companies and the large business firms that self-insure their employees—lack access to hospitals' internal records and lack data-processing capacity.

Case Payments: Diagnosis-Related Groups

Before physicians' care was highly itemized and was covered by fee schedules, some lump sum charges were devised. The doctor estimated the probable difficulty of a case, predicted the amount of work, and set a fee for the entire course of treatment. This method has been eclipsed by the more remunerative fee-for-service, but occasionally it survives in the surgical specialties. Under French national health insurance and in many American transactions, a surgeon may include both preoperative and postoperative care in the fee for the operation; obstetricians in several countries give all necessary care for a normal delivery under the overall fee. However, European countries have never tried to pay for inpatient hospital care by such case payments, since all patients were normally covered by per diems. Calculating the exact cost of an individual disease was too difficult.

Development of the Idea. The inspiration for case payments for hospital inpatient care arose in the United States. Americans for over a decade have tried to devise an "incentive reimbursement scheme"—a method of paying hospitals that would inspire restraint but avoid regulation. Per diems were thought to encourage waste by prolonging stays; charges were thought to inspire providers to multiply services unnecessarily. But American conservatives distrusted regulators who would be captured by the hospital industry and allow it to raise costs wastefully. Another alternative, payment by global budget, was not feasible in the United States, since the hospital was paid by many third parties and individuals who would not join a pool. The problem was to find the payment method that would "make the market work"—ideally, a predetermined price per unit of service, calibrated according to the economical use of resources.[23]

Meanwhile, other Americans were challenged by the idea of differentiating hospitals by case mix. Hospitals were conceived as multiproduct firms, but no two had identical outputs, and therefore no two had identical inputs. Traditional methods classified hospital by size, such as number of beds and number of patient-days, but missed the central nature of the organization in an age of scientific complexity and variety. Traditional methods of hospital finance in Europe and North America granted money by volume: revenue increased with patient-days, and allowable costs for personnel and overhead were associated with numbers of beds and of patient-days. Payment needed to be connected to the character and complexity of work performed as well as the volume.[24]

The two thrusts proceeded together in America during the 1970s. A promising idea in incentive reimbursement was to estimate the costs of appropriate care for each type of patient and then offer these amounts to the hospital. In contrast to payment units that bear no relation to clinical content, a new payment unit should be devised that motivates the most cost-effective care for each type of case. Inefficient care would cause a loss on that transaction, and efficient care would yield a profit, just as in other economic sectors. The hospital's total revenue would vary with its case mix. Its solvency would depend on its efficiency.

One of the research projects about hospital case mix during the 1970s identified types of patient by diagnosis and estimated the most common procedures and average costs for each type. It developed methods of cost finding, so that the total inputs of each hospital could be associated with each case.[25] Such intricate research was possible only in the United States. The American method of paying hospitals produced the large number of individual itemized bills providing the vast data base. America had the large-memory computers and advanced software for the clustering programs.

New Jersey. Several American states with cost-control problems during the 1970s adopted forms of rate regulation, with mixed results. A new state government in New Jersey decided to test a flat-rate incentive reimbursement system based on the diagnosis-related groups (DRGs) developed in the statistical clustering research at Yale University. By the 1980s every hospital stay in New Jersey was paid for by DRGs, and the method applied to all payers. The United States, the country of rapid innovation in clinical technology, within a few years had developed and adopted a new payment method.

In New Jersey doctors, nurses, and technicians in each hospital have continued to give the usual treatments to patients and have filled out the usual clinical records. When a patient is discharged, clerks in each hospital examine that patient's record and fill out a code sheet that lists all procedures and other clinical and financial information. At first the clerks—with the help of the physician's entries—assigned each patient to a particular diagnostic group. (A more statistically and clinically powerful system of DRGs was adopted during the 1980s. Assignment to its 467 DRGs is done most accurately by computer processing of coded information.) The costs for each patient's direct care—nursing, ancillary services, and so on—arise from the sum of cost-finding procedures within each hospital. The hospital's fixed costs—such as interest, depreciation, administration, and heating—are spread over all individual patients.[26]

The 467 DRGs included the following:

DRG number	Title	Age of patient
2	Craniotomy for trauma	18 and over
36	Retinal procedures	All
88	Chronic obstructive pulmonary disease	All
110	Major reconstructive vascular procedure	70 and over
163	Hernia procedure	Under 18
370	Caesarean section	All
410	Chemotherapy	All
etc.		

The average cost of treating each DRG throughout New Jersey is calculated from the data combined from all hospitals. Each patient is billed the cost for his DRG, rather than the unique costs for his own case.

The patient is not billed the average cost for that DRG in his particular hospital. If so, then the hospital would merely be reimbursed its historical costs trended to the current year, much as if it were reimbursed for all patient costs split up into per diems. Under such a formula, the wasteful hospitals would be paid in full and would lack any incentive to economize, whereas the efficient hospitals would get no more than their costs.

Paying every hospital the average statewide cost for each DRG would be too abrupt a change from the previous system of full reimbursement of costs. Half the hospitals would be paid less than their costs; many would be bankrupted before they could readjust. Half would be paid more than their costs, and some would get large profits.

So the New Jersey payment is a blend of hospital-specific and statewide average costs for each DRG. The intent of the DRG payment is the following. Efficient hospitals earn more than their costs on that case and use their profits as they wish. Inefficient hospitals earn less. Hospitals lose on some patients and gain on others, but if they are generally inefficient, they lose on many patients and have to become less wasteful. If they cannot become more efficient by means of fewer personnel, fewer tests, and shorter stays, they might abandon care of certain conditions that other hospitals can treat more cheaply. (The foregoing is the theory behind DRG reimbursement. As in all demonstration projects, the initial cost base in New Jersey was set high, so that no hospitals were seriously squeezed. Rates were set even higher, to enable each hospital to cover the bad debts left by medically indigent patients.)

In the design of DRGs and their use in paying hospitals, several persistent dilemmas must be faced, and they are resolved only by temporary tradeoffs:

☐ *Heterogeneity and number of groups.* No two cases are identical, and they are assigned to the same group only because they have more in common than they do with other cases. The greater the within-group homogeneity desired, the larger the number of DRGs, the more complex the system, and the greater the number of DRGs with few cases. The simpler and more comprehensible the system, the fewer and the more heterogeneous the membership of the DRGs. Areas with a small data base (such as a small American state or a small Canadian province) could generate only a limited number of DRGs, and these would inevitably be internally heterogeneous. All this makes reimbursement difficult if one tries to construct a flat rate that is highly correlated with the costs of each such case.

☐ *Uniform billing.* All members of a DRG can be billed the identical rate, or the exceptions (the "outliers" falling beyond the "trim lines") can be treated separately. Should the very expensive members of the DRG be billed more, and should the very cheap ones be billed less? The ideal of the New Jersey system and of many other American proposals is to achieve equity through the formulas, bill automatically, and avoid the capricious and corrupt involvement of regulators. But billing everyone by flat rates is acceptable to payers only in countries where all payment is done by third parties with large coverage: they willingly pay the average rates for cheap patients because those bills are offset by the average rates for expensive patients. However, America has many small third parties with cheap patients, and some bills are paid by the patients themselves. The New Jersey system was quickly bombarded by complaints over bills at the average rate when the services recorded were below average in cost. Treating outliers merely calls for new theory and methodology in a research project, but New Jersey had based its billing on a research project still in progress, and the indignant outliers were dangerous politically. So New Jersey quickly relaxed the stringency of the system and allowed the hospitals to bill almost one-third of the cases according to their costs.

☐ *Incentives.* The pressure on the more expensive hospitals is greatest when the DRGs are statewide average costs. But the New Jersey system was experimental for many years, requiring the cooperation of the hospitals and the political support of their constituencies. The designers had to consider how to phase in an incentive system. So, as I said earlier, the DRGs were a blend of statewide average costs and each hospital's own costs. In order to get cooperation, the designers started the experiment with a very high allowable cost base for all hospitals, enabling all to prosper at least as well as before; but the result was no net savings for the state's payers during the first years.

□ *Type of hospital.* In every payment system, many hospitals seek exceptional treatment on grounds that they are unique, more complex, and therefore justifiably more expensive than others. But the DRG system was supposed to answer that claim, by paying hospitals more if they had a more complex case mix. The incentives would be negated if special categories of hospitals were paid according to higher average rates. Teaching hospitals usually get special treatment in Europe, on the grounds that "teaching hospital medicine" is inherently more expensive, and they did in New Jersey. They are paid higher DRGs on the grounds that their patients inevitably have longer stays.

Medicare. The financial managers of Medicare in the United States national government—at first, the Social Security Administration and then the Health Care Financing Administration—had been the principal grantors and clients for the research and demonstrations about incentive reimbursement, hospital case mix, cost control through prospective methods, and DRGs. They had provided the funds for the development of DRGs at Yale and their use in paying hospitals in New Jersey. They had been looking for some method of controlling the annual increase in spending for Medicare, which was based on a highly permissive statute guaranteeing reimbursement of the hospital's costs and which lacked any effective regulatory scrutiny. Ideologically, the economists and managers in HCFA favored some sort of incentive reimbursement scheme that would be calculated from econometric formulas, would avoid government regulation,[27] would give the hospital managers maximum discretion and minimum complaint, and would minimize the government's own involvement in the volatile and politically troublesome health care market.

The policy makers in the Reagan administration and the financial managers in HCFA had to make an early decision and adopted DRGs, even though the New Jersey experiment had barely begun and had not yet been evaluated.[28] All Medicare patients would be paid for by DRGs, beginning in October 1983 and taking full effect in October 1986. The method differed from New Jersey's in several fundamental ways. New Jersey had an all-payers system, whereby every payer paid for every inpatient by standard DRGs. But the new scheme applied to Medicare patients alone: it was a "prudent buyer" method, whereby the purchaser (HCFA) fixed the maximum prices it would pay. The data base for DRG calculations in New Jersey was the entire inpatient care of the entire state, but the Medicare DRGs would be calculated only from Medicare patient data. The New Jersey and Yale DRGs referred to the medical conditions of all ages, but the Medicare DRGs are limited to the health care of the aged. The research office of the New Jersey Department of Health calculated the DRGs from data given voluntarily by all the hospitals, but the Medicare DRGs were calculated by a payer (HCFA) from the reports on Medicare business previously given reluctantly by the hospitals. While New Jersey mollified the hospitals and paid many cases as outliers, Medicare would apply the standard DRGs to nearly all cases, recognizing only very long stays as outliers.

An important difference was the incentive system. New Jersey permanently blended statewide and hospital-specific data, so that hospitals would not run big losses too soon and could adjust gradually. HCFA based its DRGs on averages for the entire country, with temporary blending only during the first years, so that the more expensive hospitals eventually would suffer strong pressures to economize. Since New Jersey had an all-payers system, hospitals could not avoid experiencing the incentives to economize. However, the Medicare method invited a continuation of cost shifting to other payers on a larger scale than ever. If hospitals lost more money on Medicare patients under DRGs than under the earlier rules about allowable costs, they were free to overbill other patients. Since they believe in the competitive free market, the designers of the Medicare scheme bid other payers to protect themselves by creating their own DRGs. Thus, the American mosaic would continue in a new form, with several different DRG systems, each designed by a payer unilaterally from its own self-serving data base and formulas.

The Medicare researchers calculated the average cost per case from their data and gave each DRG a relative weight. The first weights for the DRGs listed above (in the section on New Jersey) were:

DRG number	Title	Medicare weight
2	Craniotomy	3.2829
36	Retinal	0.7093
88	Pulmonary	1.0412
110	Vascular	2.9328
163	Hernia for under-18s	No Medicare cases
370	Caesarean	No Medicare cases
410	Chemotherapy	0.3527

The law required the new payment method to be "budget neutral," in contrast to the usual experience in all countries, where new methods of payment trigger great increases in spending. The expenditure for Medicare hospital care per patient was not to exceed the previous year's expenditure under cost-based daily charges, plus an allowance for inflation. The average patient cost target was set at about $2,500 for the first year of DRGs. A DRG case with the weight of 1.00 would be paid $2,500. Therefore, each case with the aforementioned illustrative DRGs would be paid:

DRG number	$2,500 × each of the following weights	Medicare pays the hospital
2	3.2829	$8,207
36	0.7093	$1,773
88	1.0412	$2,603
110	2.9328	$7,332
410	0.3527	$ 882

(The unit value was not merely $2,500 but varied by city or rural area, by regional wage costs, and by other variables. The national or regional average was not used at once; instead, hospital costs were blended during the first year. Like every other American method of paying providers, DRGs proved complicated.)

Application in Europe. Even if the DRG is not used for billing individual patients and their third parties, classifying hospitals by their case mix can be valuable in comparing their efficiency in the use of resources. French hospitals during the late 1980s will organize their records so that individual patients' diagnoses can be correlated with their procedures; detailed information about resources will be kept by centers of responsibility; and computerization of information within individual hospitals will become advanced. One can then make a comparison on case mix and on use of resources among centers of responsibility within individual hospitals and also among entire hospitals. As basic units of such comparisons, the researchers in the Ministry of Social Affairs will attempt to calculate resource use in *groupes homogènes de malades* (that is, in GHMs rather than DRGs).[29] There are several possible uses in reimbursement: regulators screening hospital budgets (a task described in Chapter Seven) might compare hospitals on case mix and conclude that some have inflated budgets while others are efficient;[30] when payment shares are distributed among French sickness funds (a task described in Chapter Eight), the shares might be weighted by the complexity of the funds' patient loads.

Research about DRGs is spreading in Holland, Britain, and elsewhere in Europe. At first the information would be used for understanding of each hospital's performance. A possible use in the British National Health Service is in facilities planning: some districts might have a more complex case mix than others.[31]

Prepayment

Prepaid arrangements between sickness funds and independent doctors were common during the nineteenth and early twentieth centuries. General practitioners agreed to treat the sickness funds' subscribers and were guaranteed a steady income through capitation fees. The doctor received a fixed amount per year per subscriber, paid in monthly or quarterly installments, regardless of utilization. From these patients he received no fees at the time of care. These "closed-panel" arrangements were common in Germany, Holland, Britain, Denmark, and elsewhere.

Great Britain. The same idea evolved in England as part of the grab bag of fund-raising methods by the managers and charitable committees of nineteenth-century voluntary hospitals.[32] Many establishments throughout the country regularly solicited funds in public places one day a week, such as "Hospital Sunday." The workers were able to make small contributions on such days, when they had cash, but could not afford to pay for care when they were sick and off payrolls. During the latter half of the nineteenth century, many voluntary hospitals started to collect small amounts from workers on their paydays ("Hospital Saturday"). Some employers cooperated by deducting the voluntary contributions from paychecks and by sending them to the hospitals or their fund-raising committees. The committees' collectors contacted other workers.

Since demand for beds exceeded supply, many hospitals admitted only patients who could present vouchers. Wealthy patrons received vouchers and distributed them to the deserving poor. Many hospitals automatically gave vouchers to their weekly subscribers. Having paid in advance, such patients often were relieved of the means test by the almoner after hospitalization, and they were charged little.

The Hospital Contributory Schemes grew in number and became more formalized. All guaranteed the hospital a flow of money, regardless of utilization. Usually the subscriber was guaranteed admission to that hospital, but he could freely go elsewhere and pay. Most Contributory Schemes were affiliated with single hospitals. In a few cities (such as Liverpool), several hospitals joined in a larger scheme, divided the revenue, and gave patients a choice of establishments.

The prepayment schemes provided no more than one-fifth of the average hospital's revenue. Contributions were small, and employers gave none. Payments dropped during unemployment. The financial weakness of the Contributory Schemes and the absence of hospital benefits from national health insurance led to Britain's adoption of full Treasury financing under the National Health Service in 1948. The Contributory Schemes were reorganized and survive as private voluntary insurance to provide hospitalized patients with cash for requirements not supplied free by the NHS, such as convalescent home care and wheelchairs.[33]

United States. A few American hospitals organized such prepayment methods, beginning in the 1890s.[34] For a fixed monthly premium, which was used in the hospital's current revenue, the person could use up to a certain number (for example, twenty-one) of inpatient days per year. Several of these schemes obtained recognition of the American Hospital Association as Blue Cross Plans during the 1930s, eventually changing to become typical insurance funds, like other Blue Cross Plans. Under insurance, the subscriber's premium goes into a fund rather than into the operating revenue of a particular hospital; the fund pays a hospital for the subscriber's charges when he is hospitalized there; the subscriber can select any hospital and is not committed to one. Prepayment for hospital care was then forgotten in the United States, although it survived in the Health Maintenance Organizations—prepaid closed panels of doctors delivering ambulatory care.

Recently some American reformers have recommended paying hospitals by capitation. As in the HMOs, the hospitals then would have an incentive to please their subscribers by keeping them healthy; they would have an incentive to be efficient and care for their subscribers within their revenue.[35] During the 1980s Blue Cross of Massachusetts and Blue Cross of North Dakota experimented with capitation payment for subscribers in ten hospitals. The hospitals received fixed amounts per subscriber and were obligated to provide all necessary care in either their own or affiliated establishments. The hospitals were supposed to absorb losses.[36] It proved difficult to keep all the hospitals in the experiment and administer it with the strictness essential to an incentive reimbursement scheme. A hospital could withdraw, receive normal reimbursement, and risk no losses. In

America—and even in Europe—hospitals usually cannot be forced to join risky experiments in which some are certain to lose.

Prospectivity

Any payment system can be administered strictly or generously. Some sort of interim pay rate is set at the start of the fiscal year—whether it is the global budget, a daily rate, or a list of charges. The question is whether these prospective rates are fixed, so that the hospital must work within that revenue, or whether the hospital can obtain increases to cover higher costs. Increases might take the form of interim revisions of the pay rates from time to time during the year. Or they might take the form of a large retroactive increase at the end of the year to cover the deficit in the cost report.

Some discussions of hospital finance depict "cost reimbursement" as a guarantee that hospitals can run up any costs and still be assured of full payment by sickness funds. However, that assumption is not correct. Cost reimbursement is the rule in developed countries, and it can be prospective and strict. The trend is to set rates on the basis of prospective budgets—that is, the anticipated costs for the fiscal year—and expect the hospital to pay for all its work accordingly.

Interim or end-of-the-year corrections were once common, but they strained the sickness funds and government budgets. The trend is to eliminate such arrangements. For example, the United States once had a very permissive system: Medicare allowed the hospital to submit quarterly corrected budgets with higher daily rates, and the end-of-the-year Medicare cost report could ask for a large adjustment for the entire year; state Blue Cross Plans usually allowed hospitals to submit corrected prospective budgets with higher rates during the year; and the hospital was free to increase its own charge list at any time. Medicare adopted DRGs in 1983 because they were a payment unit that the individual hospital could not unilaterally increase. Blue Cross began to resist notices of rate increases. Several states adopted rate regulation to make payment truly prospective.

5

■ ■ ■

Who Pays the Bill

The methods of paying hospitals differ among continental Europe, Great Britain, Canada, and the United States. These variations will reappear throughout this book. They result from these countries' differences in the evolution of third-party payment during the nineteenth and twentieth centuries. Therefore, explaining the fundamental variations today requires a summary of the past.

History of Payment to Nonprofit and Public Hospitals

Hospital revenue for centuries was a mixture of income from the farmlands and forests in the hospital endowment, from small factories operated on these lands (such as grain and lumber mills), from donations, and from sale of inpatients' property. Small gifts were solicited constantly throughout the town. Table 5-1 summarizes the revenue of a French hospital in 1450. From one hospital to another and from year to year, the distribution among sources varied.[1]

The sale of beds, clothing, and related property was the only form of patient charge in the hospital referred to in Table 5-1. Patients brought their bedding and some other property with them. When they died, the hospital took possession and sold the property in the marketplace—doubtless spreading contagious diseases inadvertently.

Gradually during the nineteenth century, hospitals had to pay out more cash for wages and supplies, had to raise it, and therefore participated more in the cash economy. The structure of revenue changed, with endowments supplying fewer provisions for direct use and for resale. Table 5-2 shows the evolution in France—namely, a growth in total revenue, declining reliance on sales of products and rental income, the rise and decline of grants from local governments, and increasing reliance on patient charges.

During the nineteenth century and sometimes earlier, patients were charged small amounts for supplies that the hospitals had to buy specifically for them, such as food, bandages, and medicines. Since donations did not keep up with costs, charges to patients were increased but, for a long time, were not equal to the whole budget.[2] Charging patients was most common in countries where hospitals had small endowments, such as the United States, Norway, and Sweden. The introduction of charges produced difficulties and disagreements within

66

Table 5-1. Revenue of a French Hospital in 1450.

	Livres
Receipts in cash:	
Rents	144
Legacies and donations	16
Sales of patients' property (beds, clothing, etc.)	11
Seignorial rights	2
Receipts in products. Some used in the hospital, some sold:	
Rents, use of land	33
Farming	
Wine	297
Wheat	170
Other grain	56
Animals	35
Wood	2
Total	766

Source: Hôtel-Dieu of Beauvais, reported in Jean Imbert, *Les hôpitaux en France* (Paris: Presses Universitaires de France, 1958), p. 19.

Table 5-2. Revenues of Public Hospitals in France.

		Percentages[a] derived from:			
	Thousands of "old francs"	Sale of Products	Rents from land and buildings	Charges by communes	Charges to or for patients
1853	65,320	21.9	14.6	14.2	20.6
1860	89,848	16.4	13.3	13.9	17.0
1872	92,176	19.5	16.3	19.1	16.9
1882	108,935	17.9	17.9	19.9	18.2
1898	140,149	12.6	17.7	18.2	20.8
1908	164,570	11.5	12.4	19.1	27.6
1922	661,877	4.5	6.2	24.3	35.0
1928	1,382,618	4.9	3.9	23.9	43.9
1938	2,583,268	3.3	2.2	27.1	43.9
1951	88,727,436	0.6	0.1	0.1	71.4

[a]The percentages sum horizontally and are proportions of each total in francs. The figures do not total 100 percent, since I have omitted miscellaneous payers.
   Source: Totals for all French public hospitals—the acute hospitals and old-age hospices owned by municipalities—in Maurice Rochaix, *Essai sur l'évolution des questions hospitalières* (Paris: Fédération Hospitalière de France, 1959), pp. 326–327.

hospitals: some owners and community supporters defended the tradition of charity and opposed advocates of more "businesslike methods"; distinct and better services were created only for the payers, they said, and nonpayers were stigmatized.[3]

Gradually during the twentieth century, charges rose, particularly for richer persons. The custom in the United States, Britain, and some other countries was to establish an unofficial range of charges for each procedure; the rich were charged more than their costs and the poor were charged less, with the hospital finance officers performing this discretionary redistribution of income. Managers, owners, and members of governing boards constantly dunned the community, the rich, and governments for money. Some gifts and grants were large, but many were small, raised from collection boxes, street solicitations, entertainments, fairs, lotteries, and the like. Hospital managers concealed rather than divulged their true financial situations; they competed for help with exaggerated predictions of impending bankruptcy.[4]

Not until well into the twentieth century did nonprofit hospitals in Europe and North America[5] balance their budgets entirely from patient charges. Not until national health insurance and national health services made coverage universal in Europe did all patients resume membership in the same class; that is, instead of being treated alike as charity cases, patients now were treated alike as payers-in-full of their hospital costs.

History of Payment to Private Clinics

Proprietary hospitals in Europe, the United States, and elsewhere have evolved differently from nonprofit and public hospitals. They have been extensions of private practice by doctors.

On the eve of modern medicine and modern medical finance, a double system existed: the poor and persons with resources were treated in different places by different caregivers. The poor depended on nursing care provided by religious orders. In a few countries, such as France, members of the religious orders visited the poor person at home or took the person to the hospital. In general, medical care for the poor was perfunctory. For others, medical care was provided by doctors and apothecaries, who charged fees. It was ambulatory or given in the patient's home, invariably paid for, and often unavailable to the poor. A hospital was a charity; it sought money to cover its costs, never accumulated profits, and rarely went bankrupt. A doctor was a businessman who sold services to customers, earned as much as he could, and used his profits to raise his personal living standards and improve his practice. A doctor could go bankrupt and could change to another career.

When new improvements in asepsis made more advanced surgery possible, doctors created cleaner and more efficient arrangements than the patients' homes; they established "private clinics" in buildings connected with their offices. Often the doctor lived in the clinic. Paying patients preferred living there for several days instead of going to nonprofit and public hospitals, which had large wards, full of the poor. The doctor's "private clinic" was part of his business, an extension of his office practice. Patients were billed for their costs as well as for the doctor's fee, and the doctor tried to make profits on both services.

Development of Third-Party Payment

People needed to give cash to the doctor at a time when illness reduced their ability to pay. Associations of workers helped their members with cash during illness. Later, special funds were created to pool risks. Originally designed to provide disability benefits and payments to doctors, these arrangements eventually extended to hospitalization.

Guilds. The principle of systematic mutual aid to alleviate individual misfortune spread among the medieval guilds in European towns. Every person in a particular occupation—masters, journeymen, and apprentices—belonged to its guild. Governments were limited to military defense, settling disputes, and monitoring the private sector. Many functions performed by modern governments were performed then by the guilds.

The guild was a solidary community, and it protected members and their families from personal misfortune. It paid members during illness, to make up for income loss. It gave the widow a lump sum upon the death of a member. It conducted the funeral of a member or gave funeral benefits to the family. Every guild had its own methods of raising and spending money. Income came from special charges (for admission to higher ranks and for other privileges), from members' dues, from fines collected from violators of regulations, and from endowments. Payments to families during illness, unemployment, and death varied among guilds and rose and fell over time.[6]

Members selected whatever medical practitioners they liked and paid fees in cash or kind, helped by the cash benefits from the guilds. A few guilds had regular relations with the more comfortable hospitals owned and managed by the Catholic Church or by voluntary associations of clergymen or laymen. In return for annual donations, the guilds were assured of satisfactory accommodations for their members. A few ancient hospital buildings in Florence and elsewhere still have friezes and frescoes commemorating their association with guilds.[7]

The guilds created the precedent for a social policy, but they did not create a system. Their funds were meager. They did not create health services but merely provided small cash benefits to members; and most of the population did not belong to them.

The guilds died out during the seventeenth and eighteenth centuries. The new central governments took over regulatory functions, new industrial and commercial classes favored freer trade, and many old crafts disappeared. In some countries, such as France, governments were captured by economic liberals, and guilds were abolished by law.

Mutual Aid Societies. While economic and political evolution eliminated or transformed the guilds, problems remained in the financing of health care, disability income, and old-age pensions. The guilds had been small associations of elites, but the Industrial Revolution created large numbers of like-minded and insecure persons. Craftsmen and industrial workers in many occupations throughout Europe created funds that performed the guilds' social functions on a much larger scale. As in the past, they paid cash to members to help them pay their doctors and fill the gaps during income loss. If a member died, they paid cash to help the widow pay for the funeral and to give the widow some transitional income.

The funds were organized on diverse bases. Some enlisted only craftsmen and merchants, but their membership was more diverse and their financial resources larger than those of each small individual guild. (Example: the *Innungskassen* of Germany.) Some enlisted all the workers in one factory and might be helped by the employers in administration and in finance. (Example:

the *Betriebskrankenkassen* of Germany.) Some were created by trade unions and political parties of the Left or by Catholic trade unions. (Many examples in Belgium and France.) Some were created by entrepreneurs for any person residing in an area. (Examples: the *Ortskrankenkassen* of Germany and the "Friendly Societies" of England.) Many early mutual aid societies were multipurpose, like the guilds, paying for old-age pensions, widows' livelihoods, funerals, disability benefits, and medical care. Not until late in the nineteenth century did the sickness benefits funds become distinct from the funds for other benefits, largely as an artifact of the national health insurance laws.[8]

During the early and mid-nineteenth century, benefits were low and uneven. Work injury and non-work-related illness of the worker were covered alike. A few European employers contributed cash and administrative assistance; others thought this was not their affair, and workers contributed alone. Some European funds paid for hospital care when a patient could not be treated at home. Commercial insurance companies were not involved. A common concern—especially among workers and physicians—was how to increase benefits and improve the finances of the funds.

In several regulatory laws during the nineteenth century, Britain already showed the signs of a different approach. It applied to the funds ("Friendly Societies") the same regulations that it imposed on commercial insurers in other fields. Instead of finding new money and expanding benefits, the funds were now required to keep premiums and benefits actuarially in balance, even if benefits must be cut. Benefits were predictable cash sums, usually not services. The British funds competed for new business and had high costs of sales and collection, like any insurance company.

National policy about work injury in Britain and North America was individualistic, as enunciated by common-law courts. Employers were nearly exempt from liability in practice. They were obligated to pay a worker only if the worker proved in court that the employer was negligent and that the worker committed no contributory negligence. Even so, the employer was not liable if the worker could be shown to have assumed the risks of the job.

No European country adopted such a sweeping policy, in legislation or in judicial practice. Doctrines such as assumption of risk and contributory negligence did not exist. Employers were supposed to maintain safe workplaces and to be considerate of their workers. Liability in Europe was ambiguous, and enforcement depended on lawsuits by the victims. Employers might be expected to pay for medical care as well as short-term and long-term disability benefits.

Workmen's Compensation Laws. In Britain and North America, the doctrines of assumption of risk and contributory negligence exempted employers from liability to such an extent that many workers and their families were financially ruined. Employers had no incentives to maintain safe premises and to avoid child labor. The Anglo-Saxon countries amended their laws around 1900 to redefine risk as one borne by the employer, who was now required to pay compensation to a worker injured on the job, the amount of compensation to be based on extent of incapacity.

Since the problem was to cover actuarially predictable rates of risk in each industry and occupation, and then to compensate with finite sums of money, Britain's large commercial insurance industry soon took over the field by offering policies to businessmen to cover the risks. Policies insured the employer against liability; they did not insure the worker against injury. Premiums were a business cost for employers. The insurance companies included in their costs considerable overheads, such as the costs involved in selling policies and in litigating against the workers' claims. Benefits paid to workers were low cash payments of a fixed amount, so that they did not necessarily cover the costs of treatment for an injury. The debate over workmen's compensation in Britain and North America did not involve other health insurance, since employers were liable to pay only cash compensation, not medical care.

In European countries work-related injury and non-work-related sickness were regarded as equally serious disasters, even if legislation for the two were not enacted simultaneously. Individualistic business interests were not as powerful in most of Europe as in the Anglo-Saxon countries; they could not delay legislation so long or keep the benefits so low. Workmen's compensation laws were on the books in Prussia as early as 1838. Usually the costs were to be borne by employers. Many laws created special funds or used existing sickness funds, with employers paying a premium per employee in advance, sometimes supplemented by smaller premiums by the workers. By delegating the administration of benefits to the sickness funds, employers could satisfy any obligations to contribute to the victims' medical care.

Health Insurance Laws. The European sickness funds needed more members and money to pay for care. Otherwise, death benefits, disability benefits, and widows' pensions would use up the money, leaving little for the doctors and very little for hospitals. Providers and unions alike sought better health insurance coverage at the time of the debates over workmen's compensation.

The improvements were linked. Several European governments simultaneously enacted health insurance laws, workmen's compensation laws, and laws governing old-age pensions—uniting employers and employees, with financial contributions from both. All workers in an industry were covered, and all employers were expected to contribute. While special machinery was needed to review workers' claims under workmen's compensation laws, the premiums and benefits in several countries were administered by their sickness funds.

By ideological principle, the sickness funds and governments in the Anglo-Saxon countries presumed that paying for health care (beyond workmen's compensation) was the responsibility of the individual. People helped themselves and exercised foresight. Paying the doctor was a private business transaction. Britain had nonprofit societies operating much like insurance companies; they tried to experience-rate their subscribers, fixing premiums and cash indemnities to defray the costs of visits to doctors. Enough doctors were impoverished in private office practice to accept closed-panel capitation agreements with some Friendly Societies. Competition kept premiums, indemnities, and fees low.

Around 1900 a national controversy over Britons' health extended to non-work-related disability. Recruitment for the Boer War revealed the poor health of the entire population, for war as well as for work. The Liberal Government in 1911 passed a very restricted law, sold on grounds that it would improve the nation's human capital, making industry more productive. Workers were required to join Friendly Societies; their employers helped to keep the workers healthy by contributing to the Friendly Societies with premiums equal to those of the workers.

The Friendly Societies still lacked the funds to pay for hospitalization and paid only the general practitioner. The voluntary hospitals still found their own money from charity and from prepaid "Contributory Schemes" for prospective patients. Under a Contributory Scheme (described in Chapter Four of this volume, in the section headed "Prepayment"), a person paid a weekly subscription charge to a hospital, the hospital received the revenue at once for current operations, and the subscriber was hospitalized with no or few charges whenever he needed to be.

Canada and the United States did not go even this far in legislation. Most of Canada relied on private health insurance until 1958. (Saskatchewan broke ranks in 1946 by adopting a provincial hospital benefits program that mixed insurance methods and general revenue methods.) The United States enacted its only compulsory health insurance in 1965, in its very limited Medicare.

Subsequent Evolution. Each European country followed a different timetable for enacting and implementing national health insurance laws. Generally, however, coverage was steadily expanded, to include more workers and their entire families. All sickness funds eventually became committed to payment for services, not merely payment of cash sums to the victims. They paid providers and not beneficiaries. Mounting costs were covered by higher premiums on both workers and employers. Workmen's compensation and national health insurance were coordinated, often merely different clauses in social security codes, with benefits often administered by the same sickness funds. NHI became a standardized, comprehensive method of covering every European population, while the Anglo-Saxon countries tried to cover their populations by a mosaic of categorical programs

In Europe small sickness funds for the workers at each factory calculated premiums according to probable costs of care (experience rating) within the limits of the workers' incomes. Larger funds arose, with members from different workplaces and neighborhoods, and members were charged average premiums for average costs (community rating). Europe has seen a steady trend toward the merger of small funds and the absorption of small overstrained ones by larger ones; community ratings for regions or even for the entire country have replaced experience ratings.

In Britain the grudging National Health Insurance Scheme of 1911 yielded too little money to improve care for the population and to provide adequate facilities and income for office doctors. The Depression destroyed charity and reduced the collections of the hospital contributory schemes; the voluntary hospitals were bankrupt. The country lacked the organization and mutual aid ideology for a system of sickness funds depending on employers' contributions. The Labour Party had always argued that—because employers were so uncooperative and workers so poor—the only solutions were extensive public ownership and management of health services, Treasury financing, and compulsory social security taxation of employers. In power just after World War II, the Labour Party did not try to redesign NHI and the Friendly Societies along European lines; instead, it established the National Health Service. Health delivery seemed so parlous and private insurance (whether commercial or nonprofit) so feeble in resources that hardly anyone has dissented, either in 1946 or since.

Transplanted to North America, the British system of owning, managing, and financing health services worked badly but not catastrophically. The problems were fewer: Canada and the United States were not so industrialized and urbanized and had much less social inequality and less misery. More persons could pay out-of-pocket. As in Britain, commercial insurers underwrote risks for employers in workmen's compensation; their customers were the employers and not the workers, and they could attract business best by minimizing payments to the workers.

At first, commercial insurers entered the sickness benefits market by covering the loss of wages during illness, a finite and predictable risk. The policies were bought by individuals or by groups of employees. Eventually, the insurance companies entered the medical expense market in the manner most consistent with traditional insurance principles, by offering fixed indemnities for each illness or injury, varying by severity. The patient's treatment costs were likely to be higher than his indemnity, and he paid the rest out-of-pocket. Medical expense insurance by insurance companies eventually became important in the United States but was displaced by other methods in Canada. The insurance companies used their customary methods of manual rating for individual policies and experience rating for groups.

In both Canada and the United States, hospitals and doctors looked for secure methods of reimbursement and developed prepayment schemes different from commercial insurance. The hospitals in several American states and Canadian provinces created Blue Cross Plans paying indemnities to patients or third-party service benefits to hospitals. Hospitals particularly needed to guarantee collection for the more expensive patients; but manual or experience rating for such persons might have deterred them from subscribing. Just as the North American hospital has always loaded parts of its higher bills onto the lower bills, Blue Cross at first community-rated its groups, standardizing rates regardless of individuals' past utilization and future risks. Eventually the Blues added group-rating methods.

Medical societies in Canada sponsored prepaid funds, to cover the costs of doctors' fees, usually for hospital care and sometimes for office work. The medical plans paid indemnities, rarely direct benefits. Similar arrangements developed slowly in the United States.

The Canadian market was too small and the subscribers' incomes too low for Canadian hospitals to match the rising facilities and service levels they saw enviously in the United States. To pay for that type of care, the national and provincial governments during the 1950s replaced all commercial insurance and provider prepayment funds with direct Treasury financing for all hospitalization.

The United States found a way to make the mixture of categorical programs work longer—namely, through nonstatutory insurance connected with employment. It thereby averted the crisis in hospital finance that requires NHI or NHS. No other country has ever adopted this method on a large scale, and it originated unexpectedly. During World War II, controls against inflation limited wage increases, but employers could offer fringe benefits. Some provided pensions and health insurance as concessions to unions and as methods of attracting scarce labor. After 1949 major industrial contracts routinely included health insurance: management earmarked money for hospital and physicians' insurance in addition to wage increases, and it turned the money over to carriers to specify the benefits and to administer payments. Blue Cross and Blue Shield got most of these assignments, they dominated health insurance, and workers' pressure for NHI legislation was absent in America. Over 80 percent of employees and their dependents now are covered by health insurance paid for in part or in whole by their employers. Benefits vary among employers. In general, however, beneficiaries have fewer benefits and more cost sharing than are provided in European national health insurance laws.[9]

Nevertheless, the American arrangement has guaranteed payment to hospitals for most patients and has provided the hospitals with an increasing flow of cash. In addition to the groups of employees, Blue Cross sold many individual policies that also delivered more money as the hospitals raised their charges. For a long time, state insurance commissioners granted generous increases in Blue Cross rates, since their mandate in all their insurance duties was to make sure that revenue was sufficient to cover costs.

Principal Types of Payers

National Health Insurance.[10] Western Europe now has insurance schemes, varying in detail. A law of the national Parliament requires nearly the entire population to join a sickness fund, usually one selected by the subscriber from several possibilities. If less than the entire population is obligated to join, the rest join voluntarily. The distribution of coverage in West Germany in 1981 is shown in Table 5-3.

Each country once had thousands of sickness funds, but the numbers have steadily diminished through mergers. In 1890 Germany had 21,173 official funds with an average of 310 subscribers apiece; by 1981 it had 1,299 with an average of 27,475 subscribers and 43,548 covered persons apiece.[11] Mergers in Holland have resulted in only one or two sickness funds in each community. Usually the sickness funds are the same private organizations that existed before the legislation, although France eventually transferred the function to new public corporations. Subscribers and their employers are obligated to pay payroll taxes to the sickness funds, as part of the social security package.

Universal coverage means that the aged and the unemployed are required to join too. They pay small premiums; and, in addition, the national government pays the sickness funds on their behalf, in lieu of an employer's payroll tax. Usually the aged and unemployed continue to be carried as full members. In a few countries, such as Holland, the aged have special accounts maintained by the parent sickness fund, so that the government subsidies are clearly earmarked for them and so that their utilization can be studied. But their benefits are the same as all other subscribers'.

The statute and administrative regulations list the minimum benefits the sickness funds must pay for their subscribers. Hospitalization, physicians' care, pharmaceuticals, and other benefits are included, with variations among countries and improvements from time to time. The basic package is the same for all sickness funds. In some countries sickness funds compete for members by

Table 5-3. Distribution of Health Insurance Coverage in West Germany, 1981.

Type of coverage	Percent of population[a]
Official Sickness Funds (*RVO-Kassen* and *Ersatzkassen*)	
Obligatory employed subscribers	33.7
Obligatory retired subscribers	16.7
Voluntary subscribers	7.4
Dependents covered under subscribers' policies	33.8
Private nonprofit insurance coverage	17.9
Not insured	1.0 (or less)
(Total population: 61,713,000)	

[a]Total exceeds 100 percent because some members of sickness funds also have private policies.

Sources: Bundesministerium für Jugend, Familie, und Gesundheit, *Daten des Gesundheitswesen—Ausgabe 1983* (Stuttgart: Verlag W. Kohlhammer, 1983), p. 199; and *Die privaten Krankenversicherung—Zahlenbericht 1981–1982* (Cologne: Verband der Privaten Krankenversicherung, 1982).

offering small additional benefits. Both the employee and his family are fully covered by his payroll taxes. (Switzerland is an exception, because of the lower funding through taxation: each family member must buy an individual policy.)

The sickness funds always pay hospitals directly, and in most countries they also pay doctors directly. In a few countries, such as France and Belgium, the doctor is supposed to bill the patient, who in turn is reimbursed by his sickness fund; in practice, however, many doctors bill the carriers directly. Cost sharing by the patient has been rare for hospitalization and physicians' care but is common for pharmaceuticals and other benefits. (During the financial crisis of the 1980s, some countries reimposed small cost sharing for hospitalization.)

National health insurance is a method of pooling and paying money, not a method of providing services. It is consistent with any method of owning and managing hospitals. The traditional forms of hospital ownership—primarily by voluntary associations and by local governments—persist.

The sickness funds are obligated to pay for care by any doctor, hospital, and private clinic that has been admitted to practice under national health insurance. Customarily included are all doctors, all nonprofit and public hospitals, and all private clinics except those with primitive facilities and those who wish to avoid public scrutiny. The patient goes to whatever hospital is selected by his referring physician.

Private health insurance survives in countries with statutory coverage.[12] Following are possibilities:

- The law obligates most persons to join official sickness funds, but others can join voluntarily. Private insurance companies offer the full benefits plus extras, such as full payment for private rooms and the fee for the specialist. Premiums exceed those of the official sickness funds. Usually these complete policies are purchased voluntarily by the rich or as a fringe benefit of employment for managers and civil servants. Examples are West Germany and Belgium.

- The law obligates certain occupations to join official sickness funds but excludes others. Those who are excluded must purchase health insurance privately and voluntarily. Once the general approach in Europe, this method has been abandoned, except in the Netherlands, where 30 percent of the population is still excluded from the statutory scheme. In practice, all buy insurance from private firms, usually as a fringe benefit of employment.

- Members of the statutory sickness funds buy supplementary policies privately, in order to pay for private rooms in hospitals and for the hospital specialists' private fees. Examples are West Germany, the Netherlands, and Belgium. In Switzerland, the same insurance companies are carriers under the statutory scheme and sell the supplementary policies.

- The law in France requires the patient to share the hospital's bill, instead of charging it completely to the official sickness fund. Private nonprofit insurance (by the *sociétés mutuelles*) enrolls about three-quarters of the population and covers the cost sharing.

National Health Services.[13] An NHS converts health care into a typical government program, like public education. Hospitals and many other health installations are owned and managed by government, either the national government (as in Great Britain) or regional governments (as in Sweden). Physicians are either salaried civil servants of government or work on contracts with government.

All investment and operating costs of health care are financed as part of the Ministry of Health's share of the government's total budget. The budget is drafted by the cabinet's financial officers and is enacted by the parliament. Every year the Ministry of Health must struggle against competing ministries for its share. The funds come not from earmarked payroll taxes (as under national health insurance) but from general tax revenue.

Every inhabitant of the country is fully covered for all benefits. Only foreigners are excluded. Benefits depend on legislation and the generosity of the health care budget. The law and the budget also determine whether the patient must share any costs.

The law usually enables every doctor to join the National Health Service, sometimes with rights to part-time private practice. Doctors may refuse to participate, but few can survive as full-time private practitioners.

Although most patients use the "free" service, some seek extra attention or prompter appointments by seeing doctors privately. Private fees usually are low, since the citizen can always get the care "free" from the NHS. Benefits not covered by the NHS, such as nursing home care, must be purchased privately. About 7.5 percent of the British people have private health insurance, obtained primarily as a fringe benefit of employment. Most British subscribers are in the upper classes. The private insurance is used to pay doctors' private fees and the surviving private clinics.[14] The British Conservative Governments of the 1980s hope that the private sector will expand, permitting economies in the NHS.

An NHS can be created suddenly by a statute that rescues the health care system from bankruptcy (as in Britain and Eastern Europe). Or, as in Sweden, it can evolve incrementally, with young doctors steadily entering salaried government jobs rather than private practice, and with the public relying on the NHS rather than private facilities. Once established, an NHS is permanent. Health care cannot be reprivatized by sale to private owners.

The fact that government is the exclusive owner, manager, and financier of hospitals facilitates capital planning and regional reorganization. No such central controls exist under national health insurance.

An NHS can be administered like a disciplined bureaucracy, as in the Soviet Union, with a hierarchy of physicians who are also officials, taking orders from the Ministry. Or it can be highly decentralized and informal, as in Great Britain, where the administrators are not civil servants controlled hierarchically by the Ministry of Health; instead, the Ministry sends money and guidelines out to the operating offices, the doctors work autonomously pursuant to contracts, and the Ministry obtains limited information from the field.

Government Financing.[15] Hospitals are principal constituencies on behalf of NHI or NHS. If insurance cannot be made universal or if premiums are not high enough to pay for hospital costs, the hospital owners turn to government for help. In Britain the owners—voluntary associations and local governments—found hospitals such a financial burden that they were willing to transfer ownership itself and all the attendant headaches to the national government. Modernization of care and of amenities seems possible only through public financing and reorganization.

In the 1950s Canada became the first country to preserve traditional ownership—by voluntary associations and local governments—and combine it with full public financing. The entire operating costs of each hospital are met by grants from the provincial Ministry of Health, shared by grants to all the provinces from the national government.

The payments come from the Ministry of Health's operating budget, which is part of the provincial government's annual budget. As in all public budgeting, the share depends on the priorities of the government-of-the-day, since health competes with other sectors. The budgetary divisions are drafted by the Cabinet's financial officers and are enacted by the provincial Parliament. The money comes from the general tax revenue of most provincial governments, supplemented in a few by earmarked payroll taxes.

Every inhabitant of a province is entitled to use hospitals and physicians' services, with costs fully covered by the grants. Foreigners alone are not covered. The benefits are defined by each province's laws and budget, but the many years of national government subsidies have made all the provinces much alike.

As in an NHS, a hospital or doctor can freely choose not to participate, but no hospitals and few doctors can survive in full-time private practice. A patient can freely patronize any doctor privately, but few are willing to pay fees rather than go where care is "free." Private fees are low, because the "free" care is always available.

Hospitals remain independently managed and continue to raise charitable donations for special programs not covered by the provincial subsidies, such as research. Compared to an NHS, government lacks full power to plan capital development and compel regionalization.

One must distinguish between labels and reality. The Canadians call their system "health insurance," because they wanted to have sufficient funding while avoiding the reality and imagery of British NHS. The doctors in particular feared infringement on their customary role of free office practitioners. But Canada has neither an NHS nor an NHI.

United States.[16] Every other developed country has abandoned self-help and the mosaic of separate categorical programs, to guarantee a generous minimum of benefits for everyone without financial barriers. The middle and lower classes, who might neglect to insure voluntarily, are always required to join sickness funds under NHI, and some countries obligate the entire population. In countries with mixed obligatory and voluntary health insurance, the remaining members of the middle and upper classes join as a matter of course. In Europe and Canada the health services were once widely unequal, but they have all been leveled upward. The rich can still buy personal attention and comforts, but everyone has equal access to good basic care.

The United States Congress has periodically considered and shelved bills for national health insurance.[17] Instead, it has preserved and propped up the patchwork of private self-help programs and government assistance that all the developed countries once possessed but have abandoned.

The difference follows from America's unique history: it has never been threatened with defeat in war, it has never had to rebuild from defeat, and therefore the rich have never had to promise the lower classes a more equitable system of social protection. While NHI and pensions have been enacted in limited forms at various times in Europe, the principal extensions and implementation have occurred during and after wars that required social solidarity. America's class conflicts have never threatened war efforts; America was never so close to defeat that the poor and minorities had to be promised a completely new arrangement; and social programs have been enacted in a succession of limited forms to alleviate specific complaints and reduce the political heat. Much of the pressure to create and preserve categorical programs rather than create general reforms comes from the service providers, since such programs seem to benefit the providers at least as much as the beneficiaries.[18] As a result, the United States has more social inequality and less social solidarity than other developed countries do.[19]

Table 5-4 shows the different methods of paying for benefits in the United States today. Table 5-5 shows the proportions of the American population with each type of coverage in 1981. Aside from the Medicaid enrollees and the completely uninsured, about 77.8 percent have some sort of third-party coverage. The percentages shown on Table 5-5 for the insured total far more than 77.8, because many people have several policies.

Because health insurance coverage is largely voluntary, it grows and diminishes erratically. Because much of it is a fringe benefit of employment, it can drop steeply during business depressions that increase unemployment. Coverage of the poor depends on public welfare programs, which are reduced when state and local governments combat their deficits. As a result, patients' bad debts may increase, and hospitals—which must constantly search for money— will be forced to seek donations and even to overcharge patients.

Table 5-4. American Payers of Hospital Services.

Constituency	Methods of enrolling for health coverage	Vendor	Benefits
Groups of employees	Fringe benefit of employment	(1) Blue Cross/Blue Shield (2) Commercial insurance companies	Basic benefits. Usually with ceiling on volume, some cost sharing
Individuals, families	Voluntary purchase	Blue Cross/Blue Shield	Basic benefits. Usually service benefits with ceiling on volume, usually with cost sharing
Individuals, families	Voluntary purchase	Commercial insurance companies	Cash payment for each illness or treatment (indemnity plans)
Groups of employees	Voluntary purchase	(1) Blue Cross/Blue Shield (2) Commercial insurance companies	Major medical costs, beyond basic benefits policy
All persons over 65 years	Automatic. Paid for by payroll taxes on workers and employees	Medicare Trust Fund of United States government	Basic benefits. Service benefits with ceiling on volume and cost sharing
Persons enrolled in social welfare programs	Automatic	Medicaid program of each state government	Basic benefits
Employees injured on job	Automatic	Workers' compensation program of each state government	Basic orthopedic and surgical benefits
Former members of armed forces	Previous military service	Veterans Administration provides care in its own hospitals	Basic benefits
Individuals		Self-payment. Includes nonpayers who leave bad debts	Basic services of hospitals and doctors

Table 5-5. Distribution of Health Insurance Coverage in the United States, 1981.

Type of coverage	Percent of population
Blue Cross/Blue Shield	
Group policies	35.2
Individual policies	2.2
Insurance Companies	
Group policies	46.0
Individual policies	11.2
Other Plans (such as HMOs)	17.8
Medicare	12.7
Medicaid	9.6
Veterans	14.1
No Coverage	12.6
(Total population: 229,307,000)	

Sources: Adapted from *Source Book of Health Insurance Data, 1982–1983* (Washington, D.C.: Health Insurance Association of America, 1983), pp. 14, 36; and from Judith A. Kasper and others, *Who Are the Uninsured?* (Washington, D.C.: National Center for Health Services Research, U.S. Department of Health and Human Services, 1981).

Because each insurance policy is incomplete, many people have several policies. In the confusion some are overinsured, with duplicate benefits or with high premiums that provide financial windfalls to the companies. On the other hand, other persons have substantial gaps in coverage, while many are not covered at all. Few persons understand their coverage, and many must pay unexpected bills. If a group in the population is persistently neglected or if a health condition is not covered by existing payers, government or private agencies often are pressed to create a special categorical program. Since the mosaic of third parties is not coordinated, the financing system becomes steadily more complex.

In other developed countries, where the middle and lower classes have standard benefits, the income of the clientele does not correlate with the solvency of the hospital. In America, however, the poor lack third-party coverage or are covered by programs (such as Medicaid) that are cut back during periods of conservative government. Therefore, the lower the class of a hospital's patients, the lower its financial margin, the greater the risk of deficits, and the lower its capacity to raise capital.[20]

The gaps in financing require the American nonprofit hospital to rely on the rich donor, as in the past. This source has disappeared in nearly every other country. But the American hospital needs gifts for new construction, for new equipment, and for the operating costs of special programs. The managers and governing board must devote much time and charm to finding and cultivating the rich. Hospitals compete in the pursuit, each offering a very large donor his name on a building, his portrait in the lobby, a seat on the board, and constant flattery at meetings.[21]

Standardization of Payment

Europe and Canada. For a long time, hospitals charged patients and sickness funds what they could. The rich paid more than the poor. But the trend has been toward standard rates for the same service. If the hospital charges a patient more, it is only for a manifestly superior service, such as a private room. All countries with organized payment systems have arrived at this practice, but by several routes:

- *Negotiating systems.* Eventually all sickness funds become cost-conscious in dealing with hospitals; they realize that hospitals might raise rates by forcing them to compete, and they create a common bargaining front. Example is West Germany.
- *Rate regulation.* Payers welcome the extension of the regulator's authority to limit their payments. Once the hospital collected different rates set in a variety of ways, but eventually the regulator fixes one for all third parties and for self-payers. Example is France.
- *Sole payer.* Sickness funds may experience a crisis, merge into a few, or be replaced by a single public granting agency. Payment by rates may then be replaced by a single global budget. Examples are Britain and Canada.

European sickness funds often compete for members and for prestige. Sickness funds regularly compete with private insurance for business. They may compete by offers of extra money to doctors, but their competition does not take the form of offering higher payment to hospitals for the same service. Rather, any competition involving hospitals takes the form of offering subscribers extra benefits, such as more inpatient days at the full rate or convalescence at spas.

Germany and Holland have competition among carriers to enroll those subscribers with choices. The middle classes in Germany can join either an ordinary statutory sickness fund (an *Ortskrankenkasse*), a special statutory fund (an *Ersatzkasse*), or a private insurance scheme. In Holland some subscribers can join either a statutory sickness fund or a private insurance scheme. The higher-status German funds (the *Ersatzkassen* and the private firms) start the competition with advantages: because of their utilization and because they impose some cost sharing, their accounts show higher revenue and lower costs. The statutory sickness funds and the private insurance companies calculate their premiums by actuarial methods in both countries but by different principles: the sickness funds by community-wide rates averaged for all subscribers; the insurance companies by experience rates rising with the age and likely costliness of each type of person. An experience rate exceeds a community rate for older and more vulnerable types of people and is lower for the younger and more affluent. Competition among funds in Germany and Holland results in adverse selection by the subscribers and preferred-risk selection by the private carriers: the older and more vulnerable persons join the traditional sickness funds, which already have an obligatory enrollment from the workers and retired; the higher-status funds get the more affluent and the healthier. With their extra money, the German *Ersatzkassen* and the private companies in the two countries offer higher fees to doctors and more benefits to subscribers, not more cash to hospitals. For instance, they pay for private rooms in the hospitals but are quite satisfied to pay the standard daily rates for all other hospital services.[22]

Hospital payment has become more standardized in Europe because of the extension of statutory health insurance, and it could become nearly complete if NHI were extended to everyone. The feasibility of such a procedure has been investigated in the Netherlands, but several obstacles deterred the government.[23] The national accounts in social security and in health would suddenly appear to increase substantially if all the previously private insurance collections and payments were added. Since health insurance taxes would rise for everyone at first, all wage agreements in the country would be upset. The government has lacked the cash to buy out the reserves of the private insurance companies. Holland recently has had to solve financial crises, and cost control in health has had priority over extending benefits.

Political pressures have successfully resisted amending the NHI laws to force enrollment in the statutory sickness funds and eliminate the option to choose private companies. Politically powerful groups, such as the business managers and civil servants, prefer the private benefits. Members of the medical profession—particularly the influential hospital specialists—earn much income from private insurance.

If national health insurance becomes universal and if everyone is enrolled in the basic sickness funds, private commercial health insurance might become very limited, as in France. But it would not disappear completely. In free societies insurance companies can still legally offer supplementary policies to cover specialists' fees and the extra charges for private hospital rooms.

In a country with NHI and automatic assignment of occupational groups to particular sickness funds, the different carriers have different incomes and different costs. But they never pay hospitals different rates. Rather, as in France, the more burdened funds levy higher payroll taxes, require higher cost sharing from their members, and offer fewer extra benefits. Serious imbalances are averted by equalization transfers from the richer sickness funds.[24]

United States. Each hospital collects different units from different payers. Each unit may be higher or lower than that hospital's estimate of its costs:

- *Medicare.* DRGs calculated from a restricted definition of allowable costs. Medicare has usually tried to exclude amortization of principal and interest in debts incurred for new buildings and equipment, charitable care for the poor, bad debts left by non-Medicare patients, malpractice insurance premiums, research, and credit and collection costs.
- *Medicaid.* Per diems calculated from a restricted definition of allowable costs.
- *Blue Cross.* Per diems calculated from a generous definition of allowable costs; or, charges for individual services, reduced by a discount.
- *Commercially insured, and affluent self-payers.* Charges for individual services.

Each hospital's mix of business is somewhat different. Medicare covers about 25 percent of the patients. Medicaid varies between 10 and 50 percent of patients, depending on region and type of hospital. Blue Cross varies between 10 and 50 percent, depending on region. Many public and nonprofit hospitals in big cities have uninsured patients who get itemized bills but leave bad debts.

In America intense competition among payers and among hospitals extends to the payment of hospitals. European governments try to impose stability on hospital finance, but American governments usually do the opposite. The public programs—Medicare, Medicaid, and workers' compensation—pay as little as possible in their definitions of acceptable costs and tacitly invite the hospitals to overcharge the private third parties and self-payers. The other payers refuse to cooperate with each other: Blue Cross tries to get discounts from hospitals, so that its costs and premiums are lower than those of commercial health insurance. If the third parties formed a common bargaining committee to obtain a standard rate from hosptials, the United States national government would break it up under the antitrust laws.[25] A few state governments (Maryland, New York, Massachusetts, and a few others) have tried to create all-payers systems by regulating hospital rates, but the national government has often interfered by delaying permission to include Medicare, insisting on differentials in the cost base, and then later canceling the permission. As a result, state all-payers systems still have some intricate "prorationing" of the allowable costs and charges among the payers.[26] Throughout the United States, the principal payers give the same hospital different amounts of money calculated by different formulas for the same treatment. Every American hospital must employ a clever chief financial officer who can distribute profits and costs among payers, so that they can detect and protest as little as possible. Most of the hospital's profits and much of the costs not accepted by the more restrictive payers must be charged surreptitiously to the others.[27]

6

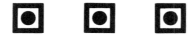

Negotiation
of Rates

The form and amount of payment can be decided in several ways. The hospital might decide its charges; patients and third parties dutifully pay. Hospitals might negotiate payment with large organized payers or with bargaining teams. Rates might be decided by impartial experts, such as a joint commission or a regulatory office of government. The organized payer might decide its payment, and the hospital must accept it. The next three chapters will describe how these methods work.

Charges Fixed by Hospitals

Every manager wants to be free to set levels of work, profit, and prestige in his own organization. But no organization is completely free. The manager must make tradeoffs between the levels of work (in both volume and complexity) and profitability (since profitability results from the operating costs and investments generated by the preferred level of work). Nor can he select an optimum level of revenue: even if he is free to select prices for his output, revenue and profits depend on the volume of sales determined by customers in the market. In the sectors discussed in the traditional economic literature, the entire income of a firm—covering both operating costs and profits—is earned from sales prices. The prices are set in accordance with the organization's strategy, constrained by the structure of that organization's production functions, competitive environment, and market.

No nonprofit or public hospital has ever earned more than a small fraction of its income from charges that the managers set themselves. Pricing freedom existed only when managers were constantly seeking funds from donors, from customers of the hospital's nonmedical production, and from patients. Managers were free to struggle. The result was organizational poverty: in markets without organized third parties, most individual patients could afford to pay little or nothing. The nonprofit and public hospitals were among the principal supporters of generous third-party coverage; their costs would be covered, and money would steadily grow. But they lost their power to fix charges unilaterally.

During the late nineteenth and twentieth centuries, only the private clinics could survive entirely on patient charges, and their prices had to be modest. The doctor-owners earned their incomes primarily from fees of medical practice. A few large and famous private clinics in Europe and America after World War I attracted rich patients and could charge more than costs, although most revenue in such establishments was absorbed by expensive staffing and amenities. Like the nonprofit and public hospitals, the private clinics in all countries have encouraged third parties, in order to increase business and cover their costs, and pricing constraints inevitably grew. Private commercial insurance usually paid indemnities to the patients for hospitalization, and the private clinics could not antagonize patients by generally charging too much above the indemnity levels. The doctors in private practice have always preferred to collect their profits from their personal fees rather than from the private clinic accounts; therefore, the clinics cannot drain off too much of the patients' cash. Some private clinics lately have been trying to develop paid-in-full agreements with some private insurers, thereby capping the rates.

The larger European private clinics, needing to keep filling many beds, have always pressed for admission to statutory health insurance practice. When successful, they often must negotiate a fixed daily charge.

Europe. In many countries today, hospital managers have no discretion in setting any charges. Even the supplements for private rooms and the outpatient fees are set by negotiations with third parties or by rate regulators. The world's hospital managers think about cost recovery, not about price setting and its possible outcomes. The problem is to find the revenue to cover costs. Even the managers of most private clinics are concerned primarily with covering their costs.

Holland is the only European country where many nonprofit and public hospitals bill the sickness funds according to charge lists as well as inclusive per diems. As I will explain in Chapter Seven, these charges are a ritual rather than a careful attempt to represent resource use and market demand. The charges are nationwide rather than calibrated to each hospital. They are set by rate regulators rather than by individual hospital managers. Revenue from the charges is combined with all other revenue to produce the break-even daily charge, but weaknesses in implementing rate regulation may allow hospitals to profit in the short run. While the hospital cannot set the price, it can increase volume of service.

United States. Only in America do hospital managers have a complete charge list that they can write. American proprietary hospitals may have a large fraction of their bills paid by such charge lists; in many states all patients in proprietary hospitals pay charges except those covered by Medicare. Fewer nonprofit hospitals collect substantial amounts of their total revenue from such charges; many hospitals collect less than a quarter, particularly in states with substantial market share by Medicare, Medicaid, and Blue Cross.

How such charges are set by the manager—when he has discretion—depends on the hospital's strategy and the structure of the market. Only a few publications have attempted to summarize the types of charge setting.[1] Following are possible management strategies:

- *Tradition.* Last year's rates, trended for cost increases, are charged.
- *Industry-wide prices.* The same rates as other hospitals' are charged, so that the local market is kept stable.
- *Cross-subsidization within the hospital.* Certain services are run at a loss, which is made up by very high charges for others.
- *Cost reimbursement.* Every patient is charged the costs of that procedure, perhaps with a markup for profit.
- *Price discrimination among patients.* Patients are charged according to their ability to pay.
- *Price discrimination among third parties.* The allowable costs and charges are identified for each third party. The utilization pattern of each third party's subscribers is identified. Charges are set for each procedure that will maximize the total revenue of the hospital.
- *Market strategy.* Charges are lowered in order to attract increased consumption or to take business away from other hospitals.

No surveys have been done across the United States to estimate the prevalence of these methods.[2] Wide variations probably exist. Following are some guesses:

- Tradition may be common for many items, once the charge list is set. But one or more of the other methods are used to create the structure. Because American medical care is highly innovative and constantly adds new procedures, each hospital often expands and sometimes restructures its list.
- Industry-wide prices may occur in some communities, but they are not the rule.
- Cross-subsidization is very common.
- Cost reimbursement may occur for some procedures in many hospitals, based on simple estimates of average costs.[3] In departments of the hospital where marginal analysis is appropriate—for example, in the laboratory and radiology, where variations in volumes of services are associated with variations in costs—methods of variable pricing to recover costs have been proposed. They can use new computer programs developed for cost finding under any reimbursement system, wherein the several components of costs for each service (such as labor, equipment depreciation, equipment interest, equipment repairs, and allocated overhead) are estimated at each postulated volume for that service.[4]
- Price discrimination among patients was common when third-party coverage did not exist or was limited to low indemnities. But it is no longer common. Some patients impose it upon the unwilling hospital by not paying their bills—possibly 5 percent of all American accounts receivable among nonprofit and public hospitals.
- Price discrimination among third parties is practiced by nearly every American nonprofit and for-profit hospital.[5] The public hospitals cannot use this strategy because they lack charge payers.
- Price cutting to expand business (market strategy) is the rule in every other sector in the highly competitive American economy. But it has never been done by hospitals, since new business is attracted by the referrals of the

affiliated doctors and by the prestige of the hospital, not by prices.[6] If doctors and the public think that higher prices result from better facilities, such a hospital has a competitive advantage, not a disadvantage. Individual patients do not comparison-shop among hospitals and gravitate to cheaper ones.[7]

During the 1980s some block purchasers (such as Health Maintenance Organizations and Preferred Provider Organizations) have been trying to force hospitals to offer lower prices in bidding for their business. As a result, American hospitals in the future might become price competitive when dealing with a few large purchasers. But such a strategy would operate like the bilateral rate negotiation that hospitals have long conducted with Blue Cross. They may never cut prices *generally* to attract *individual* customers.

The large third parties have refused to let the hospital managers fix their charges, since extra money belonged to the subscribers. The hospitals for a long time have had enough political protection so that they need not accept the dictation of the organized payers. Therefore, the two sides negotiate contracts, or government regulators act as referees.

Characteristics of Negotiation Systems

Arrangements between payers and hospitals can vary according to the following attributes:

☐ Number of tiers in the negotiations.
  - A particular hospital and the patient's third party alone. If so, whether they are backed up in some fashion by associations of hospitals and third parties.
  - In addition to the grass-roots negotiation, there is some bargaining between regional associations of hospitals and third parties. If so, how these negotiations mesh with those at the grass roots.
☐ Scope of negotiations.
  - For the individual hospital, whether the negotiations involve all payers, some, or one.
  - Whether all hospitals' pay rates are set by such negotiations. In the grass-roots bargaining, whether one or several hospitals are settled together.
☐ What is negotiated by the individual hospital and payer?
  - All or part of the hospital's cost report.
  - Unit of payment: for all payers, or only for some.
  - Contractual relations.
☐ If regional or national negotiations exist, what is the subject?
  - Contracts in general.
  - Guidelines for current grass-roots settlements.
  - Financial limits for current grass-roots settlements.
☐ Limits on the bargaining over money.
  - None: payers can press the hospitals to accept as little as possible.
  - Minima on either allowable costs or payment units.
  - Maxima on either allowable costs or payment units.

- • If there are limits, who sets them: parent associations, national bargaining over guidelines, government?
- ☐ Amount of disclosure of information to the other side.
  - • Hospital's information about its operating costs and revenue from other sources.
  - • Sickness fund's ability to pay.
- ☐ How deadlocks are settled.
  - • No contract. If no contract, two options exist:
    - — Subscribers are not reimbursed for care in that hospital.
    - — Subscribers are reimbursed an indemnity. How that figure is set.
  - • Private arbitration.
  - • Arbitration by government.
- ☐ Whether government can overrule the results. If so, on what grounds?
- ☐ Whether the outcome binds other economic transactions, such as the hospital's wage awards and the government's payroll taxes.
- ☐ Revisions of the award during the year.
  - • The hospital can increase rates unilaterally or the payer can reduce them, on grounds of necessity.
  - • Changes can be made only in a new negotiating session.
  - • No changes until the award expires—that is, each side must live within the original terms, and the hospital absorbs either its profits or its losses.

Negotiation systems in the payment of hospitals presuppose that the two sides are private, both make their own decisions, both use their own resources, and neither can have the final word. Therefore, neither the payers nor the hospitals are agencies of the national government. One cannot negotiate with a national government because it can always dictate the final results, in accordance with its larger policies on health, inflation, and taxation, and because no one can overrule it. If some hospitals are owned by governments, the owners are municipalities, and they behave in negotiations much like nonprofit establishments.

The great difficulty in negotiating with a government is evident in the payment of doctors. Negotiation of fee schedules and of salaries is the usual method of deciding doctors' pay, and medical associations insist on negotiating with national governments too, rather than accept unilaterally set rates. But such relationships are unusually conflictual. National governments usually insist on limits, particularly during budgetary stringency, and their negotiators are instructed in detail. Medical associations often make end runs to the Prime Minister or to public opinion, to put pressure on the paying agency, and noisy political controversies are common.[8]

If the payer or most hospitals are governmental, a method other than negotiations evolves. If all the money comes from government, top-down global budgeting of hospitals eventually develops. If the hospitals are governmentally owned and the payers are private or are mixed in their legal status, some sort of rate regulation develops, where the regulator exercises governmental authority to set a fair price.

Structured Bilateral Negotiation in West Germany

Evolution of Health Insurance. West Germany is the only major country where all rates of all hospitals are decided by direct negotiations between the sickness funds and each hospital. The society has a history of corporate group life, wherein group leaders influence the affairs of members, group leaders represent the members in dealing with government, and groups negotiate with each other. Sickness funds were created by private interests—by trade unions, political parties, religious associations, and employers—and most hospitals are private. The national health insurance law of 1883 (later combined with the other social security provisions in the *Reichsversicherungsordnung*, or RVO)designated the existing sickness funds as administrators of health insurance, instead of creating a special government agency. A proposal to create an Imperial Insurance Institute to administer disability benefits was blocked by the national legislature during the debates of 1881–1883, since employers, trade unions, and the existing sickness funds wished to prevent the national government from controlling health care and social security. The political compromises of 1883 merely required workers to join sickness funds. The funds set and collected premiums from workers and from their employers. Since the money did not go through government's payroll taxes and trust funds, the sickness funds and their money remained private.[9]

As in the rest of Europe, German health insurance was originally designed to pay for ambulatory and home care by doctors. For decades the sickness funds were preoccupied with employing their own doctors or paying for the services of independent practitioners. Relations were highly conflictual but were ultimately resolved privately: the funds and doctors were united in their fear of government takeovers, the funds wanted government only to ensure the collection of adequate premiums, and the doctors wanted only legislation that would strengthen their position with the funds. Eventually, the sickness funds and their doctors agreed on private collective bargaining, where the entities and procedures were spelled out in RVO.[10]

Hospitals. During the late nineteenth and twentieth centuries, German hospitals have been numerous and predominantly private. Most acute-care establishments have been owned and managed by charitable associations of laymen (many performing a religious service) or by religious orders of nuns and priests. Local governments owned and managed many hospitals, particularly those requiring the isolation of persons with contagious diseases. The local public hospitals were owned and managed by autonomous foundations; they resembled the confessional establishments in their management. As contagious diseases diminished, so did the number of public hospitals. Provincial governments (the *Länder*) owned the universities, their medical schools, and their teaching hospitals. Many doctors had small private clinics.

Development of Hospital Payment. As German hospital costs rose in the late nineteenth and twentieth centuries, managers imposed charges on patients who had money. Membership in sickness funds for extramural care implied employment and the ability to pay for intramural charges.[11] The sickness funds therefore were pressed to help their members pay hospital bills. At first the sickness funds paid the fee of a doctor who attended a worker at home, and the funds also gave the worker cash benefits to compensate for loss of wages; but he could have his hospital costs paid in lieu of these home health benefits and sickness pay.

The daily charge *(Pflegesatz)* has been very low until recently. The German hospital had remarkably few employees, paid them very little, and made them work long hours. As late as 1960, Germany's acute and specialized hospitals had 553,424 beds, only 100,665 nursing employees (not including students), and only 128,892 domestics.[12] Working hours exceeded fifty per week. Until World War II, the hospital managers were accustomed to finding much of their money from donations. Their financial accounting was primitive, and they could not estimate and prorate what a modern observer would say was the "real cost" of care. Sickness funds offered the hospital very low payments, and hospital managers—still steeped in a charitable and confessional tradition—were not yet as militant in their demands as the doctors. Until well into the twentieth century, the annual cost per sickness fund subscriber in Germany for hospital care was lower than the costs for physicians' care and for pharmaceuticals. For example, in 1907, 2.98 Marks per subscriber for hospital services, 5.22 Marks for physicians' services, and 3.31 Marks for drugs.[13] Even today proportions of all health care spending going into inpatient hospitalization are less than one-third in West Germany and between 40 percent and 60 percent in other developed countries.[14]

Organization of a Negotiating System Between Sickness Funds and Hospitals.
Regional bargaining arrangements over medical pay had to be set up between the world wars to resolve strikes and political protests by doctors against the penurious sickness funds,[15] but no formal arrangement for determining hospital pay was created until after World War II. Until then, since each hospital had its own unique costs and daily charges, the contacts with the sickness funds were local and ad hoc. Gradually the membership of sickness funds rose, and their payments could cover larger proportions of the hospitals' budgets.

A system was created after World War II, and it required legislation by the national Parliament. West Germany's federal and health care is an administrative responsibility of the province (the *Land*), but the German system enacts important decisions by united action of the national and all provincial governments via a legislature that represents both (the *Bundestag* and the *Bundesrat*). Nationwide uniformity is achieved in health care financing and in many other fields despite the federal system of government: the national Parliament enacts framework laws, and all the *Länder* implement them by means of their own laws, regulations, and bureaucracies.[16] At first sight, the hospital-financing laws did not create a private negotiating system: the original price regulation of 1954 and the subsequent legislation empowered the provincial government to scrutinize the hospital's costs and set an official daily charge, but in practice payment was decided otherwise. The hospital and the sickness funds negotiated the rates, and the provincial government's Ministry of Health or of Social Affairs issued a decree enacting the rates, almost always without change. The revisions of the law in 1984 and 1985 made the negotiating process official by spelling it out in detail. (The present governing law is the *Krankenhausfinanzierungsgesetz*, or KHG, first enacted in 1972 and extensively revised in 1984. KHG is supplemented by several regulations, particularly the *Bundespflegesatzverordnung*, or BPflVO.[17])

Disclosure. One problem of any negotiating system is each party's limited information. If the provider's organization and costs are very complicated—as in the case of hospitals—the payer understands very little. If the payer accepts the provider's claims, the provider will get too much money and the payer will ultimately be ruined. If the payer agrees to pay very little, the provider will be starved.

The law and regulations (KHG and BPflVO) require the hospital to fill out a retrospective cost report and a prospective budget every year and to send them to all the sickness funds and private insurance carriers whose subscribers make up at least 5 percent of the hospital's total patient-days. (The forms were called the *Selbstkostenblätter,* or SKB, until 1985, when they were superseded by the *Kosten- und Leistungsnachweis.*) To make sure that the cost and budget forms are reliable and can be easily read by the payers, the law requires the hospitals to fill out the forms according to certain accounting conventions (spelled out in the *Buchführungsverordnung* and the *Abgrenzungsverordnung,* two regulations implementing KHG), and they keep their books in much the same way. The forms are the basis of the funds' evaluation of the hospitals' requests for new and higher daily rates.

The Negotiating Procedure. The sickness funds form a common bargaining front, which is even more complete than their collaboration in negotiations with doctors. The more prosperous sickness funds for the middle classes—the *Ersatzkassen*—deal with the physicians separately but join with all other funds to face the hospital. Negotiation for physicians' fees is collective on both sides of the table: the same fee schedule is set for all doctors; therefore, the sickness funds face an association representing the entire medical profession. But such collective pricing is almost never attempted in hospital finance. Each hospital in Germany and elsewhere now receives a unique set of allowable charges related to its unique costs. Therefore, the German sickness funds face each hospital one by one.

Because of the complexity of hospital finance and because officials of sickness funds are specialists in insurance or in trade union affairs rather than in health care, the negotiators need expert help. The funds in all larger communities create a common office (called an *Arbeitsgemeinschaft*) with a staff that specializes in relations with the hospitals and doctors. The staff examines the hospitals' applications for rate increases and helps the joint negotiating team when it faces each hospital. In all smaller communities, the sickness funds avoid the expense of maintaining an *Arbeitsgemeinschaft* office, and the principal sickness fund in the hospital (usually but not always the *Ortskrankenkasse*) negotiates with the hospital on behalf of all.

The unity among the sickness funds and the nationwide rules about reporting and accounting permit the German negotiators to call upon a large data base. The national headquarters of the principal association of funds (the *Bundesverband der Ortskrankenkassen*) has revenue sufficient to support a data-processing system. It reads into this system all the *Selbstkostenblätter* from all hospitals in the country and sends each provincial *Ortskrankenkasse* office and each *Arbeitsgemeinschaft* tables comparing each individual hospital with the averages for all provincial and national hospitals of the same type. The *Arbeitsgemeinschaft* staff investigates the data from hospitals that are more expensive than their peer group averages and often challenges them during the negotiations.

Negotiators on the other side come with similar ammunition. A hospital must be forewarned that it is too high. All the province's hospitals encourage the very cheap ones to spend more, lest the sickness funds demand that all come down to the cheapest levels. Every provincial hospital association reads the *Selbstkostenblätter* into its own data system and generates peer group averages to help each member in its negotiations.

In Germany the statistical information now is much alike on both sides of the table, placing limits on the claims and bluffing of the negotiators. The law obligates the sickness funds to pay the costs of care in a well-run hospital, so they cannot make unrealistically low counteroffers. Of course, the two sides haggle across the table at the face-to-face meetings: as in all negotiating, the ultimate goal is to agree on one amount of money, the daily charge; the sickness fund offers to settle at slightly less than the hospital's request, and the hospital asks more; but they are usually close and quickly agree.

Each hospital in Germany has adapted its levels of services, costs, and rate applications to the resources of its locality, and it does not make wildly unrealistic requests. German sickness funds are organized with local accounts rather than with unified national accounts that would enable poor areas to bring in money from the rich.

While the financial levels differ from poor to rich localities, the decision-making procedures are identical everywhere. Normally, a federal system produces great heterogeneity in fields where the provincial governments have responsibility, such as health. The United States, as a result, is very diverse. But passage of KHG and the implementing regulations by the *Bundesrat* as well as the *Bundestag* produced uniformity in the structure and in its operating rules. Hospital leaders and sickness funds share experiences and goals throughout the country.

Settling Deadlocks. Every negotiation in Germany must end in a decision. Nonprofit, public, and most large proprietary hospitals cannot survive financially without an agreement. If a hospital had none, patients would have to pay so much out-of-pocket that they would go elsewhere; and office doctors would anticipate this reaction by referring patients only to participating hospitals.

The solution before 1972 and again since 1985 is an arbitration board (a *Schiedsamt*), a device widely used in German economic negotiations. The provincial associations of hospitals and health insurance carriers occupy equal numbers of seats. If a deadlock arises between a particular hospital and its sickness funds, the board is activated, the two sides pick a neutral voting chairman, and the board decides the daily rate.

Between 1972 and 1985, deadlocks in the negotiations were settled by the provincial government's officials, who then set the daily rate. But both hospitals and sickness funds tried to avoid this kind of settlement—the hospitals because they did not want the provincial officials to compel them to produce their books, in order to decide a rate based exactly on a hospital's costs; the sickness funds because they were afraid that the provincial government would be too sympathetic to the confessional associations and local governments that own the hospitals. As a result, hospitals and sickness funds tried to settle with each other.

Whether it is produced by negotiations or by an arbitration board, the rate must be made legally obligatory for both the hospital and its payers. The negotiators or the arbitration board notify the provincial government's Ministry of Health or of Social Affairs, and the Minister issues a decree setting a daily charge that the hospital may collect during the next year. The decree lists some or all of the following: the *grosse Pflegesatz*, which covers all costs, including physicians' salaries; the *kleine Pflegesatz* for those clinical services where part-time hospital doctors bill the sickness funds under fee schedules; the special *Pflegesatz* for newborns; the special *Pflegesatz* for unusually expensive services, such as intensive care; supplements for private rooms; and special fees for unusually expensive tests or treatments.

Limits on Bargainer's Discretion. A negotiating system can be based entirely on power bargaining: each side gets as much and gives as little as it can. Or the topics and ranges of the settlement can be prescribed.

At one time German hospital payment negotiations had few ground rules, the sickness funds paid as little as they could, and the hospitals complained about the results. The rate-setting regulation authorized the provincial government to classify hospitals in groups, with members of each group getting the same daily charge—one of the few times any country has had collective daily rates. Instead of negotiating with the individual hospital at length to learn its unique needs, the sickness funds often held rapid discussions to arrive at the offer they would give to all members of the group. The sickness funds paid low daily charges, oriented to the less advanced members of each group. The more energetic hospitals complained that their buildings were deteriorating because the funds granted them little money. The employees were said to be too few, underpaid, and forced to work fifty- and sixty-hour weeks. The hospitals were said to be lagging in technology.[18]

The hospitals obtained a complete change of the ground rules by passage of KHG in 1972. Much less was left to unfettered bargaining. The law instructed the sickness funds for the first time to grant a daily charge that would ensure "the economic security of hospitals . . . appropriate care of the population through the assurance of efficient hospitals." Each hospital would receive its own daily charge based on its unique costs, rather than a group rate. The law and its regulations listed the items that could be allowable costs and that the sickness funds must pay for. The regulations and the prospective budget forms prescribed the scheme for calculating the daily charge from the prospective cost base. Much less was left to negotiate. The sickness funds can only challenge that a hospital is asking for too much money on specific lines of the prospective budget form or in the total budget, in the light of the expected work and in the light of peer group spending.

The perennial dispute over investment funds was taken out of the negotiations. New capital for the modernization of buildings and for new equipment is not an allowable cost in the prospective budget but is supplied by the provincial governments—with contributions by the national government between 1973 and 1985. Depreciation for smaller items is an allowable cost in the prospective budget and is chargeable to the sickness funds, but it is fixed by a formula in the law.

Some Judgments About the Negotiating System. Every negotiating system has a structure and rules that give advantages and better outcomes to one side. The losers complain that the machinery is unfair and should be corrected. Even the winners may think that they miss their full desserts. An observer might list strengths and weaknesses by comparing the arrangements with some theoretical standard about how negotiations should be conducted. (In this case the starting point is the observer's belief rather than the participants' self-interest.)

□ *Detailed circumscription.* If one believes that decisions should be left to the free choice of the participants, the German system has moved in the opposite direction. Once the payment bargaining lacked a detailed scenario, but now the agenda and calculating rules are specified by law.

If one believes that hospitals should be protected, that their costs should be guaranteed, the detailed scenario now accomplishes this. During the years of power bargaining, hospitals were squeezed and employees were less prosperous.

The system produces procedural uniformity throughout the country, a common trend in unitary political systems and a difficult goal in federal countries.

Prescribing allowable costs and calculations in the law reduces conflicts. The payment of hospitals is peaceful. Less circumscribed negotiating systems sometimes have troubled periods.

The hospitals prefer the present arrangements, since they are protected better than before 1972. But some leaders of the sickness funds believe that the negotiating system is a sham and that they can negotiate very little, even after the revisions of 1985.

□ *Inclusion of items.* Investment for buildings and heavy equipment was excluded from the negotiating agenda after 1972, so that it could be funded adequately by government. It was no longer counted among operating costs. The sickness funds have been happy not to bear this cost, but the national and provincial governments have experienced financial crises and have had to limit their grants. Many leaders of hospital associations now favor adding all capital consumption to the list of negotiable items, as costs that users of hospitals should pay. But, unlike the pre-1972 situation, they believe that capital should be added to the list of costs that the sickness funds are compelled to include in their negotiations. Hospital managers would gain more money and more autonomy.[19] But, during the writing of the legislative reforms in 1984, the provincial governments blocked such a change. If the hospitals stopped relying on them for investment funds, they would lose their power in this field.

□ *Integrating rate negotiation and planning.* The sickness funds complain that they are obligated by law to pay the costs of hospitals that have been allowed to expand unnecessarily or that have been allowed to survive on a large scale while they are superfluous. The provincial governments are irresponsible in their planning, complain some leaders of sickness funds, since it is the funds and not the *Länder* that pay the operating costs. The sickness funds during the debate leading to the reform of 1984 have called for representation in the planning machinery, now controlled completely by the *Länder* governments.

The *Länder* have refused. The hospital associations—and particularly the confessional hospitals—support such refusal, since the provincial politicians protect them.

☐ *Monitoring individual hospitals.* The monitoring of individual hospitals is very difficult in regulatory systems, since the regulatory staff is small, deals with many hospitals, and has little information aside from the cost reports and prospective budgets. This is the strong point of the German system. The local offices of the sickness funds are close to the hospitals; their executives and members are users. Guidelines come from the national and provincial capitals, but the local sickness fund negotiators have the task of evaluating the performance and needs of the individual hospital. The reform of 1984 authorized the sickness funds to negotiate the service structures of the hospitals as the bases of the prospective budgets. Therefore, if the provincial government's permissive planning system allowed unnecessary capacity, the carrier could refuse to pay for it. Previously, the negotiators merely took last year's cost report and trended it upward.

☐ *Disclosure.* The weakness of a negotiating system is the concealment resulting from adversarial attitudes. The German laws require more disclosure of hospital operations than is usual in negotiating systems—and the new cost report and prospective budget forms of 1984 increased the reporting of clinical services—but the sickness funds complain that they still do not know enough. They cannot inspect the hospitals' books and must guess about too much. A leading problem in Germany is a possibly excessive number of beds kept filled by prolonged stays, but the sickness funds cannot investigate how many admissions and patient-days are unnecessary. Therefore, they cannot tell precisely how much of their money is wasted.

☐ *Conformity to public policy.* Rate regulation and public grants can be integrated with each year's public policies about controlling costs, altering the mix of services, fighting inflation, and so on. But the parties to negotiations are preoccupied with their own interests, not with implementing someone else's policies. A negotiation system presumes that the private sector is free to run its own affairs within its own resources.

Public policy affects the outcomes of negotiations only by the wording of any law. In Germany KHG and BPflVO require the sickness funds to pay full operating costs, specify the allowable costs, and prescribe the calculating methods. Much of the negotiation follows a prescribed scenario. But the sickness funds and hospitals are not required to negotiate within any limits; they are not required to follow annual economic guidelines from government or from any other source.

Faced with steep increases in costs during the late 1970s, the national government of Germany—led by the Social Democrats and supported by the sickness funds and by its own civil servants—created a national tier of negotiations to fix limits on fees. The associations of professionals (physicians, dentists, and others) meet twice a year in a forum (the *Konzertierte Aktion im Gesundheitswesens,* or KA) with representatives of the sickness funds, employers, trade unions, and local governments. They consider recommendations by the national government and other exponents of public policy. They agree on economic guidelines within which negotiations are supposed to set fee schedules.

The annual increase in total health care spending (fees and utilization) is supposed to keep within the annual increase in taxable wages (the *Grundlohnsumme*), since the wages provide the revenue of the sickness funds.

The payment of hospitals for many years was not included in the work of the KA. The sickness funds and civil servants concerned with financial policy recommended adding hospital payment to the cost-control law and to the agenda of the KA, thereby limiting hospital awards to the annual increase in the *Grundlohnsumme*. But the hospitals objected that their payment was already settled by the KHG, that they are guaranteed no less than full reimbursement of their operating costs, regardless of movements in the *Grundlohnsumme* and in the KA's recommendation about total health spending. A prolonged political deadlock ensued during the 1980s, and the provincial governments refused to allow amendment of the laws.

The legislative reforms of 1984 authorized guidelines-setting machinery that paralleled the KA. The national associations of hospitals and of sickness funds could meet and propose guidelines for all the local hospital rate negotiations. Besides their own information about personnel needs and operating costs, they could take note of the KA's recommendations about the health sector generally.[20]

□ *Arbitration.* This method of settling deadlocks hangs over any negotiation, even if it is rarely used. If the arbitrator is believed biased, the other side makes more concessions. German sickness funds believe that arbitration by the provincial government is favorable to the hospitals; the provincial government owns a few teaching hospitals and must give financial aid to the establishments owned by local governments. The sickness funds prefer an ad hoc arbitrating committee of a sort common in German private life (a *Schiedsamt*), wherein each side picks a member and the two members pick a neutral third person. Government would be excluded, and the negotiating system would become completely private. The hospitals opposed such an amendment of KHG for many years, and the provincial governments (in control of the *Bundesrat*) retained the arbitration power. Substitution of the *Schiedsamt* was one of the concessions made to the sickness funds in the package of reforms enacted at the end of 1984. The Christian Democratic/Free Democratic coalitions that ruled the national and many provincial governments accepted the reform, since it fulfilled their philosophical goal of reducing government intervention in private transactions. Because the reform strengthened the sickness funds, it promised stricter restraint over costs.

A Joint Negotiation Forum in the Netherlands

Negotiation systems develop in societies with vigorous private organizations and limited government. Of all European countries, Holland seems to have the most appropriate basis. Throughout the Dutch social structure, public services have long been created by small groups and coordinated by nationwide nongovernmental associations. Government's powers once were very limited. Many of the social networks were affiliated with religions, and Dutch society was said to function by an organized division among these sectors (called *verzuiling*). Hospitals, home care programs, sickness funds, schools, radio stations, and many other services were affiliated with these Catholic, Protestant, and secular communities.[21] Government enacted frameworks, provided a few basic services, and coped with emergencies.

For the coordination of each specialized activity, the grass-roots units joined in confessional associations; then the separate confessional associations cooperated in confederations or in committees. For example, separate associations were created for Catholic, Protestant, and other hospitals; eventually, these individual hospitals created a national hospital council. Similarly, the sickness funds were grouped in separate associations, at first cooperating and more recently merging.

Negotiations among the association headquarters have long been the common method of settling payments and work relations throughout Dutch society, with government providing guidelines and occasionally intervening during crises.[22] The payment of doctors has been settled this way: every year, the national headquarters of the sickness funds (once in a committee and recently in a unified office) has negotiated with the confederation of the several medical associations.[23] Holland has had a long tradition of social solidarity (despite the religious differences) and ethicality; in negotiations, no group was supposed to demand too much, and no one was supposed to win a great deal at someone else's expense.

Difficulties in Creating a Negotiating System. The payment of hospitals, it seemed, could not be settled by the same face-to-face bargaining as in the payment of doctors and of other workers. Doctors and other persons expected an amount above costs to produce personal income, but the number was not precise. In contrast, the negotiations over hospital pay were supposed to reimburse costs exactly, no more and no less.

Wage bargaining in every other field was simplified by collective rates. For example, the negotiated fee schedules applied to all doctors. But every hospital was to be settled individually—an immense task for the officials of sickness funds, since they were few in number, they specialized in collecting premiums and paying benefits, and they were unfamiliar with hospital affairs.

The sickness funds could negotiate over each hospital's costs only if they obtained full information. Weaknesses of any negotiating system include the paucity and unreliability of the other side's facts. Dutch hospitals would not disclose their books to the sickness funds, and the Dutch government did not enact laws requiring detailed accounting and reporting, as Germany did.

The parties to bilateral negotiations are preoccupied with their own policies and not with public policies. But a small country strongly dependent on international trade, as Holland is, requires stability and restraint throughout its economy. It had to prevent health insurance and the payment of hospitals from absorbing too many resources and from stimulating inflation; it also had to prevent the sickness funds and hospitals from making expensive agreements that would harm the economy.

A single negotiating system was difficult to construct in Holland because such a large fraction (30 percent) of the population was insured by private companies, which did not form a common front with the statutory sickness funds. The private companies created their own council, which held conversations with the medical confederation to keep private fees reasonable; but the private companies were more disposed to cooperate with the sickness funds over hospitalization, since it was much more expensive and since the private companies needed stronger protection against cost shifting by the hospitals.

Joint Commissions. Many sectors of Dutch society have standing councils that set guidelines, give advice to government, and reduce trouble. If freezes and cutbacks are necessary, these councils are available to work out agreements that everyone will accept as legitimate. The decisions are made by negotiations among the leaders of the interest groups. Such machinery was created to govern statutory health insurance, and it was extended to settle the payment of hospitals. As a result, hospital reimbursement in Holland is a hybrid, combining features of bilateral negotiation and rate regulation by a commission. But the regulator is a neutral referee, acting with a mandate from the two sides.

Monitoring all aspects of Dutch national health insurance is the Sickness Funds Council (the *Ziekenfondsraad*). The idea is not unique to Holland: neighboring Belgium has a National Institute for Health Insurance (the *Institut National d'Assurance Maladie-Invalidité,* or INAMI).[24] Each is a nominally public agency created by a law, but each really operates as a consultative body in the private sector, settling rivalries and occasionally making recommendations to government. The recommendations—about benefits, payroll tax rates, and the like—are usually accepted by government, since they represent the consensus among the private interests. The governing boards have seats for the sickness funds, the trade unions, the employers' associations, the health care providers (that is, the associations of doctors, hospitals, and others), government agencies, and a few impartial citizens. The many committees, which are staffed by civil servants employed by the commissions, include units for negotiating the payment of doctors.

Before 1941 Holland had no statutory health insurance but a variety of private schemes. Hospitals set their own rates and found the money where they could. Health insurance with limited hospital coverage became obligatory for workers in 1941 and was expanded in 1949. Price-surveillance laws were in effect until well into the 1960s, to ensure the stability of the fragile Dutch economy; and all hospitals—like other private organizations—were supposed to file their daily charges every year with the Ministry of Economic Affairs. When the price-surveillance laws were rewritten, there was a need for decision-making machinery in fields such as hospital care, which could not be deregulated completely but were too complicated for detailed examination by the ministry's small staff. The sickness funds wanted a voice in the determination of hospitals' charges, as they already had in the direct negotiation of doctors' pay.

The precedent of the *Ziekenfondsraad* was followed. The law on Hospital Charges of 1965 formally empowered the Minister of Health to prescribe the maximum rates that hospitals could charge their patrons, including the third-party payers. The Minister issued a regulation creating the Central Agency for Hospital Charges (the *Stichting Centraal Orgaan Ziekenhuistarieven,* or COZ).[25] Since it was an advisory body that brought together private interest groups and gave advice about prices paid by one set of private actors to others, it was not a governmental agency. It was a foundation (a *stichting*) under private law. None of COZ's budget came from the national government; all came from small surcharges calculated into the tariffs of institutional health services, primarily the hospitals and institutions for long-term care. (COZ was revised in 1982, but I shall describe it in its original form, when it was more of a private negotiating site than a public regulatory agency.)

The governing board of the original COZ was constructed for a bilateral negotiation agency: ten seats were held by the national hospital councils, seven by the official sickness funds, three by the private health insurance carriers, and one by the civil servants' sickness funds. The chairman and two vice-chairmen were three distinguished neutral citizens appointed by the national government. When COZ was replaced by the *Centraal Orgaan Tarieven Gezondheidszorg* (COTG) in 1982, with jurisdiction over the pay of doctors and of other providers, additional seats were added to the board from these provider associations and from the payers.

The award of daily charges to hospitals each year depended on guidelines, accounting procedures, and other rules that were negotiated between the two sides in specialized subcommissions (*kamers*) of the full board. In the hospital field, specialized *kamers* existed for general hospitals, nursing homes, homes for mental patients, and day care and family shelters. Each *kamer* consisted of about ten members of the full board, drawn from the payers and providers, with a neutral public member as chairman. Its work was reviewed and approved by the board. The full board met three or four times a year, always at COZ's offices in Utrecht. All important decisions, such as adoption of guidelines and reports, were made at plenary meetings.

The full governing board would have been swamped by all this detail. So, half its members met ten times a year as an executive board (the *dagelijks bestuur*) to review the detailed work of the *kamers* and staff. All guidelines and other rules governing payment were still approved by the full board, but this approval was usually pro forma after the screening by the *dagelijks bestuur*. Representatives of the carriers and hospitals had equal numbers of slots; the swing votes over contested issues were cast by the three "wise men" named by the government. Often, and particularly on important issues, the "wise men" voted on instructions from the Ministry of Health; sometimes they could vote as they thought best. They had considerable discretion and responsibility in working out agreements between hospitals and sickness funds.

COZ had a full-time staff of about thirty economists and accountants (plus secretaries and office workers), who performed the investigations and drafted recommendations. One senior member served as staff aide to each chamber.

Writing Guidelines. The link between public policy and the payment of individual hospitals is a set of guidelines. They protect the patient and the integrity of the health system by specifying minimum standards in facilities, staffing, and work. They protect the economy, the sickness funds, and the taxpayers by fixing ceilings on expenditure. They promote efficiency and quality by helping professionals, organizations, and patients avoid clinically unnecessary care and by encouraging doctors and hospitals to provide the necessary care in appropriate places by appropriate methods. As every country's payment system for hospitals becomes more extensive and more organized, guidelines are introduced into the decisions. Some method is developed to create the guidelines and to apply them to individual cases.

The payment of Dutch hospitals for some time has been governed by such policy guidelines (*richtlijnen*). Writing them was the principal purpose of the COZ chambers and the governing board. The individual hospital applied for rates that would cover its costs, and its papers were reviewed by the COZ staff. The staff applied the guidelines to the specific circumstances of that hospital, to cover its legitimate costs. The goal was to provide the hospital with enough money from daily charges to enable it to do its work without strain, but not to give this nonprofit organization too much. While the rate of payment of the individual hospital was not negotiated bilaterally between the carriers and hospitals, the guidelines were written somewhat adversarially. The hospital representatives in the COZ chamber asked for more, while the carriers' representatives offered less.

Separate guidelines were written for general hospitals, mental hospitals, homes for the retarded, institutions for the deaf, institutions for the blind, medical day homes for children, day homes for the handicapped, foster homes, and rehabilitation centers. Each *kamer* and its secretariat produced one or more of these sets of guidelines.

The key to the payment system was the content of the guidelines. Dozens were adopted for all components of the hospital's expected costs—for example, total maximum spending per patient-day for nursing staff for hospitals of different sizes; maximum number of occupied beds per nurse; total maximum spending per patient-day for administrative salaries for hospitals of different sizes; maximum number of administrators per hundred occupied beds; and estimated life and annual depreciation of each class of equipment and building. Nearly all guidelines dealt with the maximum numbers and spending for personnel—the component of hospital costs that was the largest and most likely to be overdone. It was assumed that other operating costs were dictated by the needs of care.[26]

The guidelines existed in some form since the 1950s, when the Ministry of Economic Affairs monitored prices throughout the country and gave hospitals advice about maximum rates. To recognize when a hospital rate was excessive, the Ministry needed formulas to estimate appropriate costs for hospitals of each size and type. Certain common conventions in Dutch hospital finance were taken over easily, such as the estimated lives of assets. Others were policy decisions, such as maximum personnel per bed. Extensive research did not yet exist then; an advisory committee collected opinions and supplemented them with experience from the members' own hospitals.

Eventually, much research was done by a special research center, the *Nationaal Ziekenhuisinstituut* (NZI), and the national hospital council (*Nationaal Ziekenhuis Raad*, or NZR) gathered views of its members systematically. Most initiatives to alter COZ guidelines came from the NZR representatives. NZR is organized into three basic sections—for general hospitals, mental hospitals, and nursing homes—and each section has a committee on charges. The committee consists of finance managers and has its staff work performed by one of the full-time economists employed by NZR. If complaints from members were common, the committee on charges investigated and might propose an increase in the guideline, the section approved, and the NZR representative in the COZ *kamer* proposed a change. The representatives of the sickness funds and private insurance carriers then took the NZR proposal back to their committees and research staffs. Eventually, the delegations from NZR and the insurers argued their respective positions, supported by their documents, in the COZ *kamer*. The *kamer* and the governing board of COZ eventually voted, usually (but not always) approving the NZR requests or working out a compromise position. The ceiling on personnel and on permissible staffing steadily rose.

A guideline coming from COZ represented a bargain between the groups most closely involved—namely, the hospitals and the insurance carriers. Few other groups were represented within COZ. But the other interested parties— particularly the employers and trade unions, who ultimately provided the money—had to be given a chance to object. The Ministry of Public Health also had to be given a voice, since the rates for individual hospitals were price regulations by government for the privately insured. The *Ziekenfondsraad* therefore examined and approved the guidelines after the passage by the governing board of COZ, since the *Raad* included the other interest groups and many government representatives, and was standing adviser to the ministry for health insurance. The *Ziekenfondsraad* review was usually pro forma and its approval quick. The Minister of Public Health then officially approved the new guideline, speaking for himself and for the Minister of Economic Affairs. In theory the two Ministers might reject a proposed guideline, but the negotiations by the interest groups had gone too far. The wording of the law sounded as if the Minister must take the advice of COZ, since the system in theory was negotiation among private parties.

As public policy problems grew, the weaknesses of the system appeared. The national government during the mid-1970s faced general problems of rapidly rising expenditures throughout the social services, mounting deficits in the sickness funds despite excessive payroll taxes, inflation, and loss of Dutch overseas markets due to excessive export prices. The negotiating system in hospital payment was subsidizing an expensive modernization of the sector and paid no attention to the economic consequences for the country. Therefore, the national government tried to curb the increases in the COZ guidelines by influencing the interest groups at the start of their negotiations. During the late 1970s, the Ministry of Public Health each year wrote and widely distributed a rolling medium-term health cost plan.[27] Several times each year, the Minister wrote formal letters to the COZ governing board about allowable hospital increases. The COZ *kamers* and governing board took note of these letters, and the COZ staff—being civil servants on special assignment—were particularly attentive. But the hospitals responded that they were obligated to provide good care, the sickness funds felt obligated to pay for it, and COZ would not subordinate its negotiating style to government direction. They treated the Ministers' letters as advice that they were not required to accept.

Rate Regulation. After COZ adopted a guideline, it was implemented by the staff members, in the review of prospective budgets of individual hospitals. The individual cases were not settled by negotiations between sickness funds and hospitals, but the staff member was a neutral regulator. I will describe the regulatory work of COZ in Chapter Seven.

Revisions of the System. The mixture of negotiations and rate regulations produced disappointing results, in the eyes of the national government and the sickness funds. Total hospital costs rose too fast, straining the fiscal capacities of the country in general and of the sickness funds in particular. Certain new hospitals were organized and built in an excessively lavish manner and had permanently high operating costs. From 1960 to 1981, Dutch hospital expenditure rose 8.4 times, one of the steepest climbs in any country.[28]

Leaving guidelines to the two sides raised costs rather than enforced restraint, ignored rather than implemented the larger public interest. Revisions of rate determination in the Law on Health Care Charges of 1981 retained negotiation of guidelines by the sickness funds and hospitals. But the outcomes must conform to public policy. If the national government sends its own guidelines, the sickness funds and hospital associations now must negotiate within those limits. With a clear legislative mandate, presumably the government will become more assertive.

The dichotomy between negotiation of guidelines by the adversaries and implementation by neutral regulators had been unsuccessful. The regulators employed by COZ did not know enough about the details of individual hospitals. The local offices of sickness funds paid the bills and heard about the experiences of their subscribers. The local sickness funds could judge which hospitals were inefficient and overstaffed and whether some utilization was padded by excessive stays. Unlike a rate regulator, who was an impartial civil servant, an official of a sickness fund could argue with the hospital's managers. The new law added negotiation to rate regulation in every individual case. The local sickness fund now receives the hospital's prospective budget and rate application; it confers with the hospital over the budget and over expected utilization. If the hospital and local fund agree, and if their budget rates fall within the guidelines, the rate regulators and the new agency (COTG) automatically accept their recommendation.

Previous decision-making methods seemed inconsistent. Doctors' contractual obligations and fees were fully negotiated, while hospital pay was settled by a mixture of guidelines negotiation and rate regulation. Doctors' pay was negotiated entirely bilaterally, without any coordinating agency. But hospitals' pay was managed by COZ. The decisions about hospital specialists seriously affected the costs of the hospitals, but the two activities were not coordinated. So the new law of 1981 replaced COZ with a Central Agency for Health Care Charges (*Centraal Orgaan Tarieven Gezondheidszorg,* or COTG), whose jurisdiction includes doctors and all other health professionals as well as hospitals. COTG can coordinate the payment of hospital specialists with the payment of the hospitals. The government's desire to make rate-setting methodology more consistent among sectors was a principal reason why sickness funds now negotiate with individual hospitals over the prospective budget.

The COZ system was highly centralizing. Everything revolved around the leaderships' negotiations in the governing board and *kamers;* investigations were handed over to the COZ staff. This practice was inconsistent with the Dutch government's attempt to decentralize and regionalize health services and many other sectors. Instead of the *verzuiling* of the past, the new Dutch society would be secularized and geographically organized. The burdens of hospital finance would depend on the local sickness funds and the individual hospitals. The sickness funds were suddenly required to build up their local staffs. The new expectations were difficult for the private commercial insurers, centralized nationwide companies that had specialized in collections and payments and had let COZ fix rates.

The old system was too cumbersome: the guidelines were written by COZ and then approved by the *Ziekenfondsraad;* individual hospital rates were fixed by the COZ finance officers and approved by the *Ziekenfondsraad.* The reason for these stages was to give a voice to the employers and trade unions, who were not represented in COZ. But the consultative rights of the ultimate payers were lost in the jurisdictional rights of the agencies. The reforms of 1981 put everything under one roof and eliminated the need for referrals. The employers, trade unions, providers, insurers, and governments make up the new COTG board. It ceases to be a bargaining site between insurers and hospitals alone. The *kamers* of COTG are still organized adversarially into the two factions of insurers and hospitals. The COTG governing board sends rate recommendations directly to the Ministry of Health, without the delays and possible reversal in the *Ziekenfondsraad.*

Every payment system produces results that please one side more than the other. Any change alters the distribution of complaints. Since the sickness funds have begun to negotiate rates directly with hospitals, the hospitals have made the usual objections to aggressive bargaining: the sickness funds are intruding into hospital management instead of confining themselves to insurance matters; they are asking too much about the internal affairs of hospitals.

Less Structured Bargaining in France

Third-party coverage of a population spreads, and basic benefits are standardized as people seek help in hospitalization coverage. The hospitals themselves are an important force for the spread of third-party coverage, since they press patients, carriers, and government for full coverage of their costs. Involvement of sickness funds as large bloc purchases leads to large-scale negotiations. A structured decision-making system of some sort evolves, to make the results fair according to clinical need. Otherwise, say the hospitals, the payers would demand full services and give less money than the hospital needs; otherwise, say the sickness funds, the hospitals would be overstaffed and wasteful. Detailed rules, neutral fact-finding, and arbitration are introduced into negotiation to avoid the one extreme of power bargaining that would work to the financial advantage of the sickness funds and the opposite extreme of accepting charge lists drafted in secret by the hospitals.

A country can have a dual system, wherein different classes of hospitals are paid by different principles decided by different methods. Such an outcome results from a long history of organizational distinction and rivalry among hospitals. They have different and perhaps antagonistic owners. A method of rate determination used for one class of hospitals (such as intrusive governmental rate regulation of municipal and charitable hospitals) is resisted by another class (such as the private clinics). The main payment system disallows certain costs and profits, which are important to some other hospitals. France has a dual payment system, with rate negotiation for private clinics. It is less structured than the negotiating methods of Germany and Holland.

A very unstructured method can exist. Each organized payer tries to strike a separate deal with each hospital. Many countries had such a method during the early twentieth century. It survives in the United States.

If hospitals are rivals, French and American experience suggests, each presses for political devices that protect itself and is happy to let the rest struggle in the "free market." Since markets in health and in all other sectors are always political as well as economic, the rival hospitals must find political help for their own advantage. The results are generous at some times and stingy at others, as in the case of negotiations between sickness funds and proprietary hospitals in France.

While each side in an unstructured bargaining system seeks political help to strengthen its own hand, both resist the introduction of public policy. Each assumes that society gains from its own victory. Or each assumes that the hospital sector should be settled by patients' "needs" and should be kept out of overriding public policies about inflation, taxation, and the allocation of resources. In contrast, structured and comprehensive negotiation systems give government leverage to influence outcomes.

Relations Between Official Sickness Funds and Private Clinics. French sickness funds are obligatd by law to cover the costs of each public hospital—and of each nonprofit "assimilated into the public service"—as defined by the regulators in the prefectures. The methods will be described in Chapter Seven. The payment of physicians' fees has evolved into a highly organized bilateral negotiating system, whereby a joint committee of the sickness funds negotiates with the medical associations. The results are a contract, a fee schedule, and prices that apply to all French physicians treating insured patients.[29] However, the private clinics owned by physicians do not fall into any of these categories. They are private enterprises that are not under the authority of the prefect. While the fees earned by doctors in their work in the private clinics are covered by the physicians' fee schedules, the clinics' other costs also must be paid for.

The statutory sickness funds and private clinics are locked into close relations, despite their preference for mutual independence. The funds have long been forced to pay the private clinics in some way, even though their leaders prefer to confine payment to the public hospitals. Free choice of doctor and of hospital (*libre choix du médecin ou établissement par le malade*) is fundamental to French medical practice. The many political compromises in enacting national health insurance included repeated enshrinement of the wording in the health insurance statutes, from the first law in 1930. The French medical profession had fought such legislation out of fear of precedents in Germany, where the sickness funds had been able to steer subscribers to their own closed medical panels and to cooperating public hospitals. Such guarantees of free choice by the patient had already long existed in French law and probably would have applied to national health insurance even if the Social Security Code had not incorporated it. For example, free choice is an article in the code of medical ethics drafted by the medical society specializing in professional discipline and issued as a decree by the Prime Minister of France. The social security laws authorize the sickness funds and *mutuelles* to create hospitals themselves, but a patient can choose to go elsewhere and receive normal coverage. Important health laws usually reaffirm the pledge. For example, the first words of the hospital reform law of 1970 are, "The right of the patient to free choice of his practitioner and of his establishment of care is one of the fundamental principles of our health legislation" (Law 70-1318, Dec. 31, 1970).

But the basic laws do not require the sickness funds to pay any level of clinic costs (whether full or partial) and do not prescribe any procedure for determining allowable costs and rates. On their side, the proprietaries practice the secretiveness common in all unregulated sectors of French private life: they will not reveal their records to the sickness funds; therefore, calculations cannot be made according to a common set of rules from a cost report, as in the fixing of French public hospital rates.

The private clinics cannot avoid heavy reliance on the statutory health insurance system, because France lacks a large amount of private commercial health insurance that would pay the higher charges of for-profit hospitals. Obligatory coverage of the population is universal; special regimes exist for the elites (the *Caisse Nationale d'Assurance Maladie et Maternité des Travailleurs Non Salariés des Professions Non Agricoles*, or CANAM, plus several special funds); and these funds follow the others in dealing with private clinics. The private firms providing extra health insurance coverage resemble *sociétés mutuelles* in their benefits and prefer to give subscribers extra cash for private doctors' fees and for extra comforts in the private clinic (such as private room fees, telephone, or special diet), but not for very high bills charged by the private clinics for their basic services. The rich can pay extra out-of-pockets to private clinics, but there are not enough rich self-payers to support the very large clinic sector: clinics operate about 37 percent of all beds. Instead of using private clinics as in the past, the chiefs of service in the modernized public hospitals now hospitalize their patients there, and the private clinics must take whatever business they can get.

In the bargaining the sickness funds pay the private clinics as little as possible. One reason is ideological. The leaders of the funds have always thought that the doctors used the clinics to profiteer and underserve; during the years when senior specialists worked at the public hospital in the morning and at their private clinics in the afternoon, the leaders of the funds thought that the specialists steered many patients into their clinics.

Another motive for the sickness funds' strict bargaining is financial. The private clinics now are owned and staffed by their own full-time doctors. (The chiefs of service in the public hospitals now work full time there.) The clinic doctors earn their incomes almost entirely from the standard fees negotiated between the medical associations and the sickness funds. Designed primarily for office doctors, the fees include a large component for office and practice expenses. If the sickness funds paid the full operating costs of the private clinics, they would pay practice expenses twice. So the sickness funds try to pay the private clinics little and force the doctors to turn over large proportions of their fees in rental to the private clinics—as all do to a varying extent. Since the private clinics and doctors do not allow research about their practice expenses, the negotiations with the sickness funds cannot be based on agreed facts but are left to power bargaining.

In this ideologically charged milieu, without a clearly structured system of rate determination and without an agreed set of facts, the sickness funds and clinics have struggled incessantly. The funds and the doctor-owners press the government for interventions to help each side. Depending on the situation in politics, the national economy, and the state of medical care, the private clinics have prospered at some times and have been squeezed at others.

Procedures. Negotiations over rates have always been conducted locally, between offices of sickness funds and clinics. The principal fund (the *Caisse Nationale de l'Assurance Maladie des Travailleurs Salariés,* or CNAMTS) usually has been the negotiator, and the others have accepted its arrangements. It is impossible to leave statutory health insurance completely to the administration of local funds, since national headquarters and the national government must levy payroll taxes and deal with deficits.

National headquarters of the sickness funds (particularly CNAMTS) have steadily increased control over the local offices. During the late 1960s, regional tiers were created to coordinate the local offices, and the regional offices (abbreviated CRAM) have dealt with the private clinics. Recently the national associations of private clinics have worked out framework contracts with the national leaderships of sickness funds, to define relationships, but prices are still settled at the local or regional levels. Since the proprietaries will not reveal their costs, the negotiators settle on a charge schedule that the sickness funds will pay, with some cost sharing by the patients.

If the hospitals are paid from social security taxes and if the economy at times is endangered by inflation, guidelines from policy makers cannot long be avoided—even in a supposedly completely private negotiation system. The hospitals seek guidelines protecting them from excessive pressure by the sickness funds. The government favors guidelines that will protect the sickness funds, taxpayers, and self-payers from excessive annual rate increases. French national governments of the Left and of the technocentric Center usually issue guidelines that limit rate increases, while governments of the Right act more generously. But the guidelines are not clear-cut, since the national government lacks direct power over private clinic rates, the clinics themselves resist regulatory help that will curb their cherished freeedom, and every guideline is the outcome of complex logrolling by many actors. The guidelines are advice to the CRAMs about their negotiating posture and are warnings to the sickness funds that government will not help them finance commitments in excess.

The guidelines emerge from discussions among the national civil servants in Paris specializing in the payment of hospitals: the Division of Hospitals in the Ministry of Health; the office in whatever Ministry (such as Labor) has jurisdiction over social security; the offices concerned with social security payroll taxes and price surveillance in the Ministry of Finance; CNAMTS; and several others. The next chapter will describe the similar but more thorough procedure for writing guidelines about public hospitals. In contrast to Holland's negotiated guidelines, French guidelines are written entirely by officials, and representatives of the associations of hospitals and private clinics do not participate in formal meetings. But, as in much of French official life, there is frequent informal communication in order to work out a consensus or to explain differences in a way that will avoid a public confrontation. The representatives of the associations of private clinics present their case for higher rates next year, and the officials tell their own intentions while they are still preparing the early drafts.

Since 1968 the private clinics in general have been allowed an annual percentage increase, matching the target increase allowed the public hospital sector. Often the annual guideline memorandum has recommended that each price charged by the private clinic during the coming year be increased by the fixed percentage allowed by the new annual cap. However, some guidelines redesign the acceptable price structures. Some guidelines vary the distribution of the increase among private clinics. For example, in 1980 not all items in all clinics were automatically raised 11.8 percent, but this was the aggregate increase for all clinics. Each price in each clinic was raised about 9.5 percent, 2 percent was given to certain clinics below their peer group averages, and 0.3 percent was reserved for correction of individual cases.

The annual guideline about payment of the private clinics is officially signed by the Minister of Health and is addressed to the prefect of each region. Officially, it is for the prefect's guidance when he issues an *arrêté* "confirming" the rates in theory discussed and agreed upon by the CRAM and by the clinics. Also, if the CRAM and the clinic fail to agree, the guideline informs the prefect of the national government's decision about the new year's official arbitrated rate for the private clinics.

The guidelines eliminate the free-for-all in a completely unorganized and decentralized system of bargaining. The CRAMs offer the annual increase, and the private clinics usually accept it unenthusiastically. More flexibility and genuine negotiation occur over distribution of any extra money in the annual cap, earmarked for special cases; truer negotiation can occur if a clinic says that greatly changed circumstances require completely new rates.

Results. The outcomes of the negotiations have varied by period.[30] Until 1968 local offices of the sickness funds negotiated with private clinics. Without guidelines from their national leaders and without full information about the clinics' internal affairs, they gave the proprietaries the benefit of the doubt. The local funds were not inhibited by financial responsibility: the revenue was determined by their leaders in Paris. Procedures and generosity varied across the country. A guideline to limit costs by introducing an objective standard had the unintended effect of increasing costs. A decree of the national government said that private hospitals should be paid charges no higher than the daily rate of the nearest comparable public hospital. But the clinics urged the sickness funds to classify them like the better and more expensive public hospitals. Besides the daily charge, the clinics increased their revenue from itemized services. The proprietaries grew in number and in income, and they competed successfully for patients with the public hospitals, which were under tighter financial control. The proprietaries' charges were profitable enough to permit them to modernize by self-financing investment.

Between 1968 and 1973, strong regional offices were created in the sickness funds, and they took over the negotiation with the proprietaries. They were better staffed and had more information than the local offices, but they still lacked verified cost reports from individual proprietaries. And they were still governed by the decree requiring the funds to treat a clinic like a nearby public hospital of similar size and function.[31] Private clinics continued to prosper. But public hospitals were now becoming attractive enough for all patients. And the public hospital doctors—now guaranteed high full-time salaries and limited private practice—viewed the private clinics as competitors rather than their part-time workplaces.

From 1973 to the mid-1980s, sickness funds and the national government became very cost-conscious. The national leaderships of the funds, in collaboration with the government, sent guidelines to their regional negotiators, recommending that the annual increases in charges granted to the proprietaries not exceed certain percentages. The custom spread of an across-the-board increase for all by the same percentage, instead of a unique award to each clinic. The clinics' charges and income rose more slowly than those of public hospitals, more slowly than the general inflation rate. Some sickess funds granted the proprietaries even less and were upheld on appeal. A proprietary could ask for additional increases, but it must substantiate its case by submitting full reports and accepting auditors' visits, which it usually feared. Even so, the sickness funds might refuse an increase. The fund was not obligated to respond within a fixed time, and the papers circulated for months, while the proprietary continued under its old rate. Therefore, the proprietaries were steadily squeezed, perhaps all ran deficits under their hospital charges, and they survived only by sharing the fees of their physicians. While the doctor-owners gained few profits from the clinics, they prospered from the fees from the more advanced medical procedures made possible by access to a clinic. At a time when the growing number of doctors strengthened the bargaining power of the sickness funds over fees, the office doctors were not as lucky as the clinic doctors.

During the 1980s CNAMTS and some civil servants groped toward a more structured method of deciding rates. The CRAMs might be monitored more closely by the national headquarters of CNAMTS, reducing the diversity in interpretation. CNAMTS might develop detailed guidelines jointly with the Ministry of Health. Private hospitals might be classified in groups ranked by clinical complexity; the more complex hospital might have a reasonable case for higher rates. But the draft reforms still did not require disclosure of the private clinics' books and still did not require the sickness funds to pay the proprietaries' costs in full. Reforms were deferred during the 1980s as the government gave priority to altering payment of the public hospitals. Hoping that the private clinics would wither away, the sickness funds and the Socialist government were not eager to adopt any methods that would protect them.

Unstandardized Bargaining with Individual Third Parties in the United States

Payers form a common front in most developed countries. But the fragmentation of the past continues in the United States. Each payer tries to get the best deal from the hospital. Negotiating an advantageous cost-based rate or advantageous charges is the typical method long used by Blue Cross.

Most payers in Europe arose as adversaries of the providers. One network of sickness funds in the Netherlands was created by general practitioners to ease the collection of capitation fees each month, but that is unusual. Most European sickness funds were created by trade unions, political parties, workers' cooperatives, and other groups interested in getting the best services at low costs. In contrast, Blue Cross Plans sprang up during the 1930s in the United States as intermediaries between hospitals and patients. The pools of money solved the hospitals' collection problems; the patients could count on help with their bills. Some state Plans began as consumer movements; others were fostered by hospitals. Since all were designed to minimize patients' out-of-pockets, all tried to make benefits equal charges, and all eventually tried to arrange direct payment to the hospital without initial expenditure by the patient.[32]

History of Negotiations. Achieving payment in full by a third party required direct agreements between Blue Cross Plans and individual hospitals. They agreed on contracts specifying relationship, eventually following models developed by the state (or regional) Blue Cross office and the state (or regional) hospital association. They also agreed on rates to be paid each hospital and created a joint reimbursement committee to handle problems and disputes. The negotiation procedures were never officially standardized: each state Blue Cross Plan has worked quite separately; a familiar American idea is that every hospital is "unique" and therefore the state Plan approaches each one in a slightly different fashion.[33] Nevertheless, the visitor to many Blue Cross offices notices similarities in hospital relations.

The communication load for Blue Cross mounted during the 1960s. Many Plans had already been persuaded by the hospitals to base their payments on a reimbursement of full costs, not on a fixed price set after quick bargaining. Cost reimbursement required study of the hospitals' financial reports and prolonged highly technical discussions. The volume of work skyrocketed. Blue Cross covered many more workers and dependents, and became the fiscal intermediary for several other programs with cost-based reimbursement—namely Medicare, the Federal Employee Health Benefits Program, the Civilian Health and Medical Program of the Uniformed Services (CHAMPUS), and some state Medicaid efforts. In the 1960s, a period of rapidly increasing hospital costs, Blue Cross experienced constant financial strains. Discussions with hospital officials continued as amiably as before, but they led to steadily more expensive commitments and annual applications to state insurance commissioners for higher premiums.

During the 1970s state Blue Cross Plans had to become more independent and more critical of hospitals. It was not possible to keep the relationship completely private, without any government intervention. State insurance commissioners no longer automatically granted higher premiums. A few specifically ordered hospitals and the state Blue Cross Plan to create negotiating machinery as a condition for premium increases and told Blue Cross to drive harder bargains over allowable costs and over rates. In particular, guidelines were issued from 1970 through 1973 to Philadelphia Blue Cross by Pennsylvania State Insurance Commissioner Herbert Denenberg. Convinced that Blue Cross had failed to confront the hospitals on the issues that raised costs, the commissioner specified topics to be covered in negotiations and contracts.[34] Where the Blue Cross Plan and the state or regional hospital association have worked out a model contract accepted by participating hospitals, most state insurance commissioners now ask that it be filed along with Blue Cross's applications for higher premiums

The Blue Cross staffs in most states—worried about pricing themselves out of the market—became conscious of the need to limit payments to hospitals. They faced price competition from growing numbers of commercial insurers, who kept premiums lower by merely reimbursing patients according to an indemnity schedule.

Procedures. In the states where Blue Cross pays the hospitals' lists of charges, the Plan's specialists in hospital relations periodically meet with each hospital to discuss its proposed increases in charges and to negotiate discounts. In some states the meetings are brief and superficial, in others more thorough.[35]

In the states where Blue Cross pays the hospitals' operating costs in a per diem with or without additional charges, a more elaborate procedure is necessary. The Blue Cross staff or someone acting for Blue Cross must see the hospital's last cost report and must discuss with the hospital the merit of proposed increases. In about a dozen states, Blue Cross supports a separate office to scrutinize the cost report and prospective budget and to negotiate the rates. The office appears to be an autonomous commission but really is a spinoff of Blue Cross. (In the other states, the Blue Cross Plan deals with the hospitals directly.) By making the office appear independent, Blue Cross can persuade more hospitals to cooperate, agree to restrain expenditure, negotiate a contract to accept direct payment in full, and avoid the out-of-contract situation when the patient pays the hospital in full and is reimbursed partially by Blue Cross.[36] Three variants are:

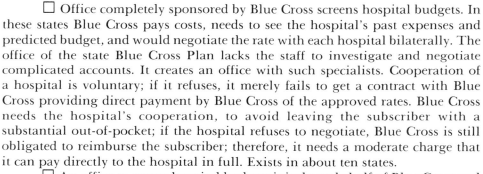

☐ Office completely sponsored by Blue Cross screens hospital budgets. In these states Blue Cross pays costs, needs to see the hospital's past expenses and predicted budget, and would negotiate the rate with each hospital bilaterally. The office of the state Blue Cross Plan lacks the staff to investigate and negotiate complicated accounts. It creates an office with such specialists. Cooperation of a hospital is voluntary; if it refuses, it merely fails to get a contract with Blue Cross providing direct payment by Blue Cross of the approved rates. Blue Cross needs the hospital's cooperation, to avoid leaving the subscriber with a substantial out-of-pocket; if the hospital refuses to negotiate, Blue Cross is still obligated to reimburse the subscriber; therefore, it needs a moderate charge that it can pay directly to the hospital in full. Exists in about ten states.

☐ An office to screen hospital budgets jointly on behalf of Blue Cross and the hospital association is maintained in Michigan. All policy decisions, budget examinations, and appeals are handled by committees with equal representation from Blue Cross and the hospital association, with a neutral chairman. Voluntary and advisory, since the individual hospital need not participate. Nonparticipants do not get Blue Cross contracts, and their patients are reimbursed by Blue Cross at less than the full rates.

☐ The hospital association of Wyoming maintains its own office to screen hospital budgets and recommend rates to be asked of payers. Voluntary and advisory. Not a program of Blue Cross alone.

Blue Cross and the hospital association have created other arrangements in a few states. For example, in Rhode Island and the area of Rochester, New York, they agree on a total revenue target for the coming year. Then Blue Cross tries to negotiate rates with each individual hospital, so that the total for all stays within this cap.[37]

Negotiating Posture. The role of Blue Cross vis-à-vis hospitals has always been ambiguous, and its role in rate setting also has been unclear. State Plans sometimes function as collection agencies for hospitals and sometimes as representatives of consumer interests. These roles have changed from time to time. It has been impossible to produce a clear and stable system for negotiations within many states, let alone a nationwide pattern allowing the sharing of experience. Often Blue Cross and hospitals have really been collaborators in negotiations for more money from state insurance commissioners. In other instances Blue Cross has been the spokesman for hospitals in negotiating health care packages with employers.

Since many Plans have tried to gain the cooperation of hospitals and since many hospital directors perceive them as collection agents who otherwise should "keep their place," many Plans have worked out reimbursement agreements on the basis of the hospitals' simple documentation, without intruding too deeply into the hospitals' files. The negotiations recently have become stricter out of financial necessity, and the Plans now have money to employ staff members conversant with hospital finance; but Blue Cross in some states still must hedge. It lacks a powerful sanction to force hospitals to agree: if no contract is signed, the patient may still go there, and Blue Cross must still reimburse him most (perhaps 80 percent) of his costs. The patient is left with out-of-pockets as a result; he will probably blame Blue Cross rather than the hospital, and he may switch to another carrier that pretends to offer more benefits. Unless the state Blue Cross Plan has a charge-based reimbursement method—that is, a definite warning to subscribers that full payment is not guaranteed—it may buy peace by giving the hospital much of what it wants. But the hospitals do not get everything.

If negotiations do not yield rates and costs that a Blue Cross Plan can meet within the rate structure allowed by the insurance commissioner and by its contracts, it must forgo its paid-in-full and direct-payment aspirations. It would offer only charge-based reimbursement to the patient or to all the hospitals, and the hospital must collect the balance from patients. If this option is adopted widely, only limited negotiations are necessary with the hospitals: they discuss the procedural clauses in contracts, and Blue Cross tells the charges it can afford to cover; the patient and hospital set the rest between themselves. As hospital costs rose during the 1950s and 1960s, some Blue Cross Plans backed away from cost-based payment-in-full and resumed primary reliance on charge policies. Of the seventy Plans responding to the American Hospital Association's survey in 1981, forty-one paid charges and twenty-four paid costs.[38] The charge payers were usually (not entirely) in states with weaker unionization, fewer group contracts, lower Blue Cross market penetration, and charge-based reimbursement for most patients. Blue Cross there must avoid expensive commitments and high premiums.

Blue Cross developed as the payer for all recognized hospitals, without discriminating among them. Therefore, throughout the country it was long presumed that Blue Cross would come to terms with them all. However, during the 1980s interest in competitive pricing and in competitively let contracts spread in American health care. Blue Cross and Blue Shield of Northeast Ohio in 1985 experimented with competitive bidding in order to press hospitals to reduce the excess capacity that kept costs high under cost-based reimbursement. Each hospital would submit a proposal to Blue Cross, and only those demonstrating the most effective cost-containment methods and the most economical rates would win contracts. Hospitals with low occupancy would have to offer reductions in capacity. If any hospitals did not win contracts, they would have to bill the patients and not Blue Cross. Blue Cross would reimburse the patient only 70 percent of his costs. Blue Cross would fully cover only emergency care there.

Disclosure. Blue Cross Plans can learn more about hospitals' accounts than negotiators in many other fields in the United States. One reason is that a great deal of information from both sides is in the public domain, because both are involved in certain governmental payment and regulatory programs. Every hospital caring for Medicare patients on the basis of full cost reimbursement must file a long annual report about costs and operations (form HCFA 2552) with the fiscal intermediary, which is usually the Blue Cross Plan itself. Blue Cross must file a complete financial statement of its own—membership, income, reserves, and expenses—whenever it seeks higher premiums from the state insurance commissioner, usually every year.

The friendly relations between the Blue Cross Plan and the local hospitals in many states result in considerable reporting. If a hospital receives prospective reimbursement consisting of last year's costs plus trend factors for prices and utilization, the contract requires submission of a full cost report to Blue Cross, usually a copy of HCFA 2552 (or an equivalent document) plus additional special pages for Blue Cross. The contract allows Blue Cross to send auditors to examine the hospital's books, a right normally absent from a payment system based on bilateral negotiation. (In contrast, Blue Shield and the Medicare fiscal intermediary cannot routinely audit every participating physician's books.)

Not all the Blue Cross Plans have such access. If Blue Cross has few subscribers in a state, a hospital does not want to tip its hand, particularly if it is a proprietary. Forgoing high Blue Cross charges or full cost reimbursement is a low price to pay for secrecy and the freedom to set advantageous charges for all its business. Often the Blue Cross Plan goes along with high charges without extensive financial reporting, since its subscribers want to use that hospital. Even in states with full cost reimbursement and extensive Blue Cross membership, the hospital can avoid the audit by not signing a contract. The patients with Blue Cross policies lose some money, and the hospitals may lose some patients, but the hospital keeps its independence.

Price Discrimination. In a private market, each payer negotiates the best deal it can. It tacitly invites the seller to find extra money elsewhere, such as from other payers. In insurance competitive advantages are thereby created for the strongest payer, since the others must collect higher premiums or offer lower benefits.

The private insurance companies complain that Blue Cross has used its market power and its special relationship with nonprofit hospitals to gain special advantages, such as discounts, exclusions of certain costs from the calculating base, and selection by most nonprofits as their Medicare fiscal intermediary. When negotiating with an individual hospital, Blue Cross alone has a large enough market share to be taken seriously. Each commercial insurer individually has only a few subscribers in that hospital. As a result, complains the association of commercial third parties (the Health Insurance Association of America, or HIAA), the hospitals undercharge Blue Cross and overcharge the commercially insured patients, a form of cost shifting now impossible in other developed countries.[39] HIAA fears that organizing a common negotiating team will be challenged as a violation of the American antitrust laws, and it has been unsuccessful in persuading Congress specifically to exempt such arrangements from the antitrust laws.[40] Blue Cross benefits from the status quo and does not wish to join forces with the commercial carriers.

Unable to form a common negotiating team with Blue Cross and with government purchasers, and unable so far to persuade the courts to declare the favorable Blue Cross contracts in violation of the antitrust laws,[41] the commercial carriers have favored state regulatory intervention as a method of putting them on the same footing.[42]

In Europe the essential facts about the negotiations are public. The procedures may be specified in law; other procedures are known to all interested persons; the hospital cost reports and other basic statistical facts are widely distributed (as in Germany) or can be viewed by interested parties (as in Holland); and the rates produced by the negotiations are published. However, in an American-style negotiation, whereby each party makes the best deal for itself, facts about each deal are secret. The American Hospital Association and the Blue Cross Association issue periodic summary reports about all the contracts in the country, and state insurance regulators obtain summary reports about each Blue Cross Plan's annual utilization and expenses; but the negotiations and rates with individual hospitals are secret. If other payers learned about the Blue Cross discounts and other concessions obtained from a particular hospital, they would demand the same. If self-paying patients learned that they were being "overcharged," they might go elsewhere. The American practice of special deals and cost shifting requires concealment.

Special Arrangements. The cordial relations between Blue Cross and nonprofit hospitals enables some Blue Cross Plans to persuade hospitals to adopt cost-saving innovations, when hospitals would make no such concessions to a combined and adversarial front of all sickness funds. The American hospital might voluntarily offer these new methods to its non–Blue Cross patients, but it might be slower, since the Blue Cross office is vigilant that its patients receive the benefits as soon as possible, while the other patients lack such an alert representative. Blue Cross and Blue Shield of Greater New York is particularly energetic in developing and persuading hospitals to implement such methods as day surgery instead of inpatient hospitalization, early discharge with home health care by the hospital, and ambulatory testing before hospitalization. Because of the flexibility of American health insurance and hospital services, Blue Cross and a hospital can experiment at once and can add the benefits widely, without official clearance from higher tiers, without amendment of laws, and without extensive discussions with other insurers and hospitals. The innovating and competitive style of the United States encourages such new benefits. In contrast, NHI abroad standardizes benefits. Experiments are possible in Europe and have become common during the 1980s, but they must be planned and authorized.

Local Negotiations in the United States

A Blue Cross Plan is one large-scale payer employing certain practices with many hospitals. In the heterogeneous American market, many smaller-scale arrangements also exist, some involving the negotiation of rates with hospitals. These methods proliferated during the 1980s, when payers began to resist hospital rate increases and when the imagery of competition and shopping became common in American health policy. Many ideas common in American business are promoted in health.

Low Private Bidders for Public Money. One method employed by a large purchaser is to direct all its beneficiaries to whatever hospital makes the lowest bid. California's Selective Provider Contracting Program, established in the 1980s, was initially planned as a competitive bidding system: the program would seek the most favorable terms and the lowest prices for the treatment of persons covered by Medicaid, the welfare program for the poor. The program's administrators would solicit bids for all or part of the Medicaid inpatient load in each community. They would then negotiate terms and prices with the lower bidders. Medicaid beneficiaries were expected to use only those hospitals. The state government's office administering Medicaid would pay the hospital the daily rates or other charges agreed in its contract.[43]

However, no American government program—particularly one offering so much revenue—is allowed to operate with great restrictions on participation and on payments. Public money implies universal access by the providers as well as by the beneficiaries. In those areas where Medicaid beneficiaries lived, the California Medical Assistance Commission within a year had signed contracts with two-thirds of their hospitals containing 70 percent of the state's beds. Traditional rate structures were accepted, primarily per diems. The negotiation method had merely obtained prospective agreements and discounts from the hospitals' usual per diems, much like Blue Cross in other states. The real innovation in California was systematic prospective rate negotiation. Medicaid costs were about 12 percent lower than the total probably incurred if the previously uncontrolled arrangements had continued during fiscal year 1983–84. Other carriers—including Blue Cross of California—also began to negotiate prospective rates with hospitals for the first time.[44]

In 1981 Arizona actually enacted a system of competitive bidding for its Medicaid business and restricted beneficiaries to the winning providers. The state had never had a full-scale Medicaid program, and the hospitals had not become dependent on Medicaid revenue; therefore, the hospitals in general did not fight restriction of business to a few. At last the dream of competitive theorists would come true. Unfortunately, the program soon crashed, because of the economic behavior that occurs in the real world, as distinct from the pure models on blackboards. Winning contractors underserviced, diverted funds improperly, sought supplements from government, and otherwise demonstrated that success in financial bidding is altogether different from efficiency in work and quality in health care. The providers assumed that, since Arizona had never committed itself to Medicaid before and now turned over the unwelcome new task to low bidders, the state was not eager to protect its poor. A payment method of low bidding therefore brought out perverse incentives on all sides.[45]

Private Agreements. Exclusive deals are possible between private payers and private sellers in health as in other sectors in America. They should not damage other sellers or raise costs to the public or else they would violate the antitrust laws. In other countries every statutory payment system must be open to every hospital and doctor, but American payers can resist.

Private group purchase arrangements exist on a small scale in American health care. A number of prepaid closed panels (Health Maintenance Organizations, or HMOs) exist for physicians' ambulatory care throughout the country. In return for the subscriber's annual fee, an HMO often promises to give all necessary inpatient as well as ambulatory care. But few HMOs own their own hospitals; therefore, many of them shop among local voluntary or for-profit hospitals, to obtain a group rate for all expected inpatient needs at a price that will enable the HMOs to break even. The HMOs' negotiators must balance their own income, expected need for hospitalization, and the rates quoted by hospitals that are available for adequate care. An unduly low rate may lead to underservicing and a loss of subscribers. An unduly high hospital rate will lead to a deficit in the HMO and to higher premiums, which might drive away subscribers. Hospitals may compete for assured business at rates lower than their usual charges if they foresee excess capacity.[46] But in most of the country at present, HMOs have too little market share to bargain effectively with hospitals, the hospitals are still prosperous enough not to need the HMO business, and the HMOs therefore save money by minimizing hospital use rather than by winning discounts.[47]

Smaller payers in the United States also seek special arrangements with individual hospitals, but the beginnings are still modest. One thrust comes from large employers who now try to control rapidly mounting health care fringe benefits by self-insuring rather than by paying Blue Cross and Blue Shield to insure all their workers. These business firms have been unable to persuade their insurance carriers to drive hard bargains with providers; and, as I will explain in the next chapter, they shrink from pressing state legislatures to regulate hospital rates. So, in keeping with the American style, these companies seek advantageous deals with doctors and hospitals for themselves. The employer or the management firm administering its benefits contracts with a hospital to care for the employees at rates lower than the usual charges. The employer's hospital costs are lower; the employee is persuaded to go to that hospital by sharing the savings, in the form of lower cost sharing. Hospitals with unused capacity—some in overbedded areas—can survive financially by filling their beds at lower rates.[48] The result for the community is either higher total utilization or a shift in business from other hospitals. As in other American negotiations, the preferential rates are kept secret, lest other payers and patients in that hospital resist the cost shifting and demand the same.

Evaluation of Negotiation Methods

Every payment method has strengths and weaknesses. But these pros and cons depend on the interests of each side. What one side considers an advantage the other regards as a disadvantage.

Advantages from the Standpoint of Payers. The third parties control what they spend in a negotiating system. They can limit payment to their own capacities.

They can refuse to pay hospitals that they deem superfluous or poor in quality. (In practice they may have to reimburse patients, but their refusal to pay some hospitals directly weakens the hospitals.)

Advantages from the Standpoint of Hospitals. Some well-connected and efficient hospitals can prosper. They can strike advantageous bargains with some third parties. They might earn extra revenue from self-payers and keep it. They cannot be forced to return profits.

Management has more discretion than under regulation. It must fill out fewer forms, reveal less about operations, perhaps submit no end-of-the-year reports to outsiders.

Advantages from the Standpoint of the Public. Hospital payment does not burden government. It stays out of politics.

Sickness funds are less likely to run deficits that government is pressed to cover.

Disadvantages from the Standpoint of Payers. Payers cannot learn much about the internal affairs of hospitals. They cannot easily bring about improvements in how their money is spent and in how their subscribers are treated.

Usually they cannot exercise much influence in planning facilities for the society generally. It is often difficult to force reductions in the sizes of wasteful hospitals.

Bargains are binding; usually the adversary refuses to reopen negotiations, and the payers cannot remedy miscalculations until the next scheduled round of negotiations. They usually cannot recapture profits that they did not plan to concede. They risk deficits in their own accounts.

Payers may refuse to form a common front. Each tries to strike individual deals with the hospital and invites the hospital to shift costs and profits to the other. Such shifting is a tactic of competition among the payers themselves, advantageous to the winners, disadvantageous to the losers, and redolent of collusion between payer and hospital.

Disadvantages from the Standpoint of Hospitals. Many are underfunded for personnel and for capital. If they run deficits, usually they cannot obtain supplements. There is no guarantee that they can obtain extra money at the next negotiating round. Hospitals can go bankrupt.

Doctors' pay is usually negotiated separately and directly with the sickness funds. Or the senior doctors have extensive private practice. Hospital managers usually cannot control the senior doctors and induce them to cooperate with the hospital's collective strategy. If the hospital is being squeezed, doctors become less involved.

Disadvantages from the Standpoint of the Public. There is no single expression of the public interest by a neutral.

If an expression of the public interest evolves from a logrolling forum of leaders of interest groups, there is no mechanism to enforce it. Negotiators at the grass roots can ignore it.

There is no reliable way to implement plans in the negotiations. If the government writes plans and tries to implement them by grants, operating costs are funded separately and possibly in contradiction. Payers may refuse to fund facilities or specific programs that have been approved in plans, or payers may continue to fund (voluntarily or involuntarily) facilities and programs that planners would like to terminate or alter.

Resources cannot be shifted from hospitals to other sectors of health care delivery or from overprovided to underprovided regions.

The hospital sector may become threadbare if payers are underfunded and stingy.

Payment of hospitals cannot be easily coordinated with payment of doctors and with payment of other providers, particularly if the third parties differ among sectors. Doctors compete with hospitals for revenue, often increasing their own incomes and office practices at the expense of the hospitals.

Trends

Negotiating arrangements begin as informal discussions between individual third parties and individual hospitals. Gradually they become more organized, as a result of pressure from all sides; and public policy guidelines are eventually introduced. At first they are designed to protect the hospitals, by guaranteeing that they cover their costs and by defining their allowable costs. Later guidelines are designed to protect the taxpayers and premium payers by limiting the annual increases in the hospitals' demands upon the third parties. Also, new guidelines may be written to coordinate health with general government policies to restrain inflation—a difficult matter, since health spending usually has risen faster than other spending.

The introduction of guidelines requires machinery to negotiate or otherwise decide them at higher tiers. A national commission might be created, with members from the associations of hospitals, insurers, and other groups. Or, if government must enact payroll taxes, subsidize deficits in NHI, and fight inflation, the guidelines come from government. Even if the guidelines come from a national commission of private associations, government gets involved, by trying to influence the outcomes in response to appeals from one or another group or because of its desire to minimize tax increases. The growing role of government is opposed by the medical association but not necessarily by the hospital association. The growing involvement of government draws hospital care into politics—supposedly avoided when decisions are made by private negotiations but probably inevitable, because of the economic importance of hospitals.

The sickness funds and the national government share common interests, particularly in health facilities planning. Eventually they cooperate, although each is touchy about relative power.

Eventually the third parties also cooperate more, by creating joint negotiating committees and all-payers methods of payment.

Payers try to learn about the hospital's entire budget and entire operations, not merely negotiate over rates. Hospitals resist such extensive disclosure and discussions but are eventually compelled by government to make such concessions to payers.

In order to challenge the more expensive hospitals, payers computerize the hospitals' billings and reports. Then, in order to make peer group comparisons, the payers cooperate and standardize practices across localities. To prepare their cases on behalf of rate increases and to anticipate challenges, the hospitals also become computerized. The national offices of the payers and hospitals grow in importance.

The trend in financing policy is to limit total expenditure, not merely the rates for individual services. Therefore, third parties and governments in many countries try to budget for each hospital and avoid cost overruns, thereby constraining utilization as well as unit prices. Ultimately, such financing implies single payers and global grants to hospitals. Where rate negotiations exist, some governments (such as Holland) try to limit total spending by calculating annual targets, giving the hospitals and sickness funds detailed guidelines, and deciding the hospitals' appeals. These actions may rob the negotiation situation of much of its discretion. The sickness funds do not complain that their role has been usurped, since they are saved money and need not worry about unauthorized deficits. As negotiators their task becomes the investigation of the individual hospitals, to cut some below the allowable ceilings.

7

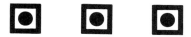

Regulation
of Rates

Where private payers face hospitals, an alternative to power bargaining is regulation. An impartial official of government investigates and sets a fair rate. He is a referee between payer and hospital, striking a balance between their competing interests.

Some might argue that regulation is superior to negotiation. Since the regulator has the authority of government, he can compel production of facts, such as the hospital records customarily concealed from the sickness funds. The regulator can employ experts to study hospital finance thoroughly, while the sickness funds usually cannot. The regulator has no personal financial stake and can set a fair rate that evokes widespread support, while bargaining is merely a victory for the stronger. Public policies about health care finance can be implemented by regulations or guidelines imposed on the regulator, whereas negotiators are free to ignore advice or instructions.

Others are skeptical about regulation, particularly in the United States. Power bargaining does not disappear under regulation, they say, but shifts to government, which determines the selection and orientation of the regulator. He inevitably becomes the captive of one side. Even if he remains independent, his agency grows too large, he loses contact with society, and he stagnates.

Characteristics of Regulatory Systems

The regulatory agency and its relations with hospitals and payers can vary according to the following attributes:

☐ Site of the agency.
  - Government line department. If so, whether the government is national or regional.
  - Autonomous government commission.
  - Private commission governed by hospitals, payers, and possibly other groups.

☐ Stability of the agency.
  • Whether it is permanent or temporary.
  • Likelihood of early amendment of its structure and powers.
☐ Whether guidelines connect the regulatory work to any public policies.
☐ If guidelines exist, their source.
  • National government officials.
  • Legislature.
  • Advisory committee from private sector. Whether associations of
    hospitals and payers are included.
  • Regulatory commission itself, formulating its own definition of the
    public interest, guided by its original statute and other sources.
☐ Scope.
  • For the individual hospital, whether the regulation involves all payers,
    some, or one.
  • Whether all hospitals' pay rates are set by such regulation.
☐ Context.
  • Each hospital receives an award appropriate to its unique costs.
  • A global amount is set for a region, and each hospital must fit within
    it.
☐ What is regulated?
  • The hospital's total prospective budget.
  • Lines within the hospital's prospective budget.
  • Unit of payment.
  • Allowable services in the budget.
  • Utilization level.
☐ Regulator's investigative authority.
  • Reports submitted by the hospital about:
    — Expenditures.
    — Personnel and services.
    — Utilization: admissions, diagnoses, discharges.
  • Hospital's internal records about expenditures, personnel, utilization.
☐ Amount of disclosure of the regulator's investigation to the payer and to the
  public.
☐ Finality of the regulator's award.
  • Appeals procedure.
  • Whether higher government agencies, the legislature, or courts can
    amend the award.
  • Whether hospital can charge more or the payers can pay less. Sanctions
    if the hospital violates the award.
☐ Whether the outcome binds other economic transactions, such as the
  hospital's wage awards and the government's payroll taxes.
☐ Whether the regulatory agency monitors the hospital during the year.
☐ Revisions of the award during the year.
  • Hospital can petition for amendments.
  • No changes are possible during the current year, but deficits are
    automatically covered by surcharges on next year's award.
☐ Relations between rate regulation and health facilities planning.

Regulatory systems usually presume that the payers are predominantly private. The hospitals can be publicly owned as well as privately owned. If publicly owned, usually they are municipal, whereas the regulatory agency is part of the national government, a provincial government, or an autonomous commission.

Each of the following descriptions of national systems will cover the foregoing dimensions of regulatory administration. The following descriptions will be detailed for several reasons. No descriptions of the structure and dynamics of hospital regulatory systems have been published previously for these countries—except for the United States—and therefore I cannot save space by referring the reader elsewhere. Each country's regulatory methods differ more or less from the others', so the readers familiar with their own situation need to understand the full arrangements elsewhere in order to grasp the possible alternatives. In particular, Americans are familiar only with their own methods, deem them unsuccessful, but need to learn how serious national systems are organized and operated. Finally, a thorough understanding of each country's methods is necessary before one can grasp the difficulties in administering regulation and before one can grasp the reasons for recent shifts toward other rate-setting methods.

This book presents systems of rate setting and not country-by-country descriptions. If a country mixes two methods, it is examined in two different chapters. For example, French public hospital rates are set by regulation (discussed in this chapter) and its private clinic rates by negotiation (discussed in Chapter Six). Holland's rate setting involves both negotiation and public regulation, and it too is mentioned in both chapters. Switzerland has rate setting for part of the hospitals' costs (discussed in this chapter) and public grants for the rest (discussed in Chapter Eight). France and Holland are now incorporating methods of global budgeting in their regulatory systems, and these developments also are described in Chapter Eight.

Government Regulation in France

For many years the rates of French public hospitals—and the private nonprofits assimilated into the public sector—have been set by civil servants, who examine the hospitals' cost reports and prospective budgets, check the arithmetic producing the rates, and officially announce the rates. Although these officials represent the public, they function primarily as referees between payers and providers. Their importance in the French system is so firm that they have been retained despite changes during the 1980s in the payment units for hospitals and in the organization of local administration.

The Hospitals. For centuries France had hospitals owned and managed by the Catholic Church in the typical European form. During the French Revolution, the new national government took over all property of the Catholic dioceses, the religious orders, and the aristocracy, including the hospitals and the lands constituting their endowments. Laws of the French national legislature and of the national executive placed ownership and management in the local governments (the *communes*). Most are owned by individual *communes,* some by two or more very small *communes.* Laws designated the mayor as chairman and several local councillors as members of the hospital's governing board. The hospitals became integral parts of the social services for the poor, which evolved during the nineteenth century. The government of the *commune* was responsible for raising funds and for paying deficits.

During the late nineteenth and twentieth centuries, operating funds increased from charging patients and their third parties. Fixing the rates by negotiation was not feasible: the hospitals were owned by governments; some third parties (such as the welfare departments of *communes*) were governments; and France has not had a tradition of private negotiation but depends heavily on official rules. Therefore, hospital rates were set by a regulator applying uniform national rules.

The Regulators. For over a century, a civil servant representing the national government in the locality has acted as regulator of local economic activities. He was called the "prefect" *(préfet)* until 1982 and is now called the "commissioner of the republic" (the *commissaire de la république*). One is assigned to each of the ninety-five *départements* of metropolitan France. The commissioner represents the Prime Minister and all other Ministries in the *département.*

The commissioner has supervisory authority *(tutelle)* over all public hospitals in the *département,* pursuant to the laws of the National Assembly, the regulations of the executive branch (some are signed by several Ministers, including the President and Prime Minister), and circulars by the Ministries overseeing health and social security. The prefect presides over a miniature Cabinet, consisting of the "external services" of the Ministries in Paris. For example, in each *département* the Ministry of Social Affairs maintains a staff to oversee health programs and to prepare the decisions for approval by the prefect. The office overseeing the hospitals is called the *Direction Départementale des Affaires Sanitaires et Sociales,* or DDASS. Financial oversight of all public agencies is performed by the public accounting office (the *Direction de la Comptabilité Publique*) of the Ministry of Finance; auditing local government agencies, such as the public hospitals, is a function of the financial Ministry's elite corps of field representatives based in the *départements* (the *trésoriers-payeurs généraux*).[1] (The names and structures of the parent Ministries are changed from time to time, but the system endures.)

After the French Revolution, the governments of the *communes* owned and managed the hospitals, included them in the social welfare parts of their operating budgets, and therefore paid the shortfalls. The financial management of the *communes* was modernized; the cost of each hospital patient and *hospice* resident was to be counted separately, so that transfers between the social welfare program and the hospital-*hospice* program would be more systematic. This procedure—counting the number of patients and assigning part of the social welfare budget to hospitals accordingly—was the forerunner of the modern daily charge (the *prix de journée*).

Arrangements were regularized for the entire country in a law passed by the national Chamber of Deputies in 1893, concerning provision of free medical care to indigents. The prefect could fix the daily charges paid by public or private welfare programs to the public hospitals, on the basis of an application by the governing board of the hospital. Subsequent decrees instructed the hospitals and prefects about procedures and methods of calculation. Since costs of clinical services varied, a decree in 1943 instructed the prefect to fix different daily charges for surgery, medicine, maternity, and the old-age *hospice*.[2]

During the twentieth century, hospitals became more attractive and more successful in their cures. In contrast to their traditional image as refuges for the indigent, they attracted workers and farmers, who were expected to pay the standard daily charges. Increasing numbers belonged to sickness funds, which paid the charges. Several hospitals maintained rooms with fewer beds than the large general wards. Decrees instructed the prefects to authorize between 10 percent and 50 percent extra for the more private rooms.

Prospective Budgeting by the Hospital. Price regulation is usually reactive. An organization requests an increase over last year's rates and files an operating cost report showing a deficit without the higher rate; the regulator studies the report and awards all or some of the application. Without a request, the regulator concentrates on other applications, and rates remain the same for that organization. Such has been the rate regulation in France for the last century.

A prospective budget of the hospital's costs and activities is the basis for the request. Every public hospital—and those nonprofit private hospitals recently "assimilated" into the public service—must fill out one every year. The format, accounting principles, and cost-assignment rules are spelled out in regulations issued by the Ministries of Social Affairs and Finance.[3] Procedures change from time to time. For example, during periods of permissive health funding, the hospital could amend its original budget upward during the year; during periods of cost containment, such as the 1980s, the hospital is forced to work within its original budget. Even though the daily charge is being replaced by lump-sum payments (global budgeting) during the 1980s, French hospitals continue to submit prospective budgets under similar rules.

The process of preparing and scrutinizing the prospective budget is supposed to follow a strict schedule each year. (The dates in practice change from time to time. I will describe the timetable during the early 1980s, with the caveat that it is not permanent.) The commissioner (formerly called "prefect") should issue the new awards by January 1, so that the first bills in the new year can be paid at the higher rates. The DDASS must have enough time to study all the hospital budgets in the *département*, reduce some lines, and calculate the recommended charges. Each hospital must have enough time to debate the DDASS's revisions. Therefore, the budgets must reach the DDASS by around November 1. Within the hospital the director must allow adequate consideration of the budget by the governing board.

The summer and early autumn are spent preparing the figures within the hospital. The director, his financial staff, and each medical chief of service prepare the budget for each center of responsibility. The director and his financial staff produce the complete prospective budget aggregated from all the centers.

Guidelines. A regulator must have a rationale for his decision, or the result is merely to replace self-interested power bargaining in rate negotiation systems by the capricious exercise of power by government. Without guidelines, the regulatory process can be captured by one of the interested sides. Merely following laws is not enough in rate regulation; laws specify proper procedure, but the rate regulator decides a level of prices, determining the payer's losses and the provider's scale of operations. Therefore, the guidelines are the heart of hospital rate regulation.

French commissioners and the "external services" (the representatives of the national Ministries in the *départements*) have always received laws and regulations from Paris designed to ensure that the laws are implemented by the same procedures. Recently several Ministries (led by Social Affairs and Finance) have jointly issued detailed guidelines to the DDASS, explaining how the economic policies of the government should be applied to the scrutiny of hospital budgets. The government's annual "Economic Budget," showing expected and desired trends in the economy, is the basis for many virtually automatic government decisions, such as the annual increases in the wages and fringe benefits of the civil service.[4] Allowable rate increases for public hospitals are one of the many decisions based on the projections of the Economic Budget. As I said in Chapter Six, CNAMTS usually agrees to increase payment to the private clinics by the same proportion.

The guidelines are formulated by the civil servants specializing in health care finance in each participating Ministry, with the drafting primarily in the Division of Hospitals of the Ministry of Social Affairs. Most details are worked out in informal interagency meetings. Disagreements may require meetings among the staffs of the Minister or even mediation by the Prime Minister's staff. The guideline memorandum is then signed by the participating Ministers. During September (according to the timetable I described above), the memorandum is mailed to all the commissioners and their DDASS.

The length and detail of the guidelines depended on the unit of payment, the regulatory methodology, and the urgency of controlling costs. Line-item budget review is potentially intricate, and the method became very detailed during the late 1970s and early 1980s, when the system was expected to limit costs very strictly. A guideline memorandum sometimes reached thirty single-spaced typed pages. Usually it began with a general statement of the government's cost-control philosophy and the recent record in controlling hospital costs. For example, the guideline in late 1979 summarized the government's goal of limiting annual increases in hospital spending to the annual rate of growth in GNP. Improvements in quality of care would continue to be possible, it said, if money were saved elsewhere in the budgets. The rest of each year's memorandum included sections for:

> Maximum percentage increases over the previous year that the prefect may grant for several account numbers. In particular, personnel. Reasons for the limit.
>
> Special problems with particular items, such as payment of doctors or inclusion of deficits from earlier years.
>
> Conditions for exceptions to the ceilings.
>
> Setting allowable costs for new services.
>
> Special cost-control instructions. For example, the circular in late 1978 set not only a maximum 10.2 percent increase for all personnel expenditures (following probable wage movements in the country) but a maximum increase of 1 percent in numbers of personnel. It urged close vigilance over creation of new posts in the medical staff.

> Arithmetic for calculating the daily charge, when that was the unit of payment. Definition of the number of patient-days used in the denominator.
>
> General warnings or urgings to the prefect, such as the need to award the hospital its new rate by January. If later, the hospital cannot send out bills at the full new rate and suffers deficits in its cash balance.

In systems with line-item regulatory review, the guideline about allowable personnel cost increases is particularly crucial. Personnel is the largest item in a hospital's budget. European regulators and negotiators find that their hands are tied on pay rates nowadays. Where most hospitals are owned by government, as in France, the pay rates for hospital workers are fixed by the civil service pay scales, established by the highest levels of the national government after consultation with the civil service unions. Where most hospitals are owned by private organizations, as in Germany and Holland, the pay rates are fixed by nationwide collective bargaining between the hospital association and the hospital workers' union. Thus, pay increases are automatically passed on in the hospitals' prospective budgets and charges. But the guidelines can determine whether the hospitals can add more workers: if the allowable increase in the personnel line does not exceed the wage increase, the hospital cannot add staff.

In addition to the end-of-the-year guidelines about evaluating the new prospective budget and fixing the daily charges, the national government also sends the commissioners a guideline memorandum every March. It originated in the need to guide the DDASS about processing the supplementary budgets during years when amendments were accepted, but now it performs many more functions. Usually it includes a progress report about the state of national hospital finance policy. It elaborates instructions that proved unclear or incomplete in the September guidelines. It clarifies items in the accounting scheme that have been troublesome. It suggests policies and procedures that might appear in the next September guideline memorandum.

If rates are set by one regulatory agency, as in Holland and in several American states, all the in-house examiners apply the rules alike. They can compare notes constantly. But the circulars on budgets and daily charges are applied in ninety-five *départements* within France and four overseas, creating a uniformity problem. Every October all DDASS directors meet at the Ministry of Social Affairs in Paris for two days. Discussion of the new circular about paying the hospital takes a half-day.

Evaluating the Lines in the Budget. The hospital sends its prospective budget on a standard official form to the office of the commissioner, along with supporting papers about recent operations, current costs, and future needs. Legally, the application asked the commissioner to approve the daily charge (the *prix de journée*)—in the years when it was the unit of payment—that ensured a balanced budget. That is, the expected costs divided by the expected number of patient-days equaled the proposed daily charge. Now the papers ask the commissioner to approve the total budget, which will be paid in installments by the sickness funds. Actually, the hospital sends the papers to the DDASS and not to the commissioner, since the DDASS will do the work.

The staff of the DDASS includes several examiners *(inspecteurs* and *secrétaires). Départements* vary in work load, and some DDASS are better staffed than others. In many DDASS two or three examiners may deal with between fifteen and twenty general hospitals. Other examiners in the DDASS review the budgets for *hospices,* nursing homes, establishments for the retarded, mental institutions, and others paid by daily charges.

The examiner's work is done in the DDASS office, on the basis of the dossier submitted by the hospital. The DDASS until well into the 1980s lacked access to any computer system with large data files showing each hospital over the years and all other hospitals contemporaneously. Therefore, during the years of close line-item budget review to calculate the daily charge, examiners could not compare the case at hand with a distribution of similar hospitals, as in Switzerland, Canada, and several American states. An examiner can complete work on a dossier in a few hours if the hospital is small, if it has not made any structural and programmatic changes since the previous year, and if its proposed increases are within the guidelines. The papers from the hospitals have never been sufficiently detailed, and the examiners have never been able to make thorough field visits to hospitals; therefore, they were not able consistently to detect all deviations in hospital practice from the strict letter of the accounting and budgeting rules under the regulations about costs covered by the daily charge. Usually, individual items were detected as excessive and inadmissible only if they produced manifestly inflated lines in the budget.

Reviews were easy for the examining staff when hospitals were given what they wanted. During the late 1970s, as guidelines tightened to reduce the annual increase in expenditures, hospitals continued to submit prospective budgets with substantial increases, and examiners studied them laboriously and cut most. Hospital directors sent elaborate justifications for why some categories— particularly personnel—should be allowed to exceed the guidelines.

The guidelines said that the hospital—except for exceptional reasons— should not increase its budget by more than a certain percentage over last year. But a certain percentage over which of two distinct possibilities—the prospective budget granted at the start of last year, or the expenditures actually made last year? For some time the increment was a proportion of the previous year's expenditures. This was a projection of the current year's spending; eight or nine months of the current year had passed at the time the hospital submitted its budget for the next year. Therefore, the hospital estimated the total for the current year at the current spending rate and claimed that it could add the guideline's percentage for that line in the budget. But, in practice, current total spending was never well controlled, because the DDASS often allowed increases during the fiscal year. Therefore, the guidelines in September 1979 abandoned the use of current rates of expenditure as the basis for the percentage increment; only the year's original prospective budget would be the basis for the increase. Examiners could approve an increase over the current prospective budget of 10.8 percent in personnel costs and 9.8 percent in all other items. Supplements during the year were suppressed, and the hospital was expected to live with the prospective budget and the daily charges approved by the prefect. The prospective budget thereafter was written and implemented more seriously.

During the years of detailed line-item review, some clauses in the guidelines memorandum used another base, such as the absolute number of jobs in the hospital organization. Use of the absolute number of jobs was often designed to guard against bypassing the simple expenditure limit: the hospital could increase personnel spending only a little for next year, could substitute many part-time or "temporary" posts within the expenditure ceiling, and then could try to convert them into full-time expensive jobs (with long-term social security and pension obligations) in subsequent years. The guideline of 1978–79 limiting the expansion of jobs to 1 percent invited more disputes than expected. The examiners had to understand the complex situation within the hospital; the structure of full-time, part-time, and temporary positions in the hospital this year and next; the merits of the hospital's claims that it had special problems, such as uncontrollable seasonal absenteeism; and the effects on the prescribed monetary and numerical ceilings from the hospital's proposed reclassifications in jobs and changes in numbers. They also had to justify cuts, so that their superiors could defend the cuts in arguments with the hospital and on appeal. The 1 percent increment guideline was easier to write in Paris than to implement in the field.

Predicting the Number of Patient-Days. Before calculating the final daily charge, the hospital's economic director and the examiners (in the later review in the DDASS office) once divided the total operating costs by the total number of patient-days. This was the cost per day, or *prix de revient prévisionnel.*

The regulations then allowed the base to be calculated either from the coverage of the last three years or (for special reasons) from an estimate of the next. When the work of hospitals seemed stable or expanded steadily, the retrospective average was common. It was an "objective" measure, designed to take calculation of the denominator out of contention. However, the three-year average proved profitable to hospitals: a figure lower than the one expected next year in the denominator of the fraction produced a total income larger than predicted. During the 1970s hospitals reduced their stays, modernization of the rooms reduced numbers of beds, patient-days stabilized and even diminished in many hospitals, and therefore the financial imbalance was reversed.

By the 1980s several DDASS seemed to accept estimates of next year's patient-days, rather than averages of three earlier years. While the aim was greater accuracy, a result was to add another issue of contention. The three-year average had the virtue of being automatic.

In practice no hospital had a single daily charge. The law authorized it to collect different rates for different services: medicine, surgery, maternity, the aged, and others on a list issued by the Ministry of Health. In practice French hospitals were long acustomed to reporting numbers of beds in different clinical specialties and applying for different daily charges. The hospital's financial accounts included crude assignments of the total operating costs to the different services with daily charges, so that the rate application would ask for enough money. The end-of-the-year cost report and the prospective budget notified the DDASS of such distribution among services.

Substitution of global budgeting for calculation of the daily charge during the 1980s eliminated the need for the hospital to perform such guesswork and eliminated the need for the DDASS to decipher it. The DDASS no longer had to verify (for example) whether the daily costs in surgery were really 382 F while the daily costs in medicine were really 310 F, whether the former could be cut while the latter could be cut less or not at all. The hospital now could install modern cost-center accounting designed to strengthen internal management, in place of the arbitrary assignment oriented toward rate applications.

Scrutiny by the Sickness Funds. The original theory of European rate regulation was that the civil servants would be trustworthy referees between the hospitals and the payers. However, as often happens in rate regulation, the French system was asymmetric in practice. The DDASS interacted with the hospital, exchanging documents and arguing about decisions, but not with the sickness funds. The sickness funds complained that the situation resulted in excessive generosity to the hospitals.

The legislative reforms in 1983 gave the sickness funds a role in the payment system. The public hospital sends its prospective budget to the regional office of CNAMTS as well as to the DDASS in the *département*. If several third parties pay the hospital, they form a commission to investigate the prospective budget and to discuss it with a representative of the hospital. Within a month of receipt of the budget, the sickness funds send their collective recommendation to the DDASS. Unlike the reforms in Holland, extensive negotiation is not intended. Regulation is not replaced by negotiation. The DDASS still has the responsibility of thoroughly examining the prospective budget and setting the final total. The intervention of the funds will make the DDASS stricter.

A drawback in both France and Holland is that scrutiny by the sickness funds adds a new step in a process already vulnerable to delay, throwing the final setting of rates further into the next fiscal year.

Examiner's Report. After consulting the supervisor and the director of the DDASS, the examiner employed by the DDASS writes a report about that hospital's application. The report first presents the previous year's approved prospective budget (under which the hospital is currently working), the maximum authorized budget for the next year under the guidelines, the hospital's request for next year, and the examiner's recommendations. Subsequent pages in the report present the examiner's assumptions and arithmetic, when he has made cuts below the hospital's requests and/or allowed items exceeding the guidelines. Certain items must be accepted without change, such as interest charges and amortization.

Debate Between Hospital and DDASS. By law the commissioner must notify the hospital of his planned award, and the hospital must have eight days to react. Otherwise, the decree awarding the new rate is illegal.

The examiner drafts a letter telling the proposed cuts in the budget, explaining the reasons, and specifying the proposed rates—such as the list of daily charges, during the years when it was the unit of payment. The letter is signed by the director of the DDASS and is addressed to the chairman of the governing board of the hospital, since it was the chairman who sent the budget to the commissioner. Within eight days the chairman sends the hospital's official letter of response to the director of the DDASS. Usually it contains a defense of the higher amount that is being cut.

During this period the hospital officials and the DDASS staff phone back and forth, and the hospital administrators visit. Even if the DDASS has only a few simple establishments in its *département*, it is strained during these weeks. If it also has several large hospitals with complex budgets, it is overwhelmed. As a result, a DDASS often misses the January 1 deadline for announcing the new year's daily charges. The guidelines sent by the Ministry of Health in September often remind the DDASS to work fast enough so that the hospitals will not have to start the new year under the old tariffs.

When the hospital agrees to the award (however reluctantly), the DDASS drafts a decree (the *arrêté*) for the commissioner's signature. The rates and the examiner's report become public. The decrees for the hospital rates are posted on official bulletin boards.

Appeals. The theoretical timetable in the past assumed few appeals and quick action, so that the hospitals and sickness funds knew very early in the year whether the daily charge proposed to the prefect would be permanent. Appeals machinery is a fundamental part of a regulatory system. In the last chapter, I said that the method of resolving deadlocks seriously affects the operations and outcomes of a negotiation system; and, likewise, the character of the appeals procedure influences the behavior and awards of the regulators.

Under the regulatory method before 1983, the hospitals always had several opportunities for appeal, both before and after the prefect issued his official decree fixing the rates. The hospitals used the appeals sparingly when the system was administered generously: the supplementary budget during the fiscal year gave the hospital opportunities for increases over the start-of-the-year rates. But during the late 1970s, when the guidelines from Paris limited annual increases in allowable costs and when the hospitals were required to live within their start-of-the-year prospective budgets, appeals skyrocketed. During the late 1970s and early 1980s, half the hospitals appealed. The appeals process became so swamped that the decrees were held up, and the decisions were not announced for months. The hospitals were forced to work within their previous year's daily charge until the decrees were finally issued, either when the appeals process was exhausted or when the hospitals surrendered. Appeals in France are heard by officials and judges, and the hospital association is not represented on any tribunal.

In appealing the proposed new budget before issuance of the *arrêté*, a hospital first presented its case to an advisory committee in the *département*, consisting of several civil servants from the prefecture and several officials from the local offices of the sickness funds. The civil servants were likely to accept the views of their colleague, the DDASS, and the sickness funds were biased against increasing the rates they would pay.

The next step was to appeal to an interministerial commission in Paris officially devoted to the improvement of hospital management (the *Commission Nationale de Rationalisation de la Gestion Hospitalière*). Until the protracted deliberations concluded—aggravated by the great increase in appeals during periods of cost containment—the decree with the new budget was still not issued, and the hospital functioned under the old rates. This was an incentive for the hospital to settle and get a new daily rate. The commission consisted of the national government's civil servants who had written the guidelines. Left alone, they might have upheld the DDASS consistently, possibly even reducing some awards.

However, the hospitals did not leave the commission members alone; instead, they used their political connections. The most effective type of appeal was a trip to Paris by the mayor of the *commune* (the chairman of the hospital's governing board) and by several local notables. Their standing with the government-of-the-day could make the commission more sympathetic this year and make the DDASS more generous next year.[5]

The appeals system had the perverse effect of destroying the intended decentralization of regulatory administration. Since the DDASS's awards could always be appealed to the commission and politicians in Paris, the DDASS did not settle the dispute locally but quickly passed every problem upward. A few leading civil servants in the national government—particularly in the Ministry of Health—ultimately made all the decisions. The need to examine so many dossiers about individual cases diverted them from their normal work of making policy and overseeing the system.

The burden rested on the commission and the Ministries because the hospitals could not appeal further. Once the commissioner (the former "prefect") issues his decree, a hospital in theory can appeal through legal channels. But its appeal will be successful only if it can demonstrate that a DDASS's application of the rules to a particular hospital is erroneous or that the DDASS failed to follow proper procedure. The regulations and economic guidelines on budget review and the daily charge have long since been upheld. The tribunals will not substitute their own judgments for the commissioner's about whether a hospital deserves more resources. As in social regulation in Europe generally, the appeals go not to courts of general jurisdiction but to a commission specializing in review of the social service programs in the *départements*, the *Commission Centrale d'Aide Sociale*. It is one of many specialized administrative tribunals supervised and partly staffed by the *Conseil d'Etat*, the chief legal adviser to the government of France.

Some Judgments About the Regulatory System. Various groups had complaints about the old arrangements. Some criticisms were directed not at the regulatory methods but at supposedly perverse effects of the *prix de journée* as a unit of paying the hospital. But some criticisms were leveled against the structure and procedures of regulation:

☐ *Excessively detailed review.* In order to fix a daily charge, the DDASS approved the hospital's expected budget and expected patient-days. To do so, the DDASS examined every line in the budget and utilization in every clinical service. Guidelines to limit costs became increasingly detailed. Understanding the internal intricacies of hospitals was beyond the training, skills, and available time of the DDASS staff. If the DDASS investigated thoroughly, the hospitals' board, managers, and doctors complained that it was exceeding its authority. If the DDASS held back, the sickness funds and the Ministry complained that it was not enforcing the guidelines and was too generous.

☐ *Limited resources and limited perspective.* Each DDASS had a few dozen hospitals in its *département*. Peer comparisons were limited to these hospitals, but (until recently) the DDASS lacked the computing capacity and statisticians to compare the hospitals even in this limited group.

☐ *Weak local responsibility.* The DDASS and the appeals machinery within the prefecture should have resolved nearly all disputes. Instead, they were happy to avoid the burden and let disputes go to Paris, thereby straining the Ministry of Health. The prospects of concessions in Paris—no matter how small—encouraged appeals and forced the DDASS to be more generous.

☐ *Lack of coordination.* The planning of hospitals was not coordinated with the payment of operating costs. This discrepancy is common in hospital finance. It might have been handled better in France than elsewhere, since both the planners and the rate regulators were civil servants of the national government. However, the planners worked in national and regional offices, while the rate regulators were in the prefecture in each *département*. The rate regulators were simply supposed to ensure that a hospital broke even. The planners could not provide any clear signals that certain hospitals should not exceed certain levels of admissions, patient-days, and beds. The DDASS had no clear authority to reduce the hospital's prospective budget on the grounds that its admissions, length of stay, and beds were excessive. The rate regulators had no authority to disallow new programs in the prospective budget until the hospital reduced its other programs.

Revision of the System. The foregoing defects are being remedied in several ways during the 1980s. One change that is not contemplated is the elimination of regulation. An impartial umpire between payers and hospitals is still considered essential in France. While the Mitterand government transferred many other functions of the prefectures to local administrations guided by regional assemblies, the DDASS's authority over the public hospital remained untouched, still derived from the Ministry of Health in Paris. Without such a regulator, national policy guidelines and health facilities planning could not be implemented.

Paying hospitals by the *prix de journée* was replaced by payment of installments of a global budget, in large part to simplify the reviews of the hospitals' prospective budget and utilization. Ultimately, the DDASS might avoid the arguments over why a hospital earned more than expected through additional patient-days, since the hospital would have to provide such additional services only within the original amount of money. The DDASS might avoid arguments over the scope and costs of new services as add-ons to all existing services, since the hospital would have responsibility to add services only while making compensating cuts in others.

The regulatory power of the DDASS was increased, since it was now authorized to reallocate levels of expenditures among hospitals. The total revenue of all hospitals each year would be capped, under an *enveloppe budgétaire* consisting of this year's total revenue, plus a percentage increase authorized by a guideline of the national government. Each hospital in the *département* would have a prospective budget approved by the DDASS slightly above or slightly below the percentage increase, so that the *département* as a whole averaged the increases. In addition, the DDASS could authorize the expenditure of 0.5 percent more in the *département*, assigned to those hospitals with worthy additional needs.

The extra 0.5 percent "margin of maneuver" was given to deserving hospitals who might have won appeals. The general tendency to appeal was reduced because the commission in Paris was abolished. The DDASS, hospital, sickness funds, and other officials are expected to resolve disputes and not overburden Paris.

New accounting and reporting methods were introduced, oriented to improved internal management rather than to calculation of a *prix de journée*. The new reports would be computerized and merged in a national data base. Both the DDASS and the individual hospital's managers could compare the expenditures and performance of that hospital with nationwide norms and nationwide peer groups.

A Regulatory Commission in the Netherlands

Rate regulation performed directly by civil servants, as in France, is possible only when the national government has field staffs. In theory the Netherlands might have developed government rate regulation, since price-control laws enacted in 1939 prevent private organizations from increasing prices to such an extent that customers are gouged and the economy inflated. Lacking a nationwide field staff, the Ministry of Economic Affairs issued guidelines about allowable increases, received lists of prices from providers (including hospitals), and questioned prices exceeding guidelines. The Ministry could order freezes and rollbacks.

This simple capping by formulas seemed badly suited to hospitals, which were supposed to provide, at full costs, whatever services were needed by the community. Unlike France, the Dutch national government did not employ specialists in hospital finance who could fix a fair amount. Doctors' fees were settled by bilateral negotiations between sickness funds and medical associations in Holland and Germany. In Germany hospital charges also were settled by negotiation. Since the sickness funds were the principal payers in Holland, they wanted a direct voice in hospital rate setting. So a new Dutch law in 1965 combined regulation and negotiation ingeniously. The national government authorized the creation of a private negotiating and investigating commission—COZ, described in Chapter Six—that performed both negotiations between hospitals and sickness funds and rate regulation on behalf of the government:[6]

☐ Rates paid by sickness funds.
  • Guidelines were negotiated between hospitals and sickness funds on the governing board.
  • Guidelines were applied to hospital budgets by examiners.
  • The rates recommended by examiners were accepted by the hospital and the sickness funds.
☐ Rates paid by self-payers and by private insurance.
  • Guidelines were set forth by the governing board on behalf of government.
  • Guidelines were applied to hospital budgets by examiners.
  • The examiners' recommendations were accepted by the governing board and sent on to government.
  • The national government announced the rates, binding on the private market.

Rate regulation was designed to protect the many privately insured and self-paying patients—constituting 30 percent of the population—from being overcharged. The Ministry of Economic Affairs protected them under the Prices Law of 1961 and adopted as price ceilings for them the COZ decisions about the hospital's basic daily rates, the hospital's private room supplement, and a general fee schedule for itemized services by all Dutch hospitals. Without legally enforceable price ceilings, the hospital could charge a privately insured person anything and could collect from him the balance over the insurance company's indemnity. Under the COZ's limits, the insurance companies could sell policies with predictable or no cost sharing. The companies preferred rate regulation to a free market.

Guidelines. Chapter Six described the structure of COZ and the writing of the guidelines by its chambers and governing board. The guidelines were designed to set upper limits on allowable items in the prospective budget. They guided the examiners, who performed two functions when doing the same work: (1) impartial investigation that would be accepted by the hospital and sickness funds in lieu of face-to-face power bargaining and (2) rate setting for the private self-payers and the private insurers.

The guidelines then and now state the maximum number of guilders that may be spent per patient per day for each category of hospital. Many guidelines deal with personnel. In addition, limits were specified on the numbers of employees per bed. For example, around 1979 the guidelines about nurses provided:

Type of hospital	Maximum guilders per day for each Class III patient	Maximum number of occupied beds per nurse
General hospitals with:		
Less than 300 beds	36.06	1.65
300 to 400 beds	36.06 to 37.05	1.60 to 1.65
400 to 600 beds	37.05 to 38.18	1.55 to 1.60
Over 600 beds	38.18	1.55
Children's hospitals	39.66	1.50
Sanitariums	18.28	3.29

Since the pay rates are set by collective bargaining between unions and the national hospital associations, wages are automatically passed into the daily charge; therefore, the regulatory agency's limits can only restrain the numbers of personnel. Separate guidelines limit the daily cost and total numbers of many different categories of personnel. Guidelines exist for several nonwage items, such as the total number of years for depreciating types of building and types of equipment. The total depreciation allowed for each hospital is included in its daily charge.

As I said in the last chapter, the Ministry of Public Health during the late 1970s added its own guidelines, to restrain the annual increases in hospital rates. They were intended to prevent the sickness funds from increasing their expenditures at a faster annual rate than their revenue, since government was then expected to pay the deficits. The Ministry guidelines were designed to dampen inflationary pressures and to protect private hospital patients from burdensome charges. Government was thereby exercising—ineffectively at first—its authority to regulate prices.

Examining the Budget Before 1982. Awarding rates on the basis of each organization's unique needs consumes enormous staff time and invites widespread disputes. But hospitals evolve in different ways, and each is supposed to get its own rates. The French solution in the past was to examine and approve each case, but a large staff was required: two to four persons in each of the ninety-five *département* prefectures, plus additional examiners to review the academic medical centers and the Paris hospitals. Standardizing performance among all these offices was very difficult to accomplish.

Holland tried to regulate hospital rates with fewer examiners—about six for the country's 240 acute and medium-stay hospitals. Coordination was easier in Holland than in France, because of the smaller number of examiners and their central location in COZ. But the few examiners would have been overwhelmed if they had tried to investigate and revise each prospective budget thoroughly. As a solution many economic sectors in many countries use a common shortcut in rate regulation: the large majority of organizations receive a standard increase over last year's rates. It is the individual cases requiring extra money that absorb most of the examiners' time. When COZ adopted this method during the late 1960s, it assumed that most hospitals would be satisfied by the standard increase and that only a few would seek special attention. However, hospital rate regulation is difficult because a great many hospitals claim to be unique and specially deserving, and a great many plead hardship during difficult economic times.

If the hospital managers wanted only the standard increase, they filled out and sent to COZ a brief and routine report about the last year's costs and work (the *calculatieschema*). Guidelines from the Ministry of Public Health and from the COZ governing board specified the percentage increase. The increase was supposed to match general cost increases for the economy in general and for the hospital industry in particular. The examiner looked at each *calculatieschema* from the two to four dozen hospitals to which he was regularly assigned, to make sure of clerical accuracy and to derive the new daily rate. Last year's costs plus the separate wage and nonwage increases equaled the approved expected expenditure budget for the current year. That total minus revenue expected from tests, private room charges, and other special charges equaled the approved net revenue budget for the current year. The revenue budget divided by expected patient-days equaled the new daily charge. The charge was announced and was paid by the sickness funds several months after the start of the year. During the first months, the hospital was presumably running a deficit, and it was supposed to break even. To the new daily charge the examiner added a surcharge, so that the entire year's business averaged out to the approved per diem.

The annual increase was dictated by the national government's calculations about annual increases in wages and market prices. Wages in the public sector—in hospitals as well as in the civil service—were limited to the average wage in private employment. When the Central Planning Bureau (CPB) calculated the average increase in the private sector's wages for last year, public employees' wages during the current year automatically rose by that percentage. In the guidelines accompanying the *calculatieschema,* COZ instructed the hospital to estimate last year's allowable personnel costs plus the increase specified by CPB. The budget lines for purchases of medical and other supplies could be last year's total plus the Central Statistical Bureau's prediction of the increase in consumer prices throughout Holland during the current year. Such an instruction in effect limited the hospital to last year's volume of purchases. By February of the new year, the government issued these index numbers,[7] COZ wrote its manual of instructions, and COZ sent the *calculatieschema* to all hospitals.

If the hospital's operations had changed and the managers wanted a higher-than-average increase, they submitted the detailed *bijlage bij individuele aanvrag,* a line-by-line expenditure report about the last two years and a prospective budget for the new year. It called for a line-item review by the examiner, using the guidelines to judge whether individual items were reasonable. After his preparatory desk work, the examiner visited the hospital to ask why certain lines in the prospective budget substantially exceeded the hospital's earlier costs. That is, the examiner asked the hospital to support its claim that it would run a deficit without an extra rate increase. The examiner also asked why some lines in the hospital's staffing or expenditure exceeded the COZ guidelines. The examiners have always been at a disadvantage, since they lack power to inspect the hospital's books. The examiner could only guess whether the hospital managers were really bluffing and could survive without reducing services or laying off staff. The examiner's information was limited to COZ's own files of *calculatieschema's* and *bijlagen,* and many may have been kited. While examiners cut back the hospitals' requests, they often gave them the benefit of the doubt. Such generosity enabled the examiners to cope with a mounting work load. At first during the 1960s and 1970s, most hospitals submitted the *calculatieschema's* and accepted across-the-board rate increases, but as costs rose rapidly during the late 1970s, each year half of the hospitals applied for special extra rate increases, swamping the examiners.

A hospital could forgo the automatic annual increase by not filing a *calculatieschema.* But that merely postponed the examiner's work rather than reduced it. Such a hospital could survive on an old rate without adjustment for inflation. Either it had successfully kited its last application, or it had reduced its service intensity and quality in ways yielding profits, or it was multiplying profitable patient-days and tests. If a hospital submitted no *calculatieschema* for five years, the examiner required it to fill out a complete individual application and investigated.

Decisions and Appeals Before 1982. For each hospital's rates, two documents resulted: COZ sent a recommendation about sickness funds' hospital payments (a *prijzenadvies*) to the *Ziekenfondsraad;* and it sent a decision about rates for private rooms and third class (a *prijzenbeschikking*) to the Ministry of Economic Affairs. The documents also listed the tests and treatments that were not covered by the daily rate and that the hospital could bill for separately. The *Ziekenfondsraad* usually routinely adopted the *prijzenadvies* as the rate to be paid by all sickness funds for all subscribers in that hospital. The Ministry usually routinely adopted the *prijzenbeschikking* as the rates to be paid by all other patients in that hospital.

Disputes and appeals did not arise from the hospitals that filed the *calculatieschema*. The hospitals themselves had filled it out and done the arithmetic. If they had wanted additional money, they would have filed *bijlagen*.

Several possible appeals channels were available to hospitals awarded less than their special application. Since several channels existed, it was never clear which was most appropriate for a particular case, officials in each channel were visibly reluctant and hoped that the hospital would switch to another forum, both COZ and the hospitals were confused, the ultimate power of COZ was unclear, and everyone was unhappy.[8] An aggrieved hospital could appeal to either the COZ governing board or to the *Ziekenfondsraad;* but both preferred to deal with general policy rather than with individual complaints, the COZ board was reluctant to reverse its own staff, and both boards consisted of rival interest groups that tried to avoid narrow issues that would incite deadlocks. The hospital could also appeal to the Ministries of Health and Economic Affairs, but the officials wished to avoid actions that would invite a flood of politically buttressed complaints to the top of the government (as in France) and wished to avoid demoralizing the regulators who were implementing their cost-containment policies. On the other hand, the hospitals were well connected with local governments, with trade unions, and with religious associations; so complaints were listened to. Even though appeals caused few reversals of examiners, the fuss was often successful because it pressed them to be more generous next year.

Charge Lists. Holland is one of the few countries where most hospitals have itemized lists of charges. Once the hospital set its own charges, but they were not numerous or high. Like the per diem for all services not charged separately, the prices were limited by government. When the hospital billed the sickness funds for tests and simple treatments, two variants existed by custom. Some hospitals included all of them in their total operating costs and daily inpatient charges (*all-in* billing). Others billed the sickness funds and insurance companies for each test, and the daily patient charge was called *all-out*. With *all-out* billing, it was often uncertain how many costs were in the bill for each act and how many were mixed into the daily charge spread over all inpatients who did and did not receive such tests and treatments.

COZ was created to make hospital payment more orderly, to relate costs to charges more clearly. COZ did not order hospitals to adopt either *all-in* or *all-out* billing. That is left to the hospital to decide. But COZ developed a standard fee schedule (the *tarievenlijst*) for the costs incurred by the hospital in performing these tests and procedures. If the hospital elected *all-out* billing for some or all of them, these acts were listed in COZ's *prijzenadvies* and *prijzenbeschikking*. They were not calculated into the daily charge. Once the hospital's rate structure was approved, it billed the sickness funds and private carriers for each test according to the *tarievenlijst*.

If the fees were truly designed to cover the hospital's costs from these tasks, they would be based on research concerning actual costs. And each hospital would have its own schedule reflecting its costs, just as each has its own daily patient charge. A little research has been done on the costs of these services in hospitals, but it quickly becomes outdated. The negotiators from the sickness funds and medical association had estimated the costs of each procedure during the years when the specialists' fees included practice costs as well as honoraria. A COZ working group from the sickness funds and NZR met during the early 1970s to develop a fee schedule for hospitals. It collected impressions from those hospital directors whose records permitted guesses about unit costs, and it consulted the participants in the negotiations between the sickness funds and specialists. COZ adopted hospital fee schedules one by one in special fields during the early 1970s and issued the first consolidated one for January 1, 1973.

COZ could not individualize fees to fit each hospital's situation, as it individualized the daily inpatient charge. For simplicity it prescribed a standard amount for each test and procedure in every hospital in the country. In most hospitals this amount probably did not cover all costs and did not constitute payment in full; some costs were mixed into the other operating costs of the hospital and were covered by the daily inpatient charge. Some other costs of the outpatient department not billed and paid directly were also ultimately charged to the sickness funds and carriers through this route. "Profits" might accrue to some hospitals and "losses" to others if the *tarievenlijst* were designed to be payment in full. But "profits" from the tests were supposed to be recaptured by the carriers by means of a higher inpatient rate.

The fees in the schedule—like the daily inpatient rate—had to be corrected for rises in labor costs and the prices of materials. For convenience COZ made such corrections every three years. Therefore, the hospital economic directors need not assimilate a completely new list every year, but a supplement to each year's *calculatieschema* instructions changed one-third of the fees. A staff member of COZ specialized in the corrections. Each fee was defined as a mix of labor costs, materials costs, and other such costs. The mix varied among procedures. The COZ economist consulted the reports about expected wage and price increases during the coming years in the Central Planning Bureau's *Macro economische verkenning*. He also investigated changes in the costs of various medical procedures. The new fee was designed to correct for errors in the predictions made three years earlier and to anticipate costs over the next three years.

For example, the new rates in effect in 1980 included compensation for an underestimation of price rises in 1977, 1978, and 1979. COZ in 1976 had estimated that prices would rise 10.4 percent over the three years, but the index of consumer prices for Holland rose 13.6 percent. The retroactive compensation for those fees, updated entirely on the basis of the price index, was 2.9 percent, since

$$\frac{1.136}{1.104} = 102.9\%$$

The Central Planning Bureau estimated a price rise of 5.6 percent for 1980. When compounded over three years, the estimated average price rise for the next three years was:

$$\frac{(1.056 \times 1.056 \times 1.056) - 1}{2} \times 100\% = 8.9\%$$

Therefore, the new fee for 1980–82 was: old fee + (1.029 x 1.089 x old fee). If the old fee was f.45.50, the new one was f.45.50 + 1.12 (45.50) = f.51.00.

In theory the Dutch charging method should not have had perverse effects. Whether a hospital got revenue from per diems or from services, it was supposed to break even on all revenue. However, a hospital manager might sense that he could amortize certain new equipment easily and earn profits on certain procedures that the doctors wanted; therefore, he might acquire and encourage high use of the equipment. He would then get automatic triennial increases of the daily charge under the *calculatieschema,* and it might be several years before COZ caught up with him in an individual rate application. During that period the hospital would be earning extra money and expanding its scale considerably. COZ would be unable to force cutbacks but would have to award new rates from the steadily higher base.

Even if a hospital earned no short-run profits from tests, it could avoid deficits, both in the short and long run. The intention of the per diem payment system was to force the hospital to reduce the costs if patient-days were fewer than predicted. Since Holland slowly reduced length of stay, many hospitals should have been cutting costs to avoid deficits. However, increased numbers of tests enabled the hospital to break even each year, even in the face of fewer patient-days. Therefore, new equipment and technicians were good investments for each hospital, even if the total health care system became more expensive in the long run.

Some Judgments About the Regulatory System. As in France, Dutch methods were thought to be too weak in controlling costs of hospitals, too burdensome in their administration, and too unpredictable in their outcomes. Government officials and sickness funds in particular favored methods that would control costs directly and that would be simpler. As in France, criticisms were directed at the daily charge as a unit of payment as well as at the method of fixing it. Following are the complaints about the regulatory methods of COZ:

☐ *Excessively detailed review.* The heart of the system was the guidelines: the examiner merely applied the formulas to individual cases. The Dutch always tried to fine-tune their methods of calculating the payment rates of health care providers, and the result in the case of hospitals was great complexity. Each guideline related an upper expenditure limit—or an upper limit on numbers of employees or resources—to variable attributes of the hospital, such as number of occupied beds, size of plant, number of patient-days, and number of employees in another category. Each guideline varied by size and type of hospital. If each guideline dictated the examination of a line in the hospital's expenditure report and expected budget, the reasoning and result would have been easily understood. But the regulators had to screen each line according to many such guidelines, particularly in judging whether personnel costs were excessive, and separate guidelines might have contradictory implications. The guidelines became steadily more complicated, since the NZR representatives in COZ argued for improvements, and since the compromises with the sickness funds often varied the improvements by size and type of hospital. The guidelines became more numerous and more complicated, since government pressed to contain costs and added its own. Uncertainty over the meaning of the guidelines invited disputes between the COZ examiners and the hospitals and between NZR and the sickness funds.

□ *Obsolescence of goals.* The original aim of regulation was to ensure that every hospital had all the resources it needed for its particular mission, but without waste. This goal called for line-item budgets, full-time impartial regulators who would meet with hospital managers, and detailed guidelines about allowable limits and norms. The content of the guidelines was strongly influenced by the hospital association, and they were steadily made more generous. When the limiting of expenditures became a growing priority for government and the sickness funds, the system proved ill suited to meeting that goal. The government and payers needed to fix lids and rollbacks. Sending guidelines to an autonomous agency was not effective. The agency was designed to be a negotiating forum between the hospital industry and the payers. The regulators were oriented toward improvements, not cuts; they were supposed to cooperate with hospitals, not fight them.

□ *Perverse effects of particular guidelines.* Certain guidelines related numbers of personnel to patient-days or to occupied beds. In order to avoid cuts and in order to grow, hospital managers tried to increase occupancy—thereby contradicting public policy goals of reducing stays and reducing admissions. The struggle to reduce the undesirable effects is summarized in Chapter Four, in the section headed "Effects on Length of Stay."

□ *Overload.* The examiners had too many individual applications. When they questioned the claims of individual hospitals, they could not debate the details of each hospital's organizational and clinical claims with the managers and leading physicians.

□ *Shortage of information.* The examiners knew little about the experiences of patients. The local sickness funds knew more but did not participate in reviewing each hospital's claim. The examiner could not verify the hospital's expenditure report and prospective budget by investigating the hospital's financial and clinical records.

□ *Comparability.* It was often difficult to judge whether a hospital differed from others in its peer group in costliness and efficiency, because the hospitals differed in budgetary structures. They also varied in the number of tests and treatments that were not included in the daily charge and were billed separately.

□ *Profits.* In theory every hospital broke even, and the calculations provided no incentive to multiply tests. However, once a break-even rate structure was set that year, the hospital might earn considerable profits from itemized services paid under the *tarievenlijst*. The hospital might earn considerable profits for several years by filing false or no *calculatieschema's*. The profits were plowed back into more technicians, equipment, and materials. When a new individual rate application was filed (the *bijlage*), the hospital had a higher cost base and higher rates of utilization, particularly in the technical services. COZ could not cut back the new cost bases substantially but had to use them in the new rate calculations. In the absence of reliable reports, no definite estimates could be made, but some officials in the Ministry of Public Health believed that such itemized tests resulted in persistent cost overruns in the entire system. Between 1976 and 1980 in all Dutch general hospitals, admissions rose by only 6 percent;

but special tests and treatments increased by 13 to 50 percent (laboratory, 50; Xrays, 17; function tests, 13; and physiotherapy, 31). Numbers of paramedical staff and auxiliaries rose around 29 percent.[9]

☐ *Inflation.* The government's guidelines forced COZ to increase allowable costs at least as high as the general wage increases and price increases in the economy. If inflation was high in the economy—as it was in Holland during the 1970s—it was even higher in the hospital sector. The guidelines guaranteed that every hospital's increase was at least as high as the general inflation rates for prices and wages, and each hospital got additional increases every few years. (The average annual increases from 1974 to 1980 were about 6.4 percent for consumer prices and about 9.2 percent for expenditures by the general hospitals.) COZ could not impose greater efficiency, since it could not formulate its own policy on hospital wages. Holland's hospital cost explosion would have been even greater if the country had had the number of nurses allowed by the guidelines; many hospitals had unfilled posts in nursing.

☐ *Expansion rather than reduction of the hospital sector.* An individual rate application was triggered only when the hospital wanted more services and more money. COZ and the payers could not force a review and reduction of any hospital on the grounds of excessive beds and excessive stays. Instead, fat hospitals always got automatic annual increases.

☐ *Lack of coordination.* The payment and employment of hospital doctors were not coordinated with the payment of hospitals. Paid directly by sickness funds under fee schedules, the doctors were motivated to order many tests and treatments and force the hospitals to bear the costs. In addition, the planning of hospitals was not coordinated with the payment of their operating costs. Hospital facilities planning was underdeveloped.

☐ *Weak local responsibility.* Everything was decided by a single agency. Local government and local sickness funds were not involved.

☐ *Appeals.* The appeals system was confusing and disorderly. It may have disposed the examiners to avoid bother by means of excessive generosity.

Revisions of the System. The new arrangement combines negotiation and regulation. Bilateral negotiation had long been common in Dutch health finance, and it was expanded in the payment of hospitals under the reforms begun in 1981. Certain regulatory features remain and have been strengthened in order to implement the public interest in controlling costs, an urgent problem in the precarious Dutch economy. Certain administrative features have been retained and strengthened; for example, COZ was converted into a more general, reorganized, and more powerful Central Agency for Health Care Charges (*Centraal Orgaan Tarieven Gezondheidszorg*, or COTG). I summarized these changes in the last chapter. In short:

☐ *Rate negotiation in the locality.* The hospital sends its last cost report and its request for new rates to the local sickness fund as well as to COTG. The funds now employ analysts. The funds and hospital negotiate over the hospital's claims about expected utilization and its prospective budget. The fund and the hospital send COTG a letter reporting the result of their negotiations. In most cases the hospital's prospective budget is approved.

☐ *Guidelines.* Some are sent to COTG by the Ministry of Public Health, primarily limiting the annual increase in total expenditure for hospitals in Holland. COTG must conform to these instructions. If a cap has been set, all hospital prospective budgets must fall within it. Other guidelines are written by chambers in COTG and are approved by the COTG governing board. They deal with limits on personnel and on expenditures for different parts of the hospital, but they will be much less detailed than in the past, since they will avoid the correlations among allowable costs, beds, and patient-days. The guidelines are designed to impose ceilings on expenditures for individual hospitals and for all hospitals.

☐ *Regulation.* An examiner employed by COTG inspects the hospital's budget. He does not perform the original work, as under COZ, but checks the recommendations of the local negotiators. He makes sure that the prospective budget does not exceed the formulas in the guidelines and does not exceed the cap for the country. He then calculates the daily charge and itemized charges, which (when multiplied by expected utilization) will yield the prospective budget.

☐ *Authority of COTG.* Upon the examiner's recommendation, COTG issues the rates. Action on behalf of the sickness fund no longer awaits approval by the *Ziekenfondsraad;* action on behalf of the privately insured no longer awaits approval by the Ministry. COTG is no longer merely a place where the hospitals and the sickness funds negotiate guidelines, as COZ was. The *kamers* still perform the identical function. But COTG also has a governing board picked by different principles and performing additional functions. Also, the COTG *kamers* have the new function of hearing appeals against the examiners. COTG's *kamers* and governing board settle the individual appeals, and the *Ziekenfondsraad* no longer considers them.

☐ *Limits.* A goal is to reduce expenditure on hospitals. A steady annual increase for all hospitals was no longer allowed; instead, all were expected to decline several percentage points in real terms during the mid-1980s. Hospitals with expenditure overruns would not receive surcharges to clear their deficits. Hospitals that reduced their costs below the prospective budget could keep the profits this year but would receive a lower prospective budget next year. Keeping both the deficit and profits was an innovation in the previously break-even Dutch payment system, and it was one of the few incentive reimbursement arrangements adopted in Europe. If the negotiators agreed to limit tests and treatments or if guidelines restricted them, tests and treatments could no longer proliferate beyond predictions.

☐ *Greater discretion by the hospital manager, less intrusion by the regulator.* Line-item review of past costs and of the prospective budget was reduced. Negotiators and regulators set limits. During the year the hospital manager could save in some spending and use it for other purposes that he deemed better for the hospital. He need no longer argue with a regulator instructed to recapture savings on some lines and prevent overruns on other lines.

☐ *Coordination with payment of doctors.* COTG had jurisdiction over both payment of hospital specialists and the payment of hospitals. Separate chambers dealt with the two, and the governing board could coordinate them if it wished. The sickness funds negotiated rates with both. The independence of specialists from hospital managements and their personal financial gains from higher service intensity had long contradicted public policies to restrain hospital costs. The national government and the COTG chambers during the 1980s searched for better methods to restrain the specialists.

☐ *Coordination with facilities planning.* Reforms in Holland during the 1980s included the establishment of regional governments, the improvement of hospital facilities planning, and the formulation of regional hospital plans by the regional commission. Hospitals' operating costs are now examined first by negotiators in the region, rather than by officials in a single national agency (such as COZ). During the 1980s the national government, the College for Hospital Planning, COTG, NZR, and the sickness funds discuss how to coordinate planning and payment at both the national and regional levels.

☐ *Reallocation.* By reducing the size of acute hospitals through expenditure restraint, the government and the sickness funds hope that more care will be given in cheaper modes, such as the hospital's outpatient department or the home health agencies. By limiting the acute hospital sector and allowing growth in others, the government hopes that homes for the handicapped will improve.

Regulators with Granting Power in Switzerland

Regulators can perform different roles. In France, Holland, and some other European countries, they have been referees between sickness funds and hospitals. In the United States, they have been spokesmen for the public interest in setting fair prices. Throughout Europe today, regulators have become spokesmen for the public interest in controlling inflation and government expenditure.

The authority of regulators can have different bases. In France, in Holland's regulation of privately paid rates under COZ, and in a few American states (such as Maryland), the regulator has a mandate from government; and his decisions are enacted as an order by a line Ministry pursuant to a price-control law. In Holland's regulation of rates paid by sickness funds and in several American states, the regulator recommends prices; and a commission representing hospitals and payers endorses the prices for future transactions.

Many a regulator dreams of backing up his awards with his own subsidies or financial penalties, but few have them. He would combine the role of regulator (either a price controller or a referee) and the role of grantor. He would control some money and would divide the operating costs between his own fund and the third-party payers. The method is a hybrid of rate regulation and grants, which will be described in Chapter Eight. An example is Switzerland, with some hints of the approach in several American states.

Evolution of Swiss Hospital Pay. Slightly more than half of Switzerland's hospitals are owned by private groups (usually nonprofit associations); the rest are owned by governments (either the cantons or the *communes*). As in other countries, a prolonged evolution has occurred—an evolution from the nineteenth-century dependence on money found by owners and toward third-party payment.[10]

But Swiss national health insurance has never become so extensive that it could cover all hospital operating costs. Business interests blocked the original legislation because it made them liable for payroll taxes for their employees' health insurance. Although the entire population eventually became insured, either compulsorily or voluntarily, most money in the accounts comes from the subscribers' own premiums. In lieu of contribution by employers, the national government since implementation of the original law of 1911 pays an annual subsidy to every health insurance carrier. But the sum is less than a full-scale payroll tax on all employers, and the need to limit national expenditures led to a cap on the subsidies in the late 1970s.

The national government's subsidy to the sickness funds is earmarked for the hospital's medical and nursing charges for the patient (the *Spitaltax*). Individuals have either compulsory or voluntary coverage, depending on their status under the varying laws of their cantons. The hospital's room-and-board charges and other nonmedical charges are personal obligations of the patient (the *Pensionszuschlag*), but usually he buys the extra coverage, and his carrier pays all hospital bills together. The distinction between medical and housing costs is made in the hospital's cost-center accounting and in rate setting, but it blurs in practice.

Every public and nonprofit private establishment covers its operating costs from a mixture of sickness fund payments, out-of-pocket patient payments, and a subsidy from the cantonal government. The proportions vary among cantons. Grants for new buildings and for substantial new equipment come either from the cantonal government (for all hospitals), from the *commune* government (for some requests from communally owned hospitals), from the owner (for nonprofit hospitals), or from special donations from private groups (for the cantonally owned teaching hospitals).

If all operating money came from daily charges billed to sickness funds, Swiss hospital pay would be decided by negotiation (described in Chapter Six) or by rate regulation (described in this chapter). Instead, the Swiss system is a hybrid.

Guidelines. As in most systems, each hospital presents a prospective budget, which becomes the basis for calculating next year's rates. But the payers do not automatically accept it, and the problem arises of how to formulate warnings to the hospitals and guidelines to the financial examiners. Switzerland lacks the centralized structure for generating guidelines, as in France and Holland. Under the country's federal constitution, the national government lacks authority in hospital affairs. The national associations of sickness funds and of hospitals are self-interested; each is engrossed in the affairs of its own sector, and they do not confer to create a national hospital policy. The cantonal governments have authority over hospitals; they meet in an interprovincial council of health officials (the *Schweizerisches Sanitätsdirektorenkonferenz*, or SDK), but they are too numerous and too diverse to work out a joint hospital policy. SDK has met and encouraged uniformity on limited but valuable technical matters, such as general adoption of the statistical reporting forms, financial reporting forms, and accounting conventions developed by the national hospital association (the *Vereinigung Schweizerische Krankenhäuser*, or VESKA).

While each cantonal government is left to instruct its hospitals and financial examiners in its own way, certain common Swiss themes arise everywhere. Articles of faith are the avoidance of inflation and the avoidance of government deficits. A universal assumption is that wage increases, annual financial obligations, and annual financial awards (such as hospital charges) should be tied to the national index of consumer prices (the *Landesindex der Konsumentenpreise,* calculated by the national government's Office for Industry and Labor). The financial examiner tries to limit entries in the hospital's prospective budget so that the new daily rate will rise no more than the probable rise in the national consumer price index. This is difficult, since—as in every other country—hospital costs rise faster than general prices.

Guidelines are supposed to make the hospitals' preparation of the prospective budget more predictable, as well as governing the work of the financial examiners. Considerable predictability is introduced by the fact that one of the payers is the cantonal government. By midyear, shortly before sending hospitals the forms and instructions to the forms, the Department of Health of the canton gets signals from the canton's Department of Finance about the probable budget next year. The Department of Health can guess about the financial resources of the sickness funds—that is, this year's spending increased by approximately the price index. The department can also guess about the increase in the biggest item in hospital costs—namely, wages. All hospital workers—both in public and in nonprofit establishments—are paid according to the civil service wage scale, which rises each year according to the consumer price index.

Around midyear the Department of Health sends all hospitals the forms for entering the prospective budget for the next calendar year. Included are guidelines *(Rechtlinien)* written by the department officials who will ultimately decide the levels of daily charges and the assignment of payment between cantons and sickness funds. The guidelines contain rules for maximum allowable entries for personnel, energy, medical supplies, and so on.

Evaluating the Budget. The hospital can fill out the budget forms early. For some time all Swiss hospitals have been keeping their accounts according to advice of the national hospital association (VESKA) and have been sending financial and organizational information to VESKA on its forms. All the diverse prospective budgeting forms are related to the VESKA conventions. I described them in Chapter Three. The fact that the national hospital association writes and collects the forms produces great similarity among the cantons in their information from hospitals and in methods of analysis.

In each canton the prospective budget is mailed to the Department of Health and is analyzed by one of its examiners for financial affairs. This role is common in all regulatory and public grants system, but the Swiss auditor is not an independent referee, as in a purely regulatory arrangement. He works for one of the payers. Therefore, he is probably more critical than if he were deciding only how others should spend their money.

The examiner approves the hospital budgets that fall within the guidelines about allowable increases. He analyzes the others in detail. The financial and organizational data about Swiss hospitals have been computerized for some time, so that the examiner can run comparisons between the hospital's new prospective budget and past costs; he can also compare that hospital with others in the same canton. Switzerland was one of the first countries making computerized peer group comparisons of hospital prospective budgets and of retrospective cost reports, in order to spot excessively expensive individual organizations.

If a hospital will greatly exceed last year's spending, the reason usually is additional personnel and additional programs. Since public money would be used, the prospective budget form asks for a full explanation, and the examiner and Department of Health must approve in advance. Several cantons, such as Bern, include in their prospective budgets sections to explain all proposed new jobs and all proposed new equipment. The applications include predictions of the consequences in operating costs if the jobs or programs are added. The financial examiner and (often) the head of the Division for Hospitals in the canton confer at least once with the hospital managers to discuss high requests and to work out compromises.

A letter is then sent by the Department of Health to the hospital, giving the amended prospective budget and explaining the cuts. The system is merely designed to fix the liability of the sickness funds and of the cantonal government for the hospital's operating costs. It is not a form of total revenue and cost control. The hospital owners can look for money elsewhere for the disallowed items.

Allocation Among Payers. The share of the hospital's operating costs assigned to the sickness funds and to the cantonal revenue is decided by a mixture of legislative definition, negotiation, and regulatory action by officials. The mix varies across the country. The national government's law says that the health insurance accounts subsidized by the *Bund* shall cover only medical care. Therefore, the *Spitaltax*—the daily rate covering medical costs—might be paid for in full by the sickness funds. The hospital's nonmedical costs—such as patients' room and board, administration, laundry, and heating—must be covered elsewhere. Patients can be billed for room, board, and nonclinical nursing; in practice the sickness funds sell an extra insurance policy for the *Pensionszuschlag*, the daily charge for nonmedical patient costs.

In practice the allocation between *Spitaltax* items, *Pensionszuschlag* items, and other hospital costs is not self-evident. What the hospital cannot collect from the sickness funds—that is, the "deficit"—the cantonal government pays. In a few cantons, such as Bern, the allocation and the size of the daily rates paid by the sickness funds are settled by bilateral bargaining between the cantonal association of sickness funds and each individual hospital. The sickness funds try to give the hospital as little as possible. However, behind the scenes stands the cantonal government: by telling the sickness funds how much of a hospital's deficit it can cover, it presses the sickness funds into offering the hospitals more. Ultimately, the cantonal grants cover general nonpatient costs not paid via the sickness funds' daily rates (for items such as administration, heating, and laundry) plus whatever patient costs the sickness funds avoided paying.

In some cantons, such as Zurich, the division is decided by officials in the cantonal Department of Health, pursuant to policies by the cantonal Parliament. After completing their evaluation of all the hospitals' prospective budgets, the officials decide the proportion of daily costs to be paid by the sickness funds and the proportion paid by the cantonal Treasury. If the awards will cause sudden disruptions for the sickness funds and the hospitals, the cantonal officials may meet with the leaders of the cantonal associations of sickness funds and of hospitals. But the officials have the ultimate legal power.

One might expect that the officials would shift costs onto the sickness funds, in order to conserve the government's budget. Such maneuvers are common in the United States: national officials limit allowable costs under Medicare and Medicaid, and hospitals then charge other payers more. But such methods are not used in Switzerland: the decisions and the detailed calculations are public and are openly debated; the sickness funds would protest if they were overcharged. Instead of shifting costs to the private payers, government officials sometimes do the opposite—that is, requiring the sickness funds to pay less than they would if they had negotiated the entire prospective budget with the hospital. For example, in Zurich during much of the 1970s, the parties of the Left dominated the cantonal Parliament and preferred that more of the costs be covered by revenue derived from progressive income taxes rather than from regressive insurance premiums. In 1977, however, strains on the government budget forced the cantonal officials—with the approval of the cantonal Parliament—to shift a larger share to the sickness funds. But the funds insisted on an objective measure. The proportion finally adopted was the average percentage between sickness funds and cantons throughout all of Switzerland.

Government Regulation to Protect the American Public

American society was created by individuals and small groups, without traditional restricting structures, such as social classes in feudal relationships. At first a small population in a huge landscape, individuals were free to move about and create farms and businesses. It was a society of immigrants, individuals who had escaped from the structures, collectivities, and rules of Europe. It was an economy of individuals. In their daily thinking as well as in their official ideology, Americans in general enthusiastically adopted the philosophy of individual rights, individual opportunities, and individual responsibilities that was merely one of the competing arguments of rival classes in Europe. Nearly all societies in Europe and the Western Hemisphere strive for order, but the United States does not.

To this day American ideology remains the individualism of the past. Proposals to face reality and base ideology and policy on the interaction of large collectivities have little influence.[11] The Americans repeatedly revive antitrust policies, criticize Big Labor, and elect to run the national government politicians who denounce that government's mere existence.

As the American economy developed, large organizations became the principal producers and sellers in some sectors; they dominated the market, dictated prices, and became very profitable. The American solution at first was to wait for new entrepreneurs to become competing producers or to offer substitute products, thus demonstrating the self-correcting nature of a market of individuals. One common European reaction to such market power when competitors do not arise promptly has been nationalization. The "natural monopolies" that might overcharge the public—such as electricity, telephone, railroads, and radio—are eventually bought out and managed by government. Another common European response is to organize a large movement of consumers or workers, who then persuade the powerful firm to moderate its prices and offer convenient services. The two sides become parts of the wider social-class movement of business and labor.

Americans cannot think and organize this way. Only in the inescapable need to organize workers to protect pay and hours have Americans created powerful movements to play a systematic adversarial role. But this exceptional trend was temporary; union membership never reached 30 percent of the American labor force, it dropped to below 20 percent during the 1980s, and the leadership of many unions stagnated. Americans have not organized the individual customers of powerful firms or the individual victims of large malefactors to fight the providers and drive down prices. Americans have rarely pressed for government takeovers of exploiters, since Big Government is deemed more threatening, more inefficient, and more corrupt than Big Business. (The rare cases of nationalization in America often have resulted from bailouts of bankrupt owners.)

In several European countries, regulation is not an alternative to consumer self-protection but aims at a fair resolution of the conflict between sellers and buyers. It prevents an excessively militant consumer movement from swinging outcomes to the other extreme and ruining the industry. But in the United States, regulation is inspired by reformers who can find no way to restrain the powerful and malevolent providers. It is the American substitute for the countervailing organizations of consumers and victims. The industry remains in private hands, but government sets rules in the name of the "public interest."[12]

Passage of such laws in America becomes an elaborate political struggle. An economic sector and particular providers must be singled out for exceptions to the rule of the free market. The law must be formulated as a reflection of the consensus of the entire "public," not merely the tactic of the provider's opposing interest groups. The law must state goals, rights, and responsibilities; it must define very elusive concepts, such as the "fair return" guaranteed providers. A regulatory apparatus must be created that will represent the "public," will not be captured by one group, will carry out the procedures faithfully, will accomplish the goals, will not infringe the rights of the regulated, and will not become a den of bureaucratic tyrants.

Critics of providers always exist; therefore, regulatory proposals always circulate on all levels of American government. But passage of such a deviation from private free-market customs requires a widespread political consensus. The coalition must be determined, since the indignant targets mobilize their political allies in opposition. Therefore, a common preparation for passage of a regulatory law in the United States is a prolonged "muckraking" campaign against the industry involved: all its providers or the principal firms are depicted as profiteers and as evil threats against the entire population. The atmosphere becomes passionate, and mutual hostilities grow. The passions are often rekindled with occasional investigations of corruption or of "regulatory capture" in the press or in the legislature.

In every American legislature—whether national, state, or municipal—every regulatory law is a compromise among political parties, interest groups, and influential individuals. Many contain diverse passages arbitrarily combined. American laws lack the clarity and brevity of those passed in other countries.

Since American legislatures do not trust administrators to carry out their intent, the laws usually contain details that in other countries are left to guidelines or to administrators' discretion. On the other hand, some American legislatures cannot create a firm consensus over the goals and criteria of regulation; consequently, an unclear statute is passed, and an independent bipartisan commission is appointed to work out policies not spelled out in the statute. Since every law has a different political history, American regulatory laws lack standardization in draftsmanship and in administrative machinery. Because of uncertainty over the goals and procedures of the laws, and because of suspicions about perversion of legislative intent, American legislative committees frequently monitor the course of regulation by oversight hearings.

While most American regulatory laws have been defensive counterattacks by the public against malefactors, a few have been designed to create order in a potentially disorderly market, to protect the public's investment in resources. In some areas, such as transportation and communication, regulatory laws evolved in practice from the restraint of rascals into the stabilization of markets, and the providers themselves came to favor regulation.

Insurance Regulation. In hospital affairs government regulation includes the licensing of establishments to open and care for persons, licensing of health care professionals, safety of buildings, adequacy of staffing, quality of facilities, the necessity of new equipment and programs, and so on. I will discuss only hospital rate regulation.

One of the first forms of regulation in any field in the United States later came to affect hospital finance. Insurance regulation by state government began in the 1850s as a typical form of protecting the public against fraudulent and irresponsible sellers. The many life and property insurance companies during the early nineteenth century assumed risks that exceeded their reserves, since they competed for business by making excessive promises and by undercutting each other's premiums. As a result, some policy holders could not collect on their protection, and companies went bankrupt.[13]

For over a century, state insurance commissioners have examined the reserves of companies, to make sure that the companies can pay their obligations. They have approved the rates of companies, to make sure that they are high enough to replenish the reserves but do not overcharge the subscribers. Originally overseeing insurance for the loss of life and property, state insurance commissions took jurisdiction over the new health insurance offerings during the twentieth century. In particular, once a year they review applications for higher community rates for individual policy holders of Blue Cross and Blue Shield.

By the late 1960s, Blue Cross's rates were increasing more rapidly than they had in the past, so that Blue Cross could pay for the accelerating hospital charges. Eventually, Blue Cross Plans in many states were asking for rate increases of 25 percent each year. The state insurance commissioners were required to grant the increases because of their obligation to protect the reserves of the Blues, but obviously Blue Cross was acting as a conduit to collect money for the hospital. The subscriber could not protect himself by changing companies, since all others sold limited indemnity policies, and Blue Cross alone offered paid-in-full coverage. So the state insurance commissioners began to intervene to protect the customer. The real overcharger was the hospitals, but the commissioners had authority only over Blue Cross, not over the hospitals. As I said in the last chapter, state insurance commissioners (first in Pennsylvania, then in Rhode Island, then in many other states) conditioned rate increases upon the adoption by Blue Cross of a strong cost-conscious negotiating policy toward the hospitals. Thereafter, rate increases were conditioned on Blue Cross's reports about how conscientiously it bargained with the hospitals.

Since the 1870s the state insurance commissioners have formed a national association and have met to compare policies, methods, and results. They were important reasons for the belated spread of consumer-oriented negotiating in the United States. Thus, rate regulation in health insurance became an indirect lever upon the rates of hospitals.

Hospital Rate Regulation. Hospitals in America have been popular, not denounced as "robber barons" whose price gouging required intervention by regulators to protect the public. Thus, a "normal" American motive for price regulation did not operate. Once hospitals were feared for contagion; safety and staffing regulations helped improve their image. American hospital users have never had powerful consumer representation, as in the European sickness funds, either to negotiate rates or to ensure that a regulator be vigorous and fair to all sides.

American hospital rate regulation arose under very peculiar conditions, to control the prices that state governments paid. American state and local governments had always had limited programs to pay health care for the poor; the programs exploded after 1965. Amendments to the national government's Social Security system offered all state governments a share of the full operating costs for generous outpatient and inpatient care for beneficiaries in certain social welfare programs and (if a state was particularly generous) for persons below certain income levels. Under Medicaid the poor were guaranteed mainstream medicine, paid in full from the operating budgets of the state and national governments. State governments administered Medicaid and were obligated "for payment of the reasonable cost of inpatient hospital services" (Title XIX, Section 1902(A), Clause 13(D), Social Security Act, Public Law 89-97, July 30, 1965). Several other payers (Medicare, Blue Cross, and several national government programs) made similar commitments to reimburse costs that the hospitals persuaded the payers were "reasonable"; the hospitals could charge other payers freely. Hospital costs rose rapidly, and Medicaid payments were obligated by the law to keep pace. During the late 1960s and the 1970s, Medicaid rose faster than any other line in every state government budget, and it became the largest line in many. By a quirk in the Medicaid law, a state government could limit payments to doctors by setting a fee schedule—even unilaterally, without negotiation—but it could not control the unit prices or the total costs of hospital pay.[14]

A few state governments then ingeniously invoked the familiar regulatory model: an agency of the state government would examine the operating costs of all public and private hospitals in the state and would set rates that ensured a fair return to the hospital. But the motive for this regulation was unprecedented: it was not designed to protect the public against exploitation and perils by malefactors; it was designed to protect the state government budget against unpredictable spending increases. The institutional form of the regulation was often peculiar: the regulatory office was located within the same state government department as the office that administered Medicaid. Without declaring the entire hospital industry a monopoly that threatened the entire public—as in other industry-wide price regulation—the state governments at first used the guise of regulation to fix only the prices that they alone paid. Gradually, as hospital cost containment became a nationwide problem, several states expanded their price regulation to other payers. A few states intended hospital rate regulation to help insurance rate regulation: state insurance commissioners could not prevent the rise in Blue Cross premiums if Blue Cross costs rose; what had been lacking was state regulatory power over the hospital costs assigned to Blue Cross. For example, the insurance commissioner in New Jersey had directed Blue Cross to hold the line on hospital costs, and Blue Cross had relied on the state hospital association to work out the rates for each hospital. Critics complained, however, that the arrangement kept costs high rather than low, and the state government itself eventually regulated the hospitals.[15] (In contrast, Blue Cross and the individual hospitals in Pennsylvania responded to their insurance commissioner by negotiating bilaterally, and state regulation has never been enacted there.)

   Structures. Of the fifty American states, less than a dozen—beginning with New York in 1969—have ever enacted any form of hospital rate regulation. Two states have repealed their laws; all others have altered their statutes, some often. The organization and techniques vary widely among states.[16] In contrast, all provinces in European federal governments adopt identical organizations and methods (as in Germany) or similar ones (as in Switzerland). The variation among states in America reflects the wide range in Medicaid spending, in the costliness of hospitals, in the popularity and political influence of hospitals, and in the political complexion of the state legislatures. The variation also reflects the fact that the national government has never enacted a policy to restrain hospital costs. If it did, the national government would enact national machinery to regulate hospital rates. Or it would enact methods to pressure or induce all states to perform similar regulation.[17]

   ☐ *Government department.* The first state laws (for example, in New York, Massachusetts, and New Jersey) conferred price-setting power upon agencies of the state government. Since regulators in the United States are not supposed to be "arbitrary," the laws set forth the methodology in considerable detail. A large staff of economists and accountants examines each hospital's last report of costs, screens out padding (perhaps in the light of utilization), and projects a rate schedule for the coming year. The regulators may have a prospective budget for the coming year, but usually they work from the last verified reports of costs and utilization. A determined government department can limit price rises more strictly than a commission.

   ☐ *Independent commission.* Fearing passage of a strict price-control system run by government officials, some hospital associations have induced state legislatures (for example, in Maryland and the state of Washington) to create autonomous rate-setting commissions, with representatives from the hospitals, representatives from payers, and miscellaneous "public representatives" named from both political parties by the governor. These independent commissions resemble state regulatory commissions in energy and in some other fields. They differ from other state commissions in their more limited reach: most lack jurisdiction over the hospitals' entire business, although Maryland and Washington finally acquired it during the late 1970s, Maryland permanently and Washington temporarily. All American commissions still must calculate different rates for different payers, since Medicare, Blue Cross, and others have different allowable costs in their laws and contracts. (Flexible rates are common in other American regulated industries, but differential burdens on classes of consumers are allowed only for good reasons.) In Europe regulation results in standard hospital rates for all payers. The American commissions work somewhat like Holland's COTG: the full board works out guidelines for the staff, the staff analyzes individual cases, and the board gives pro forma approval. Appeals are heard by the American board; in Holland they are heard by the COTG chambers but not by the full COTG board. Compared to regulation by civil servants in the line departments of American state governments, the commissions usually have experienced less turbulence—probably because the hospitals are represented in the commission, whereas the Medicaid bureau of the state is only a commission member; proposed new rates are discussed in the commission before rather than after the announcements; and the commissions are more generous to the hospitals.

Twelve other American states are often said to have "rate setting" or "regulation." But on close inspection, these are really voluntary negotiating offices created by Blue Cross, with more or less collaboration by the hospital association. I described them in Chapter Six.

A few states have "study commissions," but they lack regulatory power over hospitals' budgets and rates. Usually they were created as façades to mask the fact that state legislatures had repealed or refused to enact regulation, as in Illinois.

Objects of Regulation. An official state program focuses on one of the following:

- *Units of service.* In all cases a fair rate is set in the light of the hospital's expected total revenue. The rate usually is a mixture of per diem for basic clinical care and housing, plus charges for ancillary services, although some all-inclusive per diems exist. Since neither total revenue nor utilization is controlled, services under price regulation often exceed the predicted number, whereas unregulated services can increase in both price and volume; therefore, hospital costs may rise more than expected. Examples: Maryland, Washington, and (in the past) New Jersey.
- *Total revenue of the hospital.* The hospital managers have complete discretion in arranging their services and setting their charges. Examples: Connecticut and Maine.
- *Diagnosis-related groups.* Developed by states that were distressed to discover that regulating rates for services does not limit total hospital costs when hospitals are free to increase utilization. Examples: Maryland for some hospitals and New Jersey for all hospitals today.

Methods. The regulatory programs employ many techniques because of variety in their organizational forms and the objects of their regulation. In addition, methods vary and frequently change because of different styles in different states and because many programs got their start-up money from the national government in order to demonstrate new techniques in cost containment. Extensive summaries of the methods have been written by others.[18] Inevitably, these summaries are long and must be updated constantly. Following are a few highlights in American regulation:

□ *Reporting*. All regulatory programs require that last year's costs and utilization be reported on long line-item forms. However, some do not require full accounts of the hospital's revenue and utilization, particularly if the regulator lacks authority over all rates by all payers. The examiner usually cannot inspect the hospital's books, and hospitals are not required to standardize their internal accounts. The regulators computerize the hospital's report. A new trend in some European countries (such as France) and in some American states is for the hospital to submit a data tape rather than a written document.

□ *Budget review*. Whether the regulators ultimately announce a revenue budget or detailed rates, all examine the last cost report and some kind of prospective budget. The computer compares the hospital's past and expected expenditure—and, sometimes, staffing and utilization—with guidelines. In some states the computer compares the hospital with peer group averages. If the hospital falls within guidelines defining maxima, the regulators approve the hospital submission. Most of the regulators' time is devoted to the exceptions. (The distinction between routinely approved and specially investigated budgets also existed in Holland under COZ).

□ *Guidelines*. Guidelines—the Americans call them "screens"—are the heart of a regulatory system. They state the program's goals, the limits of expenditure (aggregate and/or specific), and the logic in cutting. European countries with rate regulation have recently developed cost-control policies, with a machinery for creating and then transmitting guidelines from national leaderships (in government and in peak associations) to the budget examiners.

American national and state governments lack hospital finance policies, but regulators are supposed to act according to some principles. The state laws were originally inspired by the need to restrain Medicaid costs; so most programs start with the enforcement of allowable costs as defined in the national government's original laws creating Medicaid and Medicare. Another goal is to protect Blue Cross from excessive strain due to inefficiency in hospital management. A common approach in guidelines is to calculate statewide or peer group averages as norms, specify a limit (a percentage over the limit or several standard deviations), and then scrutinize the outliers. Recently some guidelines explain how to find money for hospitals afflicted by many bad debts—a problem for state governments, who are responsible for ensuring health care.[19]

Guidelines are drafted initially by the agency staff or by interest groups. They are adopted by the governing board of the commission or by the advisory committee of the state department administering the regulation. These boards are drawn from hospitals, third parties, consumer activists, neutral citizens, and others. Guidelines are political compromises, constrained by the need of all states to limit their Medicaid spending.

☐ *Indexes.* Routinely approved hospitals—those falling within the guideline limits—are allowed automatic revenue increases consisting of last year's total expenditure plus an index for price and wage increases. The regulators usually take last year's total spending—not the original prospective budget—as the base. A variety of price indexes are used, measuring general consumer prices or the special market basket for hospitals.

☐ *Rates.* Some regulators approve the per diems and the charge lists, which—multiplied by expected volume—will generate the approved revenue. The regulator must apply not only the state's definition of allowable costs but also each payer's different definition. Or the regulator approves the expected revenue budget, and it is the hospital that sets the charges.

☐ *Interim submissions.* Usually the hospital can file a new application whenever it seems to run a chronic deficit or when it alters a structure. While there is usually an annual timetable for all applications in the state, a few states maintain the same rates until the hospital submits a new application. In such cases no fixed cycle exists.

☐ *Penalties.* In many states hospitals exceeding the expected revenue through high utilization suffer no consequences. A few states have groped for disincentives in the payment method, such as less than full cost-based charges next year if the hospital's excess revenue last year seemed to yield a profit. But these disincentive formulas are difficult to write and are applied gingerly. Florida during the 1980s threatened to fine and revoke licenses of hospitals that persistently exceeded their approved revenue budgets, but that is unusual.

☐ *Appeals procedures.* The machinery varies among states. As in much of government regulation in America, the commissions devote much of their time and staff work to hearing appeals. Hearings are public and adversarial: the hospital states its case against the staff's award, the staff presents its case, and any interest group and citizen can testify. The commission's orders might be further appealed within the state's executive branch. If a line department does the regulation, the state government must provide an independent appeals board. The hospital can always appeal to the general courts.

Weaknesses in American Rate Regulation. Political will is the key to health care cost containment. It has never been strong in American hospital rate regulation. I have described the weaknesses elsewhere—particularly in comparison to hospital rate regulation in Europe.[20] Following is a brief summary.

The public and politicians are not convinced that hospital costs are threatening. They wish services to improve and to be available. State governments' budgetary problems with Medicaid can be solved by methods other than controls over hospitals.

Key constituencies in every community—the elites who serve on hospital governing boards, the medical association, the workers in hospitals, and the medical supply companies—oppose controls by government. If regulatory laws are enacted—and only a small fraction of states have them—they are often permissive; otherwise, the hospitals and doctors would fight their enactment. The regulators often make concessions, lest the hospitals successfully press for repeal by the state legislature.[21]

Third-party payers do not form a strong constituency in favor of state rate regulation. They are rivals and refuse to unite in their political lobbying or in formation of an all-payers system. Some payers—such as the Medicare program under the Reagan administration—oppose rate regulation.[22] If a state lacks an all-payers system, its rate regulation has weak effects on total costs, since the hospitals can make up for limits on the regulated payers (such as Medicaid and Blue Cross) by increasing charges on the commercially insured and self-payers. But such cost shifting is possible only in hospitals with richer patients.[23]

The ultimate payers of a large share of hospital spending—business firms—cannot risk supporting strong rate regulation because of their own dependence on the large hospital market for sales. In countries with NHI, the revenue comes from taxes or compulsory premiums, the sickness funds must keep within their budgets, and the sickness funds and government finance officers are a united constituency for strong state controls. In America most health coverage is a fringe benefit of employment; business firms encounter mounting costs, and many create regional discussion groups ("business coalitions") to find solutions.[24] The bigger the company, the higher and more troublesome its health care spending. An alliance of determined large firms could easily persuade state legislatures and the national Congress to enact strong rate regulation, but business coalitions do not—partly because of their general opposition to government regulation of any business, and partly because of their vulnerability to retaliation by the hospitals. For example, during 1983 several large business firms in Arizona created the Coalition for Cost-Effective Quality Health Care, to press the state legislature for regulation of capital and operating costs. A principal member (Honeywell, Inc.) dropped out when two for-profit hospital chains suspended orders for its word processors and data processors, and when other hospitals threatened the same. Large companies elsewhere in the country long ago learned to avoid such showdowns.

Hospital rate regulation—like all rate regulation in the United States—is asymmetric. Its construction contains a bias toward the providers and against the consumers. The appeals machinery is triggered only if the hospital is aggrieved and wants more money. The regulators supposedly represent the public, and their award binds the payers. The insurance carriers cannot file an appeal for a lower hospital rate. Therefore, the appeals system either confirms the regulators' increases or adds extra money.

Regulators in most programs have limited power to compel disclosure of hospital records, fix binding rates, and reject applications for higher rates. Hospitals can easily file lawsuits in general courts that will block or amend regulations and overrule regulators' awards.[25] In several programs the regulators must automatically increase prospective budgets or daily rates by formulas (such as a hospital market-basket index plus real growth) that are more generous than Europe's. American regulators rarely can fix levels of utilization.

Sanctions are weak or absent. A hospital might charge patients and third parties more and suffer little penalty. Even if daily rates are limited in the Medicaid and Blue Cross business, the hospital may be free to raise its itemized charges for Blue Cross and other patients.

Regulatory programs are not allowed to stabilize. They are often amended, because of changes in the state or the national government, or because Americans like to tinker and "improve" things, or because the program was enacted as a "demonstration," or because the law must be periodically reenacted.

Rate regulation and facilities planning are poorly coordinated. While both are programs in state governments, they are housed in separate agencies, their managers may have quite different philosophies, and neither the laws nor the governors require them to enact and implement common programs. The planners are under much pressure to allow hospitals to expand and modernize, and the rate regulators then are obligated to authorize full coverage of operating costs—including the additional new capital costs—even though they have been trying to restrain health care expenditure.[26]

Automatic Formulas in the United States

American distrust of regulation is rooted in an image of human nature. The Founding Fathers repeated Thomas Hobbes's belief that, since humans seek gain and power, elected and appointed officials must be limited by laws and by checks and balances from other government agencies.[27] A common American assumption today is that regulatory agencies are easily captured by the industries they were supposed to regulate, that they no longer protect the public interest against venal providers but become yet another instrument for exploiting the public.[28] Other criticisms of rate regulation—of hospitals and of other sectors—are that delays and extra costs result from cumbersome procedures.

One antidote to regulation, according to conservative American critics, is to eliminate hospital rate regulation, minimize government intervention, and "make the market work."[29] An alternative American remedy is to try to make regulation automatic by prescribing formulas that allow regulators no discretion.[30] For example, hospitals might be permitted to increase their charges or total revenue each year no more than by the increments resulting from specified calculations from the previous year's figures for spending and utilization. An official agency would then be needed only to check the hospitals' financial reports, apply the computer program with the formulas, and mail the result to each hospital, as its rate or revenue limit for the next year. The same or another agency would hear appeals by hospitals claiming special reasons for more money. The agency would not negotiate with or investigate individual hospitals before setting the rates, a laborious and judgmental task performed by the normal regulatory body. The only advance negotiation would consist of meetings among the government agency, hospital association, and sickness funds to agree on a formula at the start of each year.[31]

This method was used in the Nixon administration's emergency Economic Stabilization Program in 1972 and 1973, to fix allowable revenue increases for all hospitals each year. It also was proposed in the Carter administration's Hospital Cost Containment bill of 1977 and in several substitutes by congressmen.[32]

In New York State, the method was used during the 1970s in setting prospective rates for Medicaid and Blue Cross; for a few years during the 1980s, it was extended to all payers. A simplified version was used by the Massachusetts Rate Setting Commission during the late 1970s for scrutinizing and controlling Medicaid charges, but the commission performed the normal budget review by a regulatory agency for other payers.[33] The starting point was the total costs for the last available year, plus a percentage increment that estimated rising prices and rising wages. (Wage increases resulting from collective bargaining contracts were passed through.) Several additional formulas in both states were used to provide disincentives to underutilization and excessive utilization. For example, as a disincentive to operate an underutilized hospital or to keep unnecessary beds open in New York, the number of beds for calculating the daily charge was at least 80 percent or 85 percent of full occupancy. This figure was divided into the total expected costs to get next year's daily rate. If an underused hospital could use its actual number of patient-days, then its daily charge would be higher. The formula was an incentive to reduce costs. Other formulas penalized increasing patient-days beyond the start-of-the-year expectations, and penalized number of patient-days beyond the average for hospitals of the same type.

General formulas penalized hospitals financially if they deviated too far from their peer groups. The grouping itself was created by a computer program clustering from several organizational characteristics of all hospitals. (Massachusetts changed to another formula-based method of paying hospitals after 1982. Originated by Blue Cross, it applied to all payers.)

Achievements. Formula systems focus on the annual increase in the hospital's total revenue or in its daily charge. If the formula is strict, if all (or nearly all) payers are covered, and if the appeals process is strict, annual increases can be low. The New York formulas have "ceiling penalties" that cut down the high spenders and "occupancy penalties" that restrain overcapacity and force underutilized facilities to close. There is no regulatory staff to appease indignant hospitals with individual exceptions or to be cowed by the hospital association and by the state legislature. After the system settled down, New York consistently had lower annual increases in total hospital expenditure than any other state; a number of underused hospitals closed.[34]

However, formula methods are inferior to personal regulators in cutting lines within individual hospitals and in identifying and reforming weaknesses selectively.

Difficulties. The American national and state Constitutions guarantee "due process of law" to the regulated; regulatory custom and laws guarantee to the regulated that their treatment is "fair" and "reasonable." In theory the method of automatic formulas removes all arbitrariness. In New York, for example, all sides participate in the special committees that review and approve the method; the computer applies the formulas to each hospital's prospective budget, eliminating the potentially capricious regulators. Instead of reducing complaints, however, the automatic calculations increase them. Struggles within the formula-writing committees are intense, because everything depends on their decisions. And these decisions—about whether a particular hospital (as well as many others) gains or loses—depend not only on the mathematical calculations but also on the bases to which the formulas are applied. Different outcomes result if the percentage increases are applied to costs or rates, to last year's base or to an earlier one, to the same original base every subsequent year or to a moving base.[35]

When the formula is applied to individual hospitals, the absence of a face-to-face regulator can be infuriating. When hospital managers and regulators can meet prior to a ruling for prolonged review and discussion of individual cases, the directors can be mollified, disputes (particularly over whether the hospital is a special case), can be settled, and any problems in the methodology can be revealed. Automatic application of formulas by a computer eliminates the personal adjustments between two groups of health administrators, and many disagreements have been handed over to lawyers, who escalate the issues and take them into appeals agencies and courts. At times the New York and Massachusetts systems have been swamped in litigation over the powers of the agencies, the justice of the formulas, and the effects of the calculations on individual hospitals.[36]

Constantly under attack for unfairness, the formulas are frequently "improved." Often this means merely that the representatives of one faction in the joint formula-monitoring commission have been appeased. Reading the New York State manual, one is struck by the enthusiastic descriptions of each year's revisions. The American taste for innovation and change extends to the rules of the game. After the hospital director thinks he finally understands the procedure, it changes.

At times formulas are proposed and even adopted that are unusually difficult to understand and remember (for example, essential parts of the Carter administration's Hospital Cost Containment proposals). Often these methods are designed to relate payment to volume by relating marginal cost to marginal revenue. They incorporate the econometric marginal reasoning that has been prominent in health care research in America, and they are designed to achieve appropriate equilibria in work by incentives. However, hospital managers and doctors cannot respond to incentives that they do not understand well. Some understand the formulas; others do not.

Formulas relating payment, work performed, and costs have been incorporated in European guidelines as tools of judgment by regulators when they are examining hospital cost reports and budgets. Europeans lack the American antipathy to regulators and do not pursue a mirage of automatic self-regulation by formulas. Because European payment units in the past were flat rates, marginal pricing was not possible, and the guidelines were crude. The new methods of global budgeting and aggregate grants in Europe and Canada might provide new opportunities for variable payment and incentive reimbursement schemes, using econometric formulas. But the system will continue to be monitored by regulators and negotiators, who can apply the formulas appropriately, deal with exceptions, and explain anomalies and complexities.

Evaluation of Regulation Methods

Advantages from the Standpoint of Payers. The regulatory office can employ experts who understand the subject matter of hospital care and health insurance.

Regulators can gain full access to facts that normally are hidden from payers.

Regulators can devise arrangements that will protect the weaker payers.

Divisive rivalry among payers can be eliminated.

Advantages from the Standpoint of Hospitals. Regulators can protect the solvency of hospitals.

Regulators can correct awards between regularly scheduled rounds, protecting hospitals from damage.

If public policy calls for innovations, regulators can be instructed to implement them.

An approved rate is a cachet enabling the hospital to attract patients, doctors, and lenders.

Advantages from the Standpoint of the Public. If the regulatory system is coordinated, the many awards in individual cases can be fitted together into some consistent pattern throughout the country or region.

The awards can be integrated into the national government's policies about wages, prices, efficiency, and the share of the economy devoted to social security.

The award of payment for operating costs can be coordinated with facilities plans for hospitals and for other health installations.

Regulators can penalize inefficient hospitals, press for greater efficiency, and reward the efficient.

Regulators can monitor the orderly closing or conversion of an entire hospital or of a service within one.

Better management and financial reporting can be fostered within hospitals, because of the requirements or advice of the regulators.

Disadvantages from the Standpoint of Payers. Regulators often defer to hospitals, partly because the guidelines guarantee reimbursement of costs and partly because they cannot successfully argue with hospital managers and doctors about details. Duplication, excess capacity, and inefficiencies may survive.

Hospital rates often rise generously, utilization often exceeds prediction, and some or all payers are strained. These problems can occur even in supposedly strict formula systems intended to fix caps, because of unexpected loopholes in the formulas or because the formulas perversely encourage rather than discourage utilization. If hospital revenue outruns the income of the sickness funds, government is pressed to subsidize the funds. The burden on government's budget is difficult to control.

Despite the need for stability, political campaigns may produce a new government-of-the-day that is far more generous to the hospitals than the old one. The credit goes to the new office holders; the price is paid by the third parties.

Regulators shrink from cutting wages and from reducing the number of jobs. Guidelines may mandate wage pass-throughs. In collective bargaining over wages, the hospital association may be too permissive.

Third parties cannot get full access to the hospital's accounts and plans and therefore cannot easily challenge the regulators' awards. They cannot learn enough about health care.

Disadvantages from the Standpoint of Hospitals. Much wrangling occurs with the regulators. As line-item budget analyses become more specific and as guidelines become more detailed—requiring considerable paperwork—hospital managers complain that the regulators intrude more into management. Rate regulation in other sectors of the economy usually avoids such detailed oversight of management; but hospitals are treated differently, because they are nonprofit public institutions.

Rate regulation usually eliminates or reduces the proprietary and charitable hospitals' opportunities to earn and use profits. If profits are allowed, regulators usually dictate their size and monitor their use.

In its accounting, performance evaluation, and strategy, the hospital becomes oriented to maximizing revenue under the logic of the guidelines. The hospital organization, the doctors, and the patients might be better off providing services that are less remunerative under the guidelines as applied to that hospital.

Conflicts of interest often arise between hospitals and their doctors, particularly if the doctors are paid fees separately by the sickness funds and by private patients.

Innovation may be slowed. Regulators must agree to changes, perhaps in consultation with their headquarters in the national or regional government.

Changes in the government-of-the-day can make the rules and the awards more restrictive, despite the fact that the hospital made long-range financial commitments in capital, personnel, and programs when allowances were more generous.

Hospital managers were once innocents steeped in religion and the ethics of charity. Many become devious in their cost assignments, price setting, and reporting.

Disadvantages from the Standpoint of the Public. Guidelines multiply with time. The regulatory process becomes more complex. Outcomes for individual hospitals and total outcomes for all may be difficult to understand and to predict.

If the goal is to guarantee every hospital its appropriate costs and avoid waste, government must employ a large staff, spread throughout the country. These staffs become expensive and difficult to coordinate, and may absorb an unduly large proportion of government effort.

When ceilings on awards are tight, many disputes are generated and are referred upward. Regulators pass the buck to those who wrote the guidelines and set the caps. Appeals agencies are overloaded. General courts may be overburdened.

It is difficult to reorient the entire health care system. Usually, hospital rate regulation focuses on the annual reimbursement increases in hospitals as they are traditionally defined; it does not deal with alternative health care facilities, it does not try to redirect services, it does not try to reorganize hospitals. Rate regulation is usually poorly coordinated with planning.

Rate regulation tends to freeze regional differentials; it does not shift expenditure from overprovided to underprovided regions. Rate regulators usually lack authority over investment funds.

Rate regulation of hospitals is usually poorly coordinated with the payment of doctors. It has little power to influence doctors' choices of work sites and specialties.

The rate regulator can become an unwilling party to hospital finance during wage negotiations. The hospitals and unions are happy to avoid strikes, provided the regulator guarantees new money from third parties and from the government's Treasury. The hospitals try to direct the pressures of the trade unions and political parties of the Left toward the rate regulators and toward the government. In order to avoid involvement of the regulators in labor relations and in order to avoid such maneuvers by the hospital managers, many governments index hospital wage rates and make wages an automatic pass-through in rate setting. The result is less conflict but probably higher cost.

Trends

Regulation began as an attempt to help the hospital cover some of its costs. Without official recognition of a rate, the sickness funds might try to pay much less. On the other hand, presented for the first time with funded payers, the hospital might try to charge more than its costs. A regulator was needed to protect the payers as well as the hospitals.

The regulatory task at first seemed elementary: an all-inclusive daily rate was set, and the operations and costs of hospitals were simple. Regulation steadily expanded in each European country that had it. The jurisdiction of the regulators expanded to more hospitals and to more payers within each hospital. The pay rates became standardized among all payers. The hospitals wanted full reimbursement of costs, and the sickness funds were willing, provided the hospitals got no profits. So the regulators had the difficult task of setting a unit price that in the total aggregate of expenditure and revenue would break even.

The hospital became steadily more complicated and expensive, and the task of the regulator was to keep covering costs in a dynamic situation, not to impose a freeze or a slowdown. The identification of allowable costs became more complicated, and the hospital had to adopt accounting and reporting methods that were unprecedented in health care. The hospital rate regulator had to learn more than regulators of private business rates did.

When health care cost containment became a public policy priority, regulators as well as hospital managers were suddenly subjected to contradictory instructions. The original laws and methodology of hospital rate regulation were designed to produce an expanding flow of money to keep pace with improved services, better staffing, and more normal wages. The new policy now called for limits in annual increases in revenue, for cutbacks in some attributes deemed excessive, and for critical scrutiny of any new programs. Regulators received large numbers of guidelines and had to balance competing priorities in individual cases.

At first guidelines focused on the traditional task of hospital rate regulators: limiting allowable personnel and other allowable expenditures on each line of the hospital's prospective budget. The overseers of the regulators shrank from restraining utilization of the hospital by doctors and patients, since utilization was deemed "necessary." That is, regulation was supposed to prevent waste and inefficiency, not deny care to the needy. However, utilization of the hospital steadily grew, partly because of true need by aging populations and partly because of wasteful behavior by insured populations and provider-induced demand by hospitals and doctors. Governments and sickness funds suspected that hospitals and doctors evaded rate controls by multiplying patient-days, tests, and treatments. Utilization as well as unit prices had to be restrained. Such restraint required a new type of guideline. Earlier ones had tried to limit budget lines to certain levels of utilization, but they had unexpectedly motivated hospital managers to encourage higher utilization.

New guidelines fixed caps, usually ones that moved along with national economic indexes. Gradually, the regulators overrode the older cost-raising guidelines with new cost-controlling guidelines. As a result, by the early 1980s, annual increases in hospital costs were rising only slightly faster than annual increases in general prices. However, government officials and sickness funds were suffering severe deficits during the general economic downturns of the late 1970s and 1980s, and "slightly faster" was still too much. Further, they thought that the hospital sector had become too expensive, that it was inefficient (as reflected in excessive stays), that it should be cut back, and that more care should be given extramurally. Regulatory methods were too complicated and too oriented to expansion; therefore, more direct methods must be found.

During the late 1970s and 1980s, a considerable ferment over hospital payment swept every country. Many sought lessons from abroad. Those disillusioned with rate regulation in Europe were impressed by the cost-containment records of countries—notably, Great Britain and Canada—that calculated hospitals' global budgets, paid the budgets in installments from single granting sources, and refused to reimburse cost overruns. Several countries (particularly France and Holland) then recast their regulatory systems to employ methods of global budgeting. The final result was a mixture of all the decision methodologies: the local sickness fund and the individual hospital negotiated the hospital's prospective budget; a regulator monitored the negotiations and screened the agreement to conform with national guidelines about cost containment; and the approved budget was paid in installments by the several third parties, pooled in some manner. If cost containment continues to dominate hospital finance policy, rate negotiation and regulation will eventually become the servants of global budgeting and coordinated granting.

8

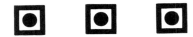

Global Budgeting
and Public Grants

Negotiations and regulation have been the methods of deciding hospital finance when finance is private: several third parties face each hospital, and the establishments are private and municipal in ownership. Hospitals have the initiative in defining services and in sending bills. Total payment results from the number of services, multiplied by the unit price—either a per diem or itemized charges—for each service. These methods can function satisfactorily only when the society's economy provides enough money to cover hospital costs via the insurance carriers.

If government pays hospitals, the system has always differed. Usually the hospital's entire prospective budget is pooled. The governmental payer does not pay the hospital claim by claim as care is rendered but, instead, covers the entire sum in installments. This form of payment is consistent with either private or governmental ownership of the hospitals.

Public payment usually originates from a crisis in financing through the private sector: hospital costs outrun the third parties' ability to pay mounting hospital costs. If the hospitals become bankrupt, government takes over their ownership as well as their financing. If the financing reforms are enacted soon enough and if the private nonprofit owners are still assertive, governmentalization of finance merely reverses mounting deficits, and ownership remains private and municipal. Therefore, government financing does not automatically produce "socialized medicine."

Characteristics

Following are some of the variants that global budgeting and direct grants might assume:

☐ Ownership and management of hospitals.
- Government: national or regional.
- Private nonprofit or municipal.

☐ Source of funds.
- Government: national or regional. If regional, whether national government subsidizes the regional government.
- Special accounts, rather than a government Treasury.

☐ Numbers of payers.
- One.
- Several, pooled together.

☐ Balance of power.
- Bottoms-up. Hospitals present their prospective budgets to the paying authority, which screens and approves. The payer is then compelled to provide the money.
- Top-down. Paying authority dictates amount of money available to each hospital.

☐ Relations between the agency that pays hospitals and other funding agencies, such as the government's Ministry of Finance.

☐ Degree of application to hospitals of standard government practices in writing budgets, controlling current expenditures, and auditing past expenditures.

☐ Reports and disclosure. Whether hospital submits a retrospective cost report and a prospective budget to the paying authority or to some other examiner. Amount of detail.

☐ Bases for annual increases in grants.
- Whatever money can be found in the government's budget.
- Formulas based on the society: changes in prices and wages, movements in the population, etc.
- Plans.
- Guidelines about the allowable costs of individual hospitals.

☐ Scope.
- Each hospital gets its own budget.
- All hospitals in the region get a share of a regional budget for hospitals.
- All hospitals in the region get a share of a regional budget for health services.

☐ Relation to wage determination.
- Payer automatically covers wage awards decided on some external basis, such as the results of industry-wide collective bargaining or increases in civil service pay scales.
- Payer lets the hospital managers award wages and hire numbers of employees within funds available.

☐ Amount of discretion by the managers in rearranging expenditure among lines.

☐ Appeals procedure, if any.

☐ End-of-the-year settlements.
- Whether hospital can recover cost overruns.
- Whether hospital can retain profits.
- Whether next year's grant is modified in light of last year's profits and losses.

Among developed countries direct public grants of the entire budgets of hospitals began in Great Britain and Scandinavia. Hospitals were financed by one government channel and managed by another, raising problems of interagency coordination. Under these public financing arrangements, hospital managers at first expected—as they usually do—that society would provide all the resources their doctors and patients "needed." Britain—the country whose methods have attracted the most attention and controversy abroad—demonstrates the inevitable development of decision-making machinery to reconcile society's resources and the hospitals' expectations. Britain also demonstrates that methods change as governments try to stabilize the place of hospital finance within larger government budgets and as they are forced to cope with new issues of cost containment. Every country with public grants to hospitals experiences a similar evolution in techniques. But each of these countries develops somewhat different methods. If such a country is federal—as Canada illustrates—each province adopts its own arrangements. But even if management details differ, one theme appears throughout public grants to hospitals: the performance of hospitals and the levels of financing are drawn into politics.

Public grants and global budgeting recently have attracted attention because of their capacity for cost containment. But a detailed investigation of Britain shows that these methods can achieve goals unrealized by other methods of payment, particularly the reallocation of resources to underserved areas and underserved groups.

United Kingdom

Evolution. At the time when hospitals and some other health establishments were taken over by the national government in the National Health Service, the British government had no single budget and expenditure account. Several public funds and expenditure budgets were designed by the Treasury, were debated within the Cabinet, and were approved by Parliament. Britain had a custom of "bids"—requests for funds for both established and new programs during the next year. These bids were initiated by operating agencies, screened by the finance and program officers of each Ministry, and then consolidated into a single Ministry bid to Treasury.

Each newly nationalized hospital submitted a prospective budget up through channels within the Ministry of Health, and the Ministry of Health submitted a total bid to Treasury. The new NHS proved more troublesome to Treasury than other government programs. Hospitals had long been underfunded, and many citizens had failed to obtain care; national policy now guaranteed liberal access and good facilities, so that utilization and costs now greatly increased. Hospitals during the late 1940s and early 1950s regularly overspent their planned budgets, and the Ministry of Health ran deficits. Each year, the hospital submitted to the Ministry a much higher prospective budget covering last year's costs plus an increment. NHS budgeting demands rose steeply. But Treasury could not reject them, since the NHS was immensely popular, the proudest achievement of the Labour Government. Nationalization had succeeded after fragmented third-party payment had failed.

Treasury, with Cabinet approval, then sent guidelines to the Ministry of Health, setting allowable annual increases in spending. But during the 1950s and 1960s, disputes were constant. The hospitals and Ministry of Health argued that they needed more money; they continued to run over their allocated budgets and asked for deficiency appropriations ("supplementary estimates") from Parliament to cover deficits. The first tightening came during the 1950s over the supplementary estimates. The hospitals could not count on automatic payment of their deficits and were expected to work within their initial prospective budgets. At first the hospitals were still able to persuade the higher ranks of NHS about the merit of their start-of-the-year requests, and the Ministry of Health often succeeded in getting generous annual increases from a reluctant Treasury and from a sympathetic Cabinet. But no government can long function this way: it must predict its expenditures in advance and keep within the limits. Britain during the 1950s and 1960s encountered two chronic problems: defense spending was deliberately increased, and therefore NHS spending had to be restrained; deficits arose in international trading accounts, and therefore deficits had to be controlled in domestic spending. Treasury and Cabinet had to settle constant struggles among Ministries for the growth money; the hospitals and NHS were always particularly argumentative. As a stopgap Britain adopted the familiar technique of across-the-board increments in the budgets of all agencies, except those given extra by Cabinet.[1]

Such an early stage of wrangling seems inevitable in publicly financed hospital payment when both sides have powers of initiative: the hospital can define its needs and propose its budget; the government's finance officers can define their priorities and set their spending limits. Ultimately, the impasse is resolved by the triumph of top-down over bottoms-up budgeting. The normal practices of government are tightened and supersede the traditional autonomy that hospitals enjoyed before finance was governmentalized.

British experience shows that, if both financing and ownership are governmentalized, hospitals inevitably become drawn into government's methods of prospective budgeting, current expenditure control, and retrospective auditing. The financial officers try to make hospitals predictable and accountable, despite hospitals' differences from line departments. As later years show in Britain, when government experiences financial crises and must improve its procedures to combat leaks everywhere, hospitals are subjected to these methods as well.

Treasury Control over the Health Service. Britain redesigned its expenditure budgeting for the entire government during the 1960s and 1970s.[2] All publicly owned hospitals and the entire NHS were automatically included. To achieve coherence, the several expenditure budgets were combined into one. The prospective budgets were enforced more strictly during the 1970s and 1980s, and the once routine supplementary estimates became few.

Since the great problems were predictablity and control, expenditure budgeting was combined with long-range planning. This innovation was intended to cope with health care, defense, and some other sectors, which had earlier placed enormous long-range costs on government by persuading Treasury and Cabinet to adopt new programs with deceptively low initial costs.

The new system of expenditure planning is called PES, since the final drafting is done for the Public Expenditure Survey Committee, an interdepartmental committee of Cabinet. The target is a White Paper on the government's expenditure plans for the next year and several subsequent years, to be introduced into the House of Commons in January, as preparation for the annual Budget speech by the Chancellor of the Exchequer every March. (In the past the PES White Paper was submitted by the Chancellor in March, but now it has become one of the planning papers debated earlier.) A year in advance, the PES cycle begins within Treasury and within each of the spending departments, such as the Department of Health and Social Security (DHSS).[3] Paying the hospital becomes merely a special case in paying the government generally.

☐ *Treasury*. One section within Treasury monitors the development of the economy. Another section forecasts tax yields, monetary trends, and the resulting effects on prices. Another section projects the effects of public finance and private transactions on the balance of payments and on exchange rates. The civil servants meet among themselves and with the political heads of Treasury (such as the Chancellor of the Exchequer and the Chief Secretary of the Treasury) to develop a consensus about the capacity of the economy to bear next year's government expenditure, and the effects of that level of public spending upon the economy.

Corresponding to each spending department is a team of civil servants within Treasury who monitor that department's program and expenditure. For example, one group within Treasury specializes in the health and social services. These Treasury teams forecast trends in spending in their sectors.

☐ *DHSS and other spending departments*. Within each Ministry many civil servants monitor existing programs, investigate the needs of the society, and plan new programs. Many new initiatives are based on the election promises of the victorious government-of-the-day, and therefore the planning involves the Minister. Another group of civil servants in each Ministry specializes in projecting utilization and costs of current programs and in projecting costs of proposed programs. Within each Ministry a consensus develops over expected future levels for current programs and priorities for new programs.

The National Health Service consists of governing boards and officials in Regional and District Health Authorities. They develop long-term and short-term plans with new schemes, some initiated to satisfy local needs and some fitting the priorities formulated by DHSS. Many of these schemes are included in the DHSS's future expenditure plans.

Gradually, the players crystallize their proposals:

- The Prime Minister, his or her inner circle, and Cabinet endorse new initiatives for programs, such as extensive new construction of hospitals or emphasis on mental health services. They endorse certain levels of expenditure in the future. And they indicate priorities in the assignment of new growth money among the Ministries.
- Treasury develops guidelines about allowable expenditure for the entire government and for individual Ministries next year.
- The finance officers of each Ministry (such as DHSS) have been developing the Ministry's bid for next year's expenditure budget, including both the

continuation of existing operations and new schemes. They write the cost projections for subsequent years.

Personal negotiations over the limits and the bids occur all year round. Before the DHSS bid is committed to paper, the civil servants of Treasury specializing in DHSS signal the probable financial limits within which the bids should be prepared; and the finance officers of DHSS make a case for higher limits. The political leaders of Treasury and DHSS also negotiate. The process becomes more formalized when the spending Ministries submit their written bids (in April), when the PES Committee begins to meet (in May), and when Cabinet starts to discuss the forthcoming budget and new programs (in June). Cabinet must fix tax levels in late July, and that sets the general limits of public spending. Government in November announces its economic policy for the next fiscal year. From December through February, Treasury and the Ministries negotiate final levels of spending in the light of political decisions and the latest estimates about the economy, and they write the final Expenditure White Paper. Treasury converts these projections into cash totals that will actually be appropriated by Parliament (the "Supply Estimates"). The House of Commons hears the Chancellor's Budget speech in March (covering taxes, new programs, and spending), receives the Supply Estimates, debates them all, and by summer appropriates money for DHSS and the other Ministries. Meanwhile, the PES cycle has been under way for the next year.

Limits. The theory behind PES was that program growth would exist and should be planned. Some growth would result unavoidably from greater utilization of public services; other growth in expenditure would result from additional programs. To distinguish between real growth and mere price inflation, until 1982 the Expenditure White Paper was written in constant money; any changes from year to year therefore reflected true changes in program levels. The Supply Estimates are always written in the money that Parliament will appropriate; therefore, its numbers combine both higher real growth in the NHS and inflation in both wages and prices.

The research within DHSS has identified a steady aging of the population and a steadily increased use of existing services within the NHS, particularly for persons over seventy-five. Therefore, the PES chapter prepared within DHSS always asks for an increase of about 0.8 percent, just to cover the higher utilization that NHS is committed to serve. This is the sort of programmatic argument that makes the Treasury staff uncomfortable: it is supposed to accept the DHSS data as authoritative, but the claim for more money is self-interested. Finance Ministries prefer fixed annual caps. DHSS supports its case with a memorandum showing all its calculations about demographic trends and differential costs.

Besides upward pressure on expenditure from the aging of the population, medical care becomes more elaborate and more expensive, particularly in the hospitals. The doctors and managers throughout the NHS constantly press for installation of new equipment, new treatments, and the technicians for the new work.

Additional growth money for DHSS depends on the priorities of the government and the fiscal capacity of the economy. As in all global budgeting through public funds, the maintenance and expansion of hospitals are caught up in the policies of the winners of the last election. Growth is supported by a mandate, but cutbacks can be also. Hospital policy is debated in national election campaigns. Under the rate negotiation and rate regulation methods described in the last two chapters, paying the hospital is omitted from national priority setting and is more likely to drift.

Different British governments-of-the-day have different commitments to health. Labour during the mid-1970s was willing to increase the NHS each year several percentage points beyond the 0.8 percent utilization growth; but the Conservatives during the late 1970s and early 1980s limited growth more strictly, since they wished to reduce the public sector in British life. (They actually imposed negative growth in housing and some publicly owned industries; but in the 1979 election campaign, they had promised not to reduce the NHS.) Labour was willing to spend more on health even if it resulted in budgetary deficits in the Supply Estimates, but the Conservatives wished to cut such inflationary deficits by enforcing stricter cash limits on annual growth. During the 1980s the Conservative Government backed away from the original PES assumption that all programs would either remain the same or grow; in their fight against inflation, the Conservatives planned annual changes in cash limits rather than in real values, thereby forcing many programs to suffer real reductions. The nationwide popularity of NHS protected it from major cutbacks, but growth for all but special programs ceased. The growth money went into services for the elderly, the physically handicapped, and the mentally handicapped (the three were colloquially called the "Cinderella services"). Under the regional allocation methods described below, growth money also went into facilities in previously neglected parts of the country.

Reelected in 1983, the leadership of the Conservative Government intended finally to apply to the NHS its commitment to reduce the public share of all British expenditure. If hospital services were reduced within the NHS, private hospitals would grow and citizens would buy private health insurance. During the first PES cycle after the election, the Chancellor of the Exchequer proposed no real growth for the NHS. A policy struggle ensued within Whitehall and ultimately in Cabinet meetings. Events were constantly leaked to the press, and DHSS aroused its constituency. Ultimately, the Prime Minister and Cabinet agreed to provide new growth money to the NHS, at first earmarked primarily for services to the elderly. In 1986, after several years of embarrassing publicity about the underfunding of the hospitals,[4] considerable new growth money was earmarked for them.

Allocation Problems. Government funding requires constant decisions about how much to spend and where to spend it. When the Ministry of Health gets its figure, it must then divide the money among its own programs and establishments. Since 1948 the Ministry has struggled to install a distributional methodology that would correct the problems that led to the original creation of the NHS.

In completely private markets, providers go where the customers are. Doctors and hospitals cluster in the cities. Doctors and private clinics cluster in the affluent neighborhoods. If hospital finance collapses and public financing comes to its rescue—as it did in Britain in the 1940s—government inherits an extremely imbalanced arrangement: the populations of the biggest cities have many beds, and the rural areas and small towns have few and primitive facilities. Government intervention usually brings an obligation to serve the public equally everywhere.

When the NHS was created, beds and specialty care were concentrated in the southeastern part of the country, particularly around London, and in certain other areas, such as Liverpool.[5] The central and northern regions were neglected. During the first decades of the NHS, the Ministry of Health was given an annual sum not earmarked by region; the total was divided into broad nationwide categories: hospital services, general practitioner services, and so on. The Ministry then had to develop its own internal procedures for distribution. As in much of public budgeting, the method was incremental: each region received the same percentage over last year's spending; individual hospitals got similar percentages. The effect was not greater equity but the reverse: since regions and installations started from greatly unequal bases, incrementalism widened the imbalances. London and the southeast absorbed a steadily growing share of NHS operating expenditure. Some figures in 1966[6] were:

	Most favored region	Least favored region
Beds per 1,000 population	13.77	7.64
Expenditure in hospitals per capita per year	£10.20	£7.22
Expenditure of nursing salaries and wages per inpatient week as a percentage of the national mean	112%	90%
Proportion of junior medical staffs born overseas	29.8%	54%

The teaching hospitals had gotten much of the country's resources for hospital care before the NHS, and they still did. They had their own autonomous Boards of Governors and were not mixed into pools with all other hospitals, under Regional Hospital Boards. In a country that reveres social position, the well-connected governors of the teaching hospitals obtained from the national government generous budget increases and special grants. Coordinating teaching and nonteaching hospitals in an area was very difficult.[7]

During the first decades of the NHS, the assumption was that regional imbalances would be cured by new investment. When sufficient funds became available for new construction during the late 1950s and 1960s, new hospitals and health centers were built in underprovided areas. Not until later was it fully realized that equalization of services requires the redistribution of operating budgets. Britain's global budgeting, successively subdivided grants, and top-down expenditure control were ideal objects for new instruments of distribution.

When the Labour Party returned to office during the 1960s, it confronted imbalances remarkably little changed from the situation that had inspired it to create the NHS in 1946. Still determined to spend more resources in the neglected (and pro-Labour) central and northern regions, the new government introduced a policy of regional equalization in all NHS services. Several stopgap formulas were designed to redirect spending, but they were not effective.[8] Tinkering with a system based on the status quo was not successful; a completely new system of distributing and managing public funds was needed.

Reorganization of the National Health Service. A new structure was created in 1974, designed in large part to reallocate expenditures.[9] England is now divided into fourteen Regional Health Authorities (RHAs), each with authority over many special programs (for example, acute hospitals, community services, and mental institutions) that once were administered and financed separately (such as a nationwide hospital service reporting to the Ministry, or a community health services administered by the local authorities).

About 70 percent of the DHSS expenditures for health is now passed to the Regional Health Authorities. (The remainder goes to general practitioners, dentists, general administration, and a few other items.) The distribution to the Regional Health Authorities is not simply incremental but redesigns health services according to the needs of the population. I will describe the method (called RAWP) on the following page.

Under the fourteen RHAs are 192 District Health Authorities (DHAs). Within each DHA are combined the acute hospitals, special hospitals, and all community health services. The management team of the DHA develops all its facilities according to the RHA above it. The RHA writes a regional plan, coordinating all the activities within its districts. The RHA distributes its funds (granted by DHSS) among the DHAs pursuant to the plans. The distribution of funds among acute hospitals and other facilities depends on the DHA plan and varies among DHAs, since no two have identical mixes of facilities and community needs. The DHA management team is not biased to overfund the hospitals, since it must run the complete mix of services. The reorganization of 1974 intentionally made the district and not the individual hospital the basic unit of management, so that the hospitals no longer would dominate financing. The once independent and powerful teaching hospitals are merely several among the acute hospitals in their districts, subject to the same constraints—including possible closure—as the others.

DHSS issues occasional guidelines about priorities that should be implemented by the DHA planners and managers. The RHA is supposed to monitor implementation. During the late 1970s and 1980s, DHSS issued several statements about expanding underdeveloped "Cinderella services," such as institutions for the mentally ill, mentally handicapped, and elderly.[10] In "annual planning reviews," DHSS checks each region's progress in pursuing these priorities in the face of the familiar pressures by grass-roots providers to preserve the status quo. As growth money became scarcer during the late 1970s and 1980s, redirecting priorities became more difficult, since it necessitated transferring money from the acute hospitals to less glamorous programs.

Reallocation of Operating Revenue Among Regions. Under usual health financing methods, the most advanced services are established in cities, and several cluster there. Distant and scattered populations get less. Thereafter, the established services—particularly the more glamorous ones and those closest to headquarters of the payers—get more of the new money. These dynamics continue, despite scarcities in other regions and despite declines of populations in the favored places. One of the most important achievements of Britain's National Health Service has been to include in its granting method devices that judge when one district is overprovided, that estimate the needs of underprovided districts, and that redirect money accordingly.

Shortly after the reorganization of the NHS went into effect in 1974, the DHSS's Resource Allocation Working Party (RAWP) recommended a new allocation formula appropriate to the new integrated arrangement. That formula has been used every fiscal year since 1976–77. The central problem is to provide services throughout the country, so that inhabitants needing care are equally likely to find them. The RAWP formulas estimate the need for care in each region. The target is then compared with facilities already available in that region. DHSS then supplies operating funds to enable the underprovided regions to move toward their targets. Eventually all regions will stand at their targets.[11]

The RAWP decided that the principal determinants of need are:

- *Size of population.* Regions with larger populations need more services.
- *Composition of population.*
     Age. The oldest and youngest need more care than others.
     Sex. Women need more services than men.
- *Morbidity.*
- *Exogenous causes of higher costs* (for example, higher wage levels in the community, which the health services must match).
- *Patient flows.* Whether persons come to that region's hospitals from elsewhere; whether that region's inhabitants go elsewhere. (NHS hospitals have no fixed catchment areas. Any patient may go to any hospital upon referral by his G.P.)

Data can be obtained easily for all variables except morbidity. The closest available description for entire regions is the condition-specific Standardised Mortality Ratio (SMR). Certain clinical conditions unlikely to lead to death are not used. For conditions of childbirth and pregnancy, an index of fertility standardized for age replaces SMR. These measures are good enough for the purpose: to decide the total level of resources needed by a region, not the specific list and the comparative sizes of specialties in that region.

Population is not weighted the same way for all the services that a region must maintain. Weighting by SMR according to the seventeen chapters of the International Classification of Diseases (ICD) is needed for nonpsychiatric inpatient care; an overall SMR weight but not separate ICD groups is possible for day and outpatient care; SMR is irrelevant to estimating a region's need for inpatient services in hospitals for the mentally handicapped. So the total regional expenditure is broken up into seven programs, and the region's need for each is calculated by slightly differently weighted populations.

When DHSS has received its PES figures for the coming fiscal year, one of its financial branches distributes the line for "Hospitals and Personal Social Services" among the regional health authorities. Some deductions are made for DHSS administration and for the few postgraduate teaching hospitals, which are paid directly by DHSS. A certain amount—the Service Increment for Teaching (SIFT)—is reserved for the extra cost of clinical education. This amount is not included in the main distribution among regions but is added at the end of the calculations, in extra payments to regions according to their numbers of medical students. After the initial deductions and the holdback for extra teaching costs, the rest is distributed according to RAWP.

The final PES figures for DHSS are not known until just before December, when the Expenditure White Paper is printed. But the essential calculations can be done earlier. The parameters for the calculating equations are known by October and November. The financial officers have developed the custom of calculating the target distribution in operating costs from last year's PES allotments, updated in this year's prices. The growth money over last year is the object of contention between DHSS and Treasury in the new PES round, and—when it is made final in December—it is distributed among the regions to bring some closer to target. But the principal allocation work can be completed earlier.

The first step is to disaggregate the total PES figure into the categories, with different methods for weighting populations. The proportions are taken from the most recent available DHSS Summarized Financial Accounts and from the Hospital Cost Summaries. For example, the proportions of the total might be as follows: nonpsychiatric inpatient services, 54.81 percent; mental illness inpatient services, 12.67 percent; community health services 9.33 percent; and so on. Each category has a slightly different formula for distributing the national total of money across each of the fourteen regions. A region will get more money if it has more people, older people, more women, and greater morbidity. It does not get more money simply because its utilization has been high (because this may have been manipulated through overuse) or because its treatment costs have been high (because this may have been inflated for years by waste). A region gets more money because it receives cross-boundary flows (that is, patients referred from other regions).

The separate categories—nonpsychiatric inpatient, mental handicap, ambulance, and so on—are then combined for each region. The four London regions (NW, NE, SE, and SW Thames) receive extra percentages to pay for their higher wages. The results are target expenditures for each region if each received a share of the national total based on its needs—see, for example, the 1983-84 figures shown in Column 3 of Table 8-1. The previous year each region actually received the amounts in Column 2. (Columns 2 and 3 are converted into the same year's prices for comparison.) Ten regions were given less than their targets, and the four London regions received more. These discrepancies appear in Column 4. They result from the past history described earlier: regardless of population size and morbidity, London received much money, and many parts of the country were underfunded. Column 3 shows the allocations if they were determined by nothing except current population, current morbidity, and the other variables summarized in previous paragraphs.

If DHSS did no more than the RAWP calculations and distributed the money according to Column 3, the targets would be achieved at once. Within one year operating funds would be redistributed from London to the rest of the country. The result would be management chaos and political bedlam: London at once would lose 8 percent of its operating funds and would have to close services; other regions at once would get larger increases in funds without the staff and other facilities to use them. The rate of progress toward the targets results

Table 8-1. Movement Toward Targets Under RAWP, 1984-85 Fiscal Year.

Regional Health Authority	1983-84 starting figure (base for RAWP calculations) £000	Target £000	Distance from target as a percentage of the 1983-84 starting figure (i.e., as a percentage of Column 2) %	Growth in 1984-85		New total after growth in 1984-85 Columns 2 + 5 £000	Postallocation distance from target (i.e., distance between Columns 3 and 7 as a percentage of Column 7) %
				Amount of money £000	Percentage of Column 2 %		
(1)	(2)	(3)	(4)	(5)	(6)	(7)	(8)
Northern	552,958	582,344	-5.31	7,743	1.40	560,701	-3.86
Yorkshire	621,309	652,195	-4.97	8,141	1.31	629,450	-3.61
Trent	734,667	780,930	-6.30	12,122	1.65	746,789	-4.57
East Anglia	315,171	333,486	-5.81	6,053	1.92	321,224	-3.82
NW Thames	649,174	597,172	+8.01	—	0.00	649,174	+8.01
NE Thames	806,429	733,953	+8.99	—	0.00	806,429	+8.99
SE Thames	715,293	668,791	+6.50	—	0.00	715,293	+6.50
SW Thames	558,782	517,923	+7.31	—	0.00	558,782	+7.31
Wessex	445,862	476,272	-6.82	8,162	1.83	454,024	-4.90
Oxford	351,283	362,910	-3.31	6,147	1.75	357,430	-1.53
South Western	541,526	547,770	-6.14	8,830	1.63	550,356	-4.44
West Midlands	863,109	909,404	-5.36	12,184	1.41	875,293	-3.90
Mersey	454,101	464,217	-2.23	3,721	0.82	457,822	-1.40
North Western	761,218	799,817	-5.07	10,199	1.34	771,417	-3.68
Total	8,370,882	8,454,184	-1.00	83,302	1.00	8,454,184	—

Data are 1984-85 cash levels. Supplements for teaching costs (SIFT) are not included.
Source: Department of Health and Social Security.

from two decisions: the total amount of growth money available to the NHS (decided by the Treasury and Cabinet) and the distribution of all operating funds plus growth money among the regions (decided by DHSS):

Total growth money	*Distributional spread among regions*	*Approach to targets of all regions*
Large	Wide	Very rapid
Large	Narrow	Slow
Small	Wide	Rapid
Small	Narrow	Very slow

Since DHSS began to use the RAWP calculations, it has lacked growth money on the large scale originally envisioned. However, during the 1970s and early 1980s, it always had some and spent it according to the second or fourth scenarios in the foregoing list: no region should lose, and each should get at least some minimum growth money. (An example was fiscal year 1983-84, shown in Table 8-1, illustrating the fourth line in the foregoing list.) During the 1970s it was decided that every region should get growth money merely to stand still: the elderly consume far more services than others; and the Finance Division of DHSS estimates that at least 0.7 percent must be added automatically to the hospital and community health services each year to care for the greater numbers of persons older than seventy-five. The regions with more elderly persons, such as London, got more of this growth during the 1970s. In addition, even the most "overprovided" regions needed extra money to deal with underprovision within their boundaries; for example, although the inner-London areas, which are losing population, may have too many facilities and too much staff, the London regions must bear the expense of transferring services to the suburbs and of expanding those services. The Finance Division of DHSS has usually rank-ordered the regions by distance from target (according to Column 4 of Table 8-1) and has given them proportionate increases by the same rank order. But giving minimum increments to every region limits the total available to the underprovided. (In 1980-81 the most underprovided regions were increased only 0.60 percent, only double the increments in London. In 1980-81 total growth money was only £5,199,023,000 - £5,174,233,000 = £24,790,000, or 0.48 percent of the previous year's operating expenditure.)

In years with more growth money, the underprovided might receive much more from DHSS. For example, in 1981-82 the increments were: Trent, 3 percent; North Western, 2.9 percent; Northern, 2.3 percent; and so on, down to 0.6 percent and 0.5 percent for the four Thames regions. The underprovided received over four times more than the better provided.

During the 1980s the Conservative Government abandoned the practice of giving every region something. Total growth money was very low, but it would go entirely to the underprovided. In 1984-85 total growth money was 1.0 percent, and the increments were: East Anglia, 1.9 percent; Trent 1.6 percent; Northern, 1.4 percent; and so on. The four Thames regions received 0.0 percent, as shown in Column 6 of Table 8-1. To maintain their community health programs, they had to cut their hospitals and reduce numbers of employees.

Gradually each year, by one or another set of increments, the overprovided regions have been squeezed downward and the underprovided have increased. Despite the severe shortage of money during the years when the RAWP formula has been in effect, regions have become more equal, primarily by leveling upward rather than by squeezing downward. At the start, during the fiscal year 1977-78, the individual RHAs ranged from 15 percent above target to 11 percent below. By 1985-86 the best-off region was 10 percent over, and the worst off was 5.6 percent below.[12]

Reallocation Within Regions. When the new regional and area boundaries were created in 1974, a census of resources discovered that provision of beds and expenditures per capita varied more widely within than among regions.[13]

The RAWP working party suggested a procedure much like the one used to allocate expenditures among regions. The basic unit would be the district. For each district, need is defined primarily by population size, weighted for age, sex, and Standardised Mortality Ratio (SMR). Need is greater or less than this figure alone, according to cross-boundary flows of patients among districts: some get many patients from outside; some treat fewer than all of their own citizens.

However, implementing the RAWP formula within each region is difficult. Data about SMRs and fertility rates are available for larger areas but are less reliable for districts. Some specific features of the RAWP calculations might be appropriate to large-scale interregional calculations but not to stable definitions of needs in smaller districts. For example, statutory boundaries of districts are not the same as catchment areas of specific health installations. Many inhabitants of a district go to installations in other districts from time to time; the installations of a district get many patients from other districts. Most of these intraregional flows are ignored when cross-boundary flows are used to correct allocations among regions; but they are very large. Interregional RAWP averages all flow together, but intraregional flows vary in size and direction among specialties. Data are not good enough to reduce error.[14]

The RAWP formula assumes a steady progression from imbalances toward equitable distribution. But such calculations are averaged across many specific cases. A district is small, important installations make up much of its budget, and its activity and finances fluctuate. In successive years a district may have "normal" progression below target, suddenly appear to drop away (if old services are shut down), and suddenly leap toward target (as new projects open). Annual expenditure allocations cannot fluctuate so eccentrically but should move steadily, in the light of the long-term events. The RAWP working party was aware of these difficulties and cautioned that a district-level expenditure RAWP formula must be applied with understanding and flexibility.

Besides the RAWP working party's advice about allocation among districts according to distance from target, the areas and districts receive other advice about priorities. For example, they are urged to develop programs of geriatric care, mental care, home care, day care, and the like. Some of these programs might require concentrations of money. Perhaps, they are told, the money ordinarily used for small annual expansions of existing services in all the districts should instead be concentrated in a few districts to develop new programs with a supra-district appeal.

On principle DHSS controls the allocation of its money to the RHAs, allows the RHAs discretion about redistribution, and knows remarkably little about the details of internal redistribution. A wide variety of methods seem to be used by RHAs, according to the few research studies of grass-roots decision making[15] and according to my own interviews:

☐ *Incrementalism.* One might increase all established programs by the same proportion every year, on the grounds that wages and market prices (the principal components of health care costs) rise at the same rate throughout the region. But this method assumes that the districts' programs remain stable, and they do not. As one gets close to the districts and units in Britain, one is struck by the great fluctuations: old installations close or are reorganized, new ones appear, programs rise and decline in size. Actual operating expenditure, reflecting work done, fluctuates. During periods of reorganization, a district may have a few years of underspending (as old programs wind down) followed by overspending (as new ones arise). The districts save during the years of underspending and carry the money over into later years. Or RHAs transfer funds back and forth while the regional aggregate appears steady. For example, they may use operating money for small capital schemes in certain areas while underspending in another DHA whose capital starts are delayed; then, they may concentrate money in the DHA with the belated new projects while underspending on maintenance and capital in the others.

Incrementalism generally does not apply to the growth money at the grass roots. The RHA has so many projects squeezed by the cash limits of recent years that it has many places to spend the growth money, instead of spreading it around.

☐ *RAWP calculations.* Increasingly, Regional Treasurers attempt to estimate the needs of their DHAs by weighted populations, as recommended by the RAWP. Often this procedure seems to provide ammunition against the management of an overspending district, rather than a means of estimating growth money to the underprovided. The relevance of the RAWP formula to district-level decisions is much disputed: those connected with teaching hospitals claim that they are national installations and that the nearby population is not the basis of their need. Some districts are very small geographically; reliable SMRs and fertility rates are elusive. Cross-boundary flows are numerous and vary by specialty. Data about health services increasingly are computerized, and some RHAs have enough staff and computing power to generate many tabulations as background information.

☐ *Plans.* The goal is to achieve a similar service mix in each region. But the districts inevitably differ. The original service mix inherited from the past results in specialization and clustering of some sort in many districts. The shortage of growth money and incrementalism in basic expenditure perpetuate the situation. If some programs are outstanding, the RHA is expected to protect them. Therefore, a division of labor tacitly is supported.

Some neighborhood-based new programs, such as home care and day care, must be spread around. But anything of a large scale, such as a home for the mentally handicapped, must be concentrated. An important part of the new organization of the NHS is a planning system: each district performs some tasks that fit into the region's plans, and the RHA distributes some of its money in targeted ways to support the district plans.

☐ *"Planning by decibels."* When it is squeezed, the RHA has little new money and requires the DHAs to work within a cap. The RHA might try to show that it has no discretion by using RAWP calculations to give no growth money to its districts that once were generously provided but now are losing population. To maintain community health services, the DHA may announce plans to cut or even close a hospital. A great uproar always follows from the community, from the doctors, and from the Opposition political party. The RHA may provide money to keep the installation open for another year, until the controversy dies down or a compromise can be devised.

☐ *Passing the money around.* A district that has been treated generously in the past is not given so much of the growth money next year. It is someone else's turn. This practice has been common among districts and units, in order to make the system seem fair to all.

The recent scarcity of funds for British government and for new social initiatives has hung over the distribution at the grass roots. Many declining but overprovided districts—like most in inner London—have had to close facilities in order to maintain existing ones and to open new ones. The "Cinderella services" for the mentally handicapped and mentally ill have not received the growth that was anticipated. Even the "Cinderella services" for the elderly have grown slowly, because the budgets of the acute-care services could not be reduced fast enough.[16] However, the British system of financial decision making demonstrates a feature that is inherent in global budgeting and global grants but is evaded in other payment methods: cost containment requires decisions about priorities and tradeoffs, and someone must be ready to take the heat.[17]

Some Judgments About Global Budgeting and Direct Grants in Britain.

☐ *Priorities.* Financing systems based on multiple sources, extensive self-payment, or insurance do not make clear cut decisions. Social priorities result from unplanned actions by many persons. Through laws and guidelines, European governments and sickness funds recently have tried to set goals and priorities.

Every public granting system—such as Britain's—must openly and decisively fix health among competing priorities. The Treasury, Cabinet, and Parliament set the share for hospitals and for all other health services, both in the government's budget and in the distribution of the society's entire resources. It is always clear that health spending can increase only if another economic sector gets less, a fact often ignored elsewhere. The British electorate makes the final decision, by reaffirming or overturning the government-of-the-day. No other payment system can convey such a mandate for its methods and outcomes.

☐ *Cost containment.* The British system sets prospective limits and can enforce them by refusing to enact Supplementary Estimates. All other payment systems produce an unplanned upward drift, usually faster than the growth of other sectors. Therefore, Britain each year contains total health care costs more strictly than any other developed country, and the differentials steadily widen. The proportions of gross domestic product spent on health by the United

Kingdom and by the other countries of the Organisation for Economic Co-operation and Development are:[18]

Year	United Kingdom	Average of 17 other OED countries
1960	3.9%	4.2%
1965	4.2	4.8
1970	4.5	5.9
1975	5.5	7.2
1980	5.7	7.4
1982	5.9	7.7

Lower spending did not lead to worse health in Britain. Throughout this period Britain surpassed most other developed countries in statistical indicators, such as lower infant mortality. However, health spending might have dampened progress. Britain steadily improved, but other developed countries improved at a faster rate, some ultimately surpassing Britain.[19]

While cost containment has not jeopardized hospitals' clinical performance, it has severely limited their amenities. Hospital services in other developed countries since World War II have been transformed in appearance and comfort, but many British hospitals remain spartan. If a DHA faces a deficit, one of its first economies is hospital maintenance.

□ *Widespread distribution or concentration.* The RAWP formula is designed to correct the extreme regional disparities of the past. The goal was to equalize expenditures and services among regions. At times it has seemed that national policy makers favored equalizing services among smaller areas; however, no official national plan said so, the planning system gave discretion to the RHAs, and DHSS spokesmen occasionally admitted that exact equalization among small districts was unrealistic. Some skeptics believe that, once underprovision is corrected, resource allocation should be based on efficiency and not on dogmatic equalization. Regional disparities cannot be eliminated, since new population shifts always occur. Cross-boundary flows of patients among regions and districts should be encouraged—not reduced—when medical services are run efficiently. It is better to transport patients to services than to spread underused services across the landscape, the critics say. Let each DHA use its grant to pay for patient care in the most efficient places: it can send some of its own patients to other districts with more appropriate services; it can develop special programs of its own for patients living within that district or originating elsewhere.[20]

□ *Reallocating resources.* In every country one hears complaints that health services are devoted excessively to acute inpatient care, with too little going into ambulatory acute care and long-term care. More than any other developed country, Britain has the machinery to reduce the acute inpatient sector and to use the money and personnel to satisfy greater needs in the same or in other districts. The same agency finances, owns, and manages the acute and other services. That agency funds both operating expenses and capital. Since the management reforms of the mid-1980s, each district has been run by general managers committed to carrying out plans and DHSS guidelines about reallocations. RHAs and DHAs do not merely write plans but can implement them, as Chapter Nine will explain further.

☐ *Teaching hospitals.* The once privileged situation of teaching hospitals has been reversed drastically since the reorganization of 1974. They are included in district budgets, and the world-famous London institutions suffer from their regions' budget cuts under the RAWP calculations. The DHAs with teaching hospitals receive a supplement—the Service Increment for Teaching, or SIFT— but the result is still the reduction of all and the threatened closing of some. Such DHAs experience constant struggles for money between the teaching hospital and other programs; the "Cinderella services" favored by DHSS cannot begin. Some critics believe that British clinical excellence and medical education can survive only if the teaching hospitals are restored to their pre-1974 special status and are funded separately.[21] In fact, a few postgraduate teaching hospitals that perform specialized services for a national patient flow have never been included under any DHA's management and budget. DHSS responds that, in practice, other teaching hospitals really perform conventional secondary and tertiary care for nearby catchment areas.

Canada

Canada demonstrates another form of public grants of global budgets: as in Britain, the money is part of the government's annual expenditure budget; but, unlike Britain's, Canada's hospitals remain owned by private associations and municipalities. Canada also demonstrates the administrative variation possible in a decentralized country.

Overview. Every Canadian province now gives each hospital a fixed sum for the year—usually an increment over last year's approved budget, adjusted according to the current expenditure trend in the entire provincial government budget. Provinces differ in methods. Some are willing to grant exceptions from the across-the-board increment; others allow few exceptions. Some add special grants for several services, while others try to include everything in the global budget. Some, such as Saskatchewan and British Columbia, retain vestiges of line-by-line evaluation. Some are more generous than others in enforcing the limits at the end of the year.

Global budgeting is payment of a total sum, and the hospital directors have discretion about using it. Such freedom motivated the hospital industry to press for global budgeting instead of line-by-line. But the discretion has limits. Quality controls by the provincial government and accreditation bodies require minimum levels of nursing and facilities throughout the hospital. The provincial government usually specifies the maximum utilization for the hospital, such as the number of patient-days to be paid by the globe. The province usually approves the list of clinical services offered by the hospital. In some provinces, such as British Columbia, the globe is broken into parts—that is, specific amounts for acute, extended, chronic, and newborn care—and the hospital is not supposed to transfer money among them.

Special Characteristics. Each Canadian hospital gets its full operating revenue from government, but the system differs from Britain's in several respects.

- The Canadian hospital continues to be owned by nonprofit associations and local governments, not by the level of government that pays—namely, the province. Therefore, hospital managers and payers are independent adversaries. While the British hospitals are managed by employees of the National Health Service, who are not in the same civil service corps as the payers in Treasury and DHSS, they are all identified with the national government.
- The basic management and budgeting unit in Canada is the individual hospital. The provincial Ministry of Health examines its prospective budget and past operating costs. All its personnel work within the hospital. In the National Health Service of Britain, the basic unit is the District Health Authority, which runs hospitals and several other programs. At times a distinct hospital budget and expenditure report have not existed in Britain: many of the activities (the laboratory, the ambulances, and so on) are shared by several facilities in the district.
- Funds cannot easily be transferred from the Canadian hospital to other worthy local activities. A reduction in expenditure is "lost" by the hospital and is resisted. In contrast, a reduction in intramural spending in a British District Health Authority can be applied to worthy local alternatives that the hospital staff can see and (however reluctantly) accept.
- Canadian payment occurs within a federal system of government. Provinces for many years followed nearly identical procedures in scrutinizing hospital budgets and making payments, as conditions for grants from the national government under the Hospital Insurance and Diagnostic Services Act of 1958 (HIDS). However, since the reduction of national financial contributions and the easing of program conditions after 1977, provinces vary somewhat. In contrast, the British system is standardized in procedures, forms, and regulations.
- Canadian provinces have had difficulty in formulating and implementing plans for the development of facilities and for operations. Britain finally has integrated management, finance, and planning.

The Route to Top-Down Governmental Finance. Like all countries at one time, Canada until 1958 had a fragmented payment system for hospitals. The average hospital collected out-of-pocket patient charges, third-party itemized fees and daily charges, local government per diems for welfare patients, and (often but not universally) subsidies from provincial and municipal governments, often calculated by number of patient-days. Canada—along with Britain and the United States—never developed universal health insurance that could cover the hospital's entire costs by daily charges. An unlikely coalition of social reformers, deficit-ridden hospital managers, and provincial government officials in Canada pressed for full hospital financial coverage in the British style without Britain's takeover of ownership. The provincial government would pay for every hospital's entire operating costs, thereby eliminating both charges for services and deficits. Since the provinces could not afford this large burden, the national government would pay for half or more of all hospital costs, by reimbursing the provincial governments.[22]

At first Canadian hospitals submitted line-by-line prospective budgets to provincial governments. Guidelines from each Ministry of Health and from each Ministry of Finance indicated the levels of staffing and cost consistent with the province's ability to pay; regulators applied the guidelines to the hospital budgets; and the Ministry of Health then paid the approved budgets in installments. A regulatory scrutiny of budgets preceded government payment. Prolonged arguments occurred, provincial governments often compromised, and Ministries of Finance complained about mounting costs. Since half the costs were shared by Ottawa under HIDS, the resistance to the hospitals by provincial Ministries of Health was weak.

Canada's widespread economic crisis throughout the 1970s led to stronger central control by finance officers over spending departments in both the national and provincial governments. Bottoms-up budgeting everywhere was superseded by top-down grants: government-wide budgets no longer were written after the spending Ministries developed and priced their wish lists; instead, the leaders of the government wrote these budgets themselves. The national and provincial governments created committees of Cabinet (called Treasury Boards or Management Boards) to plan spending, and in some provinces the agencies acquired their own Ministries and staffs.[23]

Instead of confining the debate only to money—Treasury Board could only fix arbitrary ceilings and the spending Ministry alone understood its figures—the national and many provincial governments introduced a first stage of program planning. Each spending Ministry first explained its current and future plans to a special cabinet priorities and planning commmittee and to Treasury Board; after approval of the substance of work underlying the money, Treasury Board sent each Ministry the expenditure guidelines.

The styles of bottoms-up budgeting varied among provinces earlier: some had stronger central leadership and fiscal planning than others. Likewise, top-down budgeting is implemented variously among provinces: some Treasury Boards and Premiers have less power; these provinces lack a systematic priorities and program-planning step before writing estimates; Ministries start to formulate their estimates before learning the Treasury Board guidelines; mutual fitting is still necessary between the province-wide and Ministry budgets; and Premiers make concessions to the spending Ministries and to their interest groups. However, the trend toward disciplined vertical budgeting everywhere is clear.

During the 1970s governments tried to control spending by mastering demand-driven or otherwise uncontrollable items. Hospital spending was a target because its divided structure left Ottawa with spending obligations but no authority and made provincial governments generous. Federal-provincial cost sharing under HIDS was abandoned after 1977. Certain taxing powers and block grants were transferred from the national to the provincial governments, and now the provinces pay the hospitals in full with their own money.[24] The obligation to pay hospitals' operating costs from government revenue—assumed everywhere under HIDS during the 1950s—has not been abandoned in any province, but all provincial governments experienced mounting budgetary difficulties during the late 1970s and 1980s. Some tightened their controls over the annual increases in hospital spending.

Present Procedure in Ontario. The largest province illustrates the new methods.[25] The Cabinet of the provincial government has two principal committees with overlapping membership: Management Board and Policy and Priorities Board. The fiscal year begins on April 1, and the budget cycle begins a year earlier. From the Provincial Treasurer, Management Board learns the amount of money available for expenditure during the next fiscal year. The staff of Management Board visits every Ministry (including Health) to learn the estimated costs of conducting the same programs next year. Management Board's representatives urge each Ministry's comptroller to hold the line on wages, purchases, and construction costs. The discussion at Health revolves around wages, since Health is one of the most labor-intensive agencies. The Ministry of Health usually asks for more than Management Board has in mind; it argues that its hands are tied about wage settlements and working conditions (the Ministry of Health does not negotiate them) and that productivity in health is hard to increase.

Meanwhile, Policy and Priorities Board and its committees have been meeting regularly. They hear proposals for new actions by the Ministries, modify them, and categorize them by priority. Management Board and Policy and Priorities Board gradually develop a consensus about the new initiatives. Management Board drafts guidelines for spending by each Ministry, Cabinet approves them during the summer, and guidelines are made final during November. A Ministry like Health is usually given enough to continue current operations and may have persuaded Cabinet and its Board to support new initiatives.

Each Ministry (such as Health) plans its own budget for the next fiscal year. It induces its own program bureaus to keep within the guidelines. The payment of the province's hospitals is one program in one such bureau. By the end of the year, each Ministry has prepared its detailed budget and forwarded it to Management Board, where it is scrutinized by the desk officer specializing in the affairs of that Ministry. Some Ministries exceed their guidelines, are cut back, and occasionally appeal to Cabinet. Just before the start of the new fiscal year on April 1, the Provincial Treasurer formally introduces the new budget and revenue plans on the floor of the Legislative Assembly. The legislature debates and eventually approves the provincial budget.

Before public financing, hospital managers wrote budgets toward the end of the year, in conformity with their own definitions of need. They had been officially independent and still were. They thought that the adoption of public financing simply obligated the Ministry to find the money the hospitals needed. But problems of timing accompanied the shift in power. The hospitals were required to change to the same fiscal year as the provincial government, beginning on April 1. The hospitals should know the Ministry of Health's provincial guidelines before they write their budgets, but often the guidelines are made final only after hospital financial plans are well advanced. Hospitals regularly submit to the provincial Ministries of Health prospective budgets exceeding the Ministries' ability to pay. Even if they got the guidelines in time, the managers do not wish merely to implement higher guidelines automatically; they think that they can get more money from the government if they send upward their own version of their needs, just as in the past.

No Ministry of Health in Canada denies the right of every hospital to submit a prospective budget and to present its case. The laws say that the public grants are designed to maintain adequate services. Therefore, no province simply dictates what each hospital shall get, although recent methods come close. In order to avoid wrangling over the hospitals' claims about what they need, Canadian provincial governments now rely on formulas to dispose of most of the money. During the recent years of governmental stringency, the annual percentage increase for the hospitals usually is connected to the annual percentage increase in the Ministry of Health's budget. For example, Ontario now gives every hospital a minimum percentage increase over the last approved total. The figure is known after the final meetings between Management Board and the Ministry of Health in late January or early February. The Ministry has some additional money. It does not give the identical increase to all hospitals but gives extra to those with programs it wishes to encourage. For example, the announcement for the 1980-81 budget said that a hospital could ask for 7.5 percent more than the previous year, plus:

1 percent if it had programs of chronic, convalescent, and rehabilitation care.

1.5 percent if it had an outpatient department.

1 percent in addition for outpatient care if it was located in an area that had reduced beds to the Ministry's guideline—3.5/1,000 in southern Ontario and 4/1,000 in northern Ontario.

1 percent for small hospitals with 50 beds or fewer and with a budget of less than $2 million (the extra money helped organizations with unit costs that were higher than those in larger hospitals).

Therefore, if a hospital had a chronic program and an outpatient department, it received an increment of 7.5 + 1.0 + 1.5 = 10 percent.

In late January the Ministry sends every hospital a form letter containing the financial guidelines. All the prospective budget awards and end-of-the-year expenditure reports from recent years are computerized; therefore, the Ministry can send to each hospital not only the standard form letter but also an appendix applying the calculations to that hospital.

The hospital directors prepare a prospective budget on forms supplied by the Ministry of Health. It is a detailed line-item document, filling over twenty-five pages. It is approved at a meeting of the hospital's Board of Trustees. For many (perhaps most) Ontario hospitals, it serves as the budget for internal management as well. The forms are written by the Fiscal Resources Branch of the Ministry, which sends them out in February and gets them back with an April 1 deadline. The submission is reviewed quickly by one of the three "financial advisers" in the Fiscal Resource Branch. Each official examines about eighty forms, but this volume is possible because the review is not line-by-line and is not the Ministry's final judgment. Rather, it is a quick financial screening, to advise the Ministry's Institutional Operations Branch, which monitors each hospital.

The analyst's principal task nowadays is to judge whether the hospital has any justification for asking more money than the Ministry's ceiling. The analyst looks through the forms for the new year and the last, and he notes the excesses in personnel and in materials that lead to the projected deficit. He notes any other deviations from last year's prospective budget in spending and in expected work load. Except in unusual cases, he recommends that the Ministry pay the hospital according to the Ministry's original guideline. His handwritten report notes where the hospital might cut back.

The hospital's submission, with the financial adviser's brief handwritten report, goes to the Institutional Operations Branch of the Ministry, which officially decides. An analyst in the branch examines the hospital's budget and other documents to learn its case for more staff, supplies, or other inputs. If the financial adviser in the Fiscal Resources Branch has previously noted other defects in the budget, the analyst notes them. He asks the hospital director the reasons by phoning, writing, or visiting. His goals are to make sure that the hospital has the resources to do its job, to prevent it from wasting money, and to prevent it from incurring a deficit. The Ministry has some money for adjustments; and in a few cases Institutional Operations can award more than the guidelines projected from the base. Such hospitals thereafter can work at a slightly higher scale.

Beginning on April 1, the Ministry automatically pays biweekly installments of its award, as announced in its original guideline in the January letter. If the year's guideline is very restrictive (such as the 4.5 percent in 1979-80), over 100 of Ontario's 240 hospitals appeal. The appeals committee consists of the director of the Institutional Operations Branch, a financial analyst from Institutional Operations, three members of the hospital's area team, and a financial adviser from the Fiscal Resources Branch. If the hospital loses and a large sum is at stake—at least $500,000—it can appeal to a senior committee of the top civil servants in the Ministry of Health who deal with finance and hospitals.

From there, the hospital can appeal to the Minister of Health and to the Management Board of Cabinet. In the past the directors and governing boards had many political connections. The possibility of a sympathetic hearing by the politicians made the civil servants more generous. But now the politicians are committed to limiting the provincial budget and have lost patience with the hospitals. Therefore, the civil servants hold fast, and the hospitals assume that the initial budget will rarely be increased.

Some try to overturn the prospective budget limit by overspending, pressing the Ministry to pay the deficit, and getting a higher budget thereafter. This method was common during the first years of global budgeting. However, the civil servants have become almost as strict during the end-of-the-year settlements as during the setting of the prospective budgets, and the politicians now back them up. Therefore, overspending has become risky. But some still try.

Quebec. Hospital payment in Quebec experienced the same evolution as in Ontario and other Canadian provinces. During the 1960s the hospitals wrote optimistic line-by-line budgets and asked the Ministry of Social Affairs to cover them. Meanwhile, the Ministry had to function within the provincial government budget, and its officials reviewed hospital submissions according to guidelines about allowable spending increases. The hospitals and the Ministry constantly wrangled, the Ministry compromised with the hospitals and ran deficits, and the provincial government was regularly asked to come to the rescue.

During the 1970s provincial policy planning and budgeting were tightened. Treasury Board and the Ministry interact to get the Ministry's annual figure, but the Ministry must now clearly live within it. The Ministry now warns the hospitals that the annual increase in their budgets must not exceed the increase that the Ministry itself has been able to get from Treasury Board and Cabinet.

Quebec has had one of Canada's strictest lids on acute hospitals. One reason is fiscal capacity: Quebec is one of the less affluent and one of the more crisis-ridden provinces. Another reason has been the policy of reallocating resources from acute hospitals. Until the 1970s Quebec had one of Canada's most unbalanced health care systems: Montreal had very advanced teaching hospitals, but the rest of the province (and much of Montreal itself) had few ambulatory and community services. The successive reformist governments since 1970 have tried to build up community services (such as health centers) through the Ministry of Social Affairs, but the Ministry needs to find the money from its other accounts, such as the grants to the nonprofit acute hospitals. Global budgeting through government therefore put the hospitals into competition with a government-managed program of high priority. Quebec led the Canadian provinces in the ultimately successful move to replace the federal-provincial grants earmarked for hospitals under HIDS and substitute a greater share in the national government's power to levy taxes.[26] Ottawa's grants no longer have been earmarked for the hospitals; Quebec and all other provinces have been able to spend more of the money for health centers and community services.

At the start of the year, the Ministry of Social Affairs mails to each hospital a form for a prospective operating budget in a style that the Ministry can scrutinize easily from its own perspective.[27] The Ministry sends a manual containing the guidelines about cost increases allowed by the forthcoming provincial government budget. In the upper half of the first page of the budget form, the hospital enters all its routine operating costs (*composante globale*), totaling about 85 percent of all hospital costs; that part of the budget is supposed to cover routine hospital work, which is supposed to be conducted next year in the same way and is more expensive only because of wage and price increases.

Several special programs are funded by the Ministry, by means of formulas separate from the flat increases of global budgeting; these programs are itemized in the next section of the document (the *composante détaillée*). Examples are community health programs, ambulatory health centers connected with the hospital, teaching students in nursing and in other fields, and postgraduate training. A hospital's new programs are always itemized and scrutinized carefully by the Ministry's analysts the first years and then folded into the globe during a later year when it seems to have matured and stabilized. Some years, when the Ministry suspects that its money is being used wastefully, it may ask for a separate accounting, as in the case of administrative wages in 1980.

The prospective budget document is brief and compact, since the bulk is not itemized but is in the *composante globale*. In an end-of-the-year report to the Ministry, the hospital must explain in detail how it used the money. The prospective budget includes one column—in both the *composante globale* and the itemized *composante détaillée*—for the current year's expenditures. The next column lists the hospital's requests, which can exceed the percentage increases in the Ministry's guidelines. If so, the hospital argues its case for extra money in an appendix. (Ontario does not distinguish between a short global section and a selective detailed section in its prospective budget form. Its entire document is more detailed and longer than Quebec's.)

When the Quebec hospital mails the prospective budget to the Ministry of Social Affairs, the document is automatically assigned to the financial liaison officer for that hospital, employed in the hospital service of the Ministry. Each officer has about eight hospitals and handles all financial and organizational relations between them and the Ministry. Since the prospective budgets are not line-by-line, the liaison officer can analyze them quickly. If the hospital's request in the *composante globale* exceeds the percentage allowed by the Ministry, it is asking to do the same work more elaborately and more expensively, when the method assumes that the only increases are for the wages and prices of the same inputs.

Unless the hospital can justify the increase in a detailed appendix, the liaison officer cuts it back. To learn the reasons for a proposed large increase, the liaison officer makes phone calls and perhaps visits. He agrees if the hospital can prove that an unusual increase in patient-days is imminent and is not manufactured by the hospital. Final decisions are made in consultation with the supervisors of the hospital service in the Ministry.

Usually, the liaison officer's principal work refers to the most judgmental part of the budget: any new programs or substantial expansion of existing programs, explained in appendices to the hospital's submission. These should be small-scale line-item budgets. The hospital can send them in the start-of-the-year submission or separately at any later time.

The liaison officer refers the proposal to the consulting service in the Ministry's health division, which evaluates any substantial new programs, such as new clinical services or diagnostic laboratories. The engineers, physicians, and other specialists in the service can evaluate the proposed staffing, equipment, and management of the new or expanded program. If the proposal calls for purchase of substantial new equipment, a report is also prepared by the regional health council in the hospital's area. The council comments on the need for the proposed service. The liaison officer drafts recommendations about the funding of the hospital's proposal, and these recommendations are approved or revised by higher officials in the hospital's service.

The liaison officer drafts the approved budget, consisting of the Ministry's figures in its columns in the prospective budget form originally submitted by the hospital. He also drafts the letter to be sent to the hospital by the Assistant Deputy Minister in charge of the health division. The liaison officer writes and the higher officials of the Ministry sign the order stating the hospital's budget for the coming year and instructing the Ministry's comptroller to send twenty-six biweekly installments.

Often the liaison officer meets with the governing board of the hospital, explains the cuts made by the Ministry, and discusses the hospital's spending plans during the next year, so that it can work within the grant. A large hospital merits a visit by several financial specialists from the health division of the Ministry of Social Affairs. If the hospital is very large, indignant, and prone to overspend, it is visited by the Assistant Deputy Minister.

The hospital can submit a revision of the prospective budget during the year if any events change the costs substantially. It must provide a full justification. If a new labor contract has affected all hospitals, the Ministry may issue new budgets for all of them.

Problems with Global Budgeting in Canada. Owners and managers of private hospitals welcomed full public financing with utopian expectations: they would get maximum discretion and as much money as ever. They have gotten neither. They eventually became parts of the government's system of top-down budgeting at a time of recession and austerity. Governments in Quebec and several other provinces finally acted on their conviction that too much money was going into acute care and not enough into chronic and ambulatory. Since the money was the taxpayers', government insisted on knowing and influencing how it was spent.

The individual hospital must bear more frequent and closer scrutiny in Canada than in Great Britain. The reason is greater distrust. In Canada government money is being given to private organizations with reputations for profligacy. In Britain the hospitals are owned by government itself, and its managers are pledged to public ethics and public policy.

At first during the 1960s and 1970s, the Canadian Ministries of Health allowed the hospitals to increase their prospective budgets each year by at least 10 percent. Many hospitals exceeded these limits and argued during the end-of-the-year settlements (as they had during line-by-line budgeting) that additional work had been unavoidable. Eventually, the Treasury Boards insisted on the predictability and discipline of global budgeting. The Ministries of Health then wrote not merely an exceptions procedure for covering deficits each year but also a system for evaluating hospitals' performance and systematically revising their budgets.

The greater the amount of money, the happier hospital directors are with global budgeting or with any other system of payment. As economic growth and provincial tax revenues leveled off during the late 1970s, the Ministries of Health were given only limited increases in their appropriations. Most provincial governments were bound to give the hospitals enough to cover all wage increases, but they did not give enough for both wage increases and larger numbers of employees. For all other nonwage hospital costs as well, the Ministries often granted much less than the hospitals' predictions in their global budgets. For example, during the 1977–78 fiscal year in Quebec, the hospitals asked 3.2 percent and got 0.7 percent for nonwage costs; during 1980–81 the hospitals asked 10.9 percent and got 5 percent. As a result, hospitals throughout Canada complain that they are "underfunded" and that their services have declined in quality.[28] Numbers of hospital workers were once comparable to the staffing in the United States but have increased more slowly during the 1970s and 1980s.[29]

While hospitals in most provinces now are relieved of the wrangling over specific guidelines and budget items at the start of the year, they have found that a form of line-by-line review reenters retrospectively. Government inevitably requires an end-of-the-year accounting from the hospitals, since it must account for its own expenditures to government auditors, to the legislature, and to the taxpayers. The end-of-the-year report in Quebec has over fifty pages and may be the most voluminous in Canada. To detect trouble early, many Ministries of Health also require quarterly expenditure reports.

If the hospital managers did not gain what they hoped for, neither did the planners in government. All had hoped to reallocate the Ministry of Health budgets, with less money for the hospitals and more for community services. This policy was pursued most diligently in Quebec, leading to the strongest government intervention of any Canadian province. But laymen's policies to redirect resources depend on the cooperation of the medical profession, the community elites who sponsor the hospitals, and their admirers in the general populations. Resistance by these groups has protected Quebec hospitals from excessive reductions. Shifting resources to the community health centers has been limited by the reluctance of many general practitioners—all private entrepreneurs working on fee-for-service—to join them.[30]

Incentive Reimbursement

The Holy Grail of hospital finance is a method of payment that will inspire hospitals to save money. If hospitals would save, payers would spend less money; inflation would be restrained, and society would no longer suffer the mounting transfers into unproductive medical services; hospitals would become invigorated; payers and government would forever be free of wrangling with hospital managers; politicians would be hailed for their wisdom instead of blamed for depriving hospitals and doctors of life-saving resources.

Public grants of total hospital budgets have become the principal method of using money to reward efficient hospitals and to penalize inefficient ones. Incentive reimbursement has been elusive under other systems of payment for several reasons: the per diem unit is crude; multiple payers cannot agree on incentive designs; and nonprofit sickness funds oppose letting hospitals keep profits, particularly if the gains might have been earned through underservicing.

But the Holy Grail may be a mirage under grants systems, too. Quebec and Ontario have included incentive reimbursement formulas in their global grants. Some of these methods have proved ineffective; others add complexities to a payment system that is supposed to be simple; and eventually other policy goals take precedence.

Managerial and Regulatory Pressures on Hospital Managers. If hospitals have been taken over by government, as in Great Britain, improving efficiency is a problem of public administration; efficiency is promoted by direction, not merely by payment, and civil servants are held accountable for the performance of their organizations. But most countries do not have centrally owned and controlled hospitals. Therefore, the task is how to force or inspire a decentralized sector of privately and municipally owned establishments to improve their efficiency. Most developed countries rely on detailed guidelines and rate regulators to ensure that operating costs are appropriate. Guidelines are limits set by public policy: if a hospital's nurses exceed the ratio to its beds set in the guidelines, the excess is presumed unnecessary, and the hospital's prospective budget is cut back; if the number of tests exceeds a particular margin over the peer group average, the hospital may not be paid for the excess. The rate regulator is supposed to investigate the hospital's past cost reports, meet with the managers and chiefs of service, and disallow excessive new requests. Unjustified cost overruns are not supposed to be reimbursed by retroactive increases in the per diems.

Imposing efficiency by guidelines and regulations has been difficult, as I said in the last chapter. Each hospital argues that it has special needs not apprehended by crude guidelines. Regulators must wrangle at length and are easily intimidated by managers and chiefs of service who are experts in the internal affairs of their complicated organizations. Policy makers give hospitals the benefit of doubts, lest they themselves be blamed by the public for deaths and inconveniences.

European sickness funds have usually opposed incentive reimbursement schemes, because they believe that payment should cover costs and no more. Experiments have been rare. When German hospitals were allowed to risk earning profits and suffering losses (under the reforms of 1984 and 1985), the deviations from cost reimbursement were limited and temporary. The daily charges agreed at the start of the year are expected to cover costs. If profits or losses result during the year, the negotiated rate is kept until the next year's bargaining, when either the hospital or the sickness funds may demand a revision to restore the balance. The profits or losses run only during the current year and are limited by the formulas under the "flexible budgeting" regulations: if substantial losses to the hospital and savings to the sickness funds accumulate because of large decreases in expected patient-days, the hospital may still bill the sickness funds for 75 percent of those lost per diems, representing its unavoidable fixed costs; if substantial profits to the hospital and cost overruns to the sickness funds accumulate because of large increases in expected patient-days, the sickness funds may pay the hospital no more than 25 percent of those extra per diems, representing the variable costs for the additional work.

Experiences in Quebec. Several Canadian provinces have attempted to design their annual grants to reward efficiency while not inadvertently encouraging underservicing. During the 1950s and 1960s throughout the country, hospitals often overspent their budgets, explained them at the end of the year, and received supplements from their Ministries of Health. Not only did they cover their cost overruns during the current year, but they received higher budgetary bases for the next year. During the early 1970s, Quebec and Ontario tried to break this cycle by motivating hospitals to save money. But at that time it was assumed that hospital directors and doctors were frugal and that deficits were due to unavoidable medical need. It was unthinkable to punish hospitals. Therefore, the first settlement method in Quebec under global budgeting had rewards for saving money but no sanctions for spending too much. If the hospital ran a deficit, it submitted a detailed explanation of why its volume and/or service intensity exceeded the original predictions, it argued with the Ministry of Health, and it eventually received an additional payment.

Incentive payments varied according to two types of savings: smaller ones that might not recur and large ones that resulted from a structural change and permanently lower costs in the hospital.

- For all savings, whether large or small, the hospital retained 10 percent of what it did not spend and returned the rest to the Ministry.

- The distinction between large and small savings was set by a formula applying to all hospitals in the peer group (the "cost-reduction objective")—for example, 7 percent of the hospital's global budget. If last year's savings were smaller, the hospital's prospective budget was not reduced next year. But, under the aforementioned general rule, the hospital sent 90 percent back to the Ministry.
- Large savings beyond the "cost-reduction objective" were considered evidence of permanent overestimate. As an immediate reward for having made and reported the saving, the hospital could keep 50 percent of the excess over the "cost-reduction objective," returned the rest, and suffered a permanent reduction in the global budget in the future.

The Ministry was surprised to discover that these incentives were ineffective, but the experience produced now common insights into the economic behavior of hospitals. Directors and doctors had no incentive to save money if the system allowed them to spend and expand: hospitals' deficits were paid by the Ministry during 1973, 1974, and 1975 on the grounds that the hospitals must have time to adjust to global budgeting and that nonprofit charitable organizations must not be threatened with bankruptcy. Rewarding hospitals for saving money one time is ineffective if the saving results in a permanent reduction of the budget base. Incentive reimbursement schemes deal with both short-term savings and long-term reductions in the budget base; long-term reductions are more important to hospital managers, and a successful method must include a just procedure for such cuts.

Quebec then designed a more sophisticated scheme that could distinguish between types of surplus and types of deficit—a scheme that could actually motivate desired rather than undesired behavior. Criteria were needed to identify the overruns legitimately payable by government. Similar hospitals should have similar budgets; those with bloated budgets should not be rewarded with larger increases than the efficient organizations received.

One problem was to distinguish between efficient and inefficient hospitals, between those with excessive and those with insufficient prospective budgets. A hospital's economic performance cannot be judged merely by whether it runs a surplus or a deficit. That outcome must be compared with its level of costs. A high level of spending may be associated either with waste or with a high level of work; low spending may be associated either with efficiency or with low clinical activity. An incentive reimbursement system must be administered by someone who examines both the hospital's level of costs and the balance sheet at the end of each year, someone who can make appropriate interpretations. The judgments about the performance of each hospital follow from comparing (1) the surplus or deficit at the end of the year and (2) the level of spending vis-à-vis similar hospitals:

Hospital's end-of-the-year expenditure report	Hospital's spending compared to its class average	Judgments about the hospital
Deficit	Lower	Underbudgeted
Surplus	Lower	Overbudgeted

Deficit	Higher	Either (1) Underbudgeted for high volume of work or (2) Wasteful, regardless of budget level
Surplus	Higher	Overbudgeted, wasteful

Table 8-2 shows five hypothetical hospitals with different combinations of budget outcomes (surplus or deficit on line 3) and cost levels (higher or lower than class averages on line 4). On the lowest line of the table are the policy judgments for each hospital. The line "New Budgetary Base" shows the policy action during the next year by the Ministry of Social Affairs: hospitals A and D seemed underbudgeted this year, and their next prospective budgets are increased; hospitals B, C, and E seemed overbudgeted this year, and their next prospective budgets are reduced.

The size of the increases in prospective budget depends on the hospital's performance. Hospital A gets an increase to cover its spending in full, since its level of costs was below the class average. Hospital D does not get an increase to cover the spending in full, since its costs exceeded its class average; its budget will be higher next year, but less than this year's spending.

Likewise, the sizes of the cuts in the budgets vary. Hospital E is cut more because it spent more than similar hospitals and ended the year with a surplus anyway. Hospital B ran a surplus, saved money, and therefore can operate next year with a substantially lower prospective budget, equal to this year's spending. Hospital C ran a deficit and spent more than the class average. The deficit was one element in the overspending. If the next prospective budget is cut back to eliminate the amount in this year's deficit, the hospital will still spend more than the class average, but waste will be discouraged. Hospitals C and D can be contrasted on lines 3 and 4 of Table 8-2. Hospital D runs a larger deficit but is closer to the class average in spending; Hospital C runs a smaller deficit but is much higher than the class average in spending. Hospital D is more efficient and seems in part underbudgeted; so it could use the money transferred from Hospital C.

The method is designed not merely to decide whether the hospital should get more money this year or should return overpayments. Above all, it makes permanent corrections in the annual budget, in accordance with the hospital's needs and performance. This is Quebec's great innovation. Therefore, the method is entitled "correction of the budget base."

Other countries have faced the same problem of reversing the effects of automatic across-the-board increases that unintentionally give the spendthrifts more new money than the efficient organizations. At first, one is baffled about how to reward the deserving and how to reduce overblown budgets with persuasive evidence that they are too big. Quebec's is a formula system that tries to handle these difficulties.

Following are highlights of how the concepts are operationalized and how the method is applied.[31] Details are perfected from time to time, but generally the Quebec government tries to keep the methodology stable, so that hospital managers can understand it and adjust to its incentives.

**Table 8-2. Types of Hospitals, According to Economic
Performance and Budgetary Situation.**

	Hospitals That Save Resources		Hospitals That Exceed Resources		
	A	B	C	D	E
Expenditures	10.0	20.0	30.0	40.0	50.0
Authorized budget	9.0	21.5	29.0	38.0	51.0
Surplus (+) or Deficit (–)	– 1.0	+ 1.5	– 1.0	– 2.0	+ 1.0
Higher (+) or Lower (–) than average hospital in same class	– 0.8	– 1.0	+ 2.0	+ 1.0	+ 2.0
Maximum budgetary increase (+) or reduction (–)	+ 1.0	– 1.5	– 1.0	+ 1.0	– 3.0
New budgetary base (i.e., policy action)	10.0	20.0	28.0	39.0	48.0
Policy judgment	underbudgeted	overbudgeted	wasteful regardless of budget level	underbudgeted for high volume of work	overbudgeted, wasteful

Note: Numbers in each column are millions of dollars.
Source: Gilles DesRochers, "Le financement des établissements de santé et de services sociaux," *Canadian Public Administration*, Vol. 22, No. 3 (Autumn 1979), p. 376.

☐ *Peer group classifications.* A recurrent problem in hospital financing is identifying standards for judging whether a hospital is more or less efficient, thrifty or wasteful, high or low in costs. Quebec uses the nearly universal method of comparing that hospital with others. Under line-by-line review, items in the budget were compared with statistical guidelines, but these ultimately had been derived from class averages. Under global budget review, the problem is comparison of the expenditure for the entire hospital or for part of it with others' total expenditures.

As in other federal countries, Quebec hospitals are compared with one another and not with hospitals from other provinces. All Quebec hospitals' patient discharge forms and end-of-the-year hospital expenditure reports are computerized. Quebec has been able to take full advantage of North America's large-capacity computers and advanced software. Hospitals are assigned to peer groups with similar case mix, derived form clustering programs. Cases are weighted by the complexity of care, so that peer groups are more homogeneous in service intensity.

□ *Evaluation.* Some hospitals are more expensive than peer group averages, and others are less expensive. If hospitals are more expensive, one must distinguish between those that are and are not doing more clinically necessary work than the peer group average. If hospitals are less expensive, one must distinguish between those that are and are not doing the same amount of work as the peer group average, since the former are more efficient than the latter.

Judgments are made not about the hospital's entire globe but about performance by the principal responsibility centers: nursing, operating theater, ambulatory services, laboratory, pharmacy, radiology, general administration, kitchen, housekeeping, operations of physical plant, maintenance, and several others. Wage and nonwage expenditures are identified for each responsibility center; and the individual hospital is compared with the peer group averages, both in spending and in measures of efficiency appropriate to that center. Such measures include hours per admission (when evaluating the wage costs in nursing), spending on supplies per patient-day, and many others.

For each responsibility center, the spending of the individual hospital is compared with the average spending for its peer group. The resulting number should be positive when the hospital spends too much and negative when it spends less; it should be large when it is far from the class average and small when it is close. The basic formula is always:

$$(\text{item of cost}) \times \left(1 - \frac{\text{class ratio}}{\text{hospital's ratio}}\right) = \begin{array}{l} + (\text{an excess}) \\ \text{or} - (\text{a saving}) \end{array}$$

The hospital's total performance is the sum of the results of all the equations. The several pluses and minuses in individual centers of responsibility accumulate or balance each other. The final figure may be an overexpenditure (the total has a plus sign), a saving (the total has a minus sign), or a break-even (close to zero). These figures are not the same as deficits, profits, or break-evens in the year's expenditures. Hospitals may not be budgeted according to their efficiency.

□ *Revising the next prospective budget.* The principal goal is to correct the cases of underbudgeting and overbudgeting shown in Table 8-2. Cases of deficit are distinguished easily at present by comparisons with peer groups: if a hospital did average or above-average work with a lower-than-average budget, it gets an increase in the budget base for the next fiscal year; if it did average or lower-than-average work with an average or above-average budget, it gets no increase.

Cases of surplus require subtler distinctions and decision rules. The calculations, how they are applied to individual hospitals' expenditure reports, and how the Ministry then reacts to revise the budget base (or to leave it alone) and to reclaim last year's surplus (or to leave it with the hospital in whole or in part)—all these are too involved for the overview in this book. Some hospitals experience great reductions in the budget, others, only partial cuts—depending on the sizes of the declines in their work and/or their degrees of inefficiency in their use of resources.

Similar reasoning decides the size of a budget increase for a deficit-ridden hospital that does not deserve an increase for the full amount.

□ *Payments.* Besides revising the prospective budget for next year, the Ministry must deal with surpluses and deficits registered during the last year. This is a policy problem distinct from upward and downward revision of prospective budgets in the light of past surpluses and deficits—the issues described in previous paragraphs. Between 1974 and 1979, whatever surpluses had been produced by any hospital were frozen—that is, they could not be used by the hospital, but they did not go back to the Ministry.

Treasury Board's regulation of 1980 first allocated surpluses to repay deficits incurred by each hospital during the period. This money therefore went back to the provincial government, which had already covered the deficits. This is a common fate for supluses in the payment of hospitals in every country. Each hospital's surpluses are used only for it and are not shared, unless the rule is automatic reversion of any surplus to the Treasury.

The allocation rules described on the last pages were first applied to the surpluses on deposit. The hospital obtained part according to the calculations, and the government got the rest. Allowing a private organization such as a hospital to use public money at its discretion was a novelty for Treasury Board; usually government finance officers reclaim all unspent money, making incentive reimbursement schemes impossible. Quebec's Treasury Board and the Ministry of Social Affairs set conditions for the use of the hospital's share: the project must be approved by the Ministry; the project should improve the financial performance of the hospital; it should be used for a nonrecurring expense; and it should not engender additional operating costs.

The outcomes in Quebec have demonstrated the recurrent difficulties in implementing all incentive reimbursement schemes. They presume a flexible economy. While some hospitals gain from the last year's work, others may lose; some may grow during the next year, whereas others may contract. A full test of Quebec's incentive reimbursement methods was never possible because—soon after it was perfected—the entire hospital sector of the province suffered cuts. Since all money under global granting came from the provincial government's budget, hospitals had the same reductions as all other sectors during the 1980s. All hospitals were preoccupied with operating in the face of across-the-board cuts in all grants—averaging, for example, 7 percent in 1981-82. Therefore, differential responses to the incentive reimbursement rules were masked. The system was oriented primarily to the consequences of surpluses, and managers' typical efforts now were directed to warding off deficits.

Ontario. During the early 1970s, provincial policy makers were impressed by the discussions of incentive reimbursement that appeared in publications from the United States and Quebec. Many hospitals in Toronto and elsewhere were thought to need better financial discipline. The Ministry of Health at first thought that remedies could be achieved without controls.

From 1970 to 1973, hospitals were expected to keep part of their surpluses and suffer their deficits, in ways that would encourage efficiency and discourage inefficiency. The scheme had two rewards for savings:

- "Continuous." If the hospital expected savings to be permanent, it could retain 90 percent of the difference between that year's prospective budget and expenditure report. Next year's prospective budget then was reduced to the expenditure level; or the reduction might be gradual, less than 90 percent each year but in the long run more profitable.
- "One-time." If the hospital expected savings to occur only once, it kept 10 percent of the difference between that year's prospective budget and expenditure report. The rest went back to the provincial government. Next year's prospective budget remained the same.

Both of these methods failed. When hospitals reported surpluses, very few reported them as "long term" and claimed 90 percent. The immediate gain in money was small, and the loss in budget was large. The Hospital Commission and the Ministry might have sweetened this option by guaranteeing quick increases in the reduced budget to cover rises in utilization and prices. This might have alleviated hospital directors' anxieties over a reduced scale, but the officials assumed until too late that the 90 percent in money was incentive enough.

The 10 percent retention also was not an effective motive. The money was too little, and the government did not give the hospital enough discretion in using these sums. Instead of saving money, hospitals preferred to grow. The "one-time" reward proved safest of all for the hospital, since Management Board during the early 1970s held the annual increase in global budgets several times to 7 percent or less. Any surpluses were indeed destined to be "one-time."

Eventually, Management Board scrapped the incentive award system. It was ineffective. Finance officers never like private organizations to "profit" from the taxpayer's money. The national government refused to share these amounts under HIDS, and therefore the provinces had to pay them in full.

The negative incentive in the scheme was the Ministry's refusal to pay the deficits (although it relented on some). Apparently, this strategy did restrain the increase in costs somewhat: if a hospital ran a deficit one year, it was more careful the next. Ontario hospitals had some reserves saved from the more spendthrift 1960s or available from private donors. Also, their staffing had some "fat" in numbers; some jobs could be left unfilled.

Other Ministry decisions weakened the scheme. For example, the Ministry shifted among several bases for calculating next year's prospective budget. If the Ministry projected it from this year's final expenditure report, a hospital profited from a deficit: it paid the shortfall the first year, but thereafter its budgetary base was higher.

Since 1975 Ontario has practiced a disciplined style of finance, treating the hospitals almost like government agencies. Surpluses revert to the Treasury. Hospitals get regular installments of the Net Ministry Liability (NML) fixed at the start of the year; they are expected to work within the prospective budget written to fit the NML; deficits usually do not arise, since the Ministry is not obligated to pay more than the NML, although it might pay more after thorough justification. Incentive reimbursement methods are no longer attempted. The hospitals resist them, since they foreshadow reduction of the budgetary bases. Unlike Quebec, neither Ontario nor any other Canadian province has tried to salvage and fine-tune incentive reimbursement. They have been preoccupied with fixing caps on public spending.

Emulation of Global Budgeting Under Insurance

Countries with national health insurance searched for new methods of payment during the late 1970s and 1980s. Negotiation and regulation were too conflict-ridden and too complicated. They could not be responsive to public policy simply and directly. They were associated with per diem and item-of-service payment units, and costs were exceeded, both because of higher utilization and end-of-the-year settlements. Some payers were strained.

Many governments were impressed by the stable cost control and simple procedures of Britain and Canada, and they investigated global budgeting and global grants in lessons-from-abroad research. When the health insurance system went bankrupt, Italy governmentalized the payment of hospitals in a form resembling Canada's.

The "budgeting" element of "global budgeting" was already in place under European HNI. Hospitals filled out line-item prospective budgets and submitted them to regulators, as Canadian hospitals did during the bottoms-up period of the 1960s and early 1970s. To emulate Canada and Britain, a country would have to make the following changes:

- Strict screening of the prospective budget, or the substitution of top-down grants dictated by the payer. Screening was steadily becoming more critical in European rate regulation. Top-down grants were not likely to be proposed or adopted early under NHI. Under Britain's NHS and Canadian grants, the initiative came from the hospital for over a decade, and top-down granting did not evolve until government experienced financial strain many years later.
- Hospitals could no longer run deficits and be reimbursed easily. Such settlements were diminishing under European NHI.
- Pooling of all payments into a single sum equal to the prospective budget. If several sickness funds still existed, a formula should divide the total among them.
- A single office should manage transactions with the hospital.

France. France was the first country to introduce techniques of global budgeting (*budget global*) and global grants (*dotation globale*) into a health insurance system based previously on rate regulation, guidelines to fix limits, the per diem unit of payment, and multiple payers. The innovations were intended to overcome all the defects described in Chapter Seven.

Global budgeting was one of the experiments preceding the nationwide reform in 1983.[32] In the experiment in several hospitals, preparing and screening a prospective budget followed past methods. Line-item budgets were submitted to the prefecture by the experimental hospitals. The DDASS decided whether the proposed items fell within the national government's guidelines, exactly as in all other hospitals. The only thing missing was calculation of a *prix de journée*. Important parts of the submission were the hospital's expenditure reports from the last complete year and the interim expenditure report for the year in progress.

The examiners in the DDASS needed to compare the new submissions with past spending patterns and to calculate the increments allowed by the guidelines.

The important utilization statistic was admissions and not patient-days, since the experiment avoided incentives for more patient-days. The proportion of admissions from each carrier during the last full year was calculated. The total budget approved by the prefecture was then distributed among the carriers, according to this distribution of admissions. For example, in one experimental hospital, the prefecture approved a total budget for 1980 of 147,719,223.18. F. In 1978 the distribution of that hospital's patients among third-party programs was:

CRAM, general regime	87.05%
Regime for self-employed	3.13
Regime for farmers	2.65
Government's program for war veterans	0.06
Others, such as social welfare and self-payers	7.11
Total	100.00%

Therefore, for 1980 the carriers were billed their shares of the total budget:

	Proportion	*Liability in francs*
CRAM for Paris region	87.05%	128,589,383.78
Caisse for self-employed	3.13	4,623,611.69
Caisse for farmers	2.65	3,914,559.41
National government's Ministry for war veterans	0.06	88,631.53
Self-payers, social welfare programs, and other programs were billed according to *prix de journée*	7.11	10,502,836.77
Total	100.00%	147,719,223.18

Every month, the carrier sent the hospital one-twelfth of its predicted share for the year. At the end of the year, the hospital reported its expenditures (the *compte administratif*) to the DDASS. If costs were higher than predicted, the hospital hoped to bill the sickness funds for the extra. For the first time in France, the DDASS was called upon to investigate thoroughly and critically an end-of-the-year expenditure report. The DDASS could disallow the extra claims, and the hospital could collect no more than the twelve monthly installments it had already received.

As in all payment systems, a central question was whether the payers forced the hospital to keep within the original estimate. Often experiments are sugar-coated with extra money to persuade the hospitals to cooperate. (For this reason, America's innumerable reimbursement demonstrations are always inconclusive.) But the French government regulated all hospitals; all on daily charges were being denied end-of-the-year supplements, and therefore the organizations in the global budgeting experiments had to absorb any deficits. The hospital could not find additional money by admitting more patients, prolonging stays, or generating additional services in the outpatient department.

Therefore, hospitals prepared their prospective budgets more carefully and more slowly than before.

New methods of organizing, paying, and monitoring hospitals were installed for the entire country during 1985.[33] They apply to both the public hospitals and the nonprofit hospitals assimilated into the public service. The various new methods were phased in at different times:

☐ *Structure.* Public hospitals were reorganized internally in departments.

☐ *Work plan.* Statements of the clinical work planned for the next year are made by the centers of responsibility, the departments, and the entire hospital. They are the basis for the prospective budget. These statements about goals and resources are submitted on standard forms. Therefore, the annual requests for money no longer stand alone but depend on approval of the hospital's clinical objectives and must be justified as fulfilling these goals efficiently.

☐ *Budgets.* Prospective budgets are written by each hospital. Each total budget combines individual budgets for the centers of responsibility within the hospital—the clinical departments and other units. Retrospective cost reports are kept according to the same format. Decrees of the national government specify the nomenclature and the forms.

☐ *Guidelines.* The Ministries concerned with national economic policy, governmental budgeting, hospitals, and social security continue to write and issue guidelines. These memos no longer include the details for screening line-item budgets. Rather, they focus on the annual increase that should be allowed for hospital budgets throughout the country. The increase derives from national economic policy concerning the fiscal capacity of the sickness funds, the government's capacity to subsidize the sickness funds from general revenue, and the desirable trends in the size of the acute hospital sector.

☐ *Regulatory scrutiny.* The guidelines still go to the DDASS, which still monitors the public hospitals. Since the regulatory oversight is less detailed, hospital managers have more discretion. But controls are applied in matters that Paris deems important: for example, the guidelines for 1985 instructed the DDASS to approve no new posts in hospitals.

☐ *Caps.* Every DDASS is given a limit on all hospital expenditures in its jurisdiction (an *enveloppe départementale*). For example, in 1985 all personnel expenditures during 1984 plus 5.2 percent. Some hospitals' prospective budgets could rise more and some less, but they should average to the limit. In addition, each DDASS is allowed an extra *marge de manoeuvre* (0.5 percent of 1984 expenditures) to help hospitals in deficit, or to help those with exceptionally low budgets, or to fulfill other policy goals in the guidelines from Paris. The allowable annual increase in personnel expenditures follows the annual awards in the wages of French civil servants.

☐ *Daily charge.* The DDASS must still calculate a daily charge, partly for some administrative reasons and partly for billing of anyone who does not belong to a French sickness fund, such as a foreigner.

☐ *Decree.* The commissioner still issues an *arrêté*, officially announcing the hospital's award. It tells the total allowable revenue for the next year, the shares of the official sickness funds, and the daily charges.

□ *Distribution among third parties.* A sole-source payer—such as a Canadian Ministry of Health—would pay the total in installments. But France still has several sickness funds, with unequal market shares. The shares vary among different hospitals. Distribution formulas are prescribed, as part of the regulations issued by the Ministries in Paris. The sickness funds share payment of the new global grant in ratio to their shares in the total number of patient-days in that hospital last year. In the future, calculations based on diagnosis-related groups (or similar methods) might be used to weight each payer's share by the complexity and costliness of its patient load. The specific rules for sharing are updated for announcement every year by June 1 by a *Commission Nationale de Répartition des Charges des Dotations Globales Hospitalières*, chaired by a judge of the *Cour des Comptes* and consisting of representatives of the principal sickness funds and observers of several government Ministries. The principal sickness fund in the area acts as paymaster (the *caisse pivot*). All others send it their shares each month. The principal fund sends the hospital one-twelfth of its full annual grant each month. The *caisse pivot* takes particular interest in that hospital, since it is the one that confers with the hospital over the prospective budget during the negotiations stage of rate setting.

Global budgeting and global grants were reforms in the existing system of hospital provision and hospital finance. They were designed to improve efficiency and control costs without making fundamental changes. Redistribution of hospital and health services is possible under a system such as Britain's, where regional planning guides nationally owned and centrally financed services. French facilities planning was not developed for such a task, since it was confined to identifying appropriate bed/population ratios alone. One of the most important—and one of the most politically delicate—tasks in the French reforms during the 1980s was to devise a new health care planning system. Once designed and implemented, the system will relate facilities to needs in each region. New installations will be created with public subsidies where needed, some existing ones will be redirected, and unnecessary ones will be denied operating funds. Hospitals' prospective budgets must fulfill their objectives under the regional plans. If so, the DDASS will award the operating grants requested by the hospitals.

The individual sickness funds must still monitor the hospital, despite the aggregated method of payment. The hospital notifies the *caisse pivot* of all admissions, and the *caisse pivot* notifies the patient's sickness fund. The fund must know the patient's status, since it provides other benefits directly, such as payment of fees to the doctor, payment of disability benefits to the patient, and payment of some exceptional items to the hospital. The patient's sickness fund must agree to hospitalization in that particular establishment rather than in another. The fund's control doctor may intervene to prevent unnecessary admissions and excessive stays of its subscribers. If the fund's patient-days rise excessively under the new system, it would pay a higher proportion of the hospital's revenue next year.

Netherlands. During the 1980s Holland adopted some of the arithmetic of global budgeting without paying global grants. As in France, line-item review of prospective budgets by regulators had proved too contentious, guidelines to limit expenditure became too complicated, regulators had to make expensive concessions, and the appeals system was overburdened and generous. Payment of daily charges led to cost overruns and resisted reductions. The national government and the payers have always tried to limit the annual increase in each hospital's expenditures, but now they do it directly by applying a fixed percentage. And now they try to apply the same percentage to all hospitals; the many settlements of individual claims in the past led to total overruns.[34]

Negotiation has been added to Dutch payment decisions, but the hospitals and sickness funds are not free to adopt an agreement more expensive than the allowable increase. Regulation is retained to apply the arithmetic of the new guidelines, cut back any excessive agreements by the negotiators, and announce the awards.

A detailed expenditure report (the *bijlage*) is still filled out by the hospital. One reason is to provide the sickness fund with sufficient information to develop its position during the initial round of negotiations with the hospital. Another reason is to provide the COTG examiner with the numbers to calculate the new total. The new rates are the previous year's spending plus the allowable increase. The expenditure report is subcategorized, since the annual increase is not a single percentage of the total. Different lines are increased by different index numbers: the personnel costs are allowed to rise according to the national wage index; other lines, by the national price indexes. (I described these index numbers in Chapter Seven.) The starting point for these calculations was each hospital's expenditure report for 1982. To obtain total allowable revenue for 1983, each line was increased by its appropriate index number, the new amounts were totaled, and the aggregate was increased further by 0.5 percent. The bonus was intended to appease those hospitals that complained of an abnormally low cost base in 1982, because of a shortage of nurses or for other reasons.

The national government and the sickness funds contend that hospitals were allowed too much additional money during the years of lax regulation, that a financial crisis afflicts NHI, and that the hospitals must be cut back. The limits each year consist of last year's expenditure report plus wage and price indexes. But the additional percentage becomes zero or negative: 0 percent for 1984 revenue, –1 percent in 1985, –2 percent in 1986, and 0 percent thereafter. In other words, real growth in hospital expenditure was reduced in 1985 and 1986. Hospital managers have discretion in rearranging spending, as they did not during the years of line-item rate regulation. It is hoped that the severe squeeze will motivate them to shorten stays, refer patients to home care agencies, and treat more convalescents in the outpatient department.

If the hospital and sickness fund have negotiated a global budget for next year that falls within the limits, COTG is expected to approve. If they recommend a higher figure or deadlock, the COTG examiner investigates fitting utilization to available revenue. The negotiators seem willing to reduce stays but not service intensity.

If a hospital saves money from its approved rates and approved volume, it can keep the savings. It cannot use the savings for higher wages or for hirings exceeding the guidelines for numbers of personnel. If it buys new equipment, it must get the usual license from the national planning agency, which may be reluctant. (An incentive reimbursement scheme can inspire the doctors if their savings yield benefits that they desire, such as new equipment, but the managers lack a free hand.) Next year's global budget will be calculated from this year's expenditures (reflecting the savings) and not from this year's budget. If the hospital runs a deficit, it gets no supplements. As in Quebec, a full-scale incentive reimbursement system could not be tested, because all Dutch hospitals during the 1980s were being squeezed downward; few could earn and keep substantial savings.

As in France, policy makers hope that an effective regional planning system will be installed. Then a hospital's global budget will be derived from a regional total, not automatically calculated from its individual expenditure history. Government officials hope that regional plans will continue to control costs. The hospital association hopes that regional plans will expand services to meet the population's needs. Therefore, the methods of the 1980s may be only a temporary measure during that decade's financial emergency. A struggle over the policies of global budgeting lies ahead.

Switzerland. A global grants system requires an administrative mechanism to pool the payments. If government is the sole payer, no complications arise; it merely mails the checks, as in Canada. Nor does a problem arise in Holland, which has global budgeting but not global grants: once COTG sets the revenue limit, the hospital bills the several payers according to per diems and charges, as in the past. (If Holland ever adopted global grants, most of the country now has single sickness funds, which could send monthly installments, like a Canadian Ministry.) France has global budgeting, global grants, and multiple payers, and the administrative solution is the *caisse pivot:* one sickness fund collects all others' contributions and sends single monthly installments to the hospital.

Switzerland has cantonal government grants to the hospital, as well as per diems and charges paid by sickness funds. It does not yet have full-scale global budgeting and global grants. But several French-speaking cantons have created integrated funds (*centrales d'encaissement*) that represent all carriers and the cantonal government in handling all hospital bills throughout the canton. It is the kind of pool that is ideal for the administration of global grants. Normally, each hospital in German-speaking Switzerland distinguishes among its patients according to their sickness funds and bills each carrier separately. Each fund pays all the hospitals separately, each by a different rate. Instead, the *centrale* pools all the money. It gets lists of patients, their sickness funds, and their lengths of stay. Each hospital has its own per diem. The *centrale* bills each sickness fund for all care given its patients that week (more or less) by multiplying total days by the per diems of the various hospitals. The *centrale* then sends each hospital the total lump sum in its agreed budget in weekly or biweekly installments. The cantonal government gives the *centrale* its total subsidy for all hospitals, and the *centrale* distributes it every week or two. At the end of the year, the hospital should get more or less money according to its utilization, and the *centrale* administers the reconcilement of each sickness fund's account with each hospital. Global budgeting therefore is used as an administrative convenience at present, but the *centrale* could impose stronger financial discipline and controls if the commission wished.

In the rest of Switzerland, the hospital's prospective budget is scrutinized by the officials of the governments of the cantons. In cantons with *centrales,* the *centrale's* staff examines the budget and the *centrale's* commission approves it. A *centrale* commission is more impartial than a cantonal government, since it includes representatives from both the providers (the cantonal hospital association and the cantonal medical association) and the payers (the local sickness funds and the cantonal government).[35]

Prices Fixed by Payers

The last chapters have described the gamut of payment decision methods: hospitals fix their charges unilaterally (beginning of Chapter Six), hospitals and payers negotiate (Chapter Six), a neutral regulator sets a fair price that binds hospitals and payers (Chapter Seven), and the payer dictates the payment (this chapter). Unilateral rate fixing by the payer is unusual in hospital affairs and occurs only when the payer is government. Such financial grants by the payer are customary in a national health service. Unilateral top-down granting to a privately owned hospital industry develops only after many years, when government faces a financial crisis. In the years before then, government and the hospitals worked out payment in erratic, often tense, and usually expensive negotiations, as in Canada. The governmentally dictated payment method is usually global budgeting and global grants.

American Medicare in 1965 inaugurated one of the very few arrangements wherein the payer controls only part of the hospital's revenue and the payment unit is a service rather than all or part of the hospital's total revenue. The United States lacked Europe's long experience in organized payment sytems, so Medicare was launched without any rate-setting machinery. The legislators naively thought that mere statutory language would guarantee that hospitals would bill for no more than the "reasonable cost of services." These costs were the hospital's normal per diem costs of patient care, without certain items excluded by regulations and without flagrant profits. This ambiguous standard was applied in a chaotic manner, unparalleled in a major payment commitment in any other developed country. The government did not communicate with hospitals but turned over administration to the regional Blue Cross Plan or to another fiscal intermediary. In order to limit payment and combat abuse, the United States government generated far more legislative amendments and regulations than any other developed country. Although the fiscal intermediary agreed on interim rates with the hospital at the start of the year, the negotiations were perfunctory. The hospital could repeatedly raise its rates during the year, consistently raise its operating costs, and minimize any losses on the Medicare business. Because of the American bias against regulation and the political influence of the hospitals, the national government rarely allowed state governments to include Medicare in their rate regulation. Nor did the national government enact general hospital rate regulation.[36] The day of reckoning was postponed until the 1980s: Medicare payments came from a Hospital Insurance Trust Fund whose revenue from mounting Social Security taxes was supposed to keep pace with hospitals' billings; the elderly had to share much higher proportions of the costs in the United States than in any other country; hospitals shifted some of their operating costs to other payers. The national government in 1982 enacted stricter annual price increases on the Medicare per diem payments to hospitals, but this was a temporary stopgap before a structural reform.[37]

In 1983 the United States government replaced this unique payment system with another unique one: payment of a fixed amount for each case according to the patient's diagnosis-related group. The payer sets the price on the basis of statistical research and formulas, without any negotiation with hospitals and without any decisions by regulators. The government acts unilaterally as a "prudent buyer." The DRG rates apply only to the Medicare bills, and no other patients or payers are affected. I described the methodology of DRG payment at the end of Chapter Four.

The rates are derived from formulas established by Congress in the Social Security Amendments of 1983. The hospitals and interested public groups did not participate in writing the law or determining the formulas to be used; they participated only as witnesses at hearings and as behind-the-scenes lobbyists. The law specified that the total 1984 costs of Medicare under DRGs must be no higher than the costs that would have been incurred under the controlled method of 1983 plus a market-basket cost index plus 1 percent to cover improved service intensity. The research staff of the Health Care Financing Administration performed all the prescribed calculations: the clustering of diagnoses according to prior research to produce the DRGs; the differential weights among DRGs to reflect the variations in costs from earlier Medicare data files; differentials among regions of the country to reflect wage costs; the average DRG cost in 1984 to prevent expenditure creep over 1983; and so on. Voluminous regulations were written within HCFA; they were opened for a few months of comment by the hospitals and by other interested public groups, and then they were made final.

Medicare payment had been administered permissively in the past because of the hospitals' political leverage upon Presidents and the Congress. But now it would be stricter, because Congress was worried about the impending bankruptcy of the Hospital Insurance Trust Fund. Government budgetary crises had led to top-down global budgeting and global grants in Britain, Canada, and Italy and to stricter regulation and pooled methods in France, Holland, and elsewhere. The same problem led the United States government to become a stricter payer in its own program; but the government did not define hospital finance as a public policy problem and did not opt for an all-payers regulatory system or for pooled global grants. In fact, the Medicare reform tacitly signaled hospitals to shift costs to other third parties and to private self-payers.

A formula system requires monitoring to ensure that the effects are beneficial and intended. It must be updated as medical care, the hospitals, the clientele, and the economic environment change. Committees of Congress can perform only periodic general oversight, not continuous detailed monitoring. Neither Congress, the hospitals, nor the providers to the hospitals (particularly the medical equipment industry) trust HCFA to monitor itself. The law created a Prospective Payment Assessment Commission to advise the Department of Health and Human Services. It recommends annual percentages changes in DRG rates in 1986 and thereafter. It studies the performance of the DRGs and recommends adjustments in DRG classification and weights. Its members represent principal provider groups (the nonprofit and for-profit hospital associations, several hospital administrators, the medical association, medical equipment manufacturers), other payers affected indirectly by Medicare payments (insurance companies and HMOs), and experts on health care finance. The commission provides an opportunity for private interest groups to debate the design of the DRG system. But ultimate decisions in the United States rest with Congress. Every year it fixes the percentage increases and amends some details.

The Medicare per diem payment system between 1965 and 1983 had been surrounded by rules and disputes. An important motive for the adoption of DRGs in the United States—like the adoption of grants methods elsewhere—was to reduce the rules, reduce the disputes, allow hospital managers greater discretion, and relieve the civil servants of the need to understand the intricacies of hospital management and clinical care. Better management would be inspired by fewer controls and by incentive reimbursement, a perennial American ambition. The DRG is a regional average calculated from recent data. When treating such a patient, some hospitals lose and others gain. The losers must absorb the losses, and the winners keep their savings. The gains do not revert to the Treasury. The losers have an incentive to treat that case more efficiently, probably by reducing stays; or the losers may refer such cases to other hospitals, thereby encouraging a specialized division of labor. The winners are encouraged to take more such cases. The winners can use their savings for worthy new purposes that they could not finance under the earlier break-even cost-based reimbursement. All hospitals would improve because of closer collaboration between managers and doctors. The market would work: patients would go to those hospitals that could treat their conditions most efficiently, and they would avoid other hospitals. Many Americans assume that the economically profitable are the clinically superior. Since incentives would spontaneously inspire beneficial behavior and would reduce inefficient and improper services, the Reagan administration tried to eliminate the utilization-review and quality-control machinery that had existed under the previous Medicare reimbursement—that is, the Professional Service Review Organizations, committees of local doctors with staffs, assigned to each hospital.

But a completely regulation-free incentive reimbursement scheme was too utopian. Every method has perverse incentives not fully anticipated by its enthusiastic designers. Congress reenacted the utilization-review committee to guard against venal methods of "gaming" DRGs:

- Unnecessary admissions of inpatients who could be treated in an ambulatory mode for less than the full DRG rate.[38]
- Discharging and readmitting the same patient in order to collect two DRG payments for the same case.
- "DRG creep"—that is, reclassifying the patient because of a secondary diagnosis that is more remunerative than the principal diagnosis. (A sudden increase in the complexity and costliness of recorded diagnoses of Medicare patients occurred during the first months of payment by DRGs.)[39]
- Premature discharges to save money.
- Underservicing to save money.[40]

Therefore, payments by DRGs were not as simple as intended. Many hospitals claimed that they had unique characteristics: fluctuating community utilization, their indispensability in their communities, their clinical service structures, their specialization in the longer stays within each DRG, their referral relations with other establishments, and many other characteristics. The system had voluminous rules and intricate formulas to deal with these subtle variations. The system also had rules and regulatory review by Peer Review Organizations to prevent the aforementioned abuses. Every hospital retained the American right to claim that its payments were inequitable and to appeal against both the payments and any restraints by Medicare. Government payment of private providers is contentious in every country, and every formula system is disputed. Therefore, like Medicare before, the new payment system installed appeals machinery.[41]

Experience under Medicare DRGs may show that an incentive reimbursement scheme paying fixed prices for each service or case redistributes money rather than saves it: money is initially transferred from the more expensive hospitals to the less expensive; the overstaffed and more elaborate establishments must cut back, but the thin become fatter by adding staff and programs. Payers can prevent such a redistribution by limiting annual increases for all hospitals, taking advantage of the great efficiency imposed on the formerly fat while presuming that the cheaper hospitals will stay cheaper.

Evaluation of Global Budgeting and Global Grants

Advantages from the Standpoint of Payers. Payment is predictable. Overruns cease.

Payers and regulators are no longer blamed for specific deficiencies in hospital services, as they are if they cut specific lines in each hospital's budget. They transfer to the doctors and hospital managers the responsibility for waiting lists and denials of care.

Advantages from the Standpoint of Hospitals. Detailed monitoring of management and clinical work diminishes.

Managers have an incentive to improve internal affairs within the hospital. Doctors are pressed to cooperate with the manager.

Ground rules are simpler and more understandable.

Reports are fewer and simpler.

Advantages from the Standpoint of the Public. Financing is predictable and controlled.

Disputes may be fewer—unless government is imposing serious budget cuts. Appeals machinery and courts are less burdened.

Overutilization is discouraged.

Hospitals have an incentive to become more efficient.

Hospital payment can be coordinated with health facilities planning and with public policy about spending and inflation.

If hospital payment is properly administered, resources can be shifted from hospitals to other sectors, from overprovided to underprovided regions of the country.

Disadvantages from the Standpoint of Payers. Hospitals no longer write detailed reports about their work and about services to patients. Underservicing is possible.

If there are several payers, they may disagree over their fair shares of the total.

Disadvantages from the Standpoint of Hospitals. Hospitals are tied into public budgeting, and expenditure limits eventually are tightened. Managers and doctors complain about underfunding.

Doctors must adjust to limited resources and the loss of certain capabilities in their hospital as services become regionalized.

Regulatory scrutiny does not completely disappear. It reenters during the screening of the prospective budget and during discussion of the hospital's plans; it reenters if the quality of services is monitored.

Detailed reporting does not completely disappear. It reenters in the end-of-the-year accounting to payers.

Management may lose its autonomy to regional planners.

Hospital managers may become sloppy in their internal financial accounts and in their cost finding, since they may only be held accountable for aggregates.

Disadvantages from the Standpoint of the Public. Hospital affairs become drawn into a country's national budgetary politics. Local influences are weakened.

Underservicing is possible.

Budgetary squeezes may force a local hospital to close.

Information may become sparser and less reliable. Interest may decline in performance accounting. Hospitals, regions, and countries can no longer be compared by means of reliable and copious statistics.

Trends

When global budgeting and global grants are first adopted, they are part of an effort to expand access and increase the society's expenditures in health. They are direct methods of raising and investing resources, and they make changes much faster than traditional methods of insurance, charity, and regulation. Originally, they were part of the governmentalization of hospital payment. Gradually, government's methods of deciding grants and reviewing their use were extended into hospital affairs.

Hospitals benefit when government can spend generously and when public policy gives high priority to health. But when the economy declines, government must limit annual increases in the payment of hospitals. The limits are applied quickly and shock the hospital managers and doctors, who have become accustomed to getting what they wanted and never anticipated the potential consequences of public funding. Paying the individual hospital becomes a part of larger public policies. The methods installed during periods of stringency become permanent. Top-down budgeting dictated by the Ministry of Finance and by the finance officers of the Ministry of Health replaces the earlier bottoms-up submission and discussion of prospective budgets, a method inherited from earlier financing methods. Annual increments depend on formulas tied to national economic trends or to plans, not to the wish lists of individual hospitals.

Global budgeting and global grants are direct interventions in health. During economic growth and periods of social generosity, they deliver large increases to all hospitals and particularly to underprovided areas. The same focused and direct methods also can be used for sudden reversals. The entire hospital sector can be cut back (an option not available in rate negotiation and rate regulation). Individual hospitals can be forced to close, if officials are willing to take the heat or if the granting system is so bureaucratized that indignant communities cannot find anyone to harass. Resources can be transferred out of the acute hospital sector into other services (another option not available in rate negotiation and rate regulation).

The methods of global budgeting and global grants now attract policy makers in countries with rate regulation, since the system makes it possible to enforce spending targets, resources can be moved into other sectors of health, administration is simplified, and disputes are reduced. Therefore, global budgeting and global grants are growing as a method of paying hospitals. Countries with rate regulation are adding some of these administrative techniques for calculating the entire hospital revenue and for enforcing limits. Financially troubled NHI systems are being superseded by full Treasury financing or are being rescued by large government subsidies, and inevitably public budgeting methods enter.

At first hospital managers and hospital doctors welcome global budgeting and global grants. Instead of the detailed line-item review, guidelines, and disputes under rate regulation, they will get discretion. In practice they do not long enjoy the discretion they expected—that is, the freedom to spend new money as they think best. They must account for public money. During economic downturns they are under severe constraints. Severe conflicts over spending priorities may develop between the hospital managers and the hospital doctors.

Global grants often are said to include incentive reimbursement. If managers and doctors save, they can reallocate the savings. But these schemes do not function during financial stringency, since few hospitals can find extra money. Even in easier times, managers are wary of taking the bait, lest their savings lead the payers to reduce the budget bases.

Whether hospitals have closed or open medical staffs, the doctors have placed demands on lay managers, and the managers have searched for the needed resources. Global budgeting and global grants try to make the lay hospital managers responsible to the grantors rather than to the owners and doctors alone. Grants policy often pits the acute-oriented medical profession against national policy makers with less medicalized conceptions of health care. Global budgeting and direct grants to the hospital in some countries are instruments in the gradual weakening of the primacy of the medical profession and a reorientation of its mission. But a complete change is far distant.

9

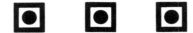

Financing
Capital Investment

Until the twentieth century, hospital capital was simple and consisted of buildings rather than extensive equipment. Patients were housed in large open wards. Buildings consisted of strong exterior walls, roofs, and a few strong interior walls. Many buildings survived for centuries: photographs during the twentieth century showed rows of beds in wards not very different from the engravings of several centuries earlier.[1] Most charitable hospitals also had endowments, consisting of farmlands, forest land, and houses for rent.

Like the construction of the buildings, the financing was simple. A rich donor gave money and/or the resources for construction (such as wood and stone) during his lifetime or in his will. The church organization or association that owned and operated the hospital might also solicit many smaller donors for contributions. Owners used their own funds in whole or in part: religious groups and private associations might sell endowments to pay for materials and labor; governments could tap their building funds. Borrowing was possible but unusual: to pay off the debt quickly, the owner had to have a regular income— such as cash income from the private owner's lands and factories or the tax revenue of local government. Massive funds were not needed: although many hospitals existed—Britain may have had eight hundred during the Middle Ages— most were small; even the very large ones in the biggest cities were constructed simply and often lasted for centuries.

During the twentieth century, medical science progressed cumulatively, innovations in medicine (as in other fields) multiplied exponentially, and an increasingly elaborate technology was introduced into hospitals. Unlike the simple technology of the past, the new equipment caused rearrangements of old buildings and extensions. The population acquired third-party coverage and began to demand the types of private and semiprivate rooms previously reserved for the rich; therefore, the old pattern of large wards became unpopular. Every country was pressed to find much new capital in a short time, to replace old buildings and to buy the new equipment. Many hospitals sold substantial parts of their endowments of land and rental buildings during the late nineteenth and early twentieth centuries to build new hospital structures.[2] But the pressure to modernize accelerated: technical improvement required replacement of new equipment within a few years of any purchase; even the new buildings had to be modified and expanded constantly.

As the demand for capital rose, by coincidence the financial capacity of charity in Europe and North America declined. As a result of the two world wars, depression, inflation, and social change, the very rich class diminished in numbers, in property, and in income after taxes. The general population became more prosperous after World War II, and the number of small donations to capital funds increased in a few countries, but not enough to keep pace with the full capital needs of all hospitals.

The old pattern of rearrangement of assets by owners was no longer feasible as a permanent source of capital. The remaining endowments of European religious and nonsectarian religious associations were destroyed completely or severely diminished by wars, depression, and inflation. To build a new hospital, private owners had nothing to sell. The only owners who could find much investment money were the local and provincial governments, who drew new money from taxes.[3]

Recent Developments in Capital Finance

New methods had to be found after World War II. The traditional private sources of investment money had been cut back. The amounts needed were much greater than earlier. The useful lives of buildings and equipment were short, and therefore a growing stream of money was needed.

One new source in several countries has been the national governments. They have taxing power over personal and corporate incomes and therefore can muster large amounts. Since they can levy income taxes and spend everywhere, the national governments have been able to redistribute resources from the rich regions to needy regions. (The traditional sources of investment money previously tended to cluster hospitals in the richer areas, particularly in the big cities.) National government grants have been common in countries where most hospitals remain privately owned, such as West Germany, Canada, and the United States. In Germany and Canada, the national money first went to the provincial governments, the provinces added contributions, and the combined grants went to the hospitals. The provincial governments screened the applications. In the United States, the national government sent the money directly to the hospitals.

A few countries have special public funds that local governments can draw on for their capital needs. Since the local governments can raise money from taxes, the funds become revolving accounts: the local governments can draw on these funds for the hospitals that they own, but they are expected to repay. An example is France.

A few countries have changed ownership as well as investment sources. The national government takes over ownership as well as funding. An example is Great Britain.

In most countries national and provincial governments replaced charitable donors. Hospital managements in a few countries found a new source that preserved their autonomy—namely, the private capital market. Examples are the United States and the Netherlands.

The postwar changes in capital financing were part of a political transformation in health. A century ago national governments had little to do with hospitals. The sector was decentralized and managed entirely by private persons and local governments, occasionally with monitoring of safety by provincial governments. The enactment of national health insurance laws in the late nineteenth and early twentieth centuries began the slow but increasing involvement of national governments in policy over hospitals' operating revenue. The new capital grants after World War II further increased the national governments' concern with how their money was used and how the public was served. By the 1980s, the national governments had become the principal conscience in hospital affairs, pressing the managers to use public resources efficiently and to provide the most appropriate care. Even in the United States— with its self-financing of capital, its insistently independent hospitals, and its decentralized federal system of government—the national government became more intrusive.

Facilities Plans

Evolution in Europe. When national and provincial governments supplied construction and equipment to all hospitals, someone for the first time questioned whether every establishment should receive all that it asked. The landscape was viewed as a whole for the first time.

In poor countries with few facilities and in the underprovided areas of developed countries, health facilities planning is concerned with the location and design of new establishments. Planning methodology estimates the needs of populations in several places, defines priorities among unmet needs, recommends the types of facilities and personnel for the higher-priority places, and estimates feasibility in costs and staffing.

The planning issues are more extensive in the developed countries. Many hospitals already exist with similar and duplicative services, siting is poorly related to catchment areas, utilization of some facilities declines, old establishments seek funds for renovation with uncertain future use, facilities do not cooperate, and gaps coexist with surpluses. Therefore, in all developed countries during the 1950s and 1960s, a considerable literature was devoted to regional health planning, whereby inherited facilities and newly constructed ones would fit together in a system. Hospitals would be arranged in hierarchies, from simpler community establishments to the most advanced in the big cities. Patients would be referred as needed. Hospitals would coordinate with ambulatory health centers and other facilities. According to plans, some existing facilities would wind down, others would expand in size and in technical level, and others would change function.[4]

Writing, adopting, and implementing such plans, affecting previously independent hospitals, are politically difficult in democracies. The managers, owners, doctors, labor unions, and communities resist reductions and conversions. However, regional hospital planning eventually has been adopted on a national scale in several European countries, such as Sweden, Great Britain,

France, West Germany, and Italy. Because of resistance by the hospitals and physicians, implementation is often slow and imperfect, but such plans have been adopted. The need to conserve money in the face of the mounting demands from medical technology eventually leads to more effective enforcement in every country. The plans are implemented by carrots and sticks: hospitals that fulfill new missions receive capital grants from government and sufficient operating revenue, either through global budgeting or rate regulation; hospitals that do not cooperate receive no new capital and suffer limits on operating revenue.[5]

The constituency for health facilities planning is the government finance officers, who must grant scarce funds to old and new hospitals. If managers of both existing and proposed hospitals found all their own money—as they did before World War II—no health facilities plans would be enacted. If managers of existing hospitals could find the bulk of their construction, renovation, and equipment money from sources other than government, only limited plans would be enacted, and the plans would be designed only to assess the needs of competing communities for new facilities.

Since hospital facilities plans have been addressed to simple issues—whether new buildings and programs should be added in a community, whether existing hospitals should be expanded—the methodology has been simple. Throughout the world the basic number has been the ratio of beds to population in an area. Number of inhabitants alone—usually not even weighted by age, sex, or morbidity—has been the definition of need. The policy decision has been choice of the threshold ratio beyond which no more beds should be added—for example, 4 per 1,000; 4.5 per 1,000; 6 per 1,000; and so on.[6] Better data and equations relating variables would be required for "comprehensive health care plans" that attempt to match service mix to the clinical needs and fiscal capacities of populations. These data and equations would be required for plans dealing with large multiinstitutional structures and the work flows among them. Such plans were seriously developed in some governments during the 1980s, requiring belated improvements in data.

Comprehensive planning requires calculating the need for advanced technology and deciding the most appropriate places for the machinery and its staff. In most countries before the 1980s, planning referred to hospital beds, but only in a few countries did it apply to equipment. Even when large equipment was inventoried separately, utilization and operating costs usually were not included in the plans.[7]

(The foregoing paragraphs and the next few are overviews of history. Details about current planning styles in individual countries appear later in this chapter.)

Evolution in the United States. The American hospital system has diverged from European development in planning and in capital investment, as in many other respects. At first, after World War II, the United States national government granted money to established hospitals for renovation and expansion and to associations wishing to create new ones. (The Hospital Survey and Construction Act of 1946 and the Hospital and Medical Facilities Amendments of 1964 were called the Hill-Burton Program.) As in the first stages of national government grants in Europe and Canada, the statutes prescribed methods for assessing the needs of communities, in order to determine where to grant new money and when certain communities had enough. Despite its voluminous literature and elegant econometric methodology—by far the most "sophisticated" in the world—American health facilities planning has never evolved much past this stage.

At first American reformers and government grantors shared the worldwide interest in regional planning and operation of the entire range of old and new facilities.[8] A showdown occurred in 1965, the year when the United States national government enacted several health laws, including national health insurance for the aged. A health-planning law was supposed to bring together in each region the health services, research centers, and educational institutions in a concentrated effort to combat heart disease, cancer, and stroke. Through exhortation (which participants would rationally accept) and through conditional grants, the Regional Medical Program (RMP) agency in Washington, D.C., would press the establishments to combine in efficient regional complexes. The American Medical Association fought the RMP bill, the rest of the 1965 health agenda (such as Medicare), and all subsequent health-planning laws, on the grounds that they would limit the discretion of doctors and of other providers. The political logrolling to obtain legislation during 1965 produced spending without constraints: to get the hospitals' support, Medicare Part A was written to please them; to reduce the doctors' anger and deprive them of political sympathizers, Medicare Part B was written to please them; to persuade the doctors to cooperate with Medicare after enactment, the American Medical Association was permitted by the President and by the Secretary of Health, Education, and Welfare to write the drafts of the RMP law. The law omitted strong presumptions that many old and new establishments should combine in systems, that a division of labor should be followed, and that recipients of grants should meet strict conditions.[9]

As in much of the American national government's legislation after 1965, RMP became merely a series of grants to apparently worthy projects, with the conditions limited to performing the proposed work and submitting final reports. The independent grantees were encouraged to cooperate, but coordination was (and remains today) completely voluntary. Not enough hospitals and other providers join in true regional systems.

Hospitals could never have survived so autonomously if an entirely new method of funding construction and equipment had not been unexpectedly developed. Almost alone among developed countries, America found an alternative to government grants. Medicare and many Blue Cross Plans guaranteed to hospitals the full costs of patient care, and an important political concession to the hospitals during the logrolling of 1965 was the inclusion of capital costs as costs of patient care. Some American hospitals had purchased buildings and equipment from loans, and the allowable capital costs under Medicare and Blue Cross included the money to amortize the loans: the interest, liberal depreciation, and some extra sums (such as "return on equity" for proprietary hospitals and a "plus factor" for nonprofit hospitals). Designed merely to help hospitals saddled with old debt, the Medicare law opened the floodgates for new debt. Since Medicare and Blue Cross coverage guaranteed the hospitals' ability to repay such debts, lenders eagerly bought hospital bonds, and hospital managers turned to the private capital market instead of to government.

Facilities planners lost whatever leverage they had to compel regionalization and—except in a few states—have had remarkably little power over new construction and the development of new programs.

RMP was followed by several national grants programs to build up planning capabilities in the states and in substate regions, and the statutes bid the agencies to encourage regionalization, but the American machinery is designed primarily to block (or redirect) the hospitals' autonomous capacity to raise their own money for duplicative facilities. Since the state and national governments are principal payers of operating costs, they want to limit new construction and equipment to the areas where they are needed. But the governments themselves are poorly coordinated to write and to implement their plans effectively.[10] The machinery is so written in statutes that the state government officials cannot make unilateral decisions but must listen to the advice of committees made up of providers and consumers, who are not payers motivated to conserve money but users motivated to encourage installation of the best new methods. The enterprising hospital can eventually get the enthusiastic endorsement of the screening committees and the reluctant approval of the planning agency.[11] In a country where hospital organizations can find and repay their own enormous investment funds, where nothing better than weak and unclear arrangements can be enacted, the chronically ineffective arrangements are periodically discredited, repealed, and replaced with much-publicized efforts that change little.

Characteristics of Capital Funding Systems

Countries differ in their methods of paying for buildings and equipment. Following are the categories at present:

☐ Objects financed.
  - New buildings.
  - Renovation of existing buildings.
  - Maintenance fund.
  - Expensive special equipment.
  - Depreciation fund to replace smaller equipment.
  - Special fund to operate an individual program.
☐ Source of financing.
  - Government grants.
    — National.
    — Provincial.
    — Local.
    — Combination, such as national-provincial shared cost programs.
  - Revolving funds created by:
    — Third parties.
    — Government.
  - Donations by private persons.
    — Large individual donors.
    — Community drives with many small donors.

- — Special private foundations that support health services or clinical research.
- — Business firms (charitable gifts or donations of equipment by medical supply companies for testing).
  - • Self-financing by hospital through:
  - — Conversion of endowment.
  - — Borrowing and repaying from operating revenue. Sources of loans.
- ☐ Hospital facilities plans. Whether a country has them. If so:
  - • Type.
    - — Coordinate an entire health services system.
    - — Guide priorities for capital grants by government or by public funds.
    - — Guide regulators in giving or denying licenses to build or licenses to buy.
    - — Educate public by estimating future requirements.
  - • Whether one or several disparate plans.
- ☐ Authors of the plans (if plans exist).
  - • Legislature.
  - • Government agency.
  - • Independent planning commission.
  - • Committee of private interest groups representing the providers, payers, and others.
  - • Hospital association.
- ☐ Content of plans (if they exist).
  - • All health services, or hospitals alone.
  - • Whether they attempt some regional coordination among hospitals.
  - • Whether they attempt to reallocate capital expenditures into:
    - — Underprovided regions.
    - — Nonacute services.
- ☐ Instruments of plan.
  - • Methods of control.
    - — Grants for approved investments.
    - — Issue new licenses. Revoke old licenses.
    - — Allow or refuse operating money.
  - • Whether instruments are applied by:
    - — The planner.
    - — Another agency on the planners' requests.
    - — Third-party payers.
  - • Relations between planners and those who negotiate, regulate, or grant operating costs.
- ☐ Enforcement.
  - • Whether new capital schemes must conform to plan.
  - • How new proposals are screened.
  - • Any sanctions against unauthorized construction or against installing unauthorized equipment.
- ☐ Methods of writing plans.
  - • Bed/population ratios.
  - • Variable relations between other definitions of needs and services.

These detailed options will appear in the descriptions throughout the rest of this chapter. The following text will be organized into the main forms of capital investment:

- Government's grants to a hospital system that it does not own and manage (Germany and Switzerland as examples).
- Loans from a special government fund (France).
- Loans from the private capital market (United States and the Netherlands).
- Government's grants to hospitals that it owns and manages (Great Britain).

Several themes will appear throughout the detailed descriptions. Several countries now finance capital through public grants; others borrow and amortize the debt from operating revenue. But public grants may be the trend in the future. Usually hospitals are owned by entities (nonprofit associations, for-profit doctors and businessmen, and municipalities) different from the grantors of capital (under public grants, the national and regional governments). Plans for regionalization and coordination are implemented only when the same level of government owns and manages hospitals, gives the capital grants, and pays the operating costs.

Government Grants to Independent Hospitals in West Germany

Whether hospitals are owned predominantly by government or by nonprofit associations, European and Canadian hospitals depend on government grants for their new construction and expensive equipment. Details vary among countries.

West Germany demonstrates that many complicated issues must be settled in any method of capital grants from government.

- ☐ If too many beds exist, how the grantors decide.
  - Exclusion of some existing hospitals.
  - Grants to other existing hospitals.
  - Substantial grants to start up new ones.
- ☐ Variations in sizes of grants.
- ☐ Basis for denying some proposals.
- ☐ Different or identical treatment of nonprofit, public, and for-profit hospitals.
- ☐ Amount of discretion that government allows owners and managers in the use of its money.
- ☐ Role of the national government in a federal system where jurisdiction is traditionally the exclusive preserve of provincial and local governments. Options are:
  - Direct national grants to hospitals.
  - Shared national-provincial programs, wherein each contributes a share to the hospital. Usually the province combines the national government's contribution with its own. All provinces have similar programs.
  - Block grants by the national governments to the provinces, which subsidize hospital investment. Each province has a different program.

- Share of the national government's taxes is collected by each province. Although the provinces promise to use the revenue for hospital investment, the level is discretionary. Amounts vary among provinces according to their fiscal capacity.
- ☐ Whether grants should reallocate resources from the rich to the poor regions.
- ☐ Coping with business depressions and severe cuts in government budgets.
- ☐ Role of third-party payers in the planning and government grants.

German experience demonstrates several important lessons. Some effort at planning inevitably accompanies grants of public money to private and municipal hospitals. The design of the planning system is a delicate outcome of a struggle among competing interests. If consensus and political will never develop, the planning is implemented in confused and contentious ways, and reforms are blocked by legislative deadlocks. Probably no country can write and implement health facilities plans without leadership by the national government and without full cooperation by the national hospital associations.

The Situation Before the Grants Programs. Before 1972, as I said in Chapter Six, German hospitals were expected to get money for construction and for new equipment from their owners, from charitable donors, or from savings from their daily charges. As a result, most hospitals were financially starved. The sickness funds refused to give much money for depreciation; therefore, hospitals could accumulate little above the costs of patient care, even for smaller equipment.[12] After Germany's succession of wars and depressions, the charitable hospitals and their owners lacked the endowments to modernize the buildings and install new equipment. The municipalities that owned some hospitals had limited funds for construction and equipment, although they had somewhat more funds than most charitable associations did. The richest provincial governments, such as North Rhine–Westphalia, gave capital grants to nonprofit hospitals, but this was not common across the country. Since the hospital sector was private and local, each hospital was autonomous, and no plans existed.

One category of hospitals boomed, because their owners were rich and generous. The teaching hospitals were affiliated with the medical schools and universities, and the universities after World War II enjoyed the highest priorities in the budgets of provincial governments. The operating and capital budgets of most teaching hospitals ranged up to several hundred million DM per year in the biggest provinces, such as Bavaria. Advanced medicine could be practiced in the teaching hospitals but not in the ordinary nonprofit public and proprietary hospitals. The teaching hospitals overshadowed all others and attracted additional funds and donations of equipment from private sources.

The underfinancing of the nonteaching hospitals pleased the office doctors, since it weakened their competitors. The medical associations had negotiated for enough money from sickness funds so that fees covered the full costs of practice, and office doctors bought considerable equipment. Fees under official health insurance and in private practices enabled owners to equip private clinics to levels equal to or better than those of the nonprofit hospitals. Therefore, much patient care that might have been done in nonprofit and municipal hospitals was done in the doctors' offices and in their private clinics.

The result was a peculiar pattern of expenditures. Hospital wage and capital costs were so low during the 1960s that less than a quarter of German personal-care spending went to hospitals; more was paid to doctors for office and clinic care, and almost as much was paid for pharmaceuticals. Not until the financing reforms of the 1970s did hospitals absorb more than a third of German personal-care spending and did hospital revenue exceed the doctors'.[13] In other developed countries during the 1970s or even earlier, hospitals used half of personal-care expenditure.

The owners of the increasingly obsolete nonprofit and municipal hospitals pressed for relief, but helping them required fundamental changes in the German political system and in its health insurance. The enormous continuing amounts of money for construction and equipment could come only from national governments, but the German Constitution confined hospital affairs to the provinces. The Constitution had to be amended to authorize national grants to hospitals, but all amendments require approval by the provinces, and the provinces opposed infringements on their jurisdiction in health.

System of Plans and Grants. The Constitution was amended in 1969, to allow collaboration between the national government (*Bund*) and the provincial governments (*Länder*) in several sectors.[14] Hospital finance was made a concurrent power of both *Bund* and *Länder* (Article 74 (19a) of the *Grundgesetz*). The hospital finance law (the *Krankenhausfinanzierungsgesetz*, or KHG) was passed by the national legislature (in the *Bundestag*) and by the provinces (in the *Bundesrat*) in 1972. This fundamentally new direction resulted from struggles and compromises. Fiscal relations among levels of government in all federal systems are constantly disputed. Therefore, the factions in Germany wrote into the law and regulations precise formulas to make automatic the amounts of money for every hospital and the shares supplied by the national, provincial, and local governments. The formulas satisfied a widespread aspiration in postwar Germany to maximize the rule of law and minimize the potentially abusive discretion by officials.

The dilemma of denying grants to some hospitals and distributing them elsewhere was settled by the introduction of facilities planning. Every provincial government writes a plan specifying its needs for hospital care, both in volume of beds and in specialties. It screens all nonprofit, municipal, and proprietary hospitals according to criteria, and it admits some to practice under its plan. An existing hospital will not be admitted if it falls below quality standards and if it is too small to be viable. If an area seems to have too many beds—a common situation in Germany—the provincial government will be stricter in admitting the smaller hospitals to the plan and will limit the number of approved beds for recognized hospitals. If a hospital is admitted to the plan, it is guaranteed capital payments from government under the statutory formulas, and the sickness funds are obligated to pay daily charges that cover the full costs of care, including depreciation.

Admission to the plan is one area of discretion in a system otherwise designed to minimize favoritism and officials' power. A hospital's admission is crucial to its survival. When substantial numbers of hospitals are omitted by officials to reduce overbedding, some hospitals mobilize communities and influential allies to win reversals.[15]

In the political struggle over the design of the system, the *Länder* got commitments for large grants to the provincial governments by the *Bund* (the *Länder* and not the *Bund* pay the hospitals), and the provinces retained complete power to write and implement the plans. Each province writes its plan according to its own literary taste and substantive priorities, so they are not standardized. But all plans must be addressed to the same general themes—that is, the needs of communities and identification of hospitals deserving construction and equipment money.[16] Under the original design of KHG, the provinces filed their plans with the national government, and Bonn then had to share in their capital expenditures. There has never been a national health facilities plan, since the *Bund* lacks authority to revise the provincial plans, to reallocate resources among the *Länder,* or to coordinate their facilities.

Germany's plans illustrate the first stage of health facilities planning: devising the baselines to decide which areas have unmet needs, which are sufficiently provided, and where new investments should be spent. Regionalization and coordination among facilities are not yet authorized by law and are not attempted. The office doctors would resist: they are paid independently of KHG, have considerable advanced technology in their offices and private clinics, and are competitors of the nonprofit and public hospitals. The private clinics would resist regionalization, since they might become subordinate to the teaching hospitals and larger urban nonprofits.[17]

Since it was in large part a formula system, the method sought clear-cut distinctions in law and in application: each investment could be placed in one of four categories, and each category was paid for by definite rules. The following categories and rules (regarding various types of construction and equipment) were followed during the 1970s and early 1980s:

☐ *Construction and equipment with an expected life of fifteen or more years.* The owners of an existing or proposed hospital wrote a proposal for such a large project and sent it to the *Land* government's Ministry of Health. No standard forms existed. There was no fixed list of eligible projects. Only hospitals officially recognized under the provincial plan were eligible to apply. The proposal was supposed to correspond to the needs of the area under the plan, as judged by the officials of the *Land* Ministry; the proposal was also supposed to be feasible for that particular hospital. The Ministry prioritized all the applications it received from hospitals each year, suggested some cuts to save money, and funded them within its budgetary capacity that year. (The procedure was specified in Paragraph 9 of KHG, abbreviated §9KHG.)

The original assumption was that the *Land* recovered one-third of its annual investment costs from the *Bund* and one-third of each project from the *commune* (from the *Landkreis* or *Bezirk*). A law controlling the *Bund's* budget—passed around 1975 with the agreement of the *Länder* in the *Bundesrat*—placed a ceiling on the *Bund's* contribution. The *Bund* contributed 30.4 percent of the *Länder* expenditures in 1973 (that is, 971,900 DM out of a total of 3,199,665 DM), but thereafter the *Bund* grants were less, and the *Bund* contributions dropped to 25.7 percent in 1975, 21.7 percent in 1978, and 18.8 percent in 1984.[18] The *Bund* tried to reduce its contribution further in 1980, on the grounds that it lacked the money. If it had succeeded, very little new construction would have been undertaken thereafter. But the Constitutional Court decided that KHG obligated the *Bund* to contribute to every project approved by the *Land* and *commune*. Recriminations over the federal-provincial shares and the financial strains on the *Bund*—far from the original expectations of a harmonious collaboration with equal shares—led to abandonment of the system in 1985.

The same financial stringencies that reduced the *Bund's* ability to pay also struck the *Länder* during the 1980s. Without extra help from the *commune* budgets, many projects could not be undertaken, and the *Bund* had fewer requests from the *Länder* for contributions. Some *commune* governments saved some projects by paying more than one-third. As in many operations of the German government, the bonds of the political parties make the system work. If the provincial government, the communal government, and the hospital are led by members of the same party, projects are more likely to be funded. One reason why the *Länder* in the *Bundesrat* insisted on automatic formulas for contributions by the *Bund* was to prevent the political party in control of the national government from discriminating among the provinces.

These large grants are the only levers for regionalization in German hospital planning at present. The *Länder* avoid supporting too many duplicating high-tech programs. They announce such grants with the hope that other facilities will refer patients there.

☐ *Equipment with expected lives of three to fifteen years.* Very large projects such as those discussed in the preceding paragraphs inevitably are created and funded at officials' discretion, even in a legalistic political culture like Germany's, where the maximum number of decisions are made according to rules. But, in the original design of KHG, small equipment was paid for by a formula. Every hospital recognized by the plan automatically received a fixed amount every year.[19]

The lawmakers looking for a simple rule at first adopted the cost of replacing a hospital bed. Research then suggested replacement costs in hospitals of different sizes and of different ages. The estimated replacement costs in Deutsche Mark per bed in the decree issued in 1979 (updating the original figure in §10KHG) were:

	Size of hospital			
Hospitals built	*Up to 250 beds*	*250–350 beds*	*350–650 beds*	*650 or more beds*
Before Dec. 3, 1950	18,529	21,760	25,234	32,183
After Jan. 1, 1951	21,545	25,303	29,342	37,421

As a rule of thumb, a hospital received per bed each year the amount equal to its amortization of that bed. Bed size was the number recognized in the provincial hospital plan; if the hospital installed additional beds, it could not include them in the calculations for the capital funds. For example, a 380-bed hospital built in 1957 received an annual capital fund of (380) (.0833) (29,342 DM) = 928,791 DM during the early 1980s. The hospital used the money for equipment and not for replacement of beds and space, but the number of beds seemed the most objective data at that time for automatic distribution formulas. This method proved troublesome and—as I will explain in later paragraphs—was amended during the 1980s.

The provincial government pays the hospital. Before 1985 it collected one-third of all its §10KHG costs from the *Bund,* and one-third of each hospital's §10KHG costs was recovered from the *commune.* The *Bund* could not reduce its contribution.

The hospital's revenue from this source was constant every year; its spending for equipment was not, but it could budget predictably. To buy an expensive item, it borrowed from a bank and then amortized the loan from its annual capital grants. It could deposit the government grants in its investment account in a bank and could spend them later.

In theory, the annual grants under the original §10KHG rules were earmarked for equipment and construction with expected lives between three and fifteen years. The *Land's* auditors could ask for an accounting of how the hospital spent the government's money. But the hospital is free to manage its affairs under the German system, and the *Land* does not challenge the hospital by intruding. The *Länder* usually accept the hospital's word. In practice in the short run, hospital managers used the money flexibly, for depreciation and other purposes. But, in the long run, at least those amounts of money were used to buy three-to-fifteen-year equipment.

In the German political and health system, each organization and interest group is sensitive to intrusions by others. Therefore, the *Land* does not allow the *Bund* to investigate how its money is used, either within the *Land* government or in the hospital. The *Land* alone has direct jurisdiction over the hospital. The rules of the game in Germany are to accept the written pledges of grantees, to presume that everyone obeys the regulations.

☐ *Equipment with lives of less than three years.* Depreciation is an allowable cost in the prospective budget submitted by the hospital to the sickness funds, as the basis for the daily charge. Each hospital makes its own case to the sickness funds, without formulas. The new laws and regulations after KHG was passed in 1972 required the sickness funds to be more generous in granting depreciation money. The hospitals have used it for small equipment and for other purposes.

☐ *Maintenance.* Preservation of all equipment is distinguished from depreciation in the payment system. Maintenance is an allowable cost in the prospective budget submitted by the hospital to the sickness funds, as the basis for the daily charge. The sickness funds must pay each hospital according to a formula, much like the method for heavy equipment under §10KHG. The formula was set by law, in the regulation concerning how the hospital and sickness funds should negotiate the daily charge (Paragraph 18 of the *Bundespflegesatzverordnung,* abbreviated §18BPflV).[20]

A supposedly well-honed system of "dual financing" was erected in 1972. Money for medium and large investments came from government, so that the cost was borne by taxpayers. Money to maintain these investments came from the sickness funds, so that the cost was borne by premium payers, subject to more regressive collections than the taxpayers. Money for small-equipment purchase also came from the sickness funds. In practice the hospital mixed all this money and spent it flexibly, although some hospital managements were more punctilious than others in segregating their expenditures.

Consequences of the Procedure. The new methods during the 1970s at first pleased the hospital owners and managers. In comparison to the previous parlous situation, the entry of government provided more capital, and hospitals could use all revenue from the sickness funds for operations. In return, they paid no price: the planning system did not burden the owners and managers at all, because it was basically a literary exercise by the provincial Ministry of Health.

The laws had defined the private clinics as hospitals eligible for inclusion in the provincial plans, and the provinces had recognized those that were larger, better equipped, and politically influential. Germany became one of the few countries providing public grants to proprietary hospitals, instead of squeezing them out of the health care system. The German clinics admitted to the provincial plans automatically have received grants for construction and equipment, and they have been guaranteed daily charges covering depreciation, maintenance, and all other operating costs. The doctors in these clinics have prospered, since they bill the sickness funds for itemized treatments under the physicians' part of NHI, while using the advanced facilities of the clinics to cover their practice costs. Other doctors must use the office equipment they have built up from their fees; or they must use the more modest private clinics that are not in the provincial plans and do not receive government capital grants.

As always, automatic formulas are complicated to administer and have unexpected (and often perverse) effects. Amending them is difficult, because changes are not merely technical matters, interest groups win and lose, and obligations shift between national and provincial governments.

The original §10KHG formulas had given hospitals more money if they were larger and newer, not necessarily when they needed it. Some hospitals got from government grants more than they spent on capital. Others with needs arising from complex work got less than they wished to spend. The problem was to devise a distribution method targeted on need that would be automatic and would not give officials authority to investigate and judge individual cases: the rules for three-to-fifteen-year equipment grants under §10KHG were changed in 1981 to classify hospitals by complexity and give them Deutsche Mark per year according to their numbers of beds:

Type of hospital	DM per bed per year
Advanced	3,666
Specialized	2,868
Routine	2,481
Basic	2,045

Each province distributed grants to its hospitals by its own definitions, billing the *Bund* for one-third of its costs.

The original formulas had tried to earmark different sets of government grants and their procedures for different types of equipment defined by expected life. But this formula ignored cost: some long-lived equipment was cheaper than some short-lived equipment. And the old method ignored the fact that the hospitals mixed their funds. The 1981 amendments made decisions less rigid. The §9KHG special proposals could be submitted and funded for expensive items with expected lives of less than fifteen years. The §10KHG money could be spent on moderately expensive items of a type with expected lives exceeding fifteen years—as managers already did in practice. Therefore, the formulas were adjusted to practice, but they were not eliminated, since the result would have been discretionary granting by officials. The 1981 amendments were stopgaps, not fundamental reforms.

The original formulas had perverse effects on the level of bedding. Since grants were calculated by payment per bed, larger hospitals got more money. KHG was written before hospital costs were high and was a principal cause of the unexpected *Kostenexplosion* of the mid-1970s: from 1971 to 1976, health costs generally increased about 15 to 20 percent per year, but hospital costs rose between 20 and 30 percent annually. During the 1970s cross-national statistical comparisons of health services were reported widely, and Germans noticed that they had by far the highest number of hospital beds of any country, about eight acute beds plus three nonacute beds per thousand inhabitants. From policy analysts in other countries came the insight that an excessive number of beds is a principal reason for excessive stays and very high costs. Germans realized too late that the formulas for paying capital under KHG discouraged the reduction of their beds, but their deadlock-prone political process postponed an alternative.

Consequences of the Amounts. Methodology in capital grants as well as in reimbursement is overshadowed by the amounts produced. If government supplies much less money than the hospitals' expectations, the managers protest and want to change the method. The German economic decline of the late 1970s and 1980s reduced the revenue of the provincial governments, and most economized by cutting capital grants to hospitals, particularly the discretionary grants for new buildings and expensive equipment under §9KHG. They could not reduce all other capital grants, since these other grants were mandated by KHG and were even increased by the change in the formulas of §10KHG in 1981. But the increases over the history of the program were much lower than the original expectations. Total capital grants for 1974 were 9.8 percent above 1973 national totals, as first expected; the totals then were the same or occasionally slightly higher until 1981; the new §10KHG formula made the 1984 nominal annual total 27.4 percent higher than the nominal figure for 1974. The total grants throughout Germany under KHG had reached only 4,473,900 DM in 1984, and most *Länder* attained their shares by pressing their *communes* to contribute more than the one-third originally envisaged.[21]

Everyone agreed that German hospitals were getting less money than they needed for new construction and for heavy equipment. Interest groups and researchers gave different estimates, ranging from 8 to 15 million DM. Many German hospitals still worked in buildings constructed before 1940.[22]

Disillusioned by public capital grants, leaders of hospital affairs called for adoption of the opposite method: self-financing rather than dual financing.[23] Hospitals would borrow in the capital market and would amortize debt as part of the allowable costs covered by the daily charge. Capital costs, like all other operating costs, therefore would be paid for by the sickness funds, and government would no longer participate. Hospital managers would be more free and more creative than under public capital grants.

Since there are few options in health care financing, the German hospital leaders came full circle. Their new proposal merely resurrected the pre-1972 arrangements that had starved the hospitals and led to passage of KHG and dual financing. Presumably, the hospitals now would insist that the sickness funds be required by law to fund amortization generously, but such a law would introduce a degree of government rate regulation that German bilateral rate negotiation was supposed to avoid.

Reforms. Every proposal sounds good. Tracing the evolution of policy can demonstrate strengths, unexpected outcomes, and weaknesses in a scheme before another country blindly adopts it. Case studies also show that the reforms enacted do not represent ideal solutions but, rather, are compromises among competing interests. Since every major hospital reform affects a significant share of the nation's economy, the debate and the solutions involve shifts in the functions of government.

Capital investment was partially redesigned in Germany after 1984, but only after a general consensus that KHG could no longer be implemented well, and only after compromise positions could be devised among the national government, the provinces, the sickness funds, and the hospital association.[24]

- *National-provincial sharing of costs.* Germany follows Canada and the United States in a cycle apparently endemic to federal systems. At first health is an exclusive provincial responsibility, but health services seem under-funded. The national government agrees to pay a fixed share of certain operating or capital costs that soon become very ambitious. The subsidized sector grows—as it was expected to do—but the national government complains about unlimited commitments and about provincial wastefulness. After much dispute the national government transfers the full program responsibility and financial burden back to the provinces. As the price for avoiding unlimited proportionate cost sharing, the national government is forced to agree to annual fixed block grants to the provinces. During a transitional period until full provincial capital funding, the *Bund* must pay fixed block grants to the *Länder* under the reforms.
- *Distribution formulas.* Distribution formulas from the German *Länder* to the hospitals were left to the discretion of the provinces. They need not give fixed amounts of capital per bed. The perverse incentives to retain excessive beds disappear, and *Länder* might even offer rewards for reductions. In plans and capital grants, Germany might develop a diversity among the provinces heretofore avoided.
- *Dual financing.* Dual financing—that is, operating costs from the sickness funds and capital costs from provincial government grants—was preserved. But the sickness funds and individual hospitals were authorized to negotiate voluntary capital surcharges on the *Pflegesätze*. This scope for innovation was another step back from the standardization of previous years.

Some Judgments About the German Approach to Planning and Capital Grants.

☐ Reliance on public funds for hospital investment grants makes some sort of planning inevitable. At the minimum, this is a method of prioritizing public grants among existing and proposed hospitals. But if the society operates normally by private enterprise and by private market relations—even a society, such as Germany, that enacts many legal rules about these relations—public planning is very limited, and its political survival is precarious. If hospital managers self-finance capital through charitable donations or user charges, no facilities planning exists.

☐ Effective planning requires consensus and political will. Otherwise, the health care system cannot be regulated and regionalized. The conditions for such systems planning are absent in Germany. Even its planning of priorities in public grants is limited and uncoercive.

☐ Effective planning requires leadership by the national government. It is possible only in those federal systems that permit strong initiatives by the national government and that have a strong multipartisan consensus for efficient regional organization in health. Germany demonstrates that federal-provincial rivalries keep planning weak: hospitals get grants with few obligations under the plans.

☐ Federal-provincial conflicts eventually work to the disadvantage of hospitals. Politicians tire of health care as troublesome. Funding suffers.

☐ Formulas cannot successfully settle the distribution of investment funds. Evaluating needs and setting priorities require judgments about health, about community resources, and about political forces.

☐ Planning formulas tend to rely on gross and familiar variables, such as bed size. If more beds bring large capital grants, the formulas discourage cooperation with cost-containment strategies that try to reduce inpatient acute capacity.

☐ Without determined government regulation, it is very difficult to reduce excess capacity in a privately owned hospital sector. Facilities plans are usually oriented toward expansion rather than reduction. Facilities planning is poorly connected to cost containment, except in the few countries where the national government directs the planning, owns and manages the hospitals, and provides money for both investment and operations. Germany is not such a country.

☐ Germany originally intended to reduce beds by admitting the larger and better hospitals to the plans, excluding the smaller and simpler, and starving the latter for capital. But these methods were ineffective. Many smaller hospitals were admitted to the plans in overbedded provinces, because they enjoyed political support from the confessional associations owning them, from their communities, and from the sickness funds. Even if smaller hospitals are excluded from the provincial government's plans, they can survive, because the sickness funds may agree to pay for inpatients' care and medical fees and because office doctors prefer to send the patients there, where they can treat their own patients and bill separately under fee schedules. In Germany, as in many other countries, facilities planning and reimbursement are not coordinated. If plans are supposed to contain costs by reducing capacity, the only direct instruments are to revoke the licenses of surplus hospitals, revise the licensed capacity of surviving hospitals, and forbid reimbursement for care.

□ Coordination with reimbursement of operating costs is essential if plans are to be implemented, excess capacity reduced, and costs contained. German government planners cannot prevent the sickness funds from paying for care in hospitals that the planners wish to starve. Under private law the sickness funds are free to contract with any hospital, including those omitted from the plans. Sickness funds are pressed by their subscribers to cover care where they want to go, and the subscribers prefer local establishments to the fancier ones farther away. Sickness funds may even prefer treatment in smaller hospitals, since the daily charges—that is, their payouts—are lower. The sickness funds feel no obligation to implement the *Länder's* plans, since they do not participate in the design of the plans and the *Länder* have persistently opposed legislation giving them a role. The *Länder* argue that planning is exclusively a task of provincial governments. The original advocates of planning and the original designers of KHG (particularly the Social Democratic Party) hoped that the system would eliminate Germany's many hospitals smaller than one hundred beds, but they have been disappointed.

□ Top-down global budgeting of capital funds is one method of integrating grants and plans and is the best method of making the government's capital grants predictable. Global amounts would be distributed among regions to match resources to needs, and to correct underprovision. But distribution within each region would require judgments by grantors. Such a system— proposed by some reformers in Germany—is incompatible with the hospitals' demands for autonomy. Major reforms in planning and granting require big changes in government and ideology.

□ If the policy goal is to locate heavy equipment in the most strategic places and to control the costs of technology, facilities planning should include physicians' office practices and not only hospitals. One reason for the prosperity of German office doctors is their ability under their reimbursement system to buy and amortize advanced equipment freely, while the nonprofit and public hospitals cannot do so. By 1984 office doctors alone or in shared arrangements owned nearly one-third of the country's CT scanners and nearly half of the country's gamma cameras.[25] Enacting laws to plan and regulate office practice— a form of small business conducted by one of society's supreme elites—is more difficult politically than imposing planning on hospitals.

Government Grants to Independent Hospitals in Switzerland

Switzerland demonstrates how certain features found in Germany recur when public money is used for investment in a privately owned hospital sector in a federal country. When government becomes a principal source of money for construction and heavy equipment, facilities planning inevitably develops. In federal systems each province asserts its traditional authority over hospital affairs, no national plans or coordination among provincial plans develop, and facilities on opposite sides of provincial boundaries are poorly coordinated.

On the other hand, Switzerland has a less legalistic political culture than Germany has, with fewer punctilious written definitions of rights and powers. (Switzerland is one of the few Western European countries not transformed under Napoleon.) The social and political systems are based on informal negotiation and consensus, harmony rather than conflicts. Public grants therefore are made by discussion and judgment, rather than by automatic formulas. Civil servants and hospital managers are not adversaries.

Switzerland has always avoided the national-provincial shared-cost programs that have proved so contentious and financially disappointing in Germany and in other federal countries. Swiss grants come entirely from provincial governments. Germany includes proprietary hospitals in the official plans and public investment grants, but Switzerland and most other countries do not.

Development of Provincial Grants. Once Swiss hospital owners and managers bought whatever new buildings and equipment they could afford. Often they found the money in advance, or they borrowed from banks and repaid interest and principal from income earned from patients. But these debts made hospitals increasingly dependent on cantonal (provincial) governments. Banks often insisted that the governments guarantee the loans, and the cantons began to audit the hospitals' finances. Deficits resulted from increased operating costs, from downturns in the economy, and from refusal of the increasingly important sickness funds to share the costs of debt service. The hospitals then sought subsidies from cantonal and local governments.

A trend is toward payment for new buildings and for substantial new equipment from cantonal funds. Decisions are supposed to be made by the cantonal officials in advance, according to priorities and on the basis of extensive documentation. Payment is made in full. (Therefore, as in all systems of public grants, no interest and amortization need appear in the budget for operating expenses. However, as I said in Chapter Three, end-of-the-year cost reports were amended during the 1980s to include depreciation as a measure of the consumption of capital.) Not all cantons have such advance screening and advance payment of large capital items, although perhaps all will in the future.

Since hospitals traditionally received philanthropic grants, they still can receive them for buildings and equipment, thus avoiding complete dependence on the cantonal government. But the cantonal officials must conclude that the investment serves the public interest, in order to allow the operating cost of the item in the prospective budget for rate setting.

Planning. After World War II, each cantonal government was pressed not merely to buy the newest buildings and equipment for its own teaching hospitals but also to install the newest buildings and equipment in *all* hospitals. If one hospital got something new, the others wanted it too. Smaller ones wished to rise to the eminence of the larger, by matching the services of the larger. Doctors wanted available the new techniques they had learned at the teaching hospitals.

The cantonal governments needed some rationale for distributing their investments and for controlling operating costs, and nearly all included planning clauses in their statutes concerning the regulation and subsidization of hospitals. By now, except for a few eastern Alpine cantons with very few hospitals, all have hospital plans. They were written by advisory commissions staffed by employees of the cantonal Departments of Health or by officials of the department with the help of outside consultants (sometimes management consulting firms) for the research. Many have been submitted to the Parliaments of their cantons (the *Grosse Rat* or *Grand Conseil*), debated, and adopted as laws. They govern how the cantons manage their own hospitals and how the cantonal Departments of Health distribute their capital grants and operating subsidies to the other hospitals.[26]

An important function of the hospital plan is stating the mission of each hospital in a coordinated division of labor within the canton. The services are specified; the personnel and types of equipment for each hospital are outlined. The goal is to concentrate expensive programs in the fewest places, rather than allowing a wide spread of expensive and underused equipment and personnel.

A weakness in hospital planning is its completely cantonal basis. The separate plans are not coordinated. The national government contributes no investment money, and there are no national plans. Two nearby hospitals can have considerable duplication, because they stand on opposite sides of a boundary between cantons.

Collecting Requests Within the Hospital. The annual cycle for preparing budgets and requests is familiar; so, as the cantonal government (during July) sends out its forms to the individual hospitals, the hospitals have already begun the calculations for next year. The finance director of the hospital has already asked the chiefs of service to submit requests for new equipment and for new construction. Small items, up to a maximum prescribed in the canton's guidelines, come out of an aggregate sum in the operating budget. Larger items must be submitted individually to the cantonal government, along with the hospital's next budget for operating costs.

As in every country with discretionary methods of allocating capital, each Swiss hospital must develop an internal system for deciding priorities. In the smaller hospitals, the director simply talks to his chiefs of service (the *chefärzte*). A more formal procedure exists in the larger hospitals—particularly in teaching hospitals, which lead in installing new equipment. The director usually sends several blank forms to each chief. The chief in turn discusses possible requests with his own medical staff. On each form one item of equipment is specified, often with the following information: manufacturer; cost; reason for purchase; and additional costs that would result for the personnel, materials, space, power, and so on. The forms do not ask about new income generated by the new equipment—such as more treatments under health insurance—but an enterprising service chief may include it in his "hard sell." In several cantons (such as Bern), the form asks the service chief to rate the priority for the item. In some other cantons (such as Zurich), the form asks the service chief to compare his total spending for new equipment for the next year and for several earlier years.

Submitting Requests to the Canton. Some hospitals screen the requests and try to send to the canton a "reasonable" total, close to the figure that the Department of Health informally confided. But in some teaching hospitals with powerful chiefs of service, such as those in Zurich, the hospital's managers pass nearly all the requests on to the cantonal government and let the officials take the heat.

Rather than burden the cantonal officials with applications for every item of equipment and construction, the hospital submits only the larger items for special funding; each item is submitted to the canton on a separate sheet, called in several cantons an *Investitionsgesuch.* For example, in Bern's preparation for the 1980 budget, individual applications had to be filled out for any new construction over Fr 25,000 and any new equipment over Fr 15,000. Everything smaller could be grouped under the miscellaneous investments category in the hospital's operating budget, totaling (for Bern canton's largest hospital) Fr 4 million. The governing board of the hospital decides which small requests go into the miscellaneous investments category. If the hospital does not use up this figure with its small requests, it can use the money to pay for a larger item, instead of submitting it separately to the cantonal government and facing possible rejection.

Most cantons pay for the larger items out of general revenue. A few have special funds earmarked for new hospital construction and for equipment. An example is Bern; between 1974 and 1986, it had a fund destined for hospital equipment and construction, accumulated from one-tenth of a percentage point added to all income taxes in the canton. Since the construction of new hospitals had stopped, this *Spitalzehntal* yielded too much money, but it could not legally be used for operating costs.

Cantons vary widely in the size of the investment subsidy from the cantonal government. Existence of a special fund enables a cantonal government to pay a larger proportion; for example, Bern pays 70 percent, and the hospital owners must find the rest. Other cantonal governments contribute half or less. The owners—that is, local governments or nonprofit private groups—pay their shares, either by raising the cash in advance or by borrowing from a bank. If the money is borrowed, the cantonal government probably and the sickness funds definitely would not allow inclusion of interest and amortization in the daily patient charges.

The canton pays for all new equipment and construction costs in the hospitals that it owns.

If the cost of reconstructing a nonprofit or public hospital is very large, the question is submitted to the electorate at the next cantonal election. But since populations want the best in health care, the proposal usually wins.

In several cantons the Division of Hospitals has an advisory commission to comment on its hospitals plan and to discuss applications by individual hospitals for cantonal subsidization of new construction and of new equipment. In Bern the *Spital- und Heimkommission* was created by the hospitals law of December 1973 and consists of leading hospital directors and architects. It is advisory—the division in Bern sets priorities and makes the grants—but ensures the fairness and technical merit of the awards. It also insulates the division from the political blame when the division turns down a request—particularly in the light of money unspent from the *Spitalzehntal*.

Every hospital sends an *Investitionsgesuch* along with its annual prospective operating budget. In addition, a few large teaching hospitals submit an interim list of requests during the year. They can add a new service or a new research project without waiting until the next year, or they can replace a machine that broke down.

Connections Between Construction and Paying for Operating Costs. A common problem in the financing of hospitals in the world is the diffusion of authority and of decisions. Hospital planners, as in the United States, may have little control over construction and cannot implement their plans. If hospitals can be reimbursed for any operating costs, plans and construction controls will be ineffective. If the same agency—for instance, the cantonal governments of Switzerland or the national government of Great Britain—pays for both the capital grants and the operating costs, that agency evaluates the investment proposal in the light of the additional operating costs. If the payers differ, the grantor of capital does not think beyond the investment grant.

Swiss Departments of Health try to fit some of these financing decisions together. If the department has refused to subsidize acquisition of a new piece of equipment, by implication it refuses to subsidize the operating costs. But not absolutely. When the auditors review an operating budget, they sometimes detect salaries and materials for the use of certain equipment that they had turned down in an earlier year's *Investitionsgesuch*. The hospital director or the chief of service had purchased the equipment and started the program with money raised elsewhere. The hospital renews its case for the program; often the canton's auditors and their superiors in the Department of Health give in and agree to subsidize those items in the operating costs.

Several French-speaking cantons have multilateral commissions that make all decisions about hospital finance and therefore can coordinate them. (One of their tasks is to direct the *centrales* described in Chapter Eight.) The members of the commissions represent the canton's hospital association, medical association, sickness funds, and government. Vaud's hospitals law in 1980 gave its commission power to write plans and pass on all applications for new construction and equipment. Even though they do not write and approve plans, the commissions in Valais and Neuchâtel are the sites for negotiating the daily rate paid by the sickness funds to the hospitals; also, they discuss the offers and responses for the cantonal governments' subsidies of the hospital deficits not covered by insurance payments and by patients' out-of-pockets.

The Valais and Neuchâtel commissions review the hospitals' applications to the cantons for grants for construction and heavy equipment, and the cantonal governments are unlikely to grant their own money without the commissions' approval. Even if the hospital looks for a private grant, it is wise to seek the commission's blessing, since the commission later must approve the hospital's operating budget.

A Public Revolving Fund in France

Almost all public capital grants programs consist of unilateral gifts. The nonprofit or municipal owner of the hospital acquires the money and becomes the owner of the new building or new equipment. The grants are not repaid. Small lines for interest and depreciation are in the prospective budget for operating costs, sufficient only for the costs of short-term bank loans to cover cash flow and purchase of small equipment with short lives. Depreciation is not allowed in prospective budgets for items bought under the public grants, since the items would then be paid for twice, once by the government and the second time by the sickness fund.

France illustrates the possibility of repayable grants for much new construction and heavy equipment. The money comes from special public funds and is given only for proposals consistent with plans. The hospital eventually returns the money, so others can use it. Amortization is recognized as a cost in the prospective budget and is included in the daily charges paid by the sickness funds. The method transfers the costs of hospital capital from the general taxpayers to the payers of social security payroll taxes.

Development of Planning. The loans are made under strict surveillance as if they were grants. As in all systems using public money for hospital construction and heavy equipment, plans govern the decisions. France evolved one of the more sophisticated methods of writing plans and one of the more effective methods for implementing them. But French experience has been disappointing, demonstrating weaknesses in traditional methods and difficulties in implementing any kind of health care planning.

Since the safety of the public has been at risk, government for many years has had the authority to examine an individual hospital's plans, to reject them, and thereby to forbid new construction or expansion.[27] These powers have been lodged in the corps of medical inspectors placed by the Ministry of Health in the region. Their judgments are reviewed by advisory commissions in the regions and in Paris. The country's health code flatly states that no new hospital may be opened (whether public or private) and no beds added without written authorization by the Minister of Health; trying to open without authorization is a crime punishable by fines and imprisonment. The statute has long given the Minister economic as well as clinical grounds for rejection: the proposal can be refused if it "does not satisfy technical conditions required or if the needs of the catchment area in health facilities, both concerning what is commonly called medical installations as well as the means for hospitalizing patients, can be viewed as sufficient" (*Code de la Santé Publique,* Livre VII, Art. L. 734-2 and 734-3). Detailed interpretations have been decided by the *Conseil d'Etat,* the country's highest court.

At first the negative powers were used sparingly. After World War II, everyone saw a need for more and modern hospital beds, but the public and private sectors lacked enough money for large growth. Old buildings were modernized inexpensively, and a few new buildings were started. A handful of researchers in the Ministry of Health began to draw up maps (*cartes sanitaires*) to identify areas of shortage, and the Ministry used its powers of authorization to direct public money into underserved areas.

During the 1960s utilization of health services greatly increased, the revenue from premiums enabled the sickness funds and *mutuelles* to pay more, public funds had much more money for investment, and health became a good investment for private banks. The principal health-planning task of the past was expansion from a low base, with differential investment, so the least served areas could be raised most. New planning problems now existed: how to identify when "enough" had been reached; how to change the flow of resources from a massively favored sector (public and private acute beds) to very different ones (such as nursing homes, ambulatory services, or home care); how to arrest the concentration of resources in the largest cities and set targets in other areas.

Payers in France were among the first in any country to believe that excessive beds produce excessive stays and financial waste, that limiting the number of beds is a key to controlling the country's hospital costs. Many communities seemed to the officials and sickness funds to have "enough" or even "too many" beds, and the rudimentary statistical indicators published by the

Ministry were said to "prove" this. The existing public hospitals and private clinics were still trying to expand—as usual, the most profitable communities for new facilities are the rich ones that are already well provided—and an entire new generation of new and technically advanced private clinics was being designed. The officials in the Ministry of Health and in the sickness funds urged the regional inspectors and the Minister to reject many construction proposals, because the statistical norms were already satisfied. Spirited debates occurred in small meetings and within the regional and national advisory commissions over the reliability of the gross statistical norms as statements of needs in general, and over their application to specific communities and to particular construction proposals. The debate raised the familiar problem of investment planning: how to make accurate forecasts for the medium-term and long-term future.[28]

The debate did not paralyze decision making. Uncertainties over the grounds for regulation can lead to court injunctions that suspend implementation in the United States, but not in France. As the private clinics grew, the Ministry turned down an increasing proportion of their proposals; otherwise, the for-profit sector would have expanded even more. About 60 percent of the proposed beds were approved from 1959 through 1964, but by the late 1960s the annual approval rate was only one-third. In particular, new expansion in obstetrics was limited—less than one-fifth per year by the late 1960s.[29] The appeals committee in the Ministry tried to condition some approvals on mergers, on the grounds that satisfactory work in each service required a minimum bed size and that small clinics were technically obsolete.

The Hospital Law of 1970 and the implementing decrees were supposed to introduce order and eliminate waste and duplication, both to improve service and to control costs. Planning became much more careful; the *carte sanitaire* used precisely delineated regional and local boundaries; a thorough inventory of present resources was made in both the public and private sectors; and enough personnel and advisory committees were created to think carefully about needs. France has been divided into 256 health districts for the inventory, each with about 200,000 inhabitants. Norms are specified by statistical indicators—that is, ratios of beds to population and other data. Planning no longer is confined to beds and buildings but includes heavy equipment, since by 1970 it was clearly capable of setting off its own cost explosion. The same logic is used as in the case of beds: installation by a private clinic of various pieces of "heavy equipment" (cobalt bombs, linear accelerators, autoanalyzers, scanners, and so on) requires the approval of the regional inspector and the regional prefect, with possible appeal to the Minister; anyone who installs such equipment in a public hospital or private clinic without authorization risks fines, seizure of the equipment, and certainly its exclusion from the *prix de journée*. The planning is implemented through a "public hospital service," which incorporates all nonprofit hospitals and takes advantage of selected capabilities of private clinics. Private nonprofit and for-profit hospitals that do not serve the planned goals of the public hospital service are expected to become marginal; they would depend on whatever rates the increasingly thrifty sickness funds would give them, and they would become so starved that they could no longer duplicate the public service. Patients still have the legal right to go to a private clinic, but the public service gets most of the investment and operating money.[30]

Creation of Proposals. The mayor and other politicians in the *commune* seek improvements in their buildings and facilities in all their sectors, including their hospitals. In the past they and the chiefs of service developed proposals unsystematically; the DDASS and the prefect approved proposals that seemed reasonably designed and financially feasible, and the mayor turned to the national government and local sources for funding. (The clinical chiefs were not always enthusiastic: if the public hospital was underdeveloped, patients with money went instead to their private clinics.) After World War II, a professionally trained cadre of hospital managers filled posts in the public hospitals; one of their tasks was writing management plans for each establishment (*plans directeurs*). The clinical chiefs became full-timers committed to modernizing the public hospitals, and every establishment developed proposals for new construction and improved programs. The proposals are approved by the governing board. New construction must conform to the *carte sanitaire*. If it does not, the prefect—who exercises legal oversight over the public hospitals—refuses to approve the minutes of the board meeting, and the hospital will not be permitted to seek funding.[31]

Requests for new equipment originate within the medical staff in France, much as they do in the Swiss hospitals described previously. Once every chief of service approached the mayor and local *notables* on the governing board separately and secretly. The chiefs competed among themselves for help in funding. The modernization of hospital management included creation of medical staff committees, one of whose tasks is to establish priorities among the applications of the individual chiefs.[32] Unusually expensive equipment must conform to the norms in the *carte sanitaire;* that is, the hospital can seek new linear accelerators, dialysis machines, CT scanners, and the like, only if the regional quota has not yet been filled, where the limit is one machine for each 10,000 or 100,000 inhabitants. Equipment not limited in the planning laws can be sought freely by the hospital. Requests for new equipment are approved by the hospital's governing board and—if they accept the board's minutes—by the DDASS and the prefect. The hospital may seek funding.

Money for Investment in Public Hospitals. Once public hospitals depended on gifts from private citizens for new buildings and new equipment, and the private nonprofits continued to do so until recently. Well-endowed hospitals ploughed the profits from farming, industry, and rents back into buildings and equipment. During the late nineteenth and twentieth centuries, the endowments were sold off for investment money. Local governments were expected to contribute, some giving more than others. Influential local politicians, such as mayors serving as national Ministers, extracted subsidies from the national government. As the sickness funds accumulated money, some gave subsidies to public hospitals to ensure good care for their members. *Communes* began to rely for investment money on loans from a larger revolving fund (called the *Caisse des Dépôts et Consignations*), created from many types of collections from the general public, including taxes; and the hospital governing boards turned to this larger fund for loans.[33] Investment funding was very unsystematic and until recently resulted in underfinancing rather than in duplication, in fancy amenities, and in waste.

By the 1960s investment money no longer came primarily from gifts and subsidies but from loans: some from the *Caisse des Dépôts* and some from the special social assistance funds of the regional CRAMs, called the *Fonds d'Action Sanitaire et Sociale*. (The CRAMs are the regional coordinating offices of the principal regime in the national health insurance system.) The CRAMs by the 1960s had decided that, if the public hospital repaid the *Caisse des Dépôts*, it could certainly repay them. Some money still came from "self-financing": the hospital's amortization under the *prix de journée* might have created a capital fund; the hospital might still earn profits from its endowment; some small transfers might be obtained from the *commune*. Enterprising hospital directors, service chiefs, and mayors might still extract subsidies from the national government if the construction project made a notable contribution to medical education, to medical research, or (sometimes) to the political popularity of the President, Prime Minister, and Ministers in that region. Money from all sources increased during the construction boom of the 1960s and 1970s, but the biggest growth came from the most flexible source, borrowing. Hospitals seemed to become such a good investment, as amortization and interest charges were automatically included in the *prix de journée*, that even commercial banks began to offer loans to the once threadbare public hospitals. Since the early 1960s, the distribution of sources for public hospitals outside Paris has been:[34]

	1962	1972	1979
Loans	25%	44%	46%
Subsidies from government	34	22	18
Self-financing by hospital	28	29	34
Sale of endowment	13	5	2
	100%	100%	100%
Total in millions of francs	(753)	(2,635)	(8,402)

As in several other countries, the self-financing under the old daily charge system and under the new global grants system furnishes the money to replace small obsolescent equipment. The loans and subsidies are for new equipment. However, the distinction blurs, since much old medical equipment is replaced by more elaborate and far more expensive items, requiring new borrowing. The amortization and depreciation covered by the pre-1983 daily charge and by the new global grants are used not only for routine small replacements but also to pay off debt.

Planning, the approval of proposals, and funding are not synonymous. The construction of facilities and the installation of heavy equipment must conform to the limits in the *carte sanitaire*, but most equipment is exempt. If the DDASS and the prefect agree to the investment proposals in the governing board's minutes, funding is not guaranteed; instead, the hospital's leadership must find it. Grantors may not provide money, and the hospital's board and managers must then decide whether they can carry additional debt in their operating costs. When screening the prospective budget, the DDASS may not agree to substantially higher operating costs from excessive debt, although the

DDASS once usually agreed to moderate increases. Even if the hospital tries to borrow, it may not find a favorable loan. Grants and loan funds fluctuate from year to year in France, depending on the state of the revenue of governments and of the CRAMs.

All buildings and equipment are depreciated at original cost by the straight-line method. The accounting regulations—mentioned in Chapters Three and Seven—give minimum and maximum expected lines for each class of items, and the hospital director chooses the figure. In cost-center accounting, capital costs are attributed to the clinical service or services that use the construction and equipment. Each year's prospective budget automatically includes amortization and interest charges for previous debt.[35]

Since amortization has been based on original costs rather than replacement costs, and since the prices of medical technology have moved up rapidly, replacement necessitates new borrowing of much greater size and therefore requires much higher revenue. The growth of outright grant money has lagged behind the growth in investment costs, and has resulted in the increase in borrowing mentioned above. Debt service was one of the several sources of hospital cost increases that the French government and the sickness funds started to combat during the late 1970s. If daily rates or global grants are kept down by public policy, hospitals deteriorate in their capital position.[36]

During the 1980s all aspects of French hospital finance, including planning and hospital investment, were rethought. Plans in the future might be implemented more directly, by direct government grants for approved projects, instead of individual repayable loans from revolving funds. Government would have not only a capital plan but a capital fund. Hospitals would no longer be saddled with debts—sometimes imprudently incurred—and capital obligations would no longer push up operating costs. Anticipating such a trend toward public grants, the CRAMs during the 1980s reduced their new loans to the public hospitals.

Money for Investment in Private Clinics. New clinics were created during the 1960s, and old ones were merged, expanded, and modernized. CRAMs were permissive in granting *prix de journée,* which covered amortization and interest. The owners usually could not get low-interest loans from the *Caisse des Dépôts* or from the CRAMs, and they relied on commercial banks. Often the individual doctors contributed investment money from family wealth or by personal borrowing from banks. Private clinics seemed a good investment during the 1960s: utilization grew, more people were covered by national health insurance, the *prix de journée* at that time guaranteed capital costs, and the fees for clinical acts and for use of the operating theater and delivery room rewarded heavy use of the most expensive equipment.

The national leadership of the sickness funds was exceedingly displeased at the prosperity of the private clinics,[37] the annual cap on charges (described in Chapter Six) was installed after 1968, and the cap tightened (with the encouragement of the Ministry of Budget) during the middle and late 1970s. The cap ensured that the *prix de journée* for the private clinics no longer rose as fast as annual replacement costs for new equipment, particularly when doctors were pressing to reduce expected lives of equipment. The private clinics could self-finance less equipment than before. Managers of the larger private clinics pressed the participating doctors for larger transfers from their gross earnings, earmarked for the investment account. This trend began to remedy the sickness funds' complaint that they had long been paying for equipment use twice—once in the private clinics' daily charges and again in the practice costs calculated under the physicians' fees.

At the same time as the reimbursement squeeze on the private clinics' investment resources, government regulators seemed to be turning down a greater number of their construction and equipment requests. But the number has not been estimated. Probably lenders were now frightened away from a sector with declining capacity to repay.

Some Judgments About French Planning. The French did not merely write plans but enacted and implemented them. Theirs was the most successful example of old-fashioned health planning. In retrospect, the method was too limited, and the French reforms of the 1980s included a new start. Following are some of the defects in the earlier approach:

☐ *Scope.* As in most countries, planning was implemented only for beds and equipment in hospitals in acute care and in a few specialized fields, such as psychiatry. The *cartes sanitaires* included numbers of professional personnel and some other facilities, but these categories were not affected by the plans themselves. France's medical profession would not cooperate. But true health care planning requires regionalization and coordination of all services.

☐ *Orientation.* The plans focused on bed/population ratios and on machine/population ratios. Such ratios are designed only to decide whether more beds and equipment should be installed in an area, or whether there were enough. The planning did not deal with flows of work.

☐ *Needs.* Size of population determined norms. French planning lacked other estimates of the population's needs. The ratio between sizes of catchment areas and large equipment was not explained; therefore, numbers of authorized machines (such as the confusing case of CT scanners) fluctuated when the Ministry of Health changed leadership.

☐ *Reductions.* The plans set limits on growth but were not addressed to reductions or closures of obsolete or excessive facilities. Criteria for reductions were lacking. Legal authority did not exist to condition new loans or grants on the closing or conversion of old facilities.

☐ *Coordination of decisions.* Planners, implementers, and funders were different people and were poorly coordinated. The planners set regional statistical norms but did not review proposals. Review of conformity to planned norms and approval of the hospital's proposals were left to each individual DDASS. The hospital had discretion about where to search for money, but final implementation was left to the priorities of the grantors or lenders. Funding might overlook highly desirable projects and go to lesser ones.

☐ *Screening method.* The screening method lacked discretion. If the bed/population or machine/population limits had not yet been reached, the DDASS must authorize the next proposal received in the mail. The planners and DDASS could not commission the best facility to undertake the project.

☐ *Individual proposals.* Each hospital developed its proposal independently and secretly. Others that could collaborate or might be better qualified were not consulted.

☐ *Coordination of clinics and hospitals.* Private clinics and the public hospitals were not coordinated under the plans. Grants and the most favorable loans went only to the public hospitals and to the private nonprofits that were accepted into the official hospital service.

☐ *Political influence.* Hospitals with influential sponsors occasionally obtained approval to build or modernize beds exceeding the norms. (Political influence was valuable even more often in obtaining funding for projects conforming to the plans.)

Self-Financing in the United States

Most developed countries finance hospital investment through public grants. France has either grants or loans from public funds that are administered much like grant programs. Grants programs invariably bring planning and public oversight, but their implementation varies with political will and with the urgency of hospital cost containment. The strictness and clarity of public oversight are weakened by diffused authority, such as the national-provincial division in Germany. Hospitals may have more success in funding their proposals if they can shop among several sources, as they can in France. Many hospital managers search for methods that will protect their autonomy and increase their revenue.

Tables are turned in the United States and the Netherlands. Hospitals have been able to raise their own money for investment and have been able to maintain independence from government controls. Planning hardly exists.

Development in the United States. Once every country had mixed financing, for capital as well as for operating costs. As philanthropy declined, all countries relied more on public grants for new construction, renovation, heavy equipment, and major new programs.

The United States at first followed these trends but then moved in the opposite direction during the 1960s. The rapid and extensive changes have made hospital capital financing one of the most volatile sectors in American health care. During the 1920s, 90 percent of the money for new construction in America came from private philanthropy and from local government.[38] After World War II, the United States had one of the first major programs of government grants for new construction.[39] But debt financing rose during the 1960s and, as Table 9-1 shows, took over almost completely by the 1980s, when government grants had nearly ended.[40]

The American development resulted from the unexpected convergence of several events during the 1960s:

- Costs of new buildings and equipment mounted. New technology had steadily shorter useful lives, and its costs were outstripping the financial capacities of philanthropy. New plant and equipment prices exceeded the hospital's depreciation based on the historical costs of the original assets.
- Borrowing became more feasible. The new cost reimbursers—Medicare, Medicaid, and Blue Cross—recognized as allowable costs interest on debts

Table 9-1. New Construction and Renovation in Community Hospitals Owned by Voluntary Associations, Investors, and Local Governments.

Sources of funds for construction	Projects completed in 1968	Projects begun in 1981
Government	23.2%	3.5%
Philanthropy	21.2	4.2
Debt	16.1	75.8
Internal operations (accumulated earnings, owners' equity)	38.2	16.5
	100.0%	100.0%

Source: American Hospital Association's biennial survey of new construction.

incurred for the purchase of equipment used in patient care, depreciation of equipment and buildings at more than historical cost, and some extras that could be deposited in the hospital's investment fund.[41] Tax rulings authorized state and local governments to help nonprofit hospitals raise money by creating special agencies that issued tax-free bonds, with proceeds earmarked for the hospitals. According to the American Hospital Association's biennial survey, such tax-exempt borrowing paid for 60 percent of all construction projects begun by nonprofit hospitals in 1981.

- Lenders judged hospitals an excellent risk, as more of the patients were covered by cost reimbursers who recognized investment costs and by charge payers who paid more than costs of care. Repayment of the revenue bonds was virtually guaranteed: the state or local government financing authority issued the bonds, the hospital pledged its revenue to retire the bonds according to a schedule, and the authority had title to the hospital until the bonds were retired.[42]

- Interest costs to the hospital were lower than if it borrowed by the usual private instruments, since owners of the bonds were exempt from income taxes on the interest they received.

- A great variety of fund-raising methods were devised—such as long-term debt, short-term debt, installment loans, and accumulated reserves—and the hospital managers could combine all of them to finance the construction and varied equipment required by a new program. Tax-exempt revenue bonds became the principal source for construction, but the funding of equipment has been heterogeneous.[43]

To survive and prosper, managers of all American nonprofit and for-profit hospitals had to develop strategic orientations different from those in any other country, except for the managers of the few large proprietary hospitals abroad.[44] European hospital managers are concerned with stability, serving the patient flow predicted in the short run, and avoiding a deficit; but the American managers are concerned with survival and growth in the long term as well as in the short, in the face of competitors who consistently challenge for market share. The American hospital manager must avoid drops in utilization and revenue since then he cannot meet his payroll or his fixed costs (particularly repayment of earlier debt), and the hospital will go bankrupt. The hospital cannot stand still, lest doctors move their practices and patients to the more modern establishments.[45] The management must keep up with a steadily accelerating technology, buying whatever new equipment and new programs seem likely to pay off by pleasing the more enterprising members of the medical staff and by expanding the numbers of patients. Each hospital management wants a free hand to develop its own strategies, to borrow and buy whatever it wants. No management is happy with subordination to facilities plans of government. None willingly joins sharing agreements with other hospitals if it can control the program or capture the market entirely by itself. As in all competitive markets, hospitals in the same catchment area rush to install identical or incrementally better technology and programs, resulting in a proliferation of the same equipment and programs inconceivable abroad.[46]

Borrowing for the new heavy equipment and for the attendant construction is prudent if the procedures will be used often enough at high reimbursement rates to amortize the debt and yield a profit. But borrowing can boomerang if the total market is too small, if the payers reimburse at low levels, or if competing hospitals install the identical programs and capture a substantial share of the market. Therefore, when they plan to purchase new construction or expensive new equipment, American managers perform formal or intuitive financial feasibility studies to estimate the size of the debt they can amortize under the revenue they expect during the life of the debt. The feasibility study highlights expected utilization by patients in the catchment area, their profitability as measured by types of third-party coverage, the willingness of local physicians to refer various types of patients to that hospital, and the prospective competition from other hospitals.[47]

The American capital market has screening mechanisms that assure lenders that hospitals are one of the best investments. Whenever a substantial new offering is made, the general bond-rating agencies—Standard and Poor's and Moody's—investigate the hospital and any public authority issuing bonds on its behalf. The agencies rank the hospital as a credit risk by the same rating system (for example, Standard and Poor's six categories from AA to BBB) used for all other firms. The rating agencies are concerned with the hospital's capacity to repay, according to the same predictors as in the hospital's own feasibility study— that is, whether the catchment area will yield high utilization by profitable patients; whether the hospital's present medical staff brings in customers; whether other doctors in the catchment area can be attracted to refer more patients; and whether other hospitals will cut into the market.[48]

Another essential part of the American hospital finance system is an equipment industry that can produce a very large number and variety of devices that will pay off, clearing the debts and earning extra revenue before their obsolescence.[49] In their operating capacity and in their potential market demand, the machines must be capable of generating very high utilization shortly after introduction, since competition in the industry generates new improvements. (The cost reimbursers—government and Blue Cross—help the American hospital cope with rapid obsolescence by accepting the accelerated method of depreciation.) An equipment industry that produced only therapeutic equipment would have a limited market for itself and could earn limited amounts for hospitals, since only the truly (or probably) sick can be treated, the patients must agree, and the more advanced treatments cannot easily be repeated on the same patients. Instead, the American equipment industry has been extremely productive in developing diagnostic machines that fit the item-of-service charging methods of hospitals and doctors. The tests can be performed repeatedly on the entire population; both patients and doctors welcome lavish testing. New versions of existing equipment seem to justify price increases; volume grows, particularly if a department has installed a new machine with new capabilities. The volume of tests with apparently modest individual prices makes radiology and pathology the most profitable revenue centers in all American hospitals.[50] In addition to testing equipment, American industry has recently begun to develop implantable medical devices (such as the cardiac pacemaker) that can be marketed very extensively and are very profitable to hospitals and doctors under present reimbursement methods.

The equipment market is very competitive and demonstrates how competition can increase rather than decrease system costs. Hospitals compete for doctors and must install the methods they prefer. The equipment companies compete to market the best and newest instruments; each claims to have the most clinically effective devices, incorporating the newest improvements. The companies must set prices to recapture their R&D, manufacturing costs, and distribution costs in the shortest time; also, they try to earn extra cash for their own debt service, reinvestment, and dividends. Since the hospitals and their leading doctors want the best and newest equipment, and since each company's product is slightly different—that is, it is a market of "monopolistic competition" rather than "imperfect" or "perfect competition"—the sellers at first are not pressed to reduce prices. (Price cuts may occur toward the end to clear inventory in the face of forthcoming better products.) The hospital reimbursement system until the mid-1980s militated against price cutting; cost reimbursers covered the hospitals' purchase and borrowing costs, and fee-for-service motivated doctors to adopt the newest methods.[51] Instead of competing by means of price reductions, companies competed by salesmanship.[52]

Because of the very large and nearly unregulated domestic market, America's medical equipment industry became the largest and most innovative in the world. In 1980 American firms had between 40 and 65 percent of the world's total sales in medical electronics, medical-surgical equipment, dental equipment, nuclear medicine, cardiac monitors, respiratory monitors, biological analyzers, and cardiac pacemakers.[53] Medical equipment manufacture became an important part of the American economy and a lucrative export. In 1982 the United States exported one-third of its domestic production of radiodiagnostic and electrical-medical equipment; from 1972 to 1982, annual increases in exports averaged 30 percent. During this period medical equipment—particularly radiodiagnostics—was one of the few sectors of international merchandise trade where the United States was in surplus rather than in deficit.[54]

Proprietary Hospitals. The for-profits cannot use some investment sources that are open only to the nonprofits—namely, philanthropic gifts, government grants, and tax-exempt bonds issued on the hospital's behalf by local government. Generally, the proprietaries must borrow in the same way that any other for-profit business does—by issuing taxable revenue bonds that will cost them three or more percentage points in interest over the nonprofits' interest costs. The bonds are rated like any other commercial borrowing. The proprietary must impress the underwriters and lenders, by generating a substantial cash flow. The government (Medicare and Medicaid) and Blue Cross for many years complied by providing all for-profit hospitals with a "return on equity" as part of their daily payments for patient care. The government's formulas were very generous.[55] In addition, charges for ancillary services are much higher and more profitable in the proprietaries than in the nonprofit hospitals.[56]

Most American proprietaries are owned by corporations with central offices. Of the 1,045 short-stay and long-stay for-profit hospitals in 1982, 668 were owned by proprietary chains.[57] To repay commercial loans, the chains use profits from sources unavailable to independent private clinics, sources completely exempt from rate regulators and health facilities planners. These sources include the many nursing homes owned by some chains (such as Humana), the extensive ambulatory and home-care programs owned by some chains (such as National Medical Enterprises), and the nonprofit and municipal hospitals that are managed (but not owned) by some chains (such as Hospital Corporation of America and Hyatt). In addition, the corporation can gain a large amount of new capital by selling stock in the stock market, the first time when the owners go public and later when they add holdings to the chain. When some independent proprietary and nonprofit hospitals faced financial squeezes during the late 1970s and 1980s, the chains bought them out, often by trading new stock to the former owners or by selling new stock for cash in the stock market.[58]

When buying goods and services, the proprietary chains often negotiate discounts because of their large volume, while independent nonprofit and proprietary hospitals cannot. Because of their managements' greater skill in business affairs, the chains may be more prudent buyers of construction services and equipment. Compared to the nonprofits' buildings, their construction more often uses standard designs, is completed more quickly, and is cheaper.[59]

The Central Role and Orientation of Managers. The American style of hospital finance is both cause and effect of the country's unusual form of hospital organization. Most doctors are preoccupied with their private office practices, have only loose affiliations with the hospital, and avoid management tasks. The governors visit only occasionally and remain committed primarily to their private businesses and charitable associations. In this structural vacuum, the full-time administrators gained control earlier than in any other country. The first professional programs in hospital administration and in institutional financial management were developed for these administrators. Each manager's career depends on the solvency, growth, and reputation of his own hospital. In contrast, most physicians have multiple affiliations and can easily switch.

American hospital managers have a far bigger voice over investment decisions than their foreign counterparts have. American doctors request new equipment and new programs, and the lay managers must please them, but the managers make the choices. Like anyone who must make investment choices in any business, hospital managers must give the highest priority to those purchases yielding revenue that will pay off the debts and produce surpluses.[60] Potential revenue is certainly in the back of every hospital manager's mind outside the United States, but in America the motive is at the forefront. The manager outside

America cannot earn much additional revenue from new equipment because the nonprofit and public hospitals cannot issue itemized bills for its use; he is not driven to think of amortizing a debt if the country's system gives him grants to buy the new equipment.

Where the medical chiefs of service share responsibility for managing the hospital, as in Europe, they insist on dominating investment decisions, since these choices determine clinical practice. The doctors fix the priority in the use of capital funds, in committees of the chiefs and in plenary meetings of the senior medical staff. Lay managers would imperil their careers if they tried to scuttle the chiefs' clinical priorities in favor of equipment that would merely bring more money into the general budget.

Facilities Planning. The first stages of American health facilities planning resembled the first stages abroad. The Hill-Burton Hospital Construction Program (1947-1974) and the Regional Medical Program (1966-1974) granted government money to nonprofit hospitals and to other nonprofit organizations. Planning agencies were created in states and localities under the national government guidelines, to identify where grants were needed and where they would be unnecessarily duplicative.

Two other health-planning efforts followed, both under the national government's initiative and with the collaboration of state governments. They were the Comprehensive Health Planning Act (1967-1974) and the National Health Planning and Resources Development Act (Public Law 93-641, 1974-1983). They were motivated by the need of the national and state governments to constrain their expenditures, to prevent the privately and municipally owned hospitals from taking too much of their money. The problem was that the hospitals did not depend on government directly for capital grants for building and equipment. But they did collect considerable government money under Medicare and Medicaid for their operating expenditure, and the operating money by statute included all interest and depreciation to repay the costs of construction and equipment. To prevent back-door government financing of buildings and equipment that government never would have paid for up-front, government would screen the investment plans in advance.

Commissions representing several groups (providers, consumers, the medical associations, and others) performed the initial screening of proposed new buildings and proposed new equipment.[61] With the help of guidelines from the national government, their staffs wrote Health Systems Plans for their localities, and the commissions approved them. If a proposed new building or heavy equipment exceeded the level of facilities needed by the area, the commission recommended that the state government—which had the legal power—not issue a Certificate of Need (CON) allowing the hospital to buy it and to charge any interest and depreciation to Medicare and Medicaid. Blue Cross might also refuse to cover the investment costs. Such a reduction in the revenue earmarked for the hospital's debt service made it unlikely that lenders would give the hospital the money to buy the disapproved item.

A Certificate of Need became pivotal to the loan. If the hospital had it, the repayment was guaranteed on time under the operating revenue from the cost reimbursers (Medicare, Medicaid, and Blue Cross) and from the charge payers (privately insured persons and self-payers). If the hospital did not have it, repayment was not guaranteed; instead, the hospital would have to piece the money together from its charge payers and donations. The project's possession of a Certificate of Need was prominently featured in the announcement of the offering, to attract lenders. The public agencies that issued tax-exempt bonds on behalf of the hospitals would do so only for projects that had received CONs. Hospitals could still try to borrow without CONs, but only with conventional mortgage loans secured by the buildings and their revenue, and their interest costs were much higher.

In a nationwide hospital environment oriented toward innovation, there was a presumption that the new project was needed and the CON should be issued. The boards of the planning commissions—under the last statute, they were called Health Systems Agencies, or HSAs—consisted of representatives of hospitals, physicians, and consumers united in favor of progress and the maximum availability of therapies. The requirement to submit credible proposals to screening panels led to better project planning: the equipment companies were expected to demonstrate that the new heavy equipment was clinically effective; the hospital had to explain and cost the project in detail. The CON application made the project more impressive, included crucial utilization and revenue-earning projections, and further guaranteed funding by lenders. Since HSAs and state agencies were more critical of expensive projects, the hospitals were pressured to obtain lower prices from the building contractors and equipment companies. The process was confined to individual districts (the jurisdiction of each HSA) and states; there was no general agency to plan for the country as a whole and to reallocate money and facilities from rich to poor areas. Free-market competition would have accelerated the widespread adoption of clinically effective and economically profitable innovations, such as CT scanners; but the CON process slowed installation, reduced duplication in neighboring hospitals, and forced manufacturers to reduce their prices. (Several companies abandoned their CT scanners, since they could not sell enough at high prices to recoup their R&D and manufacturing costs.)[62]

The HSAs and state planning agencies could not force hospitals to regionalize, but consultations within the HSAs persuaded some to logroll and form divisions of labor. Each might specialize in an advanced program, and each would get from the others support for the CON and borrowing for its own equipment and construction. But these arrangements were voluntary and sometimes only temporary, until the other hospitals could buy the desired equipment and avoid referring their business elsewhere.

American health facilities planning during the 1970s could not control the growth in American health care costs, because the planners did not distribute capital grants, did not set reimbursement rates, and could not require hospitals to share facilities and programs. Instead, the planning apparatus was merely an intermediary filter between the hospital and the source of its money in the private bond market. The methodology and strictness in issuing CONs varied widely among the fifty states.[63] The planning system did not reduce capital growth substantially across the country but only redirected it away from less utilized projects (such as the construction of new beds with uncertain demand and the purchase of duplicative equipment) to projects with an assured market.[64] Without restraint, hospitals under competitive pressure to adopt the newest innovations would have bought much imperfect, ineffective, and expensive equipment. But CONs were not issued widely for an innovation until the manufacturers had developed better and cheaper models.[65]

Therefore, the CON process reduced unwise risks for hospitals and reduced bankruptcies; it inadvertently encouraged more lending and capital growth through its cachet of probable high utilization and full reimbursement. Since American health planning merely interfered with the flow rather than the volume of investment, America has had much wider dissemination of the new equipment than any other country. For example, the numbers of CT scanners per million population in 1979 were:[66]

United States	5.7
West Germany	2.6
Canada	1.7
Sweden	1.7
Netherlands	1.4
United Kingdom	1.0
France	0.6

American facilities planning applied only to hospitals, since the hospitals spent the largest amounts of governmental and insurance money (Medicare, Medicaid, and Blue Cross) and since the medical associations have fought off planning controls even more determinedly than any other government intervention. Therefore, capital was channeled in unusual ways. Groups of office doctors could borrow and buy equipment without needing CONs, and many installed equipment that was more likely to be found only in hospitals overseas. Lest their CONs be denied or delayed, many hospital-based physicians— particularly radiologists and pathologists—created professional corporations nominally independent of their hospitals, borrowed and bought advanced equipment quickly, continued to practice as if they were still officially intramural, and billed the third parties and the hospitals. While the professional corporations had to pay higher interest for their loans, they could easily amortize in a few years from their weakly controlled fees and skyrocketing utilization. Nonprofit and proprietary hospitals happily colluded with such evasion of the planning system, often providing the professional corporations with inexpensive rental space in adjacent professional buildings. This was possible only if the doctors had prosperous practices, since lenders wanted guaranteed repayment. Hospitals with many poor and nonpaying patients and in states with strict CONs did not get some of the advanced equipment, regardless of clinical need.[67]

Like regulation in some other competitive and potentially turbulent markets (such as transportation, energy, and communication), American health planning created a more stable market in hospital affairs. As in all such regulation, it protected the established firms (the nonprofit hospitals), and it hindered new entries and expansion by risk takers (the proprietary hospitals). Since the Reagan administration favored free competitive markets in health and in other sectors and since it preferred initiatives by proprietary health providers, it eliminated the national government's role in health facilities planning and discouraged planning in the states. Raising capital would depend completely on direct approaches between hospitals and lenders.

Some Judgments About the American Approach to Planning and Capital. Other countries have identifiable systems of hospital investment applying to all or most of the industry, but the United States does not. Many countries discernibly evolve in their planning and investment payment methods, but the United States tinkers and changes. (Even among the countries that have altered their investment methods, America has been more unstable.)

The American approach has advantages as well as disadvantages, depending on one's perspective. Following are some of the advantages:

☐ There is maximum freedom for managers and doctors. The development of the hospital has depended on their priorities and ingenuity, not on planners and government grantors. But they have had to bear tradeoffs: they must devote much effort to fund raising and they bear the risks of shortfalls.

☐ Most hospitals are not tied to government budgets and do not suffer the effects of cuts. American nonprofit and for-profit hospitals can continue to modernize and grow while public hospitals languish.

☐ America's equipment industry is the world's leader in innovation and revenue. The American hospital sector is the world's testing and demonstration laboratory.

☐ Although the American public planning and licensing systems are limited and permissive, they protect the public against prematurely widespread use of some equipment with uncertain value and high cost.

☐ Organizational innovations are rewarded—for instance, the adoption of multihospital arrangements to raise capital and share expensive equipment, or the adoption of new management techniques to calculate amortization capacity and to impress lenders.

☐ The approach is adaptable to unexpected changes in the market. Faced by payers' resistance to mounting prices and admissions during the mid-1980s, hospital managers quickly redirected their expenditures into their outpatient departments and extramural programs. Because of the decentralized financing of the American hospital sector, a few could start the innovations, and many others followed in diverse forms. Some "downsized" their inpatient capacities, so that they could redirect their current expenditures without substantially increasing debt.

On the other hand, the American approach has disadvantages from some perspectives:

☐ Patient-care choices are determined by the hospital management's need to preserve the highest ratings for its bond issues. Managers prefer the patient mix that attracts much capital at low interest rates. Such a mix does not include the poor, who might leave bad debts; it does not include Medicaid patients; and it includes some Medicare patients, Blue Cross charge payers, affluent self-payers, and commercially insured. The poor and severely ill gravitate to the public hospitals, which then run operating deficits and lag in investments, burdening local government budgets.[68] In many parts of the United States, different social classes use different hospitals.

☐ Hospitals are not guaranteed survival. When investment declines, a hospital cannot make improvements to satisfy safety codes and preserve comforts, doctors treat their patients elsewhere, and the hospital can go bankrupt. But patients may find the alternative hospitals less convenient and less cordial.

☐ Faced with scarcities of capital and operating deficits, some rural counties during the late 1970s and 1980s sold their public hospitals to proprietary chains. The chains have been successful in raising capital and have completely replaced or modernized these rural establishments. Some skeptics feared that the chains might no longer serve the poor in those areas—they do not in larger communities with many alternatives—but the chains promised not to discriminate.

☐ The system is oriented entirely to increasing service intensity and costs. More expensive equipment is bought; even buildings are thought to become rapidly obsolete; new techniques require the employment of more technicians with higher pay; expertise in the equipment and amortization of its costs require increased utilization. When third parties tried to limit their payments for operating costs during the mid-1980s, hospital managers became more cautious in their investment decisions. But the system's entrepreneurial and unplanned character remained in place. If a manager thought that he could only attract doctors and patients with a new plant and if he concluded that all payers would have to cover the higher operating costs from new debt by all hospitals, he did not hesitate to proceed.

☐ Some funds are invested in amenities of the hospital building as a tactic to impress patients and doctors. These frills lack clinical value but are essential in marketing. Competing hospitals must keep pace in appearance. Historic appearances are protected in Europe but are avoided in American hospitals.

☐ If a type of hospital enjoys a vogue in the capital market for a while, it can become dangerously overindebted. By the mid-1980s the for-profit hospital companies had become one of the most highly leveraged groups in the entire American economy.[69] If the assumption of continued growth in revenue was disappointed, a crisis would occur for the holders of the bonds, for the local governments who had guaranteed the bonds, and for the patients who had counted on beds that might disappear during corporate reorganizations.

☐ Planning, investment, and reimbursement not only are not coordinated but can be used to undermine each other. CONs are supposed to prevent creation of new hospitals in already overbedded areas. But if a hospital opens without a CON and if a third party pays for patients in other community hospitals, the courts have invoked the antitrust laws to prevent the insurer from refusing payment for its patients in the new hospital.[70] Government could reconcile the conflicting laws but does not, since free competition is paramount.

☐ The national and state governments subsidize construction indirectly by "tax expenditures"—that is, the exemption from income taxes of interest on bonds. No one in the national and state governments has a chance to decide whether this kind of expenditure should be reduced or increased, compared to all other spending of public money. The only judgment on the project is issuance of a CON, taking into account only the probable volume of use. America's supposedly private capital market in health really depends on public subsidies.[71]

Self-Financing in the Netherlands

That self-financing produces both management independence and a nationwide cost explosion is confirmed by the one other country that has relied on it, the Netherlands. As in the case of the United States, self-financing became the principal method of raising money in Holland unexpectedly.

The unplanned growth of Dutch hospital services and costs did not seem possible previously. Hospitals were owned by charitable foundations with modest resources. Many hospitals had an aura of religious service and restraint. Doctors long seemed cautious in making diagnoses and in treating, in contrast to the supposedly more technically oriented and interventionist Americans and Germans. The hospital doctor's preference supposedly was to keep the patient in the bed for a long time, until (at first) he made up his mind about the diagnosis and (later) was sure the patient had recovered. Meanwhile, the patient would be helped by the combination of spiritual and physical care by the nursing staff. Many hospitals were arranged by principles of *verzuiling* (self-sufficiency of several religious communities): several parallel hospitals operated in the same area, none fancy or expensive. Many towns had three small establishments: one Catholic; one Protestant; and one secular, owned by local government.

New construction was infrequent and cheap, often based on charitable gifts. Amortization of any debt was traditionally included in the patient charges but was very low. When the laws after World War II created procedures to set the daily charges of hospitals, regulators were instructed to cover all costs, including debt service, but no one foresaw its growth. As in the United States at nearly the same time, Holland's investment source switched from grants and gifts to debt in a very short time and grew rapidly. The shift was even more extreme in Holland, because charitable donors had been wiped out during the Depression and war and because Holland's limited national government had never financed construction grants. When Holland reconstructed its hospitals, starting in the 1960s, there was no source other than borrowing and repayment from revenue.

Planning. Until the 1980s Holland never had effective facilities planning. It had no public grants program and therefore, unlike nearly every other country, did not develop a method for distinguishing between underprovided and adequately provided areas. When a hospital-planning law was enacted in 1971, the privately financed boom was under way, the planners had limited power, and they could not catch up with the extensive reconstruction.

At first, after World War II, Holland's biggest problem was to reconstruct war damage and develop communities in an orderly way. Building materials and labor were short, so building permits had to be approved by agencies of the national government. A commission on hospitals (the *Ziekenhuiscommissie*) examined applications for hospital construction, it advised the Minister of Health, and he advised the Minister of Buildings.

When building shortages eased in the late 1950s, no plans and restraints existed in hospital affairs. Hospital planning had been designed to ration new construction, but the lid came off. The hospital industry was ill prepared for the revolution in its philosophy and principles of organization; it was ill prepared for the assimilation of scientific ideas and technology from abroad. Several small installations with a family atmosphere and a religious spirit now were prized less than a merged installation with a much larger scale and with advanced technology. Because the hospital could borrow in the capital market, because it could cover debt in the daily inpatient charge, and because lenders thought that these investments were good, Dutch hospitals were transformed and became expensive.

These great changes in character and costs raced ahead before any new planning restraints were enacted. The Hospital Planning Law (*Wet Ziekenhuis-voorzieningen*) went into effect in 1971. It encountered the familiar dilemmas over how to plan in an economy with private ownership and private initiative. Rapidly imposing strict restraints was particularly difficult in a society like Holland's, which is not merely a political democracy but makes decisions by negotiation and by consensus. Some leaders might have favored a system for planning services comprehensively, but agreement could be achieved only to continue the planning of construction: a new hospital could not be built except with the approval of the Minister of Public Health. The novelty in the law was a system for writing a national hospital plan, as a benchmark for judging whether the new construction was needed. Regional plans about hospital services were to be written by the elected provincial authorities, who performed many tasks on behalf of the national government. The Minister could not tell them what to write, but he sent guidelines to the provincial authorities.[72] The guidelines were to be written by an advisory council, the College of Hospital Planning (the *College voor Ziekenhuisvoorzieningen*). The college was run by a governing board representing the sickness funds, the national hospital association (NZR), several other interest groups in health, and some impartial experts. It had a staff.

The planning machinery never went into effect. When writing guidelines for plans, one must make fundamental decisions about goals, priorities, and organization in health. One also makes decisions about priorities and allocation among a country's resources generally. As in much of the world, the Dutch could not develop a consensus about the goals and organizational methods in hospital policy. The college could not write and adopt guidelines for the provincial planners, and the planners never started work.

However, the Minister had the statutory responsibility to decide whether new hospitals should be built, and the industry was exploding. So the college staff evaluated applications and wrote reports on them for the Minister. The staff wrote several reports, some to be models for the provincial authorities' plans, others to be guides for the current approval or rejection of new construction applications.

One clause in the law (Article 18) was interpreted by the Minister as authority to approve or disapprove great changes in the clinical functions of hospitals. Therefore, he claimed power to approve certain expensive equipment for programs that would add new personnel and much higher operating costs. (Examples were renal dialysis, renal transplant, megavolt therapy, CT scanning, and open-heart surgery.) All other equipment purchases and the organizational transformation of the hospital were clearly beyond the powers of the College of

Hospital Planning and the Ministers. COZ was obligated to allow debt service for these purchases, and therefore lenders considered such loans excellent investments.

The Hospital's Initiative. The first step in towns throughout Holland was to modernize the buildings. This would have been financially difficult if Holland had remained traditionally sectarian: in each town, the Catholics and Protestants would have insisted on preserving their own social institutions. But modern health technology presumes scientific universalism, in treating patients and in pooling resources. Holland unexpectedly became secularized very rapidly during the 1960s and 1970s. One result in towns throughout the country was collaboration of Catholic hospital owners, Protestant hospital owners, and local governments in planning new acute hospitals. The small old buildings were either sold or converted to long-term care. The new combined corporation planned its new facility and then sought construction money in the private capital market, often with guarantees from the local government.

After the new hospital was established, its managers developed a list of new construction and new equipment each year. They asked the medical chiefs of service about their needs for replacements and new items. The medical director and economic manager might then discuss all the requests in one of the regular meetings of the chiefs of service. Certain items must be bought without question, such as replacement of collapsing equipment in X-ray, laboratories, surgery, the heating and electrical plant, and other life-supporting activities. The managers put the discretionary items on a priority list, for approval by the governing board. The length of this list depended on customs developed by the governing board and management and varied among hospitals:

☐ Some were cautious and tried not to increase their indebtedness. Therefore, the economic manager kept tabs on the amount of debt paid off each year, maintained credit ratings and loan guarantees that ensured favorable interest rates, and postponed requests for new investment that required too much new borrowing. This strategy enabled the hospital to balance its budget within the rates granted by COZ, without frequent special requests for new rates. Such hospitals acquired reputations for "sound" management.

☐ Some hospitals were more expansionist. The management and governing board approved new equipment requests that maintained the same level of debt plus a small increment, such as 5 percent each year.

☐ Other managers and governing boards approved many of the staff's requests for new equipment, rejecting only those that clearly would be underutilized. Their philosophy was to practice the most modern medicine, even if it was steadily more expensive. They argued that it was up to regulatory agencies (such as COZ and the College for Hospital Planning) and the government to decide any limits on new technology. Therefore, their indebtedness increased, often substantially, each year; they tailored their equipment and borrowing increases to the COZ guidelines; and they usually could get higher rates that erased past deficits and covered the new costs. While COZ "gave in" to most such requests, its regulators and the government officials concerned with cost control policy were unhappy with such hospital managements.

Like the operating budget, the capital budget was reviewed during the meetings of the triumvirate of top managers (the *directie*). Then it was passed on to the governing board.

Some hospitals had special relations with local governments. The budgets were reviewed by the municipal auditors and by the political head of the department in charge of health or social affairs. The basis for the municipal government's role varied: some customarily were overseers of the hospital's welfare, either by local statutes or by the hospital's charter; some were guarantors of the hospital's borrowing from the capital market; some loaned money if the hospital ran deficits or needed new investments. The financial requirements of the hospitals outstripped the capacities of the private credit markets, and local governments increasingly contributed, particularly to the new hospitals replacing and combining several old ones. Involvement by the local government strengthened the hospital as a credit risk in private capital markets.

Competition now ensures a minimum pace of modernization to keep pace with other hospitals in the region. When patients were loyal to sectarian communities, they could be counted on to use the local sectarian hospital, regardless of its facilities. But after Holland became secularized, the patient shopped for the best care. Since Holland is small, the patient can easily go to another city. A hospital's revenue will match its expected costs under the COZ calculations if it achieves the expected number of patient-days. If occupancy declines in one hospital, it runs a deficit and cannot pay its full payroll and fixed costs, while another hospital gains profits at the first one's expense. So each hospital must keep pace, and the community presses it to provide services matching those in distant places. Dutch competition is defensive while the American is aggressive: Dutch competition does not push the hospital to earn more cash by capturing additional market share from others, as in the United States; instead, it presses each hospital to protect the levels presupposed by the rate calculations. The Dutch system fosters modernization but not risky growth beyond the capacities of local markets, and thus little redundancy has resulted. In America the prospects of capturing markets at the expense of others lead to the risky creation of new hospitals and the expansion of established ones.

Financing Construction and Expensive Equipment. After clearance by the board and the local government, the hospital managers during the 1970s were free to prepare a prospectus and borrow from a bank, insurance company, or other institutional lenders. Until the financing controls of the 1980s, hospitals were among the better credit risks in Holland, because the reimbursement system guaranteed prompt repayment of all installments and interest. COZ was bound by law to grant daily charges that covered the hospital's operating costs, including repayment of loans and interest. The entire population was covered by official national health insurance or by private health insurance, and the hospital had virtually no bad debts. The aging of the population increased utilization, and therefore occupancy and revenue of all hospitals were high.

During the first years when each hospital was extensively renovated, it received temporary daily charges from COZ, enabling it to pay its operating costs (including debt service) at less than the occupancy level it would achieve later. After a few years, when occupancy became normal, the hospital was awarded a basic daily charge by COZ. Each year thereafter, it submitted the application for the automatic increase for all hospitals (the *calculatieschema* described in Chapter Seven), and COZ granted that year's percentage increase. The hospital's basic charge covered what might have been a large amount to amortize debt, and every year's subsequent rate included that amount plus an increment.

If the hospital rebuilt, bought, and borrowed at higher than normal rates, it incurred operating deficits. Then it filed a special application with COZ, for a higher-than-average rate increase. I described the special application in Chapter Seven. The guidelines from the COZ committees might have specified the limits for higher debt, to be allowed that year in special applications, and the COZ examiner was bound to grant the new higher rate and retroactive supplement if the hospital's expansion fell within the limits. If the hospital exceeded the guidelines, because of unavoidable necessity, sound strategy, or adventure, the COZ examiner then asked for explanations. He could more easily disallow a rate increase due to excessive payroll, and then the hospital simply conformed its operating costs by discharging workers or by reducing the hours of the part-timers. But disallowing a rate increase due to investment costs was very difficult, since the hospital managers had already placed the orders and committed themselves to the debt, and since the Dutch hospital (unlike the American) had no outside revenue to cover contingencies. So, if the hospital managers made a plausible case for the high capital costs, the COZ examiner approved.

But the hospital could not get everything it might like: there was always a risk that the COZ examiner might disallow items and that lenders might suspect the hospital managers' judgment. So hospital managers became skilled in anticipating the verdict of COZ, since it was the key to growth: if they guessed wrong and COZ did not grant the full request, the hospital was saddled with its new debt and must make compensating economies. Therefore, rate regulation had some restraining effects: the hospital did not buy equipment that would not be utilized profitably, and it did not buy so much in a year that the rates would have to increase far beyond the COZ guidelines.

Consequences. The Dutch experience shows how renovation of old hospitals can produce great increases in costs. Because several old and small hospitals were being combined into new ones, the numbers of hospitals diminished. But modernization produced small rooms instead of the large wards, increasing staffing needs. And modernization introduced new technology and specialized personnel.

From 1957 to 1978, Holland reduced the number of acute hospitals from 269 to 233 but increased numbers of beds from 50,622 to 70,291. (The number peaked in 1972 at 71,779 and has slowly declined.) The total costs of the hospitals greatly increased because of trends found in all countries (personnel, technology, and so on). These changes were felt particularly intensely in Holland, because the hospitals were so extensively transformed. Total expenditures on acute hospitals in millions of guilders rose from 355.3 in 1958 to 7,856 in 1978; guilders per patient-day rose from 20.40 in 1958 to about 355.70 in 1978. The rate of change was greater than in neighboring countries, even those (such as France) with higher inflation rates. Holland previously had one of the lower proportions of national resources going into health, but by the 1980s it had one of the highest in the world—9.1 percent of gross domestic product in 1982—because of hospital modernization and other changes. Between 1960 and 1982, share of GDP spent on health rose 2.2 times in Holland and about 1.7 times in the seventeen other members of OECD.[73]

Limits. By the late 1970s, Dutch policymakers urgently sought controls over investment as well as over operating costs. But they faced the same problem as the Americans—namely, how to control private spending when the national government paid for none of the capital and when local governments encouraged lavish self-financing by sponsoring bond issues. Even more than in America, the Dutch reimbursement system by law protected each hospital's independent growth: third parties must pay in full the costs of care for all patients, including full repayment of debt. Hospital specialists collect generous fees for treatments under both national and private health insurance in both countries, and they gain if the hospitals install the newest methods.

As in America, the Dutch for years hoped that facilities planning with appeals for moderation but without sanctions would restrain spending. But in both countries the leadership of the planning machinery included interest groups and consumers who favored the newest methods and who were lulled by the spread of the payment across many individual bills. CONs to save money-in-general are not strongly imposed.

Holland could not continue to drift. The methods of paying operating costs were revised during the 1980s, as I reported in Chapters Six and Seven. The Hospital Planning Law was amended and strengthened in 1978 and 1983. The regional divisions of government were pressed to fulfill their responsibility to write and implement health systems plans, under the supervision of the Ministry of Public Health. Investment decisions were clearly distinguished from the screening and setting of prospective budgets by the negotiators and COTG examiners. The hospital's proposals for new construction and expensive equipment were to be screened by the regional government officers and must be approved by the Ministry of Public Health. Global budgeting was introduced into investment: each region had an annual limit, and individual hospital projects would no longer be approved if they exceeded the aggregate. The Ministry gave priority to projects that implemented its policy goals, such as programs of extramural care accompanied by reductions in hospital's inpatient beds.[74]

The method was really a strict Certificate of Need ultimately administered by the national government. An essential instrument of governmental authority was missing: the Ministry still did not provide grants; the hospitals still needed to find loans in the private capital market. Perhaps this would become much more difficult, because of reimbursement constraints. A slower rate of growth was not critical, since the postwar building boom had been completed.

Grants in a Public Hospital System: Great Britain

Among all developed countries, Britain alone combines all instruments of coherent planning and investment. The owners of hospitals, the planners, the grantors of capital, and the payers of operating costs belong to the same agency—that is, the national government. No system is completely monolithic and closely integrated, and different actors belong to different offices within the national government. But, still, the British arrangement works with a degree of public initiative, consensus, and political will absent in other countries.

In all other developed countries, it is the hospitals that exercise the initiatives in the development of their programs and projects. Government waits for the proposal and gives approval either for public funding or for the hospital's own fund seeking. Governments write plans to set priorities about the locations and purposes of grants, and eventually they condition grants upon regional cooperation among grantees. Governments outside Britain may commission nonprofit owners to create facilities proposed by the planners themselves, but this is not yet done extensively in any privately and municipally owned and managed system.

Evolution of Planning. During its first decades, the National Health Service sought merely to keep existing facilities in operation. The NHS was not a disciplined vertical bureaucracy controlled by the Ministry of Health in London, but a congeries of committees responsible for managing facilities pursuant to money and guidelines from London. Because of the brevity of the guidelines and the looseness of the arrangements, the managing committees at the grass roots had considerable discretion. Each of the influential teaching hospitals retained its own well-connected Board of Governors. The other hospitals were operated in groups by local Hospital Management Committees, and the committees were coordinated by Regional Hospital Boards. All ambulatory and home services were administered and financed separately by the local governments.

Budgeting was incremental, in keeping with the aim to maintain all facilities in place. The teaching hospitals could fight off all transfers from their budgets to other programs, and they continued to absorb much of the country's resources. The creators of the NHS had intended to regionalize health services and establish new hospitals in underserved areas, but money for such growth was not available until the 1960s. A Regional Hospital Board could not reallocate its limited capital and operating money from the better-provided to the less-provided areas, since the doctors in the established hospitals pressed for the growth money and fought off cuts.[75] No methodology existed to identify needs, set priorities, and reallocate.

Organization and Planning. The reorganization of the NHS in 1974 placed all hospitals, ambulatory services, and home services under the same managers, so that they could be coordinated and redirected, in keeping with local needs. The entire NHS was organized more hierarchically, so that major reallocations could occur across the entire country. At each level, managers would write and implement rolling plans for their areas. Britain's experience shows that an effective reallocation of facilities and regional coordination require an appropriately organized national system.

All intramural and extramural facilities have been pooled under the same planners and under the same District Management Team. Between the DHA and DHSS is one of fourteen Regional Health Authorities (RHAs), which writes a strategic plan for an extensive region, in the light of the region's existing facilities, its available cash, and the policy priorities of DHSS. The department does not combine them into a single national plan. The RHA monitors implementation of its plans by all the DHAs within its jurisdiction. Since the plans deal with the operations of programs, they cover financial flows for both operations and capital. In contrast, planning in other countries refers only to the creation and modification of facilities.

Following is the planning sequence during the 1980s. (A slightly more elaborate method existed during the 1970s.)[76]

☐ DHSS notifies the RHAs of its policy priorities. It sends other guidelines about resource use.

☐ Strategic plans are drafted every five years throughout the country, with a ten-year forward look.
- Each RHA sends an outline of regional strategy to all its DHAs, emphasizing certain programs and describing each one's resources.
- Each DHA writes a strategic plan for the next decade.
- Each RHA combines the district plans in a regional plan.
- DHSS reviews and approves the fourteen regional plans. Each year it meets with all RHAs to review implementation and (sometimes) suggest amendments.

☐ Operational programs are written each year by each DHA, showing how each will carry out its strategy during the new fiscal year and the next one. Every year the RHA and each DHA meet to review the operational program.

The strategic plans include bids to higher levels—that is, each DHA's bid to the RHA and the RHA's bid to DHSS—for funding for future investments. Some investments will be created from growth money; others will be specially funded by DHSS. The strategic plans also describe the outcomes of new construction already begun. The operational plans tell how investment and operating funds are being used in the short run, and higher reviewers can confirm that capital spending conforms to policy, to resource limitations, and to ordinary standards of efficiency. The annual planning review meetings between the RHA and each DHA enable the RHA to check that capital development and program operations conform to the DHA's annual operating program and to the strategic plans. The RHA has full authority to correct deviations.

The Flow of Money. In accordance with Anglo-American practice in public expenditure, the money is appropriated each year by Parliament and must be spent or returned to the Treasury each year. The bulk of the annual appropriations for DHSS is operating funds. They are distributed among regions by the RAWP calculations described in Chapter Eight. The region then distributes the money among its districts according to the strategic and operational plans, rather than according to an automatic RAWP-type formula. The extra needs of a district are spelled out in plans, not by shortfalls from a statistical measure.

Until the 1960s very little money was appropriated for hospitals' capital, even less than under the parlous private ownership of earlier years. Of the hospital expenditure, capital spending was 16.4 percent in fiscal year 1938-39 and 3.8 percent in 1952-53.[77] Big projects to construct new hospitals or transform old ones did not exist. Each hospital got a small amount of capital funds, which it used for renovations and could use up within a year.

When substantial money became available for new hospitals during the 1960s, everyone soon discovered that health care capital expenditure did not fit the annual budgeting and appropriations cycle of government. The planning, construction, and opening of hospitals were not predictable. Payments did not parallel the course of work. Starts were delayed, and work was interrupted in unexpected ways. Plans about functions and design changed during construction. Construction costs were often exceeded. The eventual operating costs were not fully anticipated. For decades DHSS has struggled to make hospital investment more predictable, and Treasury and DHSS have struggled to make their budgeting and appropriations methods more flexible.[78]

Efforts to Control Costs and Anticipate Future Costs. A new hospital building is not merely a building. It implies a new complex of services: new programs with new, more credentialed, and more expensive staff; new and more expensive ways of delivering care. A widespread reason for the hospital cost explosion in the United States and Europe is the great increase in operating costs when a new building replaces an old one. Usually, the financial planners think only of initial construction costs and include in their presentation nothing about the effects on operating costs. Sales pitches include the utopian claim that the new technology will be "labor saving," that the new arrangements in the building will be "more efficient," that the new development will "save money." Hospital administrators and physicians avoid dialogues with sickness funds and with regulatory agencies about changes in operating costs, lest those killjoys interfere with the plans.

In Britain the Treasury and the spending Ministry pay for both construction and eventual operations. The approval of construction plans and the management of services are united. The wave of new hospital building began after the Public Expenditure Survey was in place as the method of deciding public expenditures, and a principal goal of PES was to anticipate and prevent unpleasant consequences of attractive schemes. So, during the 1960s, planners of individual hospital projects were expected to predict future operating costs, called the Revenue Consequences of Capital Schemes (RCCS).

By the start of the newly reorganized NHS in 1974, the complete planning sequence had been devised. One set of planning manuals, called CAPRICODE, has been a guide to the design and justification of expensive projects.[79] The six CAPRICODE manuals specify the steps and the forms for describing a project, the stages of work, efforts and costs at each stage, and so on. A team for each project was to be created from the regional officials at the RHA, from the area officials (when Area Health Authorities still existed), and from the district officials.

At several stages in the description of the project and in reporting progress, the project team was to estimate RCCS, numbers of new cases and patient-days, the expected stays, and outpatient visits. The forms asked about the additional staffing, equipment, and other inputs.

Including RCCS in the project planning from the start was a brake upon the planners' euphoria. English planners were constantly reminded by newspaper headlines, by parliamentary debates, and by the annual struggles between DHSS and Treasury that they lived in a country of limited resources. Hospital planners and project managers in other countries during the 1950s and 1970s were less inhibited. The RCCS estimates could be questioned by the RHA and by DHSS, and the entire project could be sent back down for cuts in its design.

When the final project proposal and its periodic progress reports were approved by the RHA and/or by the Planning and Policy Divisions of DHSS, the department was committed not only to the capital expenditure but also to the RCCS figures when the project became operational. The Finance Division's PES estimates for operating expenditures in future years included the extra RCCS figures projected by the capital projects currently under way. If new proposals would generate too much RCCS in coming years, Treasury might discourage DHSS from beginning the projects now. The negotiations with Treasury about the future year's PES estimates usually revolved around the merits and scheduling of new projects with large long-term implications. Just as Treasury and the DHSS finance officers bargained over the operating and capital expenditure allowances for the next year, so they bargained over the size and complexity of pending construction projects. After getting all it could in future commitments for RCCS from Treasury, the DHSS finance officers sometimes had to ask the planners within DHSS and the RHAs to scale down major projects or to schedule them more gradually.

This admirable system encountered difficulties. Planners in Britain—as in other countries—have underestimated not only construction costs but the future operating costs. Everyone was motivated by the hierarchical negotiation and approval system to estimate RCCS too low: the project team did not want to frighten the RHA, the RHA did not want to frighten DHSS, and DHSS did not want to frighten Treasury. DHSS could not investigate every project and was supposed to give discretion to the RHAs; in 1979, for example, it examined only projects costing over £2 million, asked to be informed of those exceeding £350,000, and left everything smaller to the RHAs. The regions implemented the planning and CAPRICODE procedures widely. Therefore, as in other countries, the costs of new hospitals and programs exceeded expectations. Committed to "protect RCCS," Treasury had to supply DHSS with larger operating expenditures than it had expected.

DHSS and Treasury then sought better methods. DHSS maintained historical statistics on forty-five new hospitals as standards for judging the estimates of the capital costs and the RCCS in new applications. The operations of the panel have been studied to learn about cost-control techniques in new hospitals. New schemes beyond a particular size (the limit rises each year because of inflation) are sent by DHSS to Treasury, where economic advisers evaluate the investment-appraisal methodology of DHSS and suggest improvements. The referrals to Treasury doubtless motivate DHSS to restrain the sizes of the projects.

As the economic limits on the health services tightened during the 1970s, RCCS was gradually folded into the total allotments to the regions for operations. Early during the decade, DHSS added to the allotments to the RHAs whatever RCCS had been approved—plus additional money for underestimates. The RCCS was limited to a short period; the RHA was expected to pay for all the operations of new hospitals after the first years, from their general allotments. Now all operations—even the first years of the region's new hospitals—are covered by the annual RAWP allotment to the RHA. The health authorities then should be motivated to design projects that will operate economically, and even to postpone them. (Although the RHA no longer gets sums specifically earmarked for RCCS, it is supposed to estimate the amounts of money when planning new projects.)

Paying for both the existing services and the new one from the same allotment has produced difficult choices. Since the managers of the services are the District Management Teams, the RHAs give them their allotments and let them resolve the dilemmas. Some DHAs decide that the new establishments should not have been built; so these establishments are left completely or partially unopened.[80] Existing services are then protected. Other DHAs wind down several old hospitals and programs a year or two before opening a new hospital, carry forward the savings, and then start up the new showcase amidst the usual cost overruns.

Capital RAWP. The decrepit condition of the capital stock and the great regional imbalances were leading reasons why all British hospitals were nationalized.[81] When new construction money was made available during the 1960s, the planners in the Ministry of Health used the familiar bed/population ratio when deciding where to build. Their goal was to provide at least 3.3 beds per 1,000 inhabitants everywhere by 1975. But this method was crude.

RAWP—described in Chapter Eight—was intended to calibrate the amounts of operating money going to each region. The method identified the regions already getting enough resources to meet their needs, the regions deserving slightly more, and the regions getting much less than the population needed. The method provided an objective rationale for differential expenditure, anticipating protests by the overprovided regions that had profited from incrementalism.

Capital—as well as operating money—needed to be redistributed across the country. The RAWP working party was asked to design an allocation formula for distributing each year's investment money. Its proposal:[82]

☐ The capital stock in each region is valued at its replacement cost, written down to reflect age and conditions. All hospitals, health centers, and other facilities are aggregated. Calculations are updated each year, to take account of improvements and closures. Facilities with inappropriate locations or obsolete functions (such as tuberculosis sanitariums) are discounted.

☐ Need (the target for the region) is defined by weighted population. Expenditure RAWP provided money for the current operating needs of each region, and the most recent population counts were used. Capital RAWP provides money for the future needs of each region, and the population forecasts in five years are used. Total capital needs are built up from separate calculations for nonpsychiatric inpatient, day patient and outpatient, psychatric inpatient, and so on, as in expenditure RAWP. Capital RAWP (like expenditure RAWP) weights population by age, sex, and SMR. For the community services component, more direct measures of need—such as consultation rates by GPs—are used. Cross-boundary flows of patients are not included in the formulas, since the goal of capital development is to eliminate them.

☐ Moving toward target is more difficult for capital RAWP than for expenditure RAWP. Hospital planning and construction take many years, and commitments must be honored from the late 1960s and 1970s; that is, DHSS must pay for some projects regardless of need defined by the RAWP formulas and by the new RHAs. To implement decisions about improved utilization, every region—no matter how "overprovided"—needs a minimum capital allotment each year for maintenance, rehabilitation, and conversions. When large, these changes must come from the capital allocation and not from the revenue allocation. Extremely underprovided regions cannot absorb large amounts of new money for capital. Because of the wide inequalities in capital stock among regions, some begin very far below target, and others far above. Formulas set floors and ceilings close to the average, but these limits disappear in successive years; meanwhile, new projects in underprovided regions and hospital closings in the overprovided move them all closer to the average.

☐ DHSS should fund separately and directly special projects, such as particular educational facilities, the high-priority health-center program, and specialized clinical centers with extraregional appeals.

RAWP went into effect during the late 1970s, when the squeeze on health services spending worsened. Much of the investment money had already been committed; therefore, little new money was available. The ratio of operating expenditure to capital allocation steadily changed, from 7:1 in FY 1970-71 to 12:1 in FY 1981-82. Whatever money has existed in each year has been distributed according to capital RAWP formulas close to those in the working party's report. Therefore, the underprovided regions have been getting new capital money under RAWP, as well as money for the completion of projects started earlier; and visitors encounter new hospitals and internal modernization of old ones. Expenditure RAWP also channels new money into these regions, so that their staffing and supplies also improve.[83]

Identifying when a region is "overprovided" is more subtle for capital RAWP than for expenditure RAWP. In the latter case, overprovision is an excess of operating money over need. But fitting RAWP reasoning to capital expenditure is quite difficult:

- *Estimating existing stock in monetary values.* Large capital stock may not be excessive if it is old and inefficient. Age does not always correlate with obsolescence. Comparing regions and districts requires standard measures, but regions and districts are diverse in the age and efficiency of their buildings.[84]
- *Future targets.* A method must be developed to combine predicted values of existing stock and additional expenditures.
- *Future targets.* Facilities plans guide present expenditures to satisfy future "needs." But assumptions about the future may be falsified by population changes, clinical discoveries, morbidity profiles, and utilization styles. For example, Britain several times has based the limitation or expansion of medical education on bad guesses about future utilization and practice patterns.[85]
- *Equalization.* The RAWP assumptions against "overprovision" may be inappropriate in capital distribution. Perhaps certain districts should consciously be made "centers of excellence." Instead of current efforts to discourage cross-boundary flows, perhaps patients should be sent to the best-endowed districts.

The allocation of operating expenditures among regions is not integrated with the allocation of capital. Both sets of formulas define a region's needs by its population size weighted by age and SMRs; the distribution of resources in the past has caused the same regions to be "overprovided" in both operating expenditure levels and in capital, and regions either grow on both or are squeezed on both. However, no formulas relate a region's new operating and new capital allotments; one cannot judge whether a region's mix is unbalanced or appropriate. The RAWP working party suggested a system of bids: if a region wished to become capital intensive, it could obtain a larger share of the total available investment money and mortgage part of its future revenue allocations; if a region wished to be more labor intensive, it could forgo some of the available investment money and get a larger share of the country's operating expenditures in the long run. This method has not yet been adopted.

Operating expenditure and investment became more closely integrated during the later 1970s by the pressures of cash limits. During the last years of Labour and during the Thatcher Government, the problem was defined as controlling each year's cash appropriations by Parliament, not ensuring the growth of the NHS. Whether the money was for operating expenditures or for investment, the problem was to limit it. Regions and areas were authorized to solve their immediate problems in operating costs by making transfers: they can transfer up to 10 percent of their annual capital grant to their operating funds at their own discretion; they can transfer up to 1 percent of their operating expenditure grant to capital at their own discretion; beyond these figures they must get the approval of DHSS, which is always given, particularly for capital-to-operating transfers. At first the transfers were from operating to capital; but as cash limits tightened, the shift was from capital to operating.[86]

1976–77	£10,320,000	Net from operating to capital
1977–78	£13,228,000	Net from operating to capital
1978–79	£ 2,925,000	Net from capital to operating
1979–80	£19,204,000	Net from capital to operating

During 1979-80, 5.3 percent of the capital allocation to the regions was transferred to operating expenditures. Throughout the country during the late 1970s and 1980s, major repairs to hospital buildings normally charged to capital funds were postponed or performed in the cheapest way. Hospital managers—particularly in areas of extreme expenditure restraint, such as London—complained that their capital stock was deteriorating.

Reallocations. The British system makes it possible not only to reduce and expand capital plant but also to regionalize and reallocate it. Operating and capital expenditures are related. The RHAs and their DHAs plan and manage both. If the DHSS national policy states that excessive inpatient capacity should be reduced and resources devoted to underdeveloped services, RHAs and DHAs are bound to pursue these goals when writing and carrying out their plans. If a region is declining in population and aging in social structure, it must reallocate without growth money, by reducing the inpatient acute sector and devoting its resources to programs for the elderly. The consolidations and redirection must be phased over many years, since the population must be served while continuing to change. Several regions and their districts have developed sophisticated plans, both regionalized in structure and dynamic in timetable. And, unlike many of the world's health plans, the plans are seriously implemented.[87]

Donations. Gifts were essential to hospitals before the spread of public grants, but they persist even today in most countries. While they can reduce pressure on grantors, gifts can complicate work of planners.

Before creation of the National Health Service, British voluntary hospitals depended on gifts and bequests for buildings and equipment. Each voluntary hospital had a circle of benefactors, often called a "League of Friends," who donated work and money. After the NHS became the principal source of investment and operating funds, Britain's long tradition of voluntary service in social affairs did not die. The leagues survived and looked for a new mission. Nearly all hospitals have individual Leagues of Friends today.

Each league still collects money by donations, bequests, memorial gifts honoring deceased persons, and (in most cases) annual subscription fees of members. Each league has it own pattern of helping its hospitals,[88] but much support is investment and enables the DHA to use its capital funds for other purposes. The leagues' money is used for interior decorating in the wards, chapel, and nurses' residence; furnishings in patients' day rooms (television sets, cinema projectors, electric organs); durable supplies such as beds, ambulances, ward lockers, and bed lights; and clinical equipment such as microscopes, gamma counters for pathology laboratories, physiotherapy equipment, and colonoscopes. Leagues of Friends donated about £12 million during the 1983-84 fiscal year, about 60 percent going for durable supplies and clinical equipment, the rest for amenities.

Several teaching hospitals have obtained major equipment—such as CT scanners, dialysis units, and organ transplant units—with the help of Leagues, business firms, and special bequests. Most items donated by leagues are small and fit into the operating and financial plans of DHAs. But the heavy equipment requires large operating expenditure, additional staffing, and new construction, which may not correspond to the plans of the DHA and RHA. The RHA usually let the DHA accept the equipment, provided that it agreed to operate the equipment within its financial plan and cash limits. However, some influential consultants launched expensive programs with outside donations and successfully maneuvered the health authorities into changing their plans.[89] During the late 1970s, DHAs began to reject donations of heavy equipment unless the donor also gave an operating endowment. The DHA then would not have to cut other services. The result has been to discourage large private donations that alter plans.

Private Hospitals. Investment in the private sector is virtually unregulated and unplanned, as in any other British private charity or private business. Any private hospital can be started, as long as it does not interfere with a nearby NHS hospital by raiding that hospital's scarce nursing personnel. The Labour Government during the 1970s required that a new private hospital with more than one hundred beds had to be approved by a Health Services Board and by the Area Health Authorities of the NHS, but smaller hospitals were exempt from review. Therefore, new private hospitals were deliberately kept smaller than one hundred beds by their creators. The Conservative Government repealed this review during the 1980s.

The private hospitals obtain their start-up investments from their owners' reserves, as in the cases of the Nuffield Provincial Hospitals Trust and the British United Provident Association. Or they borrow the funds in the private capital market. Starting a private hospital in Britain is risky, and investors are cautious.

The NHS has never been positively coordinated with the private hospitals through a planned division of labor. The private hospitals are merely a voluntary option. Patients with nonurgent surgical problems can avoid the NHS waiting lists by entering a private hospital. The privates need only maintain simpler equipment, smaller buildings, lower staffing, and (therefore) lower costs than the NHS hospitals.

Some leaders of the Thatcher Government during the early 1980s favored some contracting out of patients: the NHS could reduce beds in a district and might rent space in nearby private hospitals if the patient load exceeded the NHS capacity. The size of the NHS could be limited, and the NHS would give priority to the more serious acute cases. The private sector would have an incentive to grow. When occupancy in the private hospitals declined during the 1980s, several obtained such contracting-out arrangements, thereby warding off bankruptcy.

Summary

Planning. Hospital facilities planning in practice merely distributes buildings and equipment to less provided areas. It should set priorities in services and coordinate separate establishments, but it does so only in a few countries.

Planning is limited in design and in implementation when:

- Hospitals are owned by private groups and municipalities.
- Separate payers provide money for investment and operations.
- Hospitals can self-finance investment.
- Government is indecisive. The national government has limited authority.

Planning methodology remains remarkably backward in most countries. The barriers to improvement are intellectual as well as political. Adequate planning methods would require both theories and information about:

- Needs of populations.
- Capabilities of providers to fulfill certain needs.
- Location of providers and relations among them, in order to satisfy population needs.
- Relations between long-term strategies to short-term situations. Adaptation of the larger system to unexpected changes.
- Prediction of operating costs for different designs of programs and facilities.
- Variations in the design of programs and facilities under alternative resource caps. Consequences for delivery of services as well as for costs.

Investment. Operating and capital expenditures usually come from different sources tied to the larger economy differently:

- Operating expenditures usually are covered by entitlement programs. In case of a downturn in the economy, it is the third party (the sickness fund or the government benefit agency) that experiences the crisis. The third party has lower revenue but is obligated to keep paying providers in full, according to subscribers' demand, usually with annual rate increases.
- Capital expenditures in large part come from public grants or governmental loans. In case of a downturn in the economy, it is the hospitals that experience the crisis. As a result of governmental budget cutbacks, the hospitals lack funds for improvements and innovations. Unless generous depreciation is part of operating reimbursement, the hospitals lack funds for replacement.
- If both operating and capital expenditures come from the same source, and that source is government, both are reduced during economic downturns.
- If hospitals self-finance capital under insurance, hospitals can raise much investment money under patient revenue at all times, but only if the system for operating revenue is permissive. During economic downturns lenders might still consider hospitals a good risk. But eventually reductions in the sickness funds' revenue and general pessimism cause lenders to hesitate.

Investment practices vary according to the amount of money:

- When growth money is widespread, the entire hospital sector can modernize and innovate. Effects on future operating costs are ignored.
- When growth money is scarce, two possibilities exist:
    Across-the-board restraint. This option hurts poor areas worse than the rich, since the richer areas have had larger margins. The richer and better-connected areas can obtain exceptions.
    Selective reallocation, so that the poor areas are cut less than the rich. Perhaps the underprovided can continue to grow. This unusual case is possible only if the national government manages facilities and funding, and only if the poor areas cast many votes.

Hospital planning and hospital investment have always been oriented toward growth and modernization in individual installations and in regions. Excess capacity can be cut in overprovided areas with declining populations only if the national government owns, manages, and finances hospitals. Resources can be redirected from acute to nonacute services and from overprovided to underprovided regions only if the national government owns, manages, and finances hospitals.

Allocating investment money by formulas is a mirage. The distribution is not targeted on need, does not settle old controversies, and arouses new controversies. Construction and program development are "lumpy" rather than steady expenditures susceptible to simple calculations. There is no substitute for intelligent evaluation of needs and design of grants—that is, judgment and discussion by someone.

A new development in decisions about construction and equipment is to include prediction of their long-term operating costs. Combining calculations about both capital and operating costs is implemented seriously only when the same payer grants both investment and operating money. And this occurs only when government pays, as in Britain and Switzerland.

10

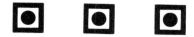

Setting Wages
for Hospital Employees

When European and North American hospitals were charities, they were staffed like charities.[1] In the many confessional hospitals, the executives and leading nurses were members of Catholic orders or Protestant religious associations. They made a lifetime commitment to serve God by unselfish service to mankind. From the religious order, they received room, board, and security during illness and retirement. The money costs of the order and of the hospitals it owned were borne by revenue from its endowment and from community fund raising; many needs (such as food and clothing) were produced by the order's own workshops. If the order did not own the hospital, it received lump-sum cash payments for its members who worked there, but the members received no individual wages. The executives and nurses lived on the hospital grounds and received free meals.

Hospitals were refuges for the sick poor, and distinctions between patients and lay employees were imprecise. Many workers lacked families and the assured occupations based on the family; the Church took care of them by providing free room and board on the hospital grounds, in return for work. Some were convalescing and former patients. Their employment was one of the charitable functions of hospitals, not to be judged by cost-effectiveness.

Other hospital workers were wage earners living at home. But they knew that they would not receive prevailing market wages, since the hospital was a charity and not a business firm. Many shared the religious motives of the executives and leading nurses. They gained secure lifetime employment in an insecure world; the women had an alternative to forced marriage. Until recently in all countries, health was an unusual market, with a downtrodden and overworked labor force.

Since workers, nurses, and junior doctors were supposed to serve and not speak, staff organization had no place. Unions belonged in factories but not in hospitals, where they violated the natural harmony. Agitation over wages and hours were thought to divert workers and nurses from their true callings. Organizing drives and strikes for higher wages and shorter hours were unnatural intrusions. Hospital staff and patients should be protected from these manipulations by outsiders.

During the twentieth century, hospital employment steadily changed. Because hospital management and staffing had long depended on affiliations with churches, the increasing number of secular hospitals—particularly those owned by government—encountered problems in recruiting competent nursing, domestic, and blue-collar staffs. Wages slowly rose and hours slowly shortened, but hospital jobs remained much less attractive than others. As I showed in Table 3-1, and in the accompanying text, until recently wages were less than half of the hospitals' running costs.[2] For example, the four public hospitals of Lyons in 1861 had 3,611 beds, 314 nursing employees, and 368 administrative and technical employees. Less than 8 percent of all expenditures went for medical, nursing, and technicians' wages.[3]

Hospital costs grew rapidly after World War II in every country, and personnel costs rose faster than nearly any other. For example, in France from 1962 to 1975 (when serious cost containment began), personnel expenditures in public short-stay and long-stay general hospitals rose at an annual average of 18.4 percent, while all other hospital expenditures rose at an annual average of about 16 percent. (General prices in France rose at an annual average of 5.7 percent.) Numbers of full-time-equivalent staff per bed rose by an annual average of 4.5 percent.[4] In every developed country, personnel now absorbs 60 to 80 percent of acute hospital budgets. (It is less than 60 percent only in the United States, where hospital employees' wages are low and the lines for capital and administration are high.) Personnel costs have risen so quickly because:

☐ Numbers of hospital employees have risen.
  • Nuns and deaconesses declined in number and had to be replaced by secular nurses.
  • Hours of work declined, and more nurses and workers had to be hired.
  • Service intensity increased.
  • Many nurses and domestics were part-timers.
☐ Wages increased.
  • Nurses and workers wanted typical civilian wages.
  • Nurses and domestics lived outside the hospital and were expected to pay for their own housing, food, and laundering.
☐ Some employees—such as junior doctors—no longer worked free but expected wages.
☐ Fringe benefits, such as employer contributions to pension and health insurance funds, had to be paid in addition to salary. Health care and retirement were no longer guaranteed by the hospital and religious order but became part of the country's social security financing.
☐ Hospitals had to create and operate additional units to please the employees.
  • Nurses' residences.
  • Cafeterias.
  • Parking lots.
  • Rooms for recreation.
  • Offices for personnel administration.

In every developed country during the 1970s, employment rose faster in health than in any other economic sector. For example, from 1970 through 1980, full-time-equivalent workers in the entire health sector rose 77.8 percent in the United States, 65.7 percent in the United Kingdom, 65.4 percent in the Netherlands, and 52.4 percent in Germany.[5] Within hospitals the growth was fastest among the technicians and administrators.[6] In many communities the hospitals became the principal employers.

Labor Relations Systems

During the twentieth century, hospitals became more typical employers, and nurses and other hospital workers became more typical employees. The modernization of hospital operating costs had already made it impossible to continue the traditional methods of unilateral fund raising by the hospitals' managers and owners. Likewise, the modernization of hospital employment made it impossible to continue the traditional methods of fixing pay and work rules, either through unilateral internal decisions by hospital management or through agreements between hospital managers and the heads of religious nursing orders.

After World War II, every advanced country developed methods to express the interests of the hospital workers and to decide their pay and working conditions. The methods everywhere were a hybrid of each country's general industrial relations and the peculiarities of hospital work. Every country was somewhat different, because of cross-national differences in industrial relations, hospital traditions, and current hospital finance. Following are the principal structural attributes that vary among countries:

☐ Spokesmen for the hospital workers, their type of organization.
  • National or regional association of all workers (that is, a class association).
  • Bread-and-butter-oriented union.
    — National or regional industrial union (embracing all hospital workers).
    — National or regional craft union (embracing only the members of a particular occupation).
    — Local plant union (embracing only the employees of one hospital).
  • Association concerned with the mission of the hospital as well as the interests of the members:
    — Religious order or confessional association.
    — Professional association.
  • Members serving in a management council of the hospital.
  • No representation, no organization.
☐ Spokesmen for the hospital.
  • National or regional government.
  • National or regional hospital association.
  • Owners and managers of the hospital.
    — Each individual hospital.
    — Multihospital chain.

☐ Agenda for negotiations.
  - Wages and fringe benefits.
  - Placing of each occupation on official wage scale decided elsewhere.
  - Work rules: hours, shifts, assignments.

☐ Whether wages and rules apply to:
  - Hospital industry alone.
    — Unique to each hospital.
    — Groupings of hospitals.
    — All hospitals in the country or region.
  - Entire public sector of the country.
  - Entire economy.

☐ Frequency of revisions.
  - Features that persist in contracts or laws for many years, such as the work rules, the structure of jobs, and the structure of the pay scale.
  - Features that are renegotiated every one or two years, such as some or all of the foregoing.

☐ Reliance on automatic formulas for:
  - Promotions in rank.
  - Pay. Type of formulas:
    — Automatic increments.
    — Cost-of-living adjustments.

☐ Reactions of hospital workers when negotiations dissatisfy them.
  - Strike.
  - General social protest.
  - Poor job performance.
  - Resignations: new jobs elsewhere in health, changes to other careers.
  - Fatalistic continuation on the job as one's duty to the sick or to God.

☐ Relations to the methods of paying hospitals for operating costs.
  - Limits: Wage and other personnel awards must fit into the prospective budget and rates that have been awarded.
  - Pass-throughs: Prospective budget and rates automatically rise to cover the new pay rates and work rules.

☐ Roles of third parties, rate regulators, and grantors in making personnel awards.

Organization of Hospital Workers

Evolution in Europe. Trade unions arose as fighters for the working class against capitalist exploiters; they usually ignored hospital workers, who were not perceived as wage workers used by industrialists for their own enrichment. Professional nurses were the only hospital employees who were organized; but their associations were small, oriented toward service ideals, and only slightly concerned with wages and hours.

After World War II, civil service unions arose, with a spirit and purposes different from those of the industrial unions. They were not fighting the capitalists for a bigger share of their own output. Wanting "fair treatment," they sought guarantees that their members would receive no worse than prevailing hours, wages, fringe benefits, and contracts. They were interested in improving working conditions and the management of public employment; in particular, they sought new laws that would regulate public and nonprofit employment. The new unions by the 1960s had added sections for hospital workers; in some countries (such as France and Switzerland), many hospital workers were public employees; in others the nonprofit hospitals seemed so analogous to public employees that the civil service unions seemed natural homes. A great many different types of unions have organized hospital workers; as a result, great rivalry and (often) a strident tone have arisen from the industrial unionism of some.

Meanwhile, other sectors of the economy in most continental European countries were moving toward nationwide multiemployer collective bargaining, sometimes even industry wide. All regional unions formed national headquarters; all national federations joined in a few national confederations. The union confederations negotiated new contracts—including wages and hours—with the national confederations of employers. Some details were added in regional negotiations, after national pacts were signed. The basic contracts and the essential supplementary details were not negotiated at the levels of company and plant.[7]

The public service unions in continental Europe negotiated for hospital workers in the same way. They sought favorable regulations and wage levels each year from the French national government, covering all employees in the hospitals owned by the *communes*. And in other countries, they sought favorable contracts with the national association of hospitals.

The principal unions are accepted as the legitimate spokesmen for worker interests throughout the industry. Exact membership size does not determine whether an officially recognized union participates in negotiations. A European union therefore need not engage in frenetic activity to make sure that it wins certification and decertification elections. If several unions have members in the hospital staffs, all are represented on the labor side of the bargaining table; the largest leads the negotiations. The unions do not depend exclusively on dues; some are subsidized by political parties or by religious associations.

Health was "taken over" by nonhealth industrial unions in Europe in a top-down fashion. These unions were interested in organizing everyone *en masse* and had little awareness of the subtle distinctions among health occupations. They combined the nurses and other hospital employees. In contrast, when health occupations organize themselves—as they did in the Anglo-Saxon countries—the leaders of each are conscious of rivalries for prestige and for jurisdiction within the hospital. In particular, the nurses with the highest education and the greatest authority in the hospital refuse to join the same craft unions or industrial unions with the lower-ranking nurses and the other hospital workers. Rivalries occur over pay, work rules, and methods during strikes.

Trade unions in Europe quickly spread to entire industries, and alliances of several industrial unions covered each country. Inclusiveness and a national scale follow from a philosophy of solidarity of the working class: all crafts and the less skilled have common interests against the same boss and thus can share the same spokesmen; unions from all sectors can join against the system and against its government. Unity was needed to exercise effective political pressures, since the unions aimed at more than improving wages and hours in individual plants.

Evolution in Great Britain. Industrial unionism came late to England and North America. The traditions of individual entrepreneurship and free price setting in the market would have inhibited the development of large-scale industrial unionism. The traditions were further reinforced by lawsuits, government pressures, and management sanctions. Unions developed locally in plants with tolerant or impotent managers and courts. Often, however, the workers refused to unite in these plant-wide unions and joined craft groups instead. The union movements in Britain and North America evolved through painstaking plant-level organization and bottoms-up amalgamation.

Hospital workers had to organize themselves rather than join a ready-made national organization. Determined male workers create the first unions in every field, and a problem in a bottoms-up evolution is how to begin organizing in predominantly female occupations. British health unionism began around 1910 among the male nurses in several mental hospitals. They obtained minimum wages for mental nurses and domestics—both male and female—in several establishments. In 1946 they merged with other unions representing nonmental nurses and domestics, to form the Confederation of Health Service Employees (COHSE). In no industry has Britain had either consistent craft unionism or consistent industrial unionism, and the fragmentation has been accentuated in a puzzling field like health. COHSE has never organized the entire National Health Service, not even hospital workers. Since many hospitals were owned by local governments before the National Health Service was created, several unions representing local civil servants organized the local authority hospital workers and then other hospital workers after the start of the NHS; that is, the administrators and clerks joined the National Association of Local Government Officers (NALGO), and the blue-collar workers joined the National Union of Public Employees (NUPE). Many nurses refused to join any union but pressed the Royal College of Nursing (RCN) to act as one. All these groups have been rivals for members, each trying to expand into the constituency of the others. They have been rivals in political ideology, in labor policy, in tactics during periods of general labor disputes with the NHS, and in detailed policies in individual hospitals. The distribution of members among the groups differs in each hospital, and definitions of problems and remedies vary with the balance of forces; therefore, many disputes must be worked out at the plant level.

The National Health Service Act written by the Labour Government in 1946 adopted for all hospitals and other installations a system of joint negotiating committees representing both public authorities and trade unions, modeled after employer-union committees to prevent strikes during World War I ("Whitley Councils"). The workers in each sector of the NHS covered by a Whitley Council had to be represented by someone; therefore, unionization was institutionalized. No longer would hospitals refuse to negotiate or to recognize one or all unions. But neither the law nor the system created a method of standardizing the structure of the unions. All the separate organizations survived, their memberships and rivalry grew, and new unions have arisen. Several belong to each Whitley Council, depending on the categories of NHS worker covered by the agenda.

Cooperation among the several unions is fragile. Some (for example, NUPE) are active in the national trade union movement (the Trades Union Congress, or TUC); others (for example, COHSE) occasionally have dropped out;

and still others (for example, RCN) have never joined. Some are militant Leftists (for example, NUPE), while others are nonpolitical (for example, RCN); some are very large (for example, NUPE and COHSE), while others are small. Several think of themselves as professional associations and look down on the others as mere labor unions; for example, when special review machinery was created in 1983 to settle nurses' contracts and wages, the Royal College of Nursing unsuccessfully opposed inclusion of any lower ranks of nurses in such agreements or in representation in the machinery.[8]

The fragmentation and rivalry among the unions and bitterness over low pay make health one of the most turbulent industries in Great Britain.[9] Usually the unions strike at different times; their members and the members of nonhealth unions in TUC may or may not support the strikers by refusing to cross picket lines. Unity is unusual and fragile, since there exists no standing union machinery to decide goals and tactics for all the unions. For example, the alliance during the strike wave of 1982 was constantly beset by disagreements and finally collapsed. The larger and more militant unions were forced to settle in 1982, when the government appeased the professional association for nurses, the union for administrators, and the union of technicians with extra wage increases and other concessions.

United States. As in British voluntary hospitals before the National Health Service, American hospitals for years were (and still are) ruled in a patronizing fashion by community elites and by the doctors. The labor forces in American hospitals were docile: as in Europe, the hospitals depended on dedicated women who worked long hours at very low pay; many blue-collar workers were unemployable elsewhere; increasing numbers of workers now are blacks and Hispanics.

The owners and managers argued that unionization and agitation would disturb the natural harmony and hurt patient care. Therefore, American hospitals have always opposed discussing anything with unions, and merely obtaining recognition has been a constant hurdle. The American national government for many years protected the unions' opportunities to win recognition in other industries, but not in hospitals. Until 1974 the National Labor Relations Act was interpreted as not covering public and nonprofit hospitals; therefore, managers did not have to recognize or bargain with unions as a uniform national policy. Each state government handled matters differently. In practice most nonprofit hospitals were allowed to resist unionization on the grounds that they were charities: they earned no profits to become objects of negotiation. Finally, in 1974 the National Labor Relations Act was extended to the private nonprofits. The National Labor Relations Board has excluded all interns and residents from coverage, by defining them as students and not employees. The national government includes in allowable costs for Medicare and Medicaid the hospital's costs in influencing employees not to join unions. (When the Health Care Financing Administration tried to reverse the policy in the 1979 edition of the *Provider Reimbursement Manual,* the American Hospital Association filed a lawsuit, and HCFA backed down.)[10]

Under American labor law, an employer is required to negotiate with a union only if the workers in an appropriate bargaining unit—one substantial occupation or the entire plant—stand behind it. Therefore, a union first must win an election making it the exclusive bargaining representative of those workers. This requirement exists in few other countries; instead, several unions often face an employer on behalf of fractions of the same group of workers. One reason for the turbulence in Britain's National Health Service is the competition among unions during the bargaining with the government over wages and conditions. In contrast, America lacks enough hospital workers unions in each plant to contest recognition elections: usually the contest is between one union and the hospital management, which tries to get out an antiunion vote by promising generous treatment without deductions for union dues.

Besides the obstacles from hospital managers and the docility of many workers, the hospital unions have had the further handicap of trying to organize while the entire American labor movement has been stagnating. By 1984 union membership among all American wage and salary workers had declined to 18.8 percent. The hospital unions did no worse, but they could not become more successful. During the mid-1970s—their first years under the protection of the National Labor Relations Act—the hospital unions won two-thirds of recognition elections. But the victory rate had dropped to 40 percent by the late 1970s. Some previously recognized unions were losing new elections in which hospital management, dissident workers, or rival unions challenged their status as exclusive bargaining agents.[11] To a European observer, an American hospital union uses an exceptional amount of energy in obtaining and keeping recognition.[12] By the 1980s fewer than 20 percent of the private nonprofit hospitals and fewer than 10 percent of the proprietaries had any union contracts. As in other industries, unions are more successful in the governmentally owned hospitals, since they can pressure elected officials to cooperate. Altogether, about 20 percent of all American hospital employees are covered by contracts. Because of the fragmentation in organization, each contract covers only some of a hospital's employees; not many hospitals have the full set of contracts covering everyone.

The leaders of the national labor federations have never tried to organize all hospital workers, either in comprehensive industrial unions or in a series of craft unions. The resulting fragmentation and rivalry inhibit serious organizing efforts among the hospital workers. Only the state nursing associations seem to have a "natural"constituency and have members in many hospitals throughout the country. Other unions are active, trying to recruit members and to negotiate with hospital managers; many are based in other industries (such as government employees and teamsters) and recruit whatever hospital workers will join; few are active beyond one region; none have a monopoly on one occupation, not even the state nurses' associations. The proliferation of organizations contributes to the disorder, the hesitation of workers to join, the limited commitment by the state and national labor leaders, and the bargaining strength of management.[13]

Winning a recognition election among hospital workers does not ensure that a union will win a contract from management. Occasional strikes occur, but many hospital employees stay at work, picket lines are crossed freely, and wage gains are modest. In other American industries, unions become influential by incorporating shared controls over work rules and job security in contracts, but hospital managements retain almost complete control over job definitions and assignments of personnel.

Wage Determination

Forms of union representation and industrial relations in health arise out of national traditions. Also, they develop according to forms of hospital ownership: control by governments, by charitable associations, or by private physicians produces somewhat different outcomes in labor representation and in negotiating styles. There is no automatic connection between the country's method of deciding all hospitals' total operating costs and the method of organizing labor relations. However, there is a connection in outcomes: if total costs are restrained more strictly by payers, wage awards to workers and new hirings are limited. If government plays a big role in deciding hospital payment—particularly in global budgeting and direct grants from the Treasury—it will be drawn into the hospitals' labor relations.

Europe. Since the 1950s and 1960s, hospital labor conditions and wages have been integrated into the familiar patterns of multiemployer collective bargaining. The one or several national unions representing hospital workers form one side. The one or more hospital associations form the other; in some countries separate associations exist for public, nonprofit private, and for-profit private hospitals, or there are separate associations for secular, Catholic, and Protestant associations. If several hospital associations exist, the unions meet first the one representing the most prosperous and/or most numerous hospitals; then they try to close the same deal with the others soon afterward. In other instances all the hospital associations form a negotiating committee, as if they were a single national confederation. In a federal system such as Germany, the national confederations representing the hospital workers negotiate basic principles with the national hospital associations; associations of both sides in each province then adopt the principles and add details in the contracts that actually bind the hospitals.

In every European country, the unions representing government employees meet the representatives of the personnel and finance Ministries every year. They negotiate the design of the salary scale for use throughout government; actually, each year they alter certain categories in the long-established scales and revise rules for assigning occupations to categories. The two sides also discuss the financial value of the basic point, which—when multiplied against the points for each category—determines the wage for each category next year.

In countries with a substantial number of public hospitals, such as France and Switzerland, the hospital workers' unions meet representatives of the Ministry of Health every year to settle job definitions and assign occupations to categories in the wage scale. Actually, they revise long-established regulations. They also revise or add many other items, such as job definitions, fringe benefits, and seniority levels. When the currency value of the basic point in the wage scale is announced by the head of government, all government employees—including all the hospital workers, employed nurses, and employed doctors—learn their pay for the year. Unitary countries such as France follow the same rules and salary scale for the entire country, but federal countries decide them provincially. The unions then try to get the same terms of service and wages from the private nonprofit and for-profit hospitals.

For example, late every year in France the leading labor confederations (CGT, CFDT, and FO) meet with the national government to settle the pay rates for the civil servants throughout France for the next year. The government team is headed by the *Directeur Général de la Fonction Publique* in the office of the Prime Minister. The negotiations give financial values to the pay scale (the *barême*), whose numbers are 150, 151, 152, . . . 320, 321, 322, . . . 808, 809, 810. Every year, the negotiations give a franc-and-centime value to each of the 661 numbers in the scale, and the next year's negotiations raise all values by a standard percentage. The unions start by asking for a large increase, and the government makes a low counteroffer. The agreement may fix a percentage for the entire year, or a low percentage may be set for the first months and a higher percentage during later months. The two sides may agree on higher additional benefits, such as the supplements for living in Paris or the supplement for each child. They do not sign a contract, but a decree is issued by the President of France. The government has the final word in case of disagreements.[14]

The other fundamental issue in the negotiations—one allowing more discretion in the bargaining—is to assign the several ranks of each occupation to index numbers in the scale. For every group of occupations in the government, specialized teams from the labor federations meet with the personnel department of that Ministry and with representatives from the *Fonction Publique*. Such special meetings are held for all the occupations in health. One task is to assign each rank in each occupation a position in the *barême*, thereby determining all salaries. These assignments essentially persist over many years, but details change. In a dynamic field like health, new jobs are created and are redefined from time to time.[15] These specialized negotiations also deal with changes in rights, working conditions, and other such matters, and can continue outside the framework of the annual negotiations over wages.[16]

Legally, French public hospital employees work for the local governments and not for the national government. Decrees of the Minister of Health and of other Ministers concerned with hospital affairs instruct the commissioners (formerly the prefects) to apply the job definitions, their scale rankings, and the work rules to the public hospitals. In the past the Minister issued a decree applying the annual values of the *barême* to the public hospitals, but now the annual decree of the President is drafted to cover them.

Most European governments have income policies or anti-inflation policies that recommend annual rates of increase. Unions and business in the private sector cooperate unevenly, but public service unions and hospitals usually are more cooperative. The government's announcements about the income limits and anti-inflation guidelines usually come at the end of the preceding calendar year; and the announcement of new civil service wages comes during the spring, in preparation for the annual national budget. The civil service pay increases are close to the guidelines, and the sickness funds everywhere automatically accept them in the public hospitals' daily charges. Rate regulators always pass through the wage awards; but they may constrain an individual hospital's personnel spending by limiting its total number of employees.

The private nonprofit and for-profit hospitals try to negotiate wage awards that stay close to the government's income or anti-inflation legislation, since anything more might be resisted by the sickness funds.

By the end of each annual round of negotiations, everyone is covered: nearly all hospitals; all jobs in them; all employees, including all junior doctors and the salaried senior medical staffs. As in the rest of the economy, negotiations and contracts do not depend on elections to designate a particular union as bargaining agent, but they proceed in order to make equitable and peacefully accepted decisons. That is, the need to decide wages, hours, and terms of service by a method other than unilateral management dictation automatically assigns to the task the principal unions for hospital workers without special recognition elections. Usually, substantial agitation occurs throughout a country when the unions first press government and the hospitals to substitute the negotiating system for management dictation. Once the system is adopted, negotiations each year are usually quiet and businesslike. However, if the hospital workers seek a big improvement in their contracts—as the junior doctors and nurses did in Germany during 1971—they may parade in the streets and strike. Street parades in Paris by the hospital workers—either alone or in association with other government employees—are a customary part of the negotiating scenario nearly every year in France.

Continental Europe's wage system has tried to eliminate flux. The hospital occupations are given parity with other public service occupations by their location on the government wage scale. Occasionally, the annual negotiations move a hospital occupation slightly upward, but relationships usually are stable. The public wage scale until the late 1970s was linked to averages of private-sector wages, which were often indexed to consumer price indices; or, in some countries, the public-sector wages were indexed directly. Annual cost-of-living adjustments enabled some countries to adopt two-year contracts for hospital workers, instead of the once prevalent annual contracts. The explosion of inflation after 1972 throughout Europe persuaded many governments to back off from direct or indirect indexing; more recently, civil servants receive raises within guidelines from the Cabinets, often influenced by negotiations with the public service unions. Regardless of the basis of the general increase, the hospital workers always move with the rest of the public service. If a hospital manager needs to economize, he must become more productive, with fewer employees; or he must substitute persons with lower skills. He cannot pay lower wages.[17]

Great Britain's Negotiation System. Europe's hospital labor relations have become increasingly structured, centralized, calm, and expensive. They have been part of a general trend throughout the economy. A drawback is the difficulty of rolling back costs in hospitals, in industry generally, and in government payrolls. Britain and the United States have resisted these trends: union representation has been split and limited; the health sector is separate from others; employers (whether nonprofit, for-profit, or governmental) have been able to resist large and automatically increasing wage awards; contracts are reopened and often extensively rewritten at subsequent negotiations; wages at times are frozen or cut. Ultimately, much conflict developed in Britain when the NHS workers believed that the employer was taking unfair advantage, treating them worse than other workers. And the conflict became a political struggle, since the employer was a national government subject to removal in parliamentary votes of confidence and in general elections.

A General Whitley Council deals with issues common to all specialized councils, such as moving expenses, annual vacations, sick leaves, discipline and dismissal, grievance procedures, unemployment payments, and retirement. Specialized councils exist for administrators and clerks; ambulancemen; blue-collar ("ancillary") workers; dental employees of local authorities; medical and hospital dental employees; nurses and midwives; opticians; pharmacists; and other professionals and technicians. In each council the intricate contracts and government regulations concerning wages, fringe benefits, job definitions, job ratings, working conditions, and similar matters are negotiated. Much of the work is done by subcommittees and ratified or amended by the full councils. The unions or professional associations represent the category of workers under the jurisdiction of that council; different councils have different lineups of unions. Representatives of the NHS health authorities and representatives of the Department of Health and Social Security serve on the management sides of all the councils; over forty unions and associations represent employees. On each council each side has a secretariat, and the two secretariats manage the council jointly.

The beginnings and ends of contracts are not coordinated throughout the British economy; therefore, the various contracts cannot be dealt with at the same time. The unions do not want such unification: if a number of contracts are coming up for renewal and the government is preaching a ceiling for all, they want a tough union (such as the miners) to go first. There is not even coordination among the contracts within the NHS: they start at different times and run for different lengths. They are not closely coordinated with the PES cycle that provides the money. However, the annual nature of government budgeting and of government wage and price policy means that wages are reexamined every year or—at most—every other year. As a result, negotiations go on all year round, peaking at the time of renewals. The few negotiators in both DHSS and the unions are overloaded and lack the time to focus on a complex new subject, such as redefining an occupational group.

When government is the employer, a chronic issue is whether true negotiations are occurring—that is, whether the management representatives have authority to make an agreement and commit the government to the concessions. The management side in the Whitley Councils consists of some civil servants from DHSS and several RHA officials, who are as eager to extract money from the Treasury as the workers are. During the early years of the NHS, the management side made wage agreements that were unilaterally reduced by the Minister of Health. Only the weakness of unions at that time permitted this. Ever since, the management side has been careful to learn what the department is able to pay, in advance of any negotiations and concessions. As expenditure planning and PES were institutionalized, the *éminence grise* on the management side was the Treasury. But the Treasury was never present in the Whitley Councils, and the unions could never debate with their true adversary. Treasury and Cabinet have often enunciated policies of restraint, often with a percentage goal for wage increases; and the NHS is not allowed to breach the limits by offering or agreeing to more, since no public or private negotiations thereafter would respect even the new percentage. The PES cycle is completed and the cash limits are set before the conclusion of the NHS wage negotiations for that year. Therefore, the wages must fit the cash limits and not the reverse. When NHS cash limits are held down, wages of NHS workers lag behind the increases in more favored public sectors and in private employment

During the 1950s and 1960s, many wage negotiations in the Whitley Councils deadlocked, and the recognized arbitration machinery was used.[18] A tribunal could make an independent judgment, using any of several criteria: giving the occupation a just relation to wages in a comparable occupation in the private sector or in the local authorities; ensuring that the NHS can recruit enough employees for the job in the future; or implementing the government's policy on inflation and on the balance of payments. (Usually arbitrators have cited the first two criteria and often have ignored the government's wage policy, because they may assume that the need for arbitration makes the case special and because they wish to demonstrate independence from government. But in practice they usually have tried to avoid aggravating a national economic crisis.)

The more resourceful occupations never agreed to participate in NHS Whitley Councils. For example, doctors' pay was decided at first by direct bargaining with the higher ranks of the Ministry of Health and the national government, more recently by an independent investigating agency. The Whitley Councils have had a smooth history in the expert and complex tasks of working rules and job ratings, but they have had a more precarious experience with the straightforward conflict of interest over wages. Despite the once moderate temper of NHS employees, wage disputes have gone outside to arbitrators more often than expected. When unions became larger and more discontented over low pay during the 1970s, the Whitley Councils were soon bypassed. Strikes and "working to rule" were called; the disputes were waged in the mass media; and the negotiations involved the higher ranks of the unions and DHSS. Special commissions were appointed to investigate the pay and conditions of service of NHS occupations and to decide what increases were appropriate. Designed to restore order, several commissions aggravated the financial havoc by awarding large retroactive pay increases that upset national wage policy and breached DHSS's cash limits.[19]

Because the NHS during the 1970s became one of the more troubled economic sectors, investigators examined the Whitley Council system and proposed remedies. One possibility is to synchronize all the separate wage agreements around central economic decisions for the entire NHS. This would require greater authority by the General Whitley Council relative to the others dealing with individual occupations. The roles of DHSS and health authority members on the management side should be defined more carefully. A formal selection method should be developed for the membership on the staff side. Conciliators and mediators should be observers in all negotiations, with a right to intervene and head off trouble. Staff-management councils should be created at regional and local tiers, so that problems can be settled promptly and at appropriate levels, instead of letting them fester and instead of overloading the national councils. Grievance and discipline procedures should be created at the grass roots.[20]

Bridging the requirements of stable industrial relations and of public expenditure planning requires ingenuity. Industrial relations in the NHS have become overheated lately, in part because contracts run for only a year.

Negotiations are always going on, and claims are constantly being filed and dramatized. Private-sector contracts for wages and conditions of work run longer in Britain. They also run longer in hospitals in Europe and North America. On the other hand, wage policy and NHS cash limits are decided every year in Britain. Unless the unions are willing to live within each year's cash limits, or unless the government is willing to pay for automatic wage increases indexed by a formula, wages and the disposition of the NHS labor force must be reexamined every year. The unions and the government are not willing to abdicate their discretion at present.[21]

Other measures to make NHS industrial relations more predictable and more stable require a reform of British industrial relations more generally. Possible changes include the restructuring and consolidation of unions, stronger authority of national leaderships over shop stewards, and legal binding to contracts of all levels within the unions. Attempts to reform British industrial relations in these directions during the early 1970s precipitated the electoral defeats of governments, the destruction of political careers, and splits within the political parties. So the possibilities of such reforms within the NHS are remote.

Great Britain's Pay Rates. Wage structure—as well as the negotiating system for hospital workers—is part of the country's larger system of industrial relations and cannot be reformed completely in isolation. The most important element in hospital finance therefore moves along with the total economy.

The NHS shares with the British economy several weaknesses in the wage system. For example, during the 1960s, when systematic cross-national comparisons of economic indicators were being produced to explain differential national growth, the figures showed a paradox: compared to the rest of Europe, English labor had lower hourly rates, shorter hours, and higher total costs. All countries were prosperous then, and a favorite explanation was that England's booming economy overstrained its labor force and required much overtime. Actually, work was being done inefficiently and expensively, with the serious consequences evident during the 1970s.

During the nineteenth century, England and Europe had large numbers of workers and low rates of pay in each plant. European industry during the twentieth century substituted capital for labor to a greater extent than Britain did. Turnover increased in Europe, employers needed to attract workers to new jobs, unions pressed for more money, and wage rates were increased. Management's authority over the job was recognized. These trends occurred more slowly in Britain. Management was slower to introduce new equipment and to reorganize the job structure. A pervasive fear of unemployment led the unions to focus on job security, making sure that workers could keep their old jobs. To spread the work, unions pressed for shorter hours. Wage rates were low, but workers might earn a higher total income by getting credit for overtime hours at a higher rate, even if all the work could have been done in the regular hours.

When British governments adopted income policies to fight inflation, they usually controlled hourly rates; unions successfully pressed employers to circumvent the policies by reducing the official workweek at the controlled hours and by paying more overtime hours, even when overtime was unnecessary. Many firms could have done the work at a fast pace with fewer workers; since many workers were underemployed, absenteeism was high. As long as British producers had foreign and domestic markets, the overmanning and low productivity did not seem weaknesses. Attempts to introduce labor-saving equipment, cut the overmanning, and limit overtime precipitated strikes, and it seemed better to buy peace through appeasement. If new equipment was installed, the tradeoff might be to retain the entire work force, formally guarantee overtime, and grant everyone "incentive bonuses" regardless of performance. The house of cards finally collapsed during the 1970s, when more efficient and less expensive foreign producers captured foreign markets and gained large shares of domestic British markets.

British hospitals before and after the creation of the NHS paid wages in this style. Rates have been even lower than those in the private sector, for all grades. As the blue-collar NHS employees (the "ancillaries") became members of unions with slightly better-paid counterparts in private firms and in local authorities, they had to be appeased by their union leaders; and one method was overtime pay. During negotiations in the 1960s over the reduction of NHS overmanning and over increasing effort by the remaining workers, "bonus schemes" were introduced.[22] In theory they were contingent on a steady increase in productivity; but actually they were an automatic guarantee of extra money for the ancillaries, supplementing their incomes from hourly pay and overtime. Outside of nursing services, many sections of many hospitals might have done their work with fewer employees and much less overtime, but customs were implanted, and the unions insisted that concessions be compensated.[23] Treasury and DHSS during the 1970s and the 1980s became more critical of overmanning, overtime payments, and the bonus payments within NHS. But, in response, the health care unions grew in membership, in militancy, and in political influence within the Labour Party. They called strikes for the first time in the history of the NHS.

One might think that an ideal solution is to take pay out of controversy, make the decisions automatic, tie health service wages to those in private business (as in other European countries), and decide all NHS wages at the same sessions. The unions favor linking with private wages—as the European health workers' unions do—but the British government does not. Particularly under Conservatives, DHSS has practiced a market strategy in offering wage increases: DHSS identifies whether unfilled jobs exist in some occupations within NHS, offers higher wages to attract persons into those jobs, but favors only minimum increases for others. For example, a widespread perception in Britain is that professional nurses are paid too little and earn less than workers in comparable occupations in both public and private employment. But DHSS responds that nurses are not truly underpaid, since the NHS can hire enough, few British nurses are unemployed, few emigrate, and the nursing market is in equilibrium.[24]

The present methods, despite the high cost in trouble, are advantageous to government (whether Labour or Conservative) because they cost less money than linking would. The "fiddles" are increments upon a low base: the basic wage rates are lower than those of private and government employees. In between the catching-up awards of much-publicized commissions (such as Halsbury in 1974-75 and Clegg in 1979-80), NHS wages lag behind wages outside of health.[25] Any linking of NHS wages to the private sector's would be inflationary, since private productivity rises while NHS productivity does not. Linking would be doubly expensive in health if there were no "give-backs" in manning, overtime, incentive bonuses, and control over the job. If NHS occupations are decided in separate negotiations, the government can strike better bargains with the more placid adversaries (such as the Royal College of Nursing and COHSE for the very large number of nurses), instead of facing a single coalition dominated by the most militant union (such as NUPE, which draws its strength primarily from the manual workers and ambulancemen). One might think that all wage increases in a year would be settled at the same percentage, but outcomes differ for several reasons: each council has a slightly different lineup of unions and negotiators; contracts are settled at different times; wage increases involve revision of contracts with intricate pay scales and job definitions, and the outcome is not clear-cut; the management teams on the councils are poorly coordinated.

The disorganized situation benefited both sides during the 1970s. The unions' agitation caused wages in the NHS to *rise* faster than average national earnings and the cost of living:[26]

	NHS salaries and wages	Average national earnings	Consumer prices (all goods and services)
1969	100	100	100
1970	119	112	106
1971	133	125	116
1972	149	141	125
1973	165	159	136
1974	233	188	158
1975	300	238	196
1976	335	275	228

But even at the end, NHS wages did not fully "catch up" with British private-sector pay, and they remained far below Europe's: a comparative study of acute-care hospitals in five Common Market countries in 1975 identified the following average monthly wages of nursing staffs in the hospitals studied. (The numbers are converted into French francs in purchasing-power parities.)[27]

	Registered nurses	Nursing assistants
Great Britain	3,242	2,482
France	3,562	3,112
West Germany	4,176	
Belgium	5,223	
Netherlands	6,222	3,759

As a result, Britain spent a lower proportion of its GNP on health than any other developed country.

Canada. The Anglo-Saxon style of unstructured industrial relations still operates in Britain, despite the national ownership of facilities, despite the

Whitley Council machinery, and despite central Treasury financing. Besides the effects of tradition and the unions' rivalry, the situation persists because the government finds the fluid situation advantageous.

Like Britain before the NHS, Canada once had hospitals that were privately owned and independent, a hospital work force that was differentiated in varied types of jobs and was nonunionized, and hospital financing that was private and heterogeneous. As I explained in Chapter Eight, financing has changed but hospital ownership has not.

Since World War II, Canadian hospital labor relations and wage determination have become more structured and more centralized, because of the following forces:[28]

- Determined political parties of the Left captured several provincial governments in the Prairies and West and enacted laws encouraging union organization and collective bargaining in all sectors, including hospitals. Other provinces followed.
- Union leaders and political parties successfully induced many hospital workers to join province-wide unions. Many were industrial unions, accepting any member who worked in health.
- Hospitals in every province after 1958 depended on operating funds from the provincial government. The working classes paid taxes and had full rights to use hospitals. Therefore, hospitals could not fight off unionization and negotiations.
- Provincial hospital associations became important in lobbying for annual grants and for favorable program conditions at the provincial Ministries of Health. Many associations developed labor policies for their members, since wages and work rules determined the financial requests from the Ministries, particularly during the years of bottoms-up global budgeting and grants.

On the other hand, complete centralization and automatic wage awards have never been adopted in Canada.

- The hospitals remain private and autonomous. Each hospital retains its right not to sign any province-wide contracts. Each seeks to work out any details in agreements with its own union locals or in its own unilateral management decisions: several provincial hospital associations and the unions negotiate framework contracts, while the individual hospital decides detailed clauses, with or without local negotiations; in some provinces hospitals negotiate their own local contracts independently of province-wide agreements.
- Provinces vary in the prevalence and authority of province-wide contracts. For example, Ontario has much less province-wide negotiation than Quebec or the Prairies.
- Wages are never linked automatically to private-sector occupations or to the civil service.
- Automatic increases in hospital workers' pay are not possible when hospital operating budgets are dictated by provincial government allowances.

Canada has Treasury financing but lacks the potential unity from government ownership of hospitals. They remain independent. Therefore, it is often difficult to determine who is in charge on the employers' side of the table: each individual hospital, the provincial hospital association, or the provincial Ministry of Health:

☐ *Each hospital.* All Canadian hospitals evolved out of the North American tradition. That is, at first each hospital management set its pay and hours unilaterally; then in discussions with committees of employees; then with provincial unions representing different categories of workers. Officially, each hospital's contract is still individual, with special details of its own, even if the provincial hospital association takes the lead in negotiating a frame contract. Unions in the most decentralized provinces—such as Ontario—take advantage of individual bargaining by getting favorable settlements from the biggest hospitals first.

☐ *Hospital association.* Provincial hospital associations become drawn into negotiations because an experienced staff and province-wide body must face the province-wide unions and the Ministry of Health. But the associations have often found the task enervating and thankless, and some have tried to back away. They lack management authority over the hospitals, cannot quickly cut deals, cannot force a hospital to conform to a compromise agreement, and are often blamed for conceding too much. They are not assured of wage pass-throughs in the form of automatically higher provincial grants; and they will inadvertently cause all their members to be squeezed if they agree to much higher wage increases than the province will underwrite in its operating grants. (This occurred in Ontario in 1974, teaching the Ontario Hospital Association extreme caution ever after.) In Quebec the hospital association has insisted that it is a voluntary professional society, but a common front was needed to face the province's energetic unions; therefore, the Quebec hospitals created a special common bargaining agent, fully empowered to negotiate province-wide contracts.

☐ *Ministry of Health.* The division that screens hospital budgets invariably avoids telling the hospitals in advance what the allowable wage increase will be. Often it does not know sufficiently in advance the money it will get from its own Treasury Board. Contracts for different classes of hospital worker expire and are negotiated at different times. If the Ministry told the hospitals the probable annual increase it expected to get from Treasury Board or the probable wage movements in the country, no hospital would be able to settle for less, and many unions would get more. By keeping everyone guessing, governments can restrain wage inflation. By staying out of labor relations, the provincial governments hope to avoid a political quagmire. But the fact that they pay the bills prevents them from standing aloof: the unions became militant during the 1960s and 1970s; they presumed that the provincial government would rarely risk refusing to pay a wage award for the eternally "underpaid" hospital workers; and the hospital managers gambled (usually correctly) that the provincial governments would underwrite any but the most exorbitant settlement.[29]

Eventually, some provincial Ministries became drawn into the negotiations to limit hospital managements' offers: in Quebec the bargaining strategy is set by the Treasury Board, and the key Ministries (Social Affairs and Treasury) join the hospital association in the management side of the negotiating committee. (In contrast, in the few other provinces where Ministries observe wage negotiations, they are only observers.)

When the provincial government clearly demonstrates that it is in charge, it becomes a political target, as it feared. For example, Quebec in 1982 had to cut expenditures to reduce the provincial government deficit. One target of its reduction was the operating grants to the hospitals. The government set a bargaining strategy to freeze many health care wages, particularly higher ones. At the negotiating sessions, the unions refused and insisted on the formula increases for 1983 that had previously been agreed. The National Assembly of Quebec in early 1983 passed a law amending the formula and canceling the increase, particularly at higher wage levels. The hospital workers throughout the province called a general strike for one day but soon surrendered: the lower ranks got small increases and stayed on the job; all realized that the province had a financial crisis; hospital workers were well paid by Canadian standards; and hospital workers were thought lucky to have jobs at times of high unemployment. The bruising dispute gave the *Parti Québecois* government an apparent victory but reduced its political strength. And the provincial government could no longer pretend that wage determination was a private transaction.

During the 1960s and 1970s, Canadian hospital finance had an internal contradiction. Wages—the most important component in costs—were decided without a central structure and rational controls. Unions pressed hospitals to pay wage increases; the unions and the hospitals persuaded the politically compliant provinces to raise grants; and the provinces could be generous, since they billed the national government for half the costs under HIDS. The consequences eventually created budgetary and economic problems on a national scale and required concerted action. The national government incurred deficits, in part because of uncontrollable federal-provincial shared-cost programs such as HIDS. Large wage increases paid by provincial governments (to teachers, hospital workers, and others) inspired higher private wages; inflation was fueled throughout the country; and Canada's international trade balance weakened.

Convinced that the permissive and unstandardized wage-determination system was unbalancing its own budget and the economy generally, the national government overrode it by direct controls over all wages, prices, and profits. Contracts beginning in 1976 in hospitals and in all other sectors were affected.[30] Wages were limited to an annual inflation rate target (8 percent in 1976, 6 percent in 1977, and 4 percent in 1978), plus adjustments for productivity and experience. Hospital workers were limited in this fashion, and the annual increases in aggregate Canadian hospital expenditures were lower. As controls came off and wage determination returned to its heterogeneous provincial patterns, wages and total nationwide hospital spending again rose. (Table 10-1 shows wage changes for general-duty nurses, but similar trends existed for other hospital employees.)

British and Canadian experiences suggest that global budgeting and direct grants alone—even by a determined single payer—are not enough automatically

Table 10-1. Wages for General Duty Nurses in Canada.

	Percentage increase over previous year	
	Average monthly salary of general duty nurses	*All expenditures in all Canadian general and allied special hospitals*
1973	8.7	13.2
1974	21.1	22.2
1975	23.6	25.7
1976	8.1	16.3
1977	6.5	10.0
1978	10.4	9.0
1979	6.3	11.1
1980	16.7	15.9
1981	13.9	16.2
1982	15.1	16.2

Source: Adapted from *Salaries and Wages in Canadian Hospitals, 1970 to 1977* (Ottawa: Health and Welfare Canada, 1980), p. 34; *Salaries and Wages in Canadian Hospitals, 1979 and 1980* (Ottawa: Health and Welfare Canada, 1982), p. 40; and *National Expenditures in Canada, 1970–1982* (Ottawa: Health and Welfare Canada, 1983), p. 33.

to place a firm lid on cost increases. The principal source of costs is personnel, and therefore restraints must reach wages and levels of staffing. Cost-restraining pressures from the top confront cost-raising pressures from the workers in each organization. The employees are a political force, and enforcing cost restraints requires confronting the political force at whatever level it is exerted, either at the local, regional, or national scene. Sometimes the hospital managers are strong enough at the grass roots and willing to take the heat locally, so that they can carry out the total budget restraints in their wage awards, overtime hiring, and total staffing. But autonomous private hospital managers (as in Canada) or public hospital managers (as in Britain) may need backup from the Ministry in the form of guidelines in order to deflect the pressures from managers of their own subordinate units and from the local unions. Significant cutbacks that create unemployment definitely require higher intervention—even when the hospitals are owned and managed by government, as in Britain—since the managers in the field try to buy peace in labor relations by preserving the status quo.

The Canadian experience suggests that cost containment over personnel under global budgeting and direct grants requires fixing full responsibility on a single payer. Until 1977 each provincial government bore the full political costs of antagonizing the hospital workers' unions. But it did not bear the full financial costs of appeasing them: half the money was supplied by the national government. Ottawa renegotiated HIDS so that it paid block grants to the provinces, abandoned proportionate cost sharing, and left the provinces with full responsibility to pay for or to economize on personnel. Some provinces continued to underwrite wage increases,[31] but clearly they were spending their own money.

United States. At present in hospital labor relations, no national pattern exists: some entire states have no unionization and collective agreements at all, and many areas even in more unionized states have none. Unions need no longer approach hospitals according to the heterogeneous laws and machinery of the states, but the 1974 NLRA amendments have not resulted in a substantial increase in unionization and collective agreements; the amendments have not produced uniform national patterns. Every individual hospital or multihospital system must develop its own job structure and its own payment policy.

The European manager has many things decided for him: he does not negotiate labor contracts, and wage awards are almost automatically passed through. An American hospital manager has more to manage. He can coordinate his wage and price decisions. If some of his employees are unionized, he must take risks, such as buying peace or chancing strikes. Usually the strikes cannot force him to pay out much, but the forlorn nurses around the front entrance are bad public relations, and too many strikes will hurt his career.

The wage outcomes are never predictable within an American hospital, since results in each place are slightly different, and the annual increases are not standard. Nurses are preoccupied with the pay and benefits in their own hospital, and they rarely form a common front for a standard package in a region. If they are displeased, the nurses' solution is the individual action of quitting and taking another job, resulting in higher turnover in the United States than in other countries.[32] Because all labor relations are resolved at the plant level, the management of the individual hospital is stronger in the United States than it is in other countries; skillful individual managers can often drive hard bargains (with individual workers in nonunionized hospitals and even with unions), subject only to the constraint of attracting enough workers. At times average hospital workers' pay in an area rises faster than that of comparable service workers; at other times it rises less rapidly.[33]

Unionization in American hospitals raises wages between 5 and 20 percent, at least initially, when the unions get their first contracts in each hospital. The effects of unions on wages vary by occupation: highest for health aides and technicians, lower for service and maintenance workers, lowest for nurses. After the first effects, American hospital unions may not be powerful enough to keep wages substantially higher than the upward trends occurring simultaneously in the minimum wage laws and in market forces.[34] The strength and effectiveness of unions vary by region; in many parts of the United States, their effect on wages and hospital costs is slight.[35] Throughout the country, unions exercise less influence over work rules in hospitals than in other industries.[36] The laws about minimum wages and maximum hours at present may be at least as important as union activity in protecting workers in this traditionally underpaid and once overworked industry, simply because these laws affect all hospitals and workers, while the unions do not.

Hospital workers' hourly wages started far below those of comparable occupations, since the hospital workers earned less money for longer hours. The wages of hospital workers since World War II in the United States—as in every other country—have *risen* faster than the wages of comparable workers.[37] But their cash still remains below that of other workers in much of the United States. American hospitals have gotten steadily more expensive, and the nonwage costs— capital, administration, medical supplies, and the like—have been rising even faster than the payrolls. As a proportion of all hospital operating costs, payrolls and fringe benefits steadily declined from 66 percent in 1960 to 59 percent in 1982, despite a growth in the number of employees.[38] In all other developed countries, the share for personnel rose steadily from less than 60 percent in the 1950s to between 66 percent and 80 percent today.

The United States therefore has managed to develop the world's most expensive hospitals in the absence of the forces that correlate most strongly with hospital costs abroad—namely, strong unionization and linking of wages. Therefore, perhaps America's biggest hospital cost explosion is still to come.

Pass-Throughs of Wage Increases

In every payment system, a fundamental question is whether increases in certain items in the hospital's costs should be covered automatically by the payer and regulator. Such items include energy, medical supplies, and capital, as well as wages. Those in favor of pass-through policy defend it on the grounds that such prices are set by higher-ups and are beyond the individual hospital's control. Those opposed to automatic pass-throughs argue that the individual hospital's managers need to bargain with their suppliers, reduce waste, and limit their costs.

As this chapter has explained, the trend in most developed countries has been to connect hospital wages to larger national patterns and to avoid industrial conflicts within the hospitals. Negotiators, regulators, and payers of hospital rates now accept these patterns as national policy decisions when once they might have protested that hospitals differed and were exempt. When these negotiators, regulators, and payers try to limit the hospitals' personnel costs, they challenge the staffing levels, use of overtime, or financial supplements, not the basic wage rates.

Negotiating Systems for Hospital Rates. If bilateral bargaining methods were unfettered, the payer would pay minimum rates and advise the hospital to pay low wages. Such was the practice in Germany until the late 1960s. The sickness funds paid low daily rates, forcing the hospitals to employ few workers, impose sixty-hour workweeks, and keep wages low. But these developments in the hospital sector contradicted the German trend toward industry-wide and nationwide collective bargaining, comparable pay and comparable hours for all workers, and social solidarity. During 1971 hospital workers struck. Hospital employment was then changed to become like employment in any other public sector. The need to pay the costs was an important reason for the hospital-financing reforms of the 1970s.

By now it is clear to both German hospital owners and the sickness funds that wage parity is public policy. The national federations representing blue-collar workers (DGB), white-collar workers (GTV), and the salaried and professional workers (DAG) speak for the hospital workers. Every spring they meet with the national government's Ministry of Interior and with the national negotiating teams of the provinces and *communes*. The two sides negotiate contracts and wage rates for all government employees, including all doctors, nurses, teachers, nursing students, and workers in the provincial and municipal hospitals. The framework contract stays in effect for many years, with occasional revisions and supplements. (An example is the framework contract for all officials, including doctors, senior nurses, and clinical teachers, the *Bundes-Angestelltentarifvertrag,* or BAT.) Specific additional framework agreements about hospital work are negotiated between the union representatives and public representatives specializing in health. Those sessions are expanded to include observers on the management side from the associations representing all public and nonpublic hospitals (such as the *Deutsche Krankenhausgesellschaft*) and representing particular groups (such as certain Catholic multihospital chains and certain private clinics). The main contracts bind all the public hospitals and— with some adaptations—are accepted by the nonprofit and for-profit hospitals. They become universal because the unions insist, because postwar Germany practices order and standardization, and because the costs are guaranteed in the *Pflegesatz* under the KHG and the associated financing reforms.

The national negotiations set forth the general framework on job structures and the average wages for the country for each position and seniority level. This is really a relative-values agreement. The country varies in prosperity and in private wages. Negotiations over specific wage scales are held within each *Land* by the provincial counterparts of the national negotiators who created the framework. Adaptations of the national framework and additional details can be settled at the *Land* level. But the essentials have been settled nationally, and local decisions are usually automatic and quick.

KHG and its regulations in 1972–1974 obligated the sickness funds to pay the full costs of care in appropriately managed and appropriately staffed hospitals. The sickness funds were expected to pay for the higher wages and the larger number of workers; they were relieved of the costs of paying disability allowances, and they could find additional funds by raising their premiums. The "cost explosion" that followed in hospital budgets during the mid-1970s startled the country and displeased the employers (who paid both the disability allowances and the higher insurance premiums). But the reform fulfilled its intentions. In their annual negotiations with the hospital over the *Pflegesatz*, the sickness funds can still challenge the size of the personnel costs in the *Selbstkostenblätter;* but the debate is now devoted entirely to possible excesses in numbers of workers. If the hospital is not adding personnel, the bargaining sessions can last barely fifteen minutes.

Rate Regulation Systems for Hospitals. Regulators review the total expenditure for personnel in the prospective budgets. They have always been supposed to be vigilant about overstaffing, and the guidelines of the late 1970s and 1980s often give maximum staff/patient or staff/bed ratios. The regulators usually do not comment on wage rates, either before or after they are negotiated. The trend toward linking hospital and other wages leaves the rate regulators no role, and the individual hospital usually must go along with regional or national agreements. So, when restraining costs in the individual hospital, the regulator tries to limit the aspect for which the hospital management is responsible: staffing.

For example, the examiner in the Dutch regulatory commission (COZ, now COTG) is supposed to limit hospital nursing costs to a certain number of guilders per patient per day. (An example appears in Chapter Seven, p. 133.) Salary rates and working conditions are decided by nationwide collective bargaining between the National Hospital Council (NZR) and the trade unions of hospital employees. The one-year or two-year Collective Labor Agreement *(Collective Arbeidsovereenkomst)* includes the pay rates for nurses and all other hospital employees. Annual increases in pay in the public sector (such as hospitals) are linked to annual increases in private wages and are granted every spring. When the Central Planning Bureau publishes the price and wage indexes, the limit on maximum nursing costs per day is automatically set: the maximum number of nurses per patient-day (set in the guideline) times the probable new wage rate equals the limit on nursing expenditure per patient-day. If an ordinary hospital exceeds the limit in a special application (described in Chapter Seven), the COTG examiner questions the number of employees. Specialized hospitals can pay premium wages, but they must justify the exceptions. The new system of initial screening of the prospective budget by the sickness funds enables the payers to check each hospital's computations and staffing. Previously, the busy COZ examiners investigated only the special applications.

In France, Holland, and other European countries with rate regulation, the prospective budget usually is examined after the next year's wage rates are negotiated. The use of cost-of-living adjustments usually makes the new total predictable, even if the new rates have not yet been announced. If wage increases are awarded later, supplementary budgets and new hospital rates automatically cover them. The guidelines also provide automatic pass-throughs of prices for other uncontrollable items, such as heating oil.

Basic wage rates are automatically approved, but supplements are not, since they are awarded by each hospital management. Extra salary and amenities to managers and technicians might be justified to attract scarce labor and inspire superior performance. But they may result from self-dealing by insiders, and the sickness funds should not have to pay them. Trying to attract other hospitals' managers, nurses, and technicians by extra pay disrupts the others and does not improve the performance of the health care system. Special regulations and decisions by the appeals courts specify the criteria for distinguishing between legitimate extra payments and benefits and those considered *abusif*.[39] The DDASS in France can strike illegitimate payments from the hospitals' prospective budgets, but detecting them requires investigation.

The more amorphous styles of rate regulation and labor relations in the United States sometimes drag rate regulators into wage negotiations, but not invariably. A payer or a regulator is someone who says "no," and unions prefer to face only persons who say "yes." In states without rate regulation, unions demand more money from hospitals, oppose having to listen to negative arguments from payers at wage-bargaining sessions, and let the hospitals charge the payers more. A few states introduced rate regulation because Blue Cross and other insurers were too generous or because hospitals passed along mounting costs to patients. Hospitals then had a new argument against wage settlements when bargaining with unions: allegedly draconian regulators would forbid them to pass along increases to third parties and to patients. Everyone at the wage-bargaining table needs to know the regulators' position, but the regulators— although the *éminence grise* in wage settlements—refuse to attend. The unions oppose advance announcement of regulatory limits: they wish to obtain generous settlements, let the hospitals bear the burden of making the case to the regulators, and present the regulators with a *fait accompli*. One solution has been to prolong negotiations over wages for months: the hospital and union converge on a settlement, the hospital tells its probable labor costs to the regulators, the regulators decide to underwrite some or all of the costs, and the union and hospital then sign a final contract. Another solution is to sign a contract with a "subject-to" clause: the hospital agrees on a wage level subject to a sufficient revenue award by the regulators.[40]

If the American regulators are a line department under the governor, as in New York, the unions then try to persuade the governor to allow a sufficient rate increase to cover the "subject-to" wage settlement. The governor gains votes, and third parties pay the costs. Such political concessions undermine the integrity of a supposedly neutral regulatory system and demoralize the administrators. After a decade of intermittent generosity, New York's governor in 1984 refused to signal such generosity to settle a prolonged strike among all of New York City's nonprofit hospitals. The union had gambled on his intervention and suffered its worst defeat.

An American state regulatory commission occasionally intervenes to influence labor contracts, so that hospitals become more efficient. Wages might be linked to greater productivity or to the general cost of living. The union is offered a particular wage increase for a particular number of employees, so that the total hospital costs do not exceed a target. Such intervention occurs in American states, such as Maryland, where the commission's mandate is to improve the efficiency of hospital care, not only to limit costs and set rates.[41]

When personnel trends in the regulated American states are analyzed statistically, the result is much like that in other countries: rate regulation restrains the growth in numbers of workers more strictly than it limits increases in wage rates.[42]

Global Budgeting. When the payer is also the owner of the hospitals, it cannot avoid full responsibility for negotiating contracts and wages. It grants only what it can afford. In Great Britain, for example, the Ministry of Health's negotiators must limit wage concessions to the appropriations they can obtain from the Treasury.

This presumes a degree of Treasury authority and interministerial coordination that was not always attained during the early years of Britain's NHS, as I reported on previous pages. PES and other expenditure reforms were introduced so that DHSS and other Ministries could make current decisions (for example, about wage rates) in the light of probable future funding levels. Under the pooling of services and expenditures in the NHS at present, DHSS can decide to improve morale or buy peace with higher wages, but it must make compensating cuts in services.

If the British Cabinet has appointed a special commission to restructure compensation in general or to settle a particular dispute, the Cabinet and Treasury are obligated to supplement the expected allocation to the NHS. Special commissions are unusual, appointed only when the Whitley system has broken down or when an occupation has convinced Parliament and the public that its situation is chronically unfair. A permanent arbitration commission of this sort—the Review Body on Doctors' and Dentists' Remuneration—has long decided the payment of professions that were not included in the regional or district health authority's operating budgets for hospitals.[43] The Cabinet and Treasury nearly always agree to payment in full, by adding the money to the DHSS expenditures. The awards have been reduced—or, more often, postponed—

only if the Prime Minister pointed to an exceptional budget crisis. A similar independent Review Body was created in 1983 for regular recommendations about the payment of all nurses and midwives in NHS. Therefore, the largest category in the hospitals' operating costs would be settled by arbitrators rather than by bilateral negotiation in the Whitley Councils. The Cabinet and Treasury were expected normally to provide the money, as they do for the doctors and dentists.

In contrast to Britain, global budgeting and public grants in Canada are associated with private and municipal ownership of the hospitals. It is the owners and not the payers who negotiate the labor contracts. The provincial governments—except for Quebec, described earlier—play no role in the negotiations. The governments expect the hospitals to keep down labor costs by all methods.

The annual cycles for labor contract renewals, government budgeting, and hospital rate regulation coincide in Europe, so that rate setters know the forthcoming labor costs. But in Canada the annual budget-setting cycles for the provincial governments and Ministries of Health usually do not coincide with the cycles of labor negotiation between the unions and the hospitals. No system exists: in much of Canada, several unions represent workers, and a hospital often faces them at different times during the year. The methods of negotiation change, in some provinces more often than others. For example, Ontario gravitates between individual hospital and province-wide negotiation; the bargaining unit varies among occupations.

At times a provincial Ministry makes clear its allowable wage increases, particularly if it has given the annual global budgets before the time for the labor renewal negotiations; at other times it leaves unclear the percentage increase that it will cover. (A Ministry of Health's deepest secret is the size of the contingency fund it maintains to cover overruns of individual hospitals at the end of the year and to cover over-ceiling wage agreements that it will reluctantly accept). At times a Ministry adds money to the installments of each global budget to cover an individual wage award since the start of the fiscal year; at other times it collects all the settlements and then underwrites a total figure that may or may not cover every award.

Limiting Numbers of Workers

Total cost containment in labor-intensive enterprises such as health requires limiting numbers of workers as well as wage rates. As wages rose under European collective bargaining and pay linking, rate regulators enforced guidelines that limited numbers of hospital workers to the volume of work. The regulators could cut back the personnel lines in prospective budgets if numbers of nurses, domestics, and other personnel were excessive. Examples are cited in Chapter Seven.

The initial theory of global budgeting presumed that such detailed oversight was unnecessary. For example, in Britain's National Health Service, each DHA got a lump sum and had discretion to use it most effectively. Since the DHA could not hire cheaper labor, it was supposedly motivated not to overstaff. But if overmanning had been customary before, many DHAs have retained the existing personnel instead of reducing them, thereby failing to free resources for new or expanded services. DHSS thought that financial limits would inspire beneficial economies and reorganization at the grass roots, but the manager in the field shrank from fights with his workers.[44] Since British workers and their unions resist transfers to new jobs, openings were often filled with new workers, even if the DHA and its hospitals were overmanned. DHSS could not cut the annual RAWP awards to some regions—such as the London regions during the late 1970s—if numbers of employees remained the same. Therefore, DHSS in 1983 began sending guidelines to all RHAs, requiring specific reductions in personnel. Between March 31, 1983, and March 31, 1984, each RHA was asked to reduce total staff by 0.75 percent to 1 percent. Blue-collar and domestic posts were to be reduced between 1.35 percent and 1.8 percent. RHAs submitted quarterly summaries of total manpower to DHSS, which then could monitor the reductions. Each RHA would monitor implementation by its DHAs.

During 1984 and 1985, DHSS judged that certain RHAs were overprovided and overmanned, and it specifically instructed them to reduce jobs by certain numbers. (For example, the North West Thames RHA was instructed to reduce beds by 2,000 and jobs by 5,000 during the next decade.) Since the RHA plans were supposed to be comprehensive, embracing long-term and short-term changes in services and personnel as well as in facilities alone, the plans were supposed to spell out the anticipated reductions in personnel while maintaining services to satisfy the populations' needs.[45] The controls succeeded. During 1984 the number of employees in the National Health Service dropped for the first time.

During the mid-1980s, the Thatcher Government was unable to make the NHS a public corporation or a partially private enterprise, as it preferred. But it applied its philosophy of privatization to several departments of hospitals with reputations for overmanning and "fiddles." Instead of maintaining full staffs of NHS employees to perform the work, DHAs were expected to place cleaning, laundering, maintenance, and several other tasks out to private tender. Private business firms would do the work for fixed and predictable sums, and the workers no longer would be employed by the NHS. Exempt from Whitley awards and political pressures, the private firms were expected to lower labor costs and speed the work pace.

Fiscal restraints from global budgeting alone may not force personnel cuts when jobs are filled and unions protect their members from unemployment. British experience suggests that other instruments must be added. However, if jobs are unfilled, the pressures of global budgeting may eventually lead hospitals to eliminate them from the organizational structure, so that the available money will be used for other purposes and will not be recaptured by the payers. For example, persistent openings were finally eliminated from hospital rosters in British Columbia.[46] Therefore, global budgeting ultimately resulted in a permanently lower staffing level and higher productivity—just as it was supposed to do.

Summary

The trend in developed countries is to assimilate nurses and other hospital workers into the general labor movement. After a period of low membership in unions and fragmentation among their organizations, they are included in the larger national union federations. Negotiation of their contracts and wages often is part of larger negotiations covering public employment. They are organized into rank structures that are placed in the general public structures of ranks and pay. Even if they are not included in such larger negotiations, hospital workers are covered by nationwide or regional bargaining for the hospital industry alone. Dictation by each hospital management has disappeared, except in the United States. During the initial stage of plant-level decisions and fragmented organization, hospital labor relations are turbulent, but eventually national organization and linkage introduce stability.

In most countries the distinctions between professions and ordinary workers blur. Junior doctors, nurses, and the remaining hospital workers think of themselves as a common labor force seeking better positions and pay in the same hierarchy. However, in some countries the nurses belong to a long professional and charitable tradition; their professional association refuses to cooperate with the blue-collar unions; and hospital owners can deal with them separately. One result is lower pay.

In wage negotiations the identity of the true leader on the management side often is difficult to discern. Particularly when hospital revenue is governed by rate regulation or by global grants, the Ministry of Finance has the final word. But the unions face the owners and not Finance in the bargaining. The trend is to settle the uncertainty by tying hospital wages to civil service wages, by connecting the hospital workers to the public service unions who negotiate with a government team that includes Finance. Therefore, Finance is obligated to approve the NHI payroll taxes and the general revenue grants that cover the hospital's wage increases.

At one time junior doctors, nurses, and hospital workers had long hours, inconvenient shifts, low pay, and heavy reliance on psychic and religious gratification. Now the trend everywhere—even in the United States—is toward normal schedules, normal pay, and overtime pay. In many countries wages are settled nearly automatically because they are linked—by formula or by usage—with wages in private employment. Linking and national negotiations minimize conflicts and strikes in individual hospitals.

In the first stage of this evolution, the improvement of workers' situations increased costs and numbers of personnel in hospitals. Eventually, wages were settled above the level of the individual hospital, and awards were included automatically in the prospective budgets approved by negotiators, regulators, and payers. Sickness funds were pressed to find more money each year. When cost-containment efforts were begun, they usually had little effect on wage awards, since they were directed at the individual hospitals that no longer decided pay rates. Instead, cost containment has pressed hospitals to limit and even reduce numbers of workers.

In return for the higher personnel costs, the hospitals and payers obtain greater harmony, higher morale, and lower turnover. Better-paid workers are more likely to cooperate in improving the efficiency of the hospital. Decentralizing hospital labor relations and trying to dictate to the workers cause health care to pay a high price in low morale, periodic disputes, and high turnover. Handling labor relations entirely autonomously magnifies the role and income of the individual hospital's management, as in the United States.

11

⊡ ⊡ ⊡

Arrangements
for Paying Physicians

The payment of doctors affects the costs of hospitals, since now in every country some or all of a hospital's doctors are paid under the operating budget. Wages have become the principal cost of hospitals, and doctors constitute small but growing fractions. Doctors also affect the costs of hospitals because they generate the hospital's work. A payment method might increase costs by stimulating greater output or by inspiring waste.

Doctors have always been a different sort of hospital worker. The others have always been employees, until recently very subordinate to management. The medical profession in all countries has usually consisted of self-employed entrepreneurs. With the rise of scientific medicine and the improvement of their education, the medical profession gained control over clinical practice. Governments recognized the self-regulating authority of their guilds and professional associations; these associations and governments excluded unqualified practitioners from medicine.

As hospitals evolved from the custody of the unfortunate to the cure of the sick, they invited doctors to practice inside as well as to continue their private practices outside. Some doctors used hospitals as sites to train students. The numbers of doctors who visited hospitals slowly grew. During the nineteenth century, when the middle and upper classes entered nonprofit and public hospitals, they were treated by these doctors privately or by their own personal physicians; the doctors collected fees from the patients or, eventually, from the patients' insurance carriers. Some specialists created their own small hospitals (the private clinics) and charged fees.

In all these arrangements, doctors differed from other hospital employees. The doctors were in charge of medical care. Other hospital workers were subordinates and took orders from the doctors. Only the hospital managers were not totally subordinate.

Ordinary hospital employment evolves in comparable ways in developed countries. But the relations between hospitals and doctors vary, and so do the

291

methods of paying them. Following are the principal organizational options today:

☐ Medical staff structures of hospital.
  • Closed or open.
  • Full time or part time. If doctors are part time, do they spend their extramural practice in:
    — Their own offices.
    — Competing hospitals.
  • Hierarchical or egalitarian.
  • Mechanisms to monitor clinical performance.
☐ Do hospital doctors have an ambulatory practice?
  • If so, its magnitude.
  • Within the hospital or elsewhere.
  • Same or different payment units and payment rules for inpatient and outpatient practices.
☐ Who pays the hospital doctor?
  • Hospital.
  • Public agency that owns or manages the hospital.
  • Sickness fund.
  • Patient.
  • Junior doctors paid by senior doctors from senior doctor's total practice income.
☐ Unit of payment.
  • Salary.
  • Fee-for-service. If so, whether rates are set by:
    — Fee schedule applying to all.
    — Individual doctor.
  • Case, diagnosis-related group.
  • Share in revenue of:
    — Entire hospital.
    — Doctor's own department.
☐ Unit of payment is decided by:
  • Same negotiations between hospitals and unions as those for all other hospital employees.
  • Same negotiations between sickness funds and medical association as those for all other doctors.
  • Special arbitration machinery.
  • Each doctor's own decisions.
☐ Whether the payment and employment arrangement creates solidarity or conflicts of interest between the hospital doctor and:
  • Hospital.
  • Payers.
☐ Whether the payment and employment arrangements bear incentives to:
  • Increase or decrease certain tests and treatments.
  • Increase or decrease effort.
  • Increase or decrease time spent in the hospital.

- Prefer certain types of patients.
- Prefer teaching and research over care of patient.

Medical Staff Structures

Evolution in Europe. Doctors traditionally have been self-employed small businessmen. They diagnose and treat, rather than work for organizations that practice medicine. Policy leaderships and quality control emanate from the profession as a whole, through associations' influence upon individual doctors.

For centuries, nearly all doctors practiced outside the hospital, seeing private patients in the patients' homes. During the nineteenth century, doctors acquired more equipment and saw more paying patients in offices, usually connected with doctors' own homes; surgeons and obstetricians treated patients for stays of several days or weeks in their private clinics.[1]

Hospitals have always employed nurses, domestics, and laborers, but doctors were not regular members of their organizations until the eve of the nineteenth century. Since hospitals were previously custodial rather than effective therapeutic establishments, doctors could contribute little and hospitals could not use them effectively. Some members of male religious nursing orders tried to practice medicine on the hospital patients until the sixteenth century, when the papacy ordered them to cease. Hospitals aspiring to cure patients—and not merely house them—invited doctors, but appointments were not permanent or standardized. The hospital lacked funds to pay a private doctor to visit regularly; either a private foundation was enlisted to donate an honorarium or the municipality had to assign its salaried physician. Doctors were few in number; until the nineteenth century, the largest cities had only a few hundred apiece. Most doctors stayed with the private patients who paid fees, and most avoided the contagious hospital environments. A few professors at medical schools observed hospital patients as part of their research and bedside teaching, but this practice did not become common until the nineteenth century. During epidemics some city governments hired doctors to examine hospital patients and devise remedies, but these arrangements were limited to a few places and were temporary.[2]

When medical therapy became feasible during the nineteenth century, the medical profession in nearly every European country was composed of independent private office practitioners. It became customary for every urban nonprofit hospital to hire one doctor or, if the hospital was large and had several specialized clinical services, one doctor for each service. During the years before national health insurance guaranteed payment for every treatment, the medical profession was expected to provide uncompensated care for the indigents who filled the wards. The hospital doctor received at most a small annual honorarium. Each morning the doctor observed patients on his rounds and prescribed medicines, bandages, and diet; surgeons and obstetricians performed some operations. The doctor spent the rest of his day in his main work: private practice in his private clinic or in private patients' homes. The hospital appointment was desirable despite the low pay, since it represented public recognition of professional eminence, and the doctor attracted more private patients. A few doctors had such hospital appointments as early as the seventeenth century, but the arrangement did not become common until the nineteenth.[3]

Large and hierarchical medical staffs began in the teaching hospitals of Paris, the creators of the nineteenth century's new forms of clinical education. The professors were salaried members of the Faculty of Medicine and received no payments from the teaching hospitals. For teaching, each was given use of an entire service in his specialty, consisting of an office, a classroom, several dozen beds, operating and delivery room, and some of the hospital's employees. Undergraduate medical students listened to the professor in the classroom and on bedside rounds. Recently graduated doctors needed additional hospital experience before being certified as specialists. They became assistants to the professor, caring for patients under his orders and helping teach the students. These "interns" competed for the appointments and depended on the professor for instruction, their credentials, and their later senior hospital appointments. The hospital and the medical school paid the interns little or nothing.[4]

As the numbers of qualified specialists grew and as medical practice became differentiated into more specialties, the numbers of professors in each teaching hospital grew, and the numbers of chiefs of service in the nonteaching hospitals also grew. Each was assisted by full-time assistants who carried out orders and who were on duty during the long periods when the professors and chiefs were outside in their private practices. The assistants were younger doctors who had already completed postgraduate internships; they in turn were assisted by interns. Larger hospitals and busier specialties added a few senior specialists who helped care for inpatients and outpatients, and helped the professors teach the interns and medical students. The largest and most differentiated staffs of senior and junior doctors clustered at the university teaching hospitals, but such hierarchies also developed at other nonprofit and public urban acute establishments. The growing staffs did not burden the hospital budgets, since the senior doctors continued to get only small honoraria, the assistants received small salaries, and the interns were paid little or nothing. The house staff often complained about excessive responsibility, since senior doctors were often absent. Few doctors of any rank were dedicated members of their organizations; each was using the hospital for his own career interests. This pattern predominated in Europe until well after World War II.[5]

In the nonprofit hospitals during the late nineteenth century, payments by patients and their sickness funds grew. Some patients could pay the professor and chief of service out-of-pocket, to ensure that they would receive personal care instead of being turned over to the house staff. In the contracts they exacted from the hospital, the professors and chiefs obtained a few private beds for these private patients.[6] But most of their private practices were conducted in their offices and private clinics elsewhere in town. The doctor preferred to channel private patients to his private clinic, since he—and not the hospital—earned the daily rate in addition to his fee. Sickness funds were pressed by their subscribers and by the medical associations to cover the private clinics.

By the 1960s urban hospitals had closed medical staffs distinct from the large numbers of doctors in the communities:[7]

☐   Nonprofit and public hospitals. Staffing of each clinical service.
- •   Chief of service. In a teaching hospital, usually he was also a professor in the medical school. A part-time job in practice, since the duties were ambiguously defined and required him only to be available rather than present at all times. He had unlimited rights of private practice during the rest of his workday and during weekends. The chief saw most of these patients in his private office and private clinic. He saw a few in his office in the hospital and in the private beds in his service.
- •   Licensed specialists. Other licensed specialists might also work in a large service at the pleasure of the chief. Like him, they received small salaries and devoted most of their time to private practice outside. As in the case of the chief, the appointment was a valuable form of advertising for private patients. A hospital affiliation gave the specialist an advantage in the competition for chief of service when a post opened in that hospital or elsewhere.
- •   Full-time house staff. Aspiring specialists ranging from recent medical school graduates ("interns") to more experienced physicians at various stages of credentialing in their specialty (assistants, "attachés," and other ranks and titles). University teaching hospitals had many junior doctors, distributed among many ranks. Some countries required hospital internships of all doctors before licensing. House staffs were paid low salaries.

☐   All other physicians in the community.
- •   Licensed specialists. Worked in their offices. Many worked in private clinics, owned by themselves or by other physicians. Earned fees paid either by patients privately or by the sickness funds.
- •   General practitioners. Worked in their offices and in the patients' homes. Earned fees paid either by patients privately or (more often) by the sickness funds. Some had part-time or full-time capitation or salaried arrangements with sickness funds and other organizations.

While closed medical staffs became the rule in the cities, rural hospitals throughout Europe had open staffs. Specialists preferred urban to rural life, because of amenities and money. Rural hospitals lacked the budgets to hire medical staffs. A town had one or only a few doctors, and they were general practitioners with offices but (usually) no private clinics. If the GP hospitalized his patient, he continued to attend the patient entirely by himself in the rural hospital.

European Medical Staffs Today. Hospitals were reorganized and modernized throughout Europe during the 1960s. Governments pressed for improved services to the public, for greater accountability in performance and in expenditure. Sickness funds expanded in coverage and wanted improved services for their subscribers, as good as the care available to private patients. Care in nonprofit and public hospitals would be raised to the levels previously associated with private practice.

One reform has been to convert the post of chief of service to a full-time position. Since the chiefs are expected to spend the full workday in the hospital, without outside affiliations for private practice, hospitals have had to offer them full-time salaries equal to the incomes previously earned in private practice. In a few countries, the chiefs are still given contracts allowing them to see a few private patients in the hospital, so that they retain control over a few private beds in their services. Full-time salaried posts were also created for other fully credentialed specialists in the larger services. If the part-time senior doctors refuse the bait of higher salaries, they are not forced to become full-timers; but when they retire, they are replaced by full-timers.[8]

The hospitals were rebuilt after 1960 and were given new equipment, so the chiefs were willing to spend their time there instead of in the more comfortable and more advanced private clinics. The proprietary hospitals became the work sites of those doctors without appointments in the nonprofit and public hospitals. Paying patients and sickness fund members now were willing to come to the nonprofit and public hospitals instead of to the private clinics alone.

The junior medical staffs had long been unhappy, claiming they had been doing the chiefs' hospital work while the chiefs enriched themselves in private practice. The reforms after 1960 included paying the junior doctors much higher salaries, as I reported in the last chapter. The junior doctors, the nurses, and other hospital employees in several countries were paid according to the government's civil service scales, even if the employers were charitable associations rather than government.

Throughout Europe the trend has been toward more full-time salaried practice, toward the final closing of the closed medical staff structure. The evolution is slow, since the chiefs must voluntarily agree to sign full-time contracts and give up their private hours outside. As the younger doctors who never had private practices move into the senior posts, entire staffs in urban hospitals eventually become full-time salaried.

France illustrates the trend. Among the credentialed hospital specialists above junior assistants in the nonuniversity public acute-care hospitals, the proportions are:[9]

	1964	1974	1979
Full-time	21.7%	58.3%	70.0%
Part-time	78.3	41.7	30.0
	100.0%	100.0%	100.0%
Total number of doctors	(8,450)	(12,992)	(17,345)

Lingering issues are the size and structure of a service. Continental Europe traditionally divided services into general categories—"surgery," "medicine," "obstetrics," and so on—and the chief of a busy service controlled many beds and many junior doctors. The larger the number of beds and assistants, the greater his power and fame. But as subspecialties grew, the chief could not know all of them; therefore, a number of experienced senior doctors were needed, but they would not accept subordination to a single chief. One solution in several countries is to create services in several subspecialties, each with its chief. This greatly increases the size of the medical staff and the operating costs of the hospital. France's plan in 1985 was to replace the many services with a few departments, such as a department of surgery or a department of child medicine: several coequal senior subspecialists belong, no permanent chief exists, and the members elect a chairman every four years.

The earlier, more open hospital staffing survives in the smaller cities in specialties lacking the volume of patients to cover a full-time salary. Examples are opthalmology, orthopedics, and dermatology. The local specialist has a contract for salaried hours to treat the hospital's in- and outpatients. For the rest of his time, he may have a salaried agreement with another hospital. More often he continues to practice from a private office, collecting fees from insured or private patients.

Open medical staffs remain in towns and rural areas of Europe and Great Britain. The rural hospitals provide basic surgical and medical care to the average patient and long-term custodial care to some elderly; patients with more specialized and more difficult conditions are referred to urban establishments. As in the past, the small low-budget hospitals have no full-time salaried specialists. Rather, the local general practitioners see their patients in the hospitals and continue to collect item-of-service fees or (in Holland and Britain) capitation fees. The trend is to eliminate the acute services in the rural hospitals, refer acute patients to the nearest urban hospital, and convert the rural hospitals into extended-care facilities for the elderly.

(The variation in types of hospitals among countries makes impossible any comparative doctor/bed statistics. Teaching hospitals have much larger medical staffs—seniors and especially juniors—than nonteaching hospitals. Town and rural hospitals do not have true medical staffs, since they are open.)

Private clinics in Europe always had closed medical staffs. The owner of the very small private clinic in the past and present has been the only doctor. The larger private clinics built more recently have fixed numbers of partners or (in a few cases) several doctors on contract to the doctor-owner. None of these physicians—except for a few junior housemen for standby and emergencies—receive salaries. All earn fees from national health insurance and from private practice. They use the private clinics as their offices to see their entire ambulatory practice as well as to treat inpatients.

Doctors in private clinics are the elite of the office doctors. Both categories rely on item-of-service fees from national health insurance and from private practice, but only those affiliated with private clinics can perform the more complex and more profitable procedures. The large majority of doctors earn lower incomes from performing simpler procedures on ambulatory patients in their offices. If a patient needs more complex inpatient care, the office doctor without practice rights in a private clinic must refer him to the salaried medical staff in the nonprofit or public hospital, and the office doctor earns nothing.

Table 11-1 shows the distribution of doctors resulting from the structure of employment in West Germany in 1978. The large majority of the fully credentialed doctors are entirely office-based. A number of junior doctors are learning specialties as members of house staffs, but they will subsequently practice in offices.

Evolution in Great Britain. Urban hospitals in the National Health Service also have predominantly closed medical staff, increasingly with full-time practice by senior specialists. But they never were constructed in the hierarchical

Table 11-1. Distribution of Doctors in West Germany, 1978.

	Number	*Proportions*
Full time in hospitals		
Chiefs of service	9,176	7.0%
Juniors	50,388	38.6
Office doctors with part-time hospital appointments *(Belegärzte)*	6,061	4.6
Office doctors		
Specialists. A few have admitting privileges in private clinics	25,407	19.5
General practice	27,568	21.1
Administration and research	11,814	9.1
Total	130,414	100.0%

Source: Adapted from Bundesminister für Jugend, Familie, und Gesundheit, *Daten des Gesundheitswesens* (Stuttgart: Verlag W. Kohlhammer, 1980), pp. 213, 248.

fashion of European hospitals, with a single chief of service for an entire specialty. Britain has always had several coequal "consultants" in a large specialty, each helped by several junior doctors, and each with rights to hospitalize patients in beds reserved for them.

Specialization arose in Britain during the nineteenth century and grew during the twentieth century. Today a division of labor exists: the specialist monopolizes acute hospital practice; the general practitioner gives ambulatory primary care and sees routine medical cases in the smallest community and geriatric hospitals; neither invades the other's turf. But this stable distinction is a result of the NHS. Before that, doctors were competitors, and many specialists were insecure.

Until the NHS most specialists earned item-of-service fees from private patients, whom they treated either in the pay beds of voluntary hospitals, in private hospitals, in their offices, or in patients' homes. Many specialists had "honorary" appointments at voluntary hospitals, treating the poor without charge; the appointments were advertisements to attract private patients. Some specialists had full-time or nearly full-time salaried appointments in local authority hospitals, but most had to search constantly for individual patients.

Considerable rivalry pitted GPs against the specialists. Many GPs tried to treat patients in hospitals rather than refer them to consultants. Most specialists did primary care too. Specialists wooed for referrals those GPs who were not interested in specialty work, such as those with a full panel of patients yielding capitation fees under National Health Insurance. Flattery, gifts, and split fees were common methods of courting the GPs.[10]

The hospital service was designed to commit the specialists to support the NHS. Each consultant would be economically secure and no longer dependent on the GPs for livelihood. The "firm" structure of the voluntary hospital was combined with the salary structure of the local authority hospital. Each consultant would have a certain number of sessions at a hospital, and he cared for patients in his specialty in a fixed number of beds. Some of his sessions could be spent seeing NHS patients in the outpatient department. All consultants were paid salaries according to a scale common to all specialties. General practitioners no longer served on hospital staffs. A consultant had a contract with a Regional Hospital Board or with the Board of Governors of a teaching hospital; to make up as many sessions as he wished, he could work only in one hospital or be part-time in several. He could choose less than a full-time contract and could see private patients, either in the NHS hospital or in a private hospital.

Beneath the consultant, in his "firm," are several junior physicians. All are full-time and salaried. They range from the trainees just out of medical school to the consultant's principal assistants, the "registrars" and "senior registrars." The registrars wait for openings in that specialty somewhere in the country, due either to an expansion of the hospital service or to the retirement of an incumbent. The applicants for the job are interviewed by the Medical Executive Committee in the area, and the winner is formally invited to sign a contract with the RHA. At times in the past, openings have not arisen quickly enough, and junior doctors have dropped out into general practice or have emigrated.[11]

As in Europe, the senior posts have slowly developed from part-time to full-time appointments. When the NHS was first created in 1949, 25.2 percent of the 5,189 consultants chose full-time contracts. By 1964 the proportion was 30.6 percent out of 8,161.[12] By 1977 the 12,504 consultants included 51.5 percent who were full-timers without private practices; an additional 24.3 percent had "maximum part-time" contracts allowing nearly full-time salaried hours but also unlimited private practice rights.[13] (In 1980 the full-time posts were made more attractive by adding limited rights of private practice.) The private inpatient care is given in the consultant's private office outside the NHS hospital, in a nearby private clinic, or in the pay beds of the NHS hospital.

Table 11-2 shows the distribution of doctors in the United Kingdom, resulting from the structure of employment. The numbers are clinical practitioners in 1978 and omit those in full-time teaching, research, and administration.

United States. Many American nonprofit hospitals were created by religious and charitable associations that accompanied their national immigrants. A few were created when the country was still ruled by the British. During the eighteenth and nineteenth centuries, hospital organizations and medical practice in America were a melting pot of European and British methods. American society was less stratified and less unequal than Europe's and Britain's, and hospitals did not seem so repugnant to the American middle classes. Earlier than in Europe, farmers and urban artisans were willing to stay in the hospital, and hospitals charged fees. The patients' private doctors continued to see them in the hospitals, and the doctors steered their patients into certain ones.

The European model of a teaching hospital controlled by a few faculty members was emulated only in a few American establishments, usually owned by municipalities. America eventually developed a different conception of a teaching hospital, to fit its pattern of graduate medical education: young physicians training for specialty credentials performed prolonged "residencies" with considerable clinical responsibility but without close supervision by

Table 11-2. Distribution of Doctors in United Kingdom, 1978.

	Number	Proportions
Specialists in hospitals:		
Consultants	13,206	19.3%
Medical assistants	1,124	1.7
Junior hospital doctors ("registrars" and "house officers")	23,000	33.7
General practitioners:		
Without hospital appointments	25,251	37.0
With hospital appointments	2,070	3.0
Community and school health	3,621	5.3
Total	68,272	100.0%

Source: Royal Commission on the National Health Service, Report (London: Her Majesty's Stationery Office, 1979), p. 218.

professors and chiefs of service. Therefore, America classified many hospitals as "teaching hospitals," staffed by residents and interns with extensive responsibility over nonpaying patients and with routine surveillance over the paying patients on behalf of the patients' personal doctors. The patients' doctors spent most of their time in office practice outside.

The dichotomy between hospital practice and office practice grew in Europe but disappeared in America: in 1982, 91.4 percent of all American patient-care physicians had admitting privileges in a hospital, and the average doctor was affiliated with 2.4 hospitals.[14] Hospitals automatically accept nearly all applications for affiliation, rejecting only 8.2 percent during 1981.[15] The attending physician has complete clinical responsibility for his patient, and he leaves orders with the house staff and nurses. The hospital usually has no salaried doctors with general clinical responsibility; therefore, the office doctor does not lose control over his own patients. Fewer than a quarter of all senior patient-care doctors receive any salaried payments from hospitals, and these are small amounts covering limited administrative and charitable clinical work, rather than care of insured patients.[16] (Physicians doing teaching and research at academic medical centers get full-time or nearly full-time salaries for their academic duties rather than for patient care.) The personal physician's bill combines both his inpatient and extramural services during that patient's spell of illness, usually calculated as item-of-service fees. The hospital bills the patient for all inpatient services, except for the work of his personal physician.

American voluntary hospitals therefore have evolved like the large European private clinics, except that each American establishment has many more doctors with admitting privileges. Across all American acute-care hospitals (nonprofit, public, and for-profit), there is one affiliated doctor for every bed. The largest and busiest hospitals with 500 or more beds have an average of 373 doctors with admitting and treatment privileges.[17]

American hospital-doctor relations are much alike in nonprofit and for-profit hospitals, while European nonprofit and for-profit hospitals differ in staff structure and in financial dynamics. Mutual dependence develops between the American hospital and doctor. Instead of financing and managing very expensive equipment in private offices and in private clinics, the American doctor lets the hospital buy, amortize, and staff it. American hospitals compete for busy doctors who bring in many patients.[18] The hospitals prefer that the most expert and productive doctors keep the equipment fully occupied and offer them consulting rooms for nominal rent. The radiologists, pathologists, and anesthesiologists were the first to become "hospital-based" private practitioners. As their work revolves around expensive equipment and staffs concentrated in the hospitals, leading surgeons, cardiologists, and others are gradually giving up outside private offices to spend all their time within the hospital's wards, treatment rooms, and professional office building. The doctors continue to earn all or nearly all their incomes by fees; they bill the patients directly, not as part of the hospital's bill; the hospital does not influence their rates. In their legal status and billing, those doctors are indistinguishable from the private practitioners based in outside private offices. Almost no hospitals adopt closed medical staffs: most of their doctors continue to be independent businessmen, many of them in one-person professional corporations or in small incorporated groups.

Paying the Hospital Doctor by Salary

Full-Time Salaries. Since World War II, junior hospital doctors nearly everywhere have been full-time salaried professionals. Arrangements for the senior physicians have been mixed:

- *National health services.* Government owns the hospitals and employs the physicians. Senior doctors have been salaried from the start, either full time or part time. Any fees are from private practice and not from official payers. Examples: Great Britain and the Soviet Union.
- *National health insurance.* Private persons (associations or individuals) and municipalities own the hospitals. Sickness funds pay the providers. At first senior doctors collected part-time salaries from the hospitals and fees from the sickness funds for their extramural work. The trend—not fully completed anywhere—changes the doctor from an entrepreneur to an official. In a fee-service practice, the doctor bills the sickness fund for each procedure. The trend is toward payment of the hospital by the sickness fund at a higher rate than before; the doctor's salary is included in the total amount, and the hospital doctor and sickness fund no longer deal with each other.

When doctors become fulltime salaried employees, the hospital and its owners are no longer concerned only with paying the doctor an arbitrary sum of money. The hospital job becomes the doctor's career, and the employer must devise an advancement ladder, guarantee retirement benefits, offer health and disability funds, and so on. Doctors in independent fee-for-service practice—even under national health insurance—must provide all this themselves from their gross revenue.

In order to pay full-time salaried doctors, the hospital and its owners must find substantial new money. Under the previous mix of part-time salaries and unlimited private practice (under both the NHI fee schedules and unconstrained private fees), the medical chiefs of service were the best-paid workers in the country. To persuade them to become full-time salaried employees, the hospitals and their owners must pay the chiefs at least as much as they previously made. Medical salaries in the prospective budget rise, but the increase has been gradual, since the trend toward full time has been slow in most countries. During the bargaining to write the model contracts for full-timers, the chiefs' representatives in most countries have obtained rights of limited private ambulatory care. But some chiefs seem to have more private patients and higher total incomes than originally expected. (The hospital managers dare not monitor the chiefs' work and outside income, no surveys are done, and the facts are not known.)

Most salary systems are designed especially for the hospital doctors and apply to no other occupations, even in countries where all other hospital employees are integrated into wage scales applying to the entire public service. This exception enables the doctors to think of themselves as a special elite occupational group. The exception enables the chiefs of service to get higher salaries than anyone else, including the highest civil servants.

Salaries distinguish the hospital doctors from the larger number of practitioners in offices and private clinics, who are paid by fee-for-service and capitation fees. Usually—but not always—hospital salaries are negotiated at a different time than the other doctors' fees, by different procedures, and with different spokesmen.

The senior and junior doctors have conflicts of interest. The juniors wish higher pay, even if less money is available for the chiefs. The juniors still complain that the chiefs delegate too much of the hospital's work to them and pursue their private practices. The juniors sometimes demand rules to give them shares of the chiefs' private earnings. Some strikes by junior doctors—in Britain, West Germany, and occasionally elsewhere—are directed against the chiefs as well as against the hospitals. In salary negotiations chiefs and junior doctors usually are represented separately and often (not always) meet the hospitals separately.

The contracts and salary scales in each country are very complicated for several reasons: many concessions are made to the hospital doctors in order to avoid antagonizing them and to persuade them to become full-timers; every country is in transition and retains earlier arrangements until their incumbents retire; medical staffs have many ranks; and the teaching and nonteaching hospitals have different structures. Following are brief overviews of a few countries.

Salaries in France. The French public hospital system was reformed during 1958-1961, and a fundamental change was to stabilize the medical staff structure and to induce the physicians to work in the hospital for long periods each day.[19] The numerous compromises worked out in the laws and regulations distinguish the hospital doctors from other public employees: they are *agents du service publique* and not *fonctionnaires;* they do not "work a full schedule" but "dedicate the whole of their professional activity to the hospital"; they receive *émoluments* and not ordinary *salaires*. They serve according to obligations and privileges spelled out in laws and regulations.

French hospital doctors are represented by many special associations, speaking for different ranks and for different clinical specialties. Most associations belong to the umbrella organization of the French medical profession, the *Confédération des Syndicats Médicaux Français* (CSMF), but each deals with the government directly. The Ministry of Health has a Division on Health Professions that writes the drafts of regulations and conducts meetings with the associations. Major decisions, such as the writing of the first regulations and major revisions, involve the Division of Hospitals, the Minister of Health, and (if disputes spill into the media) the Prime Minister. The Division on Health Professions meets the hospital doctors' associations throughout the year to consider detailed changes in the terms of service.

As I said in the last chapter, all other public hospital employees are ranked on the scale (the *barème*) for the entire public service, are included in the same annual wage negotiations, and receive the same annual wage increases. While doctors' pay also rises every January 1, their pay scales have different structures, and they meet the government representatives separately.

Table 11-3 shows a few ranks in the larger nonuniversity hospitals. Within each category, pay rises by seniority.

The differentials, job definitions, positions of jobs on the hierarchy, and extra benefits are negotiated, but the actual money is not. The annual increases are automatic. Every year, the national government increases the pay of all its employees by a percentage across the board, and the Ministry of Finance during the 1970s and 1980s—as part of the effort to control health care costs—insisted that the doctors get no more. So the entire pay scale for all hospital doctors automatically increases by the same percentage. As in very few other countries, public budgetary and anti-inflation policies control the incomes of doctors.

Often the union representing one group of hospital doctors tries to increase its pay by narrowing the differentials between that rank of doctors and better-paid ranks. In their discussions at the Ministry of Health, the association pictures the heavy reponsibilities and unjust treatment of its members. But change would make the lower rank nearly as well paid as beginners in the higher rank. The civil servants who labored on the statutes are reluctant to reopen their essential structure merely to satisfy one group's interests. The other groups of hospital doctors also resist special concessions and usually agree only on a general rise for everyone. The increase in the hospitals' wage bills resulting from restructuring distresses the financial officers in government and in the sickness funds, so the automatic annual increase for everyone becomes the fallback position.

Salaries in Great Britain. I have described the British salary structure and the method of deciding it elsewhere.[20] The following paragraphs present only highlights.

The National Health Service began with the assumption that the payment of all its personnel, including doctors, would be settled through bilateral negotiation in Whitley Councils. Both the hospital consultants and the general practitioners refused and negotiated directly with the Ministry of Health. As befitting an elite, the Royal Colleges representing the consultants often bypassed

Table 11-3. Doctors' Pay in Nonuniversity Hospitals in France.

Rank	Seniority	Francs per year Nov. 1, 1984 through Oct. 30, 1985
Chief of service	14 years and over	379,365
	9–14	333,667
	4–9	284,919
	Start to 4	235,589
Deputy chief	19 years and over	287,440
	14–19	255,014
	9–14	229,780
	4–9	204,553
	Start to 4	190,382
Assistants	3 and over	190,382
	1–2	169,982
	Start	149,762

Source: Each year's salary scale is published in the Journal officiel. In early 1985, 1 F = $0.10.

the civil servants to "have a word" with the Minister, and they occasionally bypassed the Health Minister to persuade the Prime Minister and the Chancellor of the Exchequer.

Bilateral negotiations between the Royal Colleges and the civil servants in DHSS are still used in settling the job structures, working conditions, and career lines of hospital doctors. The basic contracts were settled long ago and are amended occasionally. Major disputes sometimes arise—such as during the mid-1970s—and extensive revisions are finally adopted.

This unsystematic and sometimes conflictual method fit badly the requirement of annual or bienniel increases in pay, and it was replaced during the early 1960s by arbitration by a Review Body on Doctors' and Dentists' Remuneration. The agency resolves the dilemma that no occupation can engage in true negotiations with a central government employer, since government always has the final word. The Review Body consists of eight independent and public-spirited persons who investigate every year the financial situation of consultants, general practitioners, and dentists. For hospital doctors' pay, the Review Body considers written and oral testimony by representatives from DHSS, from the sections of the British Medical Association concerned with consultants and junior doctors, and from any other groups speaking for the senior and junior doctors. The Review Body is aided by its own research staff, seconded from the civil service. The Review Body makes recommendations to the Prime Minister; they are accepted unless the government can demonstrate "clear and compelling" reasons to reduce, postpone, or reject them.

The salary structure and methods of deciding them differ from those in the rest of the NHS, the rest of government, and the private sector. The Review Body uses its own criteria, often contradicting those used by the government-of-the-day in its other wage awards. For example, the Review Body will give large awards to particular ranks of hospital doctors if it believes that higher pay is necessary to motivate more conscientious work, more applicants, and greater retention. The Review Body takes evidence about the government's economic policies but is bound not by them but by its interpretation of the staffing requirements of the NHS. Therefore, several times during the 1970s and 1980s it precipitated conflicts with a government-of-the-day that was trying to maintain strict cash limits on the NHS and strict wage-price limits on general inflation. If the Cabinet reduced or postponed an award, a dispute over the Review Body's authority resulted, and the doctors protested; if the Cabinet accepted a large award, all the hospital workers demanded higher wage increases than Cabinet was imposing on them.

The Review Body made Britain one of the few countries where all doctors' pay rates are decided together. Normally this is possible only when everyone is paid according to a universal fee schedule negotiated between medical associations and sickness funds. When hospital doctors are salaried (with part-time private practices) and the office doctors earn fees, they are often competitors; they bargain with different payers (the hospital owners and the sickness funds); their negotiations occur at different times; and the medical association may not represent both. However, the British Review Body decides the awards for consultants and general practitioners at the same time, uses similar criteria, and probably links their pay unofficially. Deciding all the pay rates together is possible only because of the division of labor and remuneration methods: consultants have a monopoly on hospital work, GPs have a monopoly on office care, and neither the NHS nor private health insurance pays a large number of office-based or clinic-based specialists.

Consultants have never been integral members of British hospitals. Before the NHS they visited only to treat their patients, while the nursing staff and a few administrators managed the organization. Even though the consultants now have become full time or nearly full time on site, they are still oriented toward patient care and let others worry about the hospital's operation and financing. Each consultant has his own firm and patients; no chiefs of service and no medical hierarchies control personnel, distinct parts of the building, and expenditure. The consultant does not feel dependent on the hospital, because it does not pay him; he is not part of its budget and personnel roster; and he is not even paid by the DHA. At the time the NHS was created, the consultants opposed any hint of subordination to local lay officials; their contracts are with the Regional Health Authorities, and their paychecks come from the RHA budgets.

For the past decade, DHSS has searched for methods of motivating the consultants to feel responsible for managing and economizing in the hospital, instead of continuing their prior habits of expecting to be served. Some consultants joined management teams in each district after the NHS reorganization of 1974, but their practice styles were not affected. Committee members could not control the work of other consultants, since all were coequal. While nurses, pharmacists, and others were assigned "functional budgets" and were expected to fulfill their missions within those resources—each was called a responsible "budget holder"—no "clinical budgets" were created for the individual consultants. They continued to expect the other employees managing the resources to deliver whatever the doctors deemed medically necessary. Instead of becoming more committed to the performance of each hospital and district, the doctors complained that excessive committee work distracted them from care of patients.[21]

Salaries in West Germany. West Germany is one of the few countries where the contracts and wages of the hospital doctors are connected with those of other occupations, but only in general principles.[22] During the series of negotiations about payment of German public employees described in the last chapter, the administrative civil servants and professionals are represented by the *Deutsche Angestellten-Gewerkschaft* (DAG). In association with this federation, the senior and junior hospital doctors are represented by the *Verband der angestellten und beamteten Ärzte* (colloquially called the *Marburger Bund*). Doctors never agree to be represented by any body of laymen; therefore, the *Marburger Bund* works closely with DAG as an equal collaborator, but it is not a member. The hospital doctors are not represented by the same organization as the other hospital workers (who belong to trade unions) or the office doctors (who belong to special associations of their own called *Kassenärztliche Vereinigungen,* or KVs).

All administrative and professional employees of the national, provincial, and local governments are covered by a contract for work schedules, job classifications, fringe benefits, career stages, and other matters. This contract (the *Bundes-Angestelltentarifvertrag,* or BAT) was first negotiated in 1961 between DAG and the representatives from the national, provincial, and municipal governments. In their annual spring meetings, the two sides occasionally amend BAT. All doctors in municipal hospitals, provincial hospitals, and medical schools are covered by BAT. The *Marburger Bund* and the government negotiators work out additional contracts about the work of the hospital doctors. For example, major changes in 1972 gave the junior doctors fixed hours, extra pay for overtime, a definite promotion sequence, and many other rights.[23] The *Marburger Bund* and the government negotiators meet occasionally to work on new issues. For example, a persistent question during the late 1970s and 1980s concerned weekend duty schedules of junior doctors. (After prolonged deadlocks in the negotiations and an appeal by several junior doctors to the Federal Labor Court, a compromise settlement was devised in late 1982. But the *Marburger Bund* contended that the hospitals were not implementing it, and negotiations resumed.)

The negotiations often produce important concessions on both sides. For example, at one time the chiefs of service in public and nonprofit hospitals were given private beds for private inpatients, who paid considerable shares of their total incomes. The negotiations during the 1970s aimed at making the chiefs full-timers in inpatient hospital practice, so that they would not be diverted by private inpatient care in outside private clinics or in their own hospitals. In order to give up private inpatient beds, the chiefs wanted more than large salary increases. They were compensated in addition by creation of a special pension fund, with benefits comparable to those of the highest civil servants. The private beds clearly became part of the hospital's bed capacity, and the hospital could collect surcharges on the daily rate. The patients could still pay the chiefs privately for medical care, if the chiefs' individual contracts with the hospitals allowed it; but the scale of private inpatient care diminished, and the chiefs were less independent of the hospital organization. The chiefs retained their rights of ambulatory private practice in their hospital offices. Considerable private practice survived, not only because the chiefs insisted but also because government officials had a vested interest in it: noncontributory private health insurance is a fringe benefit of the civil service.[24]

BAT created a standard pay structure for all its occupations. An example is:

Occupational level	Age of incumbent					
	23	25	27		41	43
I	3,619.41	4,007.63	4,395.82	. . . . .	5,821.16	6,024.77
Ia	3,290.21	3,625.15	3,960.06	. . . . .	5,265.49	5,451.98
Ib	2,991.46	3,278.80	3,566.16	. . . . .	4,844.95	4,921.04
II	2,719.35	2,964.82	3,210.29	. . . . .	4,275.94	4,373.04
.	.	.	.			
.	.	.	.			
.	.	.	.			
.	.	.	.			
IX	1,257.15	1,302.87	1.348.59			
X	1,167.35	1,204.91	1,242.47			

The foregoing numbers are Deutsche Mark per month, paid to employees in hospitals owned by *communes* during 1985. Occupations are assigned to each level by negotiators from DAG and the public employers. The more responsible and more educated occupations are assigned to higher levels. The greater the number of subordinates, the higher the level and the higher the pay: chiefs of service with large numbers of assistant doctors receive higher rankings, thereby getting an incentive to overstaff and to keep the junior doctors busy.

During the annual spring negotiations described in the last chapter, the bargainers for the public employees—the team includes the *Marburger Bund*—obtain from the levels of government *(Bund, Land,* and *Gemeinde)* an agreement to raise all public pay. For example, they may agree on a 6.5 percent raise beginning in May 1981. Therefore, every number in every box in all the matrices rises 6.5 percent. The negotiators also agree on rates for overtime pay, Sunday and holiday pay, cost-of-living supplements around the country, fringe benefits, and so on. Perhaps they also amend BAT.

The *Marburger Bund* meets with representatives of the public hospitals to agree on the new pay rates for the doctors. The illustrative matrix that I presented contained one year's monthly pay for hospital doctors; their pay rates are always spread among occupational levels I, Ia, Ib, and II. The *Marburger Bund* makes a case for more money but must settle for the general increase during periods of cost containment. The negotiators meanwhile are often working on changes in the special supplements to BAT concerning the doctors.

BAT and its supplements are framework agreements applying only to the national, provincial, and local hospitals. The *Marburger Bund* also negotiates with other major associations of hospital owners (Catholic *Caritasverband,* the

Evangelical Protestant Association, and others) to persuade them to adopt framework agreements containing all or most of BAT and its supplements. By now the routine is familiar. The costs of BAT's rules, wage rates, and other benefits are passed through to the sickness funds in the daily rates, but the public hospitals have more money from government subsidies, allowing them to pay higher wages and fringe benefits. So, with the nonprofit hospitals, the *Marburger Bund* usually must settle for slightly lower pay scales for doctors' salaries and lower contributions to their pension funds.

These framework agreements are not final contracts. Hospital doctors are free professionals, not civil servants governed by any legislative enactment of BAT. The decrees issued by the national government in France have no counterpart in Germany. Each hospital doctor tries to negotiate his own contract with his hospital and tries to get more than the rights and pay levels under BAT. He tries to get other concessions (such as equipment and assistants) that BAT and its supplements do not cover. Therefore, implementation of contracts and of pay rates is diverse.

Professors and leading chiefs of service have considerable leverage in getting more pay, staffing, private practice privileges, equipment, and other advantages, particularly during periods of generous resources, such as the 1960s in the provincial academic medical centers and the mid-1970s in other urban hospitals. Unlike countries where one owner controls all hospitals (such as Britain) or one class of owner controls most (such as France), Germany has many owners. Germany's federal system of government decentralizes authority to the provinces, and the *Länder* compete to build leading teaching hospitals and medical services. Hospitals compete for referrals and for private practice, in order to survive in an overbedded country; and they need to attract and retain leading doctors. Since private practice brings much additional revenue, the hospitals do not restrict an energetic chief, but the contract may press him to share his revenue with the hospital budget and with the junior doctors who helped him. (The contracts with hospitals are secret; therefore, no surveys have ever been done about the chiefs' work schedules, private practice, sharing with juniors, and so on.)

Part-Time Salaries. Until recently, the chief of service throughout Europe spent only part of the morning in the hospital, and the honorarium was a token compensation for this sacrifice from his private office practice. Often he ran a competing private clinic.

Public policy in many countries has offered carrots and occasional sticks to convert the hospital jobs into full-time salaried positions. Modern hospital finances provide sufficient revenue. But it is not possible to make all hospital staffs full time and make the hospital economical and efficient; it is not possible completely to isolate the hospital from outside ambulatory practice. Not all medical specialties have sufficient work to justify full-time hospital appointments. For example, in all but the biggest cities, orthopedists, ophthalmologists, and some others lack enough inpatients for a full-time schedule in one hospital. Therefore, their contracts provide certain numbers of hours per week at the normal pay rates for chiefs of service, and they spend the rest of their time in private practice for fee-for-service, either in private offices or in private clinics.

Such part-timers *(Belegärzte)* provide a substantial amount of the hospital services in Germany. Of the 65,625 hospital doctors in 1978 (shown in the first three lines of Table 11-1), 9.2 percent were *Belegärzte*, 14 percent were chiefs, and the rest were juniors. Normally, only the full-time office doctors in Germany can bill for services under official national health insurance; the full-time hospital doctors cannot. (The hospital doctors can bill only private health insurers.) But a *Belegarzt* works in both worlds. Since he is primarily án office doctor, he belongs to the payment agency for NHI (the KV), and he can bill it for his inpatient care. The sickness funds pay a reduced daily rate to the hospital (the *kleine Pflegesatz*, which includes the hospital's daily rate minus the costs of the average principal doctor), and they pay the *Belegarzt* directly according to the standard NHI fee schedule.

Like Germany, France has replaced part-time by full-time practice. France differs in some respects. Its central government designed the reforms; in Germany a consensus of national officials, provincial officials, hospital reformers, and sickness funds designed the new arrangements. French government is organized to implement a reform quickly and extensively, but the reform has evolved more slowly in Germany and has cost more in concessions. France now has fewer part-timers than Germany.

France has replaced part-timers by two groups. Full-time appointments have increased in number; when an older part-time chief retires, the post is advertised as full time, and many young specialists apply. If a hospital needs additional specialized work, it hires outside doctors on a sessional basis, rather than giving anyone a formal contract for a substantial fraction of the week. These *attaché* arrangements were always common in teaching hospitals: the professor needed extra help, he hired his young alumni, and often he paid the *attachés* personally from his private earnings. In theory an *attaché* is added only to introduce a specialty not provided by the fulltime staff, but there are now so many fulltime staff members that duplications of specialties must occur. The DDASS is supposed to disallow unnecessary additions. The *attaché* now receives a lump sum without fringe benefits from the hospital budget for each session. Young doctors take the jobs because competition in office practice is growing, a hospital affiliation is a good advertisement, and keeping close to the chief may help them get a senior appointment when one opens. Of the 37,098 fully licensed doctors in French hospitals in 1979, 32.7 percent were full time (including the senior doctors and the members of the house staff), 14 percent were part time, and 53.3 percent were *attachés*.[25] The arrangement strengthens the senior full-time staff and makes the hospital more cohesive. The *attaché* is too junior to attract patients away from the hospital into his own practice, as part-timers often were supposed to have done.

Paying the Hospital Doctor by Fee-for-Service

Europe. Fee-for-service continues to be the principal method of paying hospital doctors in European private clinics. The private clinic is simply an extension of traditional private office practice, where the doctor bills by fee-for-service. Sickness funds under statutory health insurance and private commercial health insurance pay the private clinics' inpatient bills by itemized charges rather than by all-inclusive per diems, and they pay the doctors separately according to the negotiated fee schedules. The doctor sees his ambulatory patients in the private clinic's consulting rooms as well as in the wards during hospitalization, and the billing office usually handles all his claims. In accordance with the doctor's contract with the private clinic, the billing office retains some of the sickness funds' payment to cover practice costs. The doctor would have incurred such practice costs if he were still equipping and staffing his private office, and nowadays the medical staffs use the private clinics as their full-time practice sites. Sickness funds usually refuse to pay profits among the private clinics' allowable costs, and the owners must earn their profits by sharing in the fees of their medical staffs. Examples are common in France and West Germany.

Private clinics compete with the nonprofit and public hospitals for patients. Clinic patients pay both doctors' fees and hospital charges, while the nonprofit and public hospitals charge an all-inclusive rate, including the full-time doctors' salaries. Therefore, the private clinics try to lower their staffing and operating costs, so that patients will have enough money to pay the doctors' fees.[26] When negotiating with private clinics, the French and German sickness funds try to pay low daily charges, so that they can save money and so that the clinics press the doctors to share higher proportions of their incomes for practice expenses.

I have described elsewhere the structure of fee schedules applying to hospital doctors and the methods of negotiating them in Holland, Belgium, Switzerland, and Canada (for all hospital doctors), and in France and Germany (for those in private clinics).[27] When the senior hospital doctor bills the sickness funds under official national health insurance, he must accept the standard negotiated rate and cannot extra-bill the patient. The rules are the same as in office practice. When the patient pays privately out-of-pocket or is covered by private commercial health insurance, the hospital doctor often bills what he likes. The patient can recover only an indemnity from the commercial carrier. But no insurance can long tolerate unlimited extra-billing by doctors, and the commercial carriers urge voluntary restraint. The private health insurance companies in Germany ask the hospital chiefs to charge their beneficiaries no more than six times the NHI fee schedule for each procedure. Many doctors charge more, but events in all these separate transactions are not known. The German interest group representing the doctors who practice outside NHI (the *Hartmannbund*) opposes any fixed rates and recommends that doctors and patients settle their own finances in each case. No European private carrier has full-scale rate negotiations with a medical association comparable to the determination of NHI fees.

Sickness funds, governments, and some hospitals complain about large financial windfalls for specialists earning inpatient and outpatient fees within the hospital.[28] Payers urge hospitals to collect much higher rental payments from their chiefs of service than the current nominal amounts. But hospitals shrink from demanding more, since they compete to attract outstanding chiefs, and the specialists are just now becoming so numerous that it is they who compete for appointments. If the chief's original contract with the hospital provided low rentals for his use of the facilities and personnel for his private practice, that approximate amount remains unchanged until his retirement.

United States and Canada. North American hospitals' open medical staffs have never been paid even part-time salaries for their clinical work. American and Canadian physicians have always been office based, treating personal patients both outside and inside the hospital and billing patients and third parties for the entire course of treatment. If an inpatient has been treated by several doctors— such as his own family physician, a specialist, an anesthesiologist, a radiologist, and an emergency-room doctor—each bills the third party separately on an itemized fee-for-service basis. In European nonprofit hospitals, all medical services are aggregated as part of the total inpatient costs, and every claim includes the average medical salaries as part of the unit of payment; therefore, every patient's third party is billed for an average share.

Billings by hospitals and doctors in the United States are kept separate. The doctor's office bills the patient or his third party directly, and the hospital never knows the varied charges of its numerous doctors. The hospital cannot share in the doctors' personal revenue. The doctors must collect their own bad debts.

Alone among the medical professions in the world, the Americans have avoided basing fee-for-service on binding fee schedules. Only a few programs have fee schedules (Medicaid in half the states and workers' compensation), and American doctors avoid them. Both in hospital and ambulatory work, the doctor prices his fees as he likes. Medicare and Blue Shield in half the states employ an involved "usual, customary, and reasonable charge" methodology, which pays for each claim either the fee customarily charged by that doctor or the prevailing charge among all other doctors in that area.[29] To control its own costs, Medicare has been constraining its annual increases by an economic index, to the outrage of the doctors, who have preserved their incomes by extra-billing the patients.

Case Payments. Hospital doctors almost always are paid by salaries or by fee-for-service. But some fees are really all-inclusive case payments. For example, an obstetrician in private practice may quote a total amount that includes periodic examinations before hospitalization, the delivery, and subsequent checkups. Surgeons often do the same. Under NHI the fee schedules are highly itemized, and such global fees are replaced by detailed claims.

The American government in 1985 seriously considered paying for the inpatient physician's charges by a surcharge on the DRG.[30] The diagnosis of the patient at admission would determine Medicare payments for both the hospital and the doctor(s). Like the DRG for hospitals, the figure is an average of all physicians' payments for that case throughout the country. Each patient would be covered by the average charge, not the charge that each doctor would like to make. Doctors who previously earned more for that type of case now would receive less; the more restrained doctors now would earn more. Like the method of paying hospitals by DRG, it is an incentive reimbursement scheme: the doctors who give more treatment than the average for that diagnosis would no longer profit from overtreating. The proposal was launched at a time when many Americans thought that wide regional variations existed in treating the same case and that excessive clinical interventions should be discouraged.[31]

Shares of the Hospital's Revenue. Radiologists and pathologists run departments within hospitals and differ from the usual American model of predominantly self-employed practice out of the doctor's own office. But the

United States has never developed standard methods of employing and paying the hospital-based doctors, leaving them to work out individual arrangements with their hospitals.[32]

Until the mid-1960s, most American hospitals billed patients and third parties for the diagnostic work in radiology and pathology, and most paid the chief radiologists and pathologists percentages of the gross receipts. The doctor usually lacked a second affiliation, and his entire income came from the arrangement. The system resembled business; the doctors had strong incentives to increase output, and the many small claims produced steadily larger incomes for both hospital and doctors.[33] Except in some private clinics, no European hospitals have paid doctors by such revenue-based formulas.

American Medicare was written as two separate programs, Part A for hospitals and Part B for doctors; and payment for the two providers was separated. Hospitals might have continued to mix the payment of radiology and pathology with the reimbursement of the physicians for all the non-Medicare billing, but they abandoned division of receipts. Today in America nearly all hospital-based radiologists bill by fee-for-service, while their European counterparts are becoming salaried. Now nearly half the American hospital-based pathologists are salaried, while the others bill fees. Other hospital-based specialists have evolved recently—for instance, anesthesiologists—and they are paid almost entirely by fee-for-service. The payment method's incentives are to increase work and to raise the hospital's costs.

Instead of becoming increasingly integrated into the hospital organization, some American hospital-based practices have developed in opposite fashions. Departments that perform the doctors' work are sometimes converted into autonomous corporations managed or even owned by radiologists, pathologists, anesthesiologists, emergency-room doctors, pulmonary specialists, and others. Legally free of Certificate of Need planning restraints, these arrangements can buy or lease more equipment, and the total hospital budget avoids the ceiling restraints under some forms of state and Medicare reimbursement formulas. (No research has been performed about the prevalence and consequence of these arrangements.)

Implications for Management and Costs

Part-Time Salaried Arrangements in the Past. Earlier salaried methods in Europe placed the chief of service in conflict with the hospitals and with statutory health insurance. If the chief in the voluntary or public hospital earned the bulk of his income by fees in his private clinic and private office, he was motivated to give the patient better care in those sites. The patient might be covered by statutory health insurance and have no out-of-pockets if he went to the voluntary or public hospital. But most of his care would be given by the junior staff. No research ever was done about the subject, but it was believed in many countries that chiefs spotted possible paying patients during initial outpatient screening and assured them of personal attention only in their private clinics.[34] The practice perpetuated the stereotype that voluntary and public hospitals got only the working classes.

To eliminate the conflict of interest, countries invested heavily in hospitals and in health insurance after 1960. The chiefs would be willing to spend all their time in the voluntary and public hospitals if the buildings were modernized, the full-time salaries were equal to the revenue from private practice, and the chiefs were given opportunities to see private ambulatory patients in the hospital. Meanwhile, public regulations and stiff rate negotiations by the sickness funds made the private clinics less profitable. The reforms were also designed to improve the organizational capacity of the hospitals. Previously in all countries, hospitals were ramshackle organizations; the central figure, the chief of service, meandered in and out. He thought of the hospital as a tool for his own interests.

Full-Time Salaried Arrangements. Spending much more time in the hospital under the reforms, the chiefs became interested in strengthening its clinical ability and appeal, instead of keeping it a weak competitor of private clinics. They tried to build up its technology and staff and do technically advanced work there. The chiefs' professional reputations became bound up with the performance of the hospitals, and they personally monitored the junior doctors, employees, and patients in their services. Previously they had delegated supervision to the chief medical residents.

As new construction, renovation, and new equipment became more expensive and more complicated, the several chiefs of service in every public and nonprofit hospital had to form governing committees. Investment could no longer be a free-for-all, as it had been before the 1970s, with each chief sending proposals to the hospital's governing board and looking for money independently in the community or among business firms. Investment money now comes from outright government grants (as in Germany and Switzerland) or from loans from special public funds (as in France). The specialties' wish lists exceed resources. Therefore, the procedure requires official applications, the setting of priorities within the hospital, and careful financial scrutiny of each scheme. Cohesive medical staff organizations are required to write priority lists. Each service chief in the hospital develops a proposal for new equipment or for new construction, either at any time or in response to an annual notice from the lay director; using prescribed forms or informal papers, the service chief and the hospital's finance officer prepare a detailed summary and an estimate of the costs; the entire senior medical staff in plenary session or the governing committee of service chiefs discusses the merits and need of the proposal and lists them by priority; if the money is fixed by the government grant or by the hospital's borrowing capacity, the medical staff sends the hospital's governing board only a short list within that total; the governing board sends the serious proposals (including contingencies) to the grantor or lender.

This procedure has made the service chiefs much more knowledgeable about the costs of acquiring new programs and new equipment. They must think about each other's disciplines, too, because of the hospital-wide prioritizing. In practice in many hospitals, each chief is allowed a certain investment total each year, and he must think about tradeoffs—that is, whether several smaller items will benefit his program more than certain expensive ones. The procedure could make the chief sensitive to long-term operating costs from each scheme; but only a few grantors, lenders, or planning agencies (such as several Swiss cantonal governments) require the applications for the new acquisition to estimate future results.

The chief is someone whom the lay director and financial officer can talk to about operational budgeting and about controlling operating costs, not merely about proposals to acquire heavy equipment. As I said in Chapter Three, several countries have developed cost-center accounting, where the hospitals' total operating costs are assigned to the clinical services that originated them. Some Swiss hospital managers inform each service chief of the prospective budget and end-of-the-year cost report for his service; so he is aware of the magnitude and budget lines of overruns. Monthly and quarterly reports can be generated by large hospitals with good computers; so the chief can head off trouble—either by making economies or by finding more revenue.[35]

Involving the chiefs and medical staff more deeply in hospital management can erect obstacles to public policy as well as benefits. The doctors may be able to resist attempts to cut down hospital beds by keeping them filled. The hospital's managers have little authority over admissions and discharges; these decisions are made by the doctors. Germany has more beds than other developed countries but little empty capacity, and an important reason may be that the chiefs work at a rate slower than necessary. The *Belegärzte* keep the small hospitals of under one hundred beds filled and apparently essential, when many critics wish to shut them.

Diffuse Medical Staff Structures. Its medical staff structure is probably a principal reason for America's higher hospital costs. Within the United States, the hospitals with more compact medical staffs and more focused work are less costly. On the other hand, when a hospital has more affiliated doctors, each doing a limited amount of work within the organization, each hospital bids for doctors by offering the newest equipment, more staff, office space, and few controls. Each doctor orders work without much understanding of the consequences to the hospital and to the payer.[36] The hospital's house staff and nurses must cope with a great variety of habits in clinical technique, in length of stay, and in costliness.[37]

During the late 1970s and 1980s, American doctors became targets of educational campaigns to make them more cost-conscious, to urge them not to order unnecessary tests and treatments. The American Medical Association appealed with publications and manuals for cost-consciousness sessions in local medical societies. Blue Cross developed educational literature and motion pictures for doctors. Medical journals ran articles. Hospitals devoted medical staff meetings to cost problems and methods of avoiding waste, and they showed doctors the patient bills that they had ignored before.[38]

These were consciousness-raising efforts, but the cost-raising structures and motives remained in effect. Several observers concluded that, since hospital costs were determined by doctors, the only solution was to create new medical staff structures that would make the doctors responsible for the financial solvency of the hospitals and of health insurance.[39]

Such reforms imply smaller and more hierarchical medical staffs, as in Europe. Most office doctors would be excluded. The result would be a revolution in the organization of American medical practice and a revolution in hospital economics. The office doctors oppose such a change, the hospital managers have other priorities, and government shrinks from touching off disputes. The office doctors can successfully block such widespread loss of hospital practice privileges, and hospitals cannot survive without their referrals. The few community hospitals with closed and cohesive staffs either surrender or lose out to new competitors that the office doctors easily set up.[40]

As long as Medicare, Blue Cross, and other payers spent steadily more, both the attending physicians and the hospital managers could pursue their cost-raising aims, and each side gained from the other's activities. But the payers tried to save money during the 1980s: all encouraged extramural care; the Medicare DRGs had ceilings. Cost controls were directed against hospital managers rather than against the doctors, who were the ultimate cost raisers. A considerable literature and many workshops arose to guide managers and doctors in joint efforts to evade these restrictions by finding new methods of raising revenue.[41]

Fixing Individual Responsibility. Merely providing a final cap—whether a global budget or a DRG—does not convince every doctor to work within it. The public grantor deals with the hospital managers and never with the hospital physicians, and the doctors think that it is the managers' task (not theirs) to operate within the caps. Even after twenty years of global budgeting, Canadian hospitals still have not integrated their physicians into their organizations or even developed methods to control the doctors' diverse practice styles. Canadian hospitals—like the American—still have affiliated medical staffs consisting of office doctors who admit and treat their own inpatients. Most Canadian doctors have hospital-admitting privileges, but they are office based and not hospital based. Canadian provincial governments fail to coordinate financing: each pays hospitals and doctors in two uncoordinated programs. Doctors submit bills for their own ambulatory and inpatient care, and they are paid by fee-for-service. Quebec had some hospitals with partially salaried medical staffs paid from the global budgets during the 1960s and 1970s; but, when the Ministry of Social Affairs began to squeeze the hospitals' total grants, the specialists insisted on substitution of fee-for-service from the separate medical care financing channels.

The Canadian hospital-financing system has constrained the hospital managers' ability to satisfy the doctors' clinical demands. Unlike the American hospital, the Canadian did not depend on a constant stream of admissions and itemized charges to survive; therefore, they did not compete so intensely to please the community's doctors. The Canadian doctors—unlike the American—could not force each hospital to acquire a profusion of new equipment in a competitive race, since big-ticket capital was not an allowable cost under the Ministries' global grants. The Ministries decided on the number and sites of expensive new programs in their direct capital grants to hospitals, independent of the operating grants. Regardless of the hospital doctors' wishes, they had to work with the available hospital personnel, since steady tightening of global budgets prevented Canadian hospitals from keeping pace with the personnel increases in the United States. Numbers of doctors have risen much faster than the numbers of beds allowed by the Ministries' grants and budget scrutiny, and doctors have had to fit their admissions and stays within a constrained supply; beds per active civilian physician dropped from 4.4 in 1970 to 3.6 in 1980.[42] Hospital directors have had constant struggles with the amorphous medical staffs, to persuade them to avoid waste and not create deficits. Earlier than in the United States, Canadian hospitals had cost-consciousness campaigns, supplementing what their doctors read in their professional journals and daily newspapers.[43]

Frustrated by the stricter squeeze on their workplaces during the 1970s and 1980s, specialists throughout Canada were outraged when the provincial Ministries also limited the accounts that paid their fees. Fees rose more slowly than Canada's high inflation, and therefore doctors' real incomes dropped.[44] (Meanwhile, their unconstrained role models south of the border were increasing net real incomes.) Specialists in much of Canada reacted by extra-billing their patients for both inpatient and ambulatory care, either by (1) opting out of the official fee schedule in provinces allowing it (as in Ontario, where the patient paid the doctor his full bill and recovered the official fee from the Ontario Health Insurance Plan), or by (2) sending the patient a second bill in addition to billing the provincial plan in provinces allowing it (as in Alberta). A confusing mosaic resulted: doctors in some provinces (such as Quebec and British Columbia) were forbidden to extra-bill; but half in some other provinces (such as Alberta and Nova Scotia) did so. Where extra-billing existed, charges per patient were low, and doctors' income was less than 5 percent from the extra-billing. Extra-billing varied among specialties and among communities.[45]

Extra-billing contradicted traditional national policies and the wishes of all political parties in the national government, but Ottawa lacked constitutional authority to forbid it. The provinces paid the doctors and alone could regulate them. But the national Parliament devised an ingenious and eventually successful lever. Under the Canadian Health Act of 1984, the national government could withhold one dollar in Medicare grants to a province for every dollar that patients paid to doctors out-of-pocket. In early 1985 Ontario was losing $4.4 million per month. Ontario's party alignments changed in an election fought over this and other issues. The new coalition Cabinet ended extra-billing in 1986. (The law was implemented after the Ontario Medical Association called and lost one of the longest strikes of doctors in any country's experience.)

Even a closed, governmentally employed, and salaried hospital staff has problems of cost containment under global budgeting if the staff structure fails to involve the senior physicians in the crucial decisions and then fails to fix responsibility for implementation. An example is Great Britain, where the consultants have never been "budget holders." They define their task as patient care, while the other staff provide the means. As a result, some wasteful practice styles have persisted for many years in individual hospitals, unknown to superiors and not fully understood by others in those hospitals.[46] (Wide variations in practice styles can be identified in other countries with salaried medical staffs, despite the supposedly standard financial incentives.[47]) Statistical peer comparisons among all British hospital consultants would have revealed the differences, but they are never done. The DHA might have used the wasted resources for other purposes, but the lay managers had no method of forcing or persuading any consultant to practice differently.

Britain during the 1970s adopted a familiar device, a committee of the consultants in each hospital as a channel of communications between managers and doctors and as a forum to discuss each organization's needs.[48] But a committee does not change staff structures or styles of practice. It meets only occasionally, and many doctors are not involved.

The problem is to make the hospital doctors responsible for the use of resources. In Britain a method called "clinical budgeting" has been proposed to make the traditional hospital "firm" responsible for planning, assignment of resources, and financial discipline. This arrangement would not necessitate the unlikely transformation of British medical staffs into services or departments. The DHA would negotiate a "Planning Agreement with Clinical Teams" with each of its consultants at the start of each year. Each consultant would learn the total resources available to the DHA and would have to fit his wish list into his share. The consultant would have to specify his intentions and resource needs; in the tradeoffs he might be persuaded to do some things more efficiently. He would use various central hospital services up to expected limits (for example, certain expected levels of radiodiagnosis and supplies), rather than controlling such services himself. During the year he could make economies and use the savings for other activities. In contrast to all previous experiences, the method would ensure that every consultant is constantly involved in planning, financial implementation, and tradeoffs.[49]

Effects of Fee-for-Service on Hospital Costs

Does fee-for-service generate more self-interested and more unnecessary work than salaries? Does fee-for-service inspire faster and more efficient work? Virtually no research has ever been done comparing the work of doctors paid by different methods and isolating the doctors' hospital work from their work in office practice. Therefore, the precise effect of fee-for-service on inpatient work is difficult to estimate.

Hardly any statistics can be inferred from hospital records for such comparisons; a purpose of salaried payment is to eliminate detailed economic records about work. Germany is one of the few countries where salaried and fee-for-service payments are used for the same hospital work—that is, for work performed by the salaried chiefs, the *Belegärzte,* and private clinic doctors. But no detailed data exist to compare them, and the KVs would not cooperate with any research testing a hypothesis that fee-for-service motivates too many treatments.

A widespread hypothesis is that fee-for-service encourages more services, and some evidence confirms it. In the countries where the doctors in proprietary hospitals collect fees for laboratory tests, both the hospital organization (that is, the doctor-owner) and the pathologist may be motivated to order many tests. The tests are paid for under the fee schedules negotiated between the medical association and sickness funds to pay the individual doctor. But the pathologist usually works in a proprietary hospital or medical group, and he personally or his organization can buy an autoanalyzer (which automatically generates many tests on the same sample, whereas a manual tester would perform fewer). During the 1970s the number of tests skyrocketed all over Europe, and the pathologists' income rose.[50] In order to reduce perverse incentives and financial windfalls, the joint committees of sickness funds and medical associations reduced the fees for tests. Likewise, diagnostic tests are important sources of income for American doctors and American for-profit hospitals,[51] but American payers lack the regulatory and negotiating machinery to force down doctors' fees and proprietary hospitals' charge lists. At the most, American payers can prevent the hospital managers and residents from ordering tests indiscriminately themselves; they can place that responsibility on the attending physician; and they can remind the doctor to order only those tests he deems necessary. For example, under the Medical Necessity Program of several state Blue Cross and Blue Shield Plans, the hospital and doctor are paid for a diagnostic admission battery only when the attending physician specifically orders it.[52]

It is widely suspected that fee-for-service encourages surgery. American and Canadian hospital surgeons collect fees, whereas British and Swedish surgeons are salaried. The American and Canadian populations have twice the surgery rates as the British and Swedes. The average American and Canadian surgeon operates more often.[53]

The practice styles of physicians and the mere number of doctors can counteract the effects of payment systems. For example, the average rates for several surgical procedures are higher in fee-earning America than in salaried Britain and Norway, but the frequency in each country varies widely among communities; some British and Norwegian communities have higher rates than American communities.[54] Perhaps fee-for-service provides greater opportunities for provider-induced demand. In the United States, the highest rates for surgery occur in the districts with the most surgeons. To maintain income, surgeons in overdoctored areas not only can increase their activity but—because America lacks fixed fee schedules—can raise their charges.[55]

If fee-for-service payment coincides with certain pressures from hospital employment, the utilization and costs of the hospital greatly increase. For example, Holland is one of the few European countries where senior hospital doctors are paid entirely by fee-for-service rather than by salaries. As a condition for his appointment to a hospital post, the specialist must pay "good will" to his predecessor. Usually he borrows and pays off the debt from future earnings. As Dutch specialty practice became more remunerative during the 1960s and 1970s, and as the competition for hospital posts intensified, the prices for "good will" and the debts rose substantially. Specialists were under pressure to increase work and (once they were appointed) to fight against creating additional senior hospital posts.

The situation was a principal reason for the great increase in Dutch hospital costs during the 1970s. As often happens during such an intense work pace, the specialists overshot their targets and earned very high net incomes. The Ministry of Public Health imposed a ceiling on the gross revenue of the entire Dutch specialty sector: as total annual national spending approached the ceiling, COTG ordered cuts in individual fees. The specialists protested and in early 1986 called a one-day national strike.

Fee-for-service increases services if doctors can use hospital facilities that allow or encourage greater utilization. For example, most inpatient surgery on German patients under NHI is given in hospitals where the sickness funds pay *grosse Pflegesätze* and the surgeons earn salaries. Those surgeons can earn fees only from ambulatory private patients and from occasional private surgical inpatients. The alternative hospitalization occurs in Germany's many private clinics: third parties under both NHI and private health insurance pay fee-for-service to the surgeons; the private clinics benefit from charges and *kleine Pflegesätze*. This competition with salaried hospital care may be an important reason for Germany's high rate of appendectomies; that is, the higher surgical rates may arise from the private clinics.[56]

Fee-for-service increases the total cost of the health care system by combining with certain medical practice styles to increase use of the hospital. Under open-staff systems, as in the United States and Canada, doctors can treat their patients either in the hospital or in the office. Hospital work gives them the chance to bill for more remunerative procedures. If hospital and physicians' insurance is separated, the doctors may not be billed for practice costs by the hospital but must cover them only in their own offices. The bias toward inpatient hospitalization even for simple work such as testing was formalized in the United States and Canada when health insurance became widespread and generous first for hospital care and only later for ambulatory services.[57]

Because it is the doctors who make the hospitals' clinical decisions, fee-for-service can counteract the effects of cost-containment efforts directed at the hospitals' internal affairs. For example, as Chapter Eight demonstrated, Canadian provincial governments try to use global budgets and close monitoring to reduce unnecessary service intensity and unnecessary patient-days. But the provincial governments at the same time pay doctors by fee-for-service in the separate Medicare system. Unlike the doctors in much of Europe, Canadian doctors do not belong to salaried closed hospital staffs. When granting operating funds, the provincial governments face the hospital administrators and not the medical staffs. Because of the divided and possibly contradictory payment system, Canada's hospital costs may not be limited as strictly as they might. Length of stay increased in Canada during the 1970s, while dropping everywhere else.[58]

A chronic problem in reimbursement policy is finding the right balance. Changing a payment method may substitute new difficulties for old ones. For example, while fee-for-service encourages high productivity, salaries may foster excessive slowdowns. The waiting lists for beds in Britain's National Health Service—discussed in Chapter Eight—may be due in large part to the salaried consultants' preference for an orderly and constant work flow. Only fee-for-service could motivate them to speed up and clear the waiting lists. The queues are usually attributed to shortages of resources, but increasing the numbers of salaried consultants might increase rather than reduce waiting lists.[59]

Summary

The trend in developed countries is to make the hospital a more organized facility. Once occasional visitors, doctors are becoming members of management, with full-time schedules, defined obligations, and salaries. As the hospital's clinical work becomes more complicated and more expensive, the senior doctors become a decision-making collective, prioritizing purchases of heavy equipment. As cost containment becomes more important, the chiefs become involved in the efficient operation of the hospital. Junior doctors are no longer merely students or employees of the chiefs; they now hold ranks in a salaried medical staff.

As the senior doctors become full-timers, their outside practices disappear. They no longer run private clinics to the disadvantage of the nonprofit or public hospital. The distinction between hospital practice and office/clinic practice widens.

Public policy can control such hospitals through interventions by governments and sickness funds. But American hospitals are far more independent, since they continue to be workshops designed to serve all the office doctors in their community. American hospitals do not employ, pay, or control the medical staffs; and the doctors force the hospitals to compete to please them.

The trend in Europe for doctors as well as for other hospital employees is to make their salaries part of a large salary structure in the public sector. The specialists often suceed in obtaining special contracts with a special salary scheme. To persuade them to become full-time hospital workers, the government hospital associations, and sickness funds must guarantee them very high salaries, equivalent to what they would have earned in the mixed intramural and extramural practice of the past. The specialists usually succeed in retaining some limited rights of private practice. The result is profitable for the doctors and expensive for the payers, but hospitals become more stable.

12

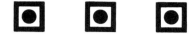

Responsibilities
of Hospital Management

In the days when hospital owners found all the operating funds, the manager was a subordinate, responsible for housekeeping, paying small bills, and managing some employees. In religious hospitals the managers often were leading members of the nursing order. When hospitals started to collect fees from patients and third parties, new managerial specialists were added to find money and calculate cost reports. Hospitals became more elaborate in capital, personnel, purchasing, and collections. By now, in every country, the lay hospital managers—specializing in finance and in organizational maintenance—have become prominent and well paid. The boards representing the owners have become the managers' helpers rather than their rulers. The lay managers have become the experts in the crucial relations with new groups that eclipse the owners—that is, the payers of operating revenue, the payers of capital grants, and the regulators in government.

The organizational structures of hospitals and the roles of managers have changed with the evolution of hospital finance. Every country is groping with several central issues today. This chapter will summarize the principal alternatives in handling a few key topics:

- How to persuade the managers of individual hospitals to cooperate with public policies. Chapters Six through Nine described how regulations, grants, and exhortations are directed at hospitals. The next problem is implementation: whether the training, roles, and rewards of managers result in more or less conformity.
- Relations between the physicians and administrators. Roles of the physicians in management.
- Roles of managers and their effects on efficient services and on hospital costs. As in the cases of the hospital workers and physicians—described in Chapters Ten and Eleven—certain roles and personal aims of managers can greatly increase hospital costs. Other roles and career ambitions can be cost controlling.

- Machinery to restrain wasteful utilization. Machinery to prevent undesirable effects of the financial system on quality of care. How the delicate confrontations are managed among doctors, hospital administrators, and payers.

As in earlier chapters, I will describe several principal arrangements in detail, since alternative outcomes cannot be judged without a full understanding of the inputs.

Committing Managers to National Policies

Hospitals until recently have been totally oriented toward their local communities. Many hospitals were owned by local groups. Even when they were owned by multihospital associations, such as religious orders, few guidelines and controls came from headquarters, gifts came from the locality, and the hospital served patients primarily or entirely from the local catchment area.

The traditional methods of selecting and promoting the lay managers of confessional, secular voluntary, and secular public hospitals limited their horizons to the individual hospital and its parent associations. In nearly every country, the lay hospital administrators came from commercial training courses. When selecting this career, they knew that they were entering a lifetime of community service and that they were something other than businessmen. They were hired by the incumbent senior administrators and governing boards of each hospital. After promotion to senior posts, they stayed until retirement or (in occasional cases) until invited to a senior post in a more famous hospital.

As modern medical care advances technically and as modern financing expands, such arrangements can become excessively expensive. Each individual organization and each multihospital group responds to the doctors' pressure for new facilities and responds to owners' and managers' aspirations for prestige. Considerable duplication results. But policies such as containing costs and developing a division of labor among hospitals require from managers of individual installations a much wider orientation. They must think of the system as a whole; they must ask themselves how their establishments serve the public interest.

A National Corps of Hospital Administrators. France has developed a method of orienting hospital managers toward the needs of the larger system, while continuing to administer individual installations. French hospital management was staffed and oriented in the aforementioned traditional fashion for centuries, with merely a change of ownership from private associations to local governments during the Revolution.[1] During the 1960s national planning was begun, to produce a coherent system, raise standards, and eliminate waste. But national hospital plans usually are ignored by lay managers and doctors. Normally in almost all countries, hospital administrators cannot easily be reached, since they are autonomous. A general reform in hospital management was possible in France because the national government may set standards for the civil servants employed by local governments.[2]

As in many other sectors of French life, the national government created an elite corps of administrators in health, trained at a special graduate school (the

Ecole Nationale de la Santé Publique) and based in an office of the national Ministry of Health. Posts in public hospitals throughout France are filled by the Ministry after consulting the governing boards. After graduation young members of the corps fill lower administrative positions. To be promoted, they apply for higher jobs opening in their current hospital or (more usually) elsewhere in the country. The administrator ultimately becomes a hospital director after service in several locations. He can then compete for openings as director in more desirable places. Other administrative employees who did not graduate from the school can still work their way up—now also moving from place to place; but the tone is set by the others.

The administrator is evaluated formally on the basis of his dossier in the Ministry and informally in the grapevine. On the one hand, he must excel in implementing national policies, such as running hospitals efficiently and economically. On the other hand, he must also please his hospital's governing board and the local community. Each board is headed by the mayor and includes members of the community council and other local notables. The manager must mollify the hospital's medical staff. An administrator who can accomplish all this successfully will rise in the competition for better posts.

The administrator's job is to fit local interests into national policies. Compared to administrators in other countries, French hospital administrators seem more cooperative with the rate regulators, who are other civil servants from the Ministries of Health and Interior in the local prefecture. They seem less aggressive in pushing proposals by doctors for new services that would duplicate those in other hospitals; and they appear to be more cooperative with plans for regional divisions of labor among hospitals. They also seem more cooperative with national cost-containment policies, such as closing beds and limiting personnel to the ratios in the Ministry's guidelines.

Collective Professional Influences. No other country has anything like France's methods of selecting, training, assigning, and rewarding hospital administrators. Until recently the principal lay administrator of each hospital was a minor official; the finance officer was no more than a bookkeeper. Lay management grows everywhere in importance and size, because every hospital becomes bigger, more complicated, and more involved with external payers and regulators. Training programs for students of hospital administration are recent and produce limited numbers of students. Postgraduate courses and special training institutes are offered by hospital associations in many countries, and they are growing in number and in prominence. But they are still short in duration and voluntary in participation. One method of widening hospital directors' orientations—used by the Swiss hospital association (VESKA) and the Dutch hospital research institute (NZI)—is to bring together regularly the managers of the hospitals in each peer group created by the rate regulators. At their meetings the managers discuss national policies and evaluate each other's performance from comparative statistical profiles.

An energetic hospital association—as in Switzerland, Germany, and the Netherlands—can help the previously disparate managers develop considerable esprit de corps and awareness of public policies. The associations clearly convey messages about the public good and the collective interests of the hospital industry, not the tactics of each individual's winning out over everyone else.

Having mobilized a strategically situated nationwide profession, the hospital association then becomes a great political force, represented in national discussions about hospital policy. The question of orientation then moves to a higher plane: Do the leaders of the hospital association then seek only the maximum financial gain and the maximum freedom for the hospitals alone, or do they try to help solve the problems of the economy and of health services more generally?

Only Germany has a mechanism for involving the hospital association in such policy making. Under the national cost-containment law of 1977, the Minister of Labor calls a semiannual conference of the health care providers and payers. Such a coordinating body (*Konzertierte Aktion im Gesundheitswesen,* or KA) was necessary to set pricing policy, since all the providers and payers were private and set prices by direct negotiation; at the same time, Parliament was unwilling to confer nationwide pricing powers upon the national or provincial governments. The KA consists of the national representatives of the doctors, dentists, sickness funds, employers, trade unions, provincial governments, and local governments. Several federal Ministers also participate. The secretariat, consisting of civil servants employed by the Ministry of Labor, prepares data for the conferees about the performance of the health care system and the trends in the economy. The conferees receive recommendations from the national Ministries and from the interest groups. The KA deliberates and makes recommendations about annual increases in fees for doctors and other providers, as well as predictions about utilization. These guidelines are supposed to keep health care costs within increases in the fiscal capacity of the sickness funds (the *Grundlohnsumme* yielding the premiums). The actual decisions about increases in fees are made in negotiations between the associations of insurance doctors and sickness funds (and between other providers and sickness funds) in each province. But the negotiations in practice usually conform to the KA recommendations.[3]

The national hospital association was always represented in the KA, but the law did not give the KA power to adopt strict guidelines about hospital finance. In particular, the original law and later amendments did not give the KA power to recommend that annual increases in hospital rates should stay within the *Grundlohnsumme.* The hospital association argued that each hospital should be free to develop its costs according to its individual needs and should negotiate freely with the sickness funds. While the KA nearly stabilized the growth in physicians' payments, hospital rates grew, and stays were not adequately reduced. After years of uncertainty, Parliament clearly gave the KA authority—beginning in 1985—to recommend improvements in the economic efficiency of the hospital industry as a whole, to recommend desirable utilization standards, and to recommend reasonable average increases in the *Pflegesatz.* Therefore, the national hospital association must develop an economic policy proposal, must negotiate KA guidelines with representatives of the sickness funds and other groups, and must persuade all the country's hospital managers to settle close to the annual guideline figures. The individual hospital manager is still autonomous in preparing his prospective budget and seeking a new *Pflegesatz,* but now he must be aware of a national policy. If he deadlocks with the sickness funds, he knows that the arbitrator will follow the KA guidelines.

For many years medical associations and sickness funds have settled fees and conditions of service by nationwide collective bargaining. The office doctors remain private and independently managed, but many of their decisions are made collectively. Germany is the first country to begin extending this idea into hospital financial management.

Ownership and Management by the National Government. Hospital finance policies—whether to expand and redirect resources or to contain costs—are formulated by national governments. The simplest method of implementation—giving orders to all the hospital managers—is possible only if the national government owns and controls all the hospitals and employs all the managers. Such central ownership and control through an administrative hierarchy is very unusual. It exists in the Soviet Union and in a few Middle Eastern countries where all health services are run by the army. Everywhere else, tradition, community pressures, and the resistance of the doctors keep the hospitals under local management. Nearly every developed country has a mixture of municipal and private ownership.[4] The methods described earlier in this chapter evolved because most national governments can only influence rather than directly order hospital managers.

Great Britain has achieved considerable central authority over the individual hospital's management, but the evolution has been prolonged and is still incomplete. Before the enactment of the National Health Service, the hospitals were owned by voluntary associations and local governments. The wartime national coalition government proposed an NHS with voluntary takeovers by government of some hospitals and Treasury grants to those remaining private and autonomous.[5] The postwar Labour Government nationalized all municipal and voluntary hospitals, in order to save them from bankruptcy, to redirect resources into underserved areas, and to secure the livelihoods of the specialists. But, as in every democratic country, concessions were made in hospital governance, leaving them quite independent for over twenty more years. The noted teaching hospitals remained under their individual Boards of Governors, whose distinguished members and consultant medical staff could press for new programs and resist cutbacks. The smaller hospitals were coordinated by Hospital Management Committees, recruited locally.

The structure of management within each hospital changed during the first years of the NHS. Before creation of the NHS, the administrative hierarchy in every voluntary hospital was based on the only authority structure within the organization—that is, the nursing staff. The matron was really the hospital director, in charge of all housekeeping as well as care of patients. The consultants were office based and visited only to treat their patients in their beds. A clerk ran the business office.

Under the NHS the clerk became the "secretary" of the teaching hospital and the "secretary" of the Hospital Management Committee. The secretary gained jurisdiction over each hospital's infrastructure—buildings and grounds, the kitchen, the laundry, and the supply room. Therefore, the matron was no longer director of the hospital.

The secretary and the governing councils were expected to carry out guidelines from the national Ministry of Health, but conflicts between national and local obligations did not arise often. During the 1950s and 1960s, both

Labour and Conservative Governments merely tried to maintain the NHS, all hospital budgets were increased incrementally, and hospital managements were not forced into new directions. The hospital secretaries were employees of the National Health Service and were responsible to their governing committees; they were not civil servants employed by the Ministry of Health in London. Guidelines and funds passed down from London through successive committees until they reached the individual hospitals.[6]

This ramshackle structure was reorganized during the 1970s, to make the individual hospital more responsive to national policy.[7] The policies themselves became more restrictive: Labour Governments wished to limit new funding for the teaching hospitals and for London and to direct resources into deprived regions; Conservative Governments wished to cut back spending on the NHS everywhere and to close hospitals in overbedded areas. Regional Health Authorities replaced the Regional Hospital Boards and Boards of Governors; they were expected to make and carry out facilities and operating plans. I described these policies and their implementation in Chapters Eight and Nine.

The reform presumed that the NHS would be managed better, but creation of a coherent management structure foundered over several dilemmas. One problem was whether the national government or the locality was in charge. The utopian hope was that both Whitehall and every district would be satisfied simultaneously and that priorities enunciated by both DHSS and the DHA would be fulfilled. The DHSS sent down guidelines and growth money that was targeted selectively by RAWP. Planning was bottoms-up, and the mix of services and expenditure was supposed to reflect local needs. Regional plans written by the RHAs were supposed to synthesize all the district plans and priorities and to add special regional tasks. The district was expected to work within plans and expenditure levels approved by the region, but the DHA really held the initiative in setting the missions. A few DHAs precipitated showdowns with DHSS and their RHAs by refusing to economize, arguing that all services were needed by the patients, spending their allocations before the end of the fiscal year, and demanding that DHSS cover the deficit. The Secretary of State had to take drastic action—splashed embarrassingly across the newspapers—by temporarily replacing rebellious DHA governing boards with appointed commissioners and then reinstating the boards with some new members.

Instead of one person in charge of the hospital—a leading consultant, a matron, or a lay administrator—everyone was now in charge. For nearly a decade, the watchword was "team management." Every organization and the district itself were to be managed by a committee representing all principal actors. Every such team decided by consensus. The District Administrator (the successor to the secretary of the Hospital Management Committee) provided secretarial support and was responsible to his NHS superiors only for ensuring that every management team got through its agenda. The District Administrators performed their ambiguous jobs in an unexpectedly wide variety of styles. Every team devoted much effort to negotiating decisions, particularly the cuts and reallocations required by stringent funding. The easiest course of action was to preserve existing programs, particularly since the consultants favored keeping and developing acute services, even if DHSS guidelines encouraged new directions. The consultants complained that meetings were too numerous and diverted them from their patients. The system was said to be "overadministered" and "undermanaged."[8]

The NHS was again reformed in 1984, to assign managers to each organization, to each DHA, and to each RHA. The managers are responsible for implementing policies from higher levels and for making economies and reallocations. Instead of the delays and compromises of team management, each individual manager is supposed to be quick and willing to take actions unpopular with clinicians and with the community. Each hospital (and every other unit) has a general manager, assisted by managers for financial services, planning, quality assurance, and clinical services. The DHA appoints the managers, and the managers are accountable to the DHA rather than to higher levels. But the managers' qualifications and performance are monitored by special management training and oversight agencies in DHSS. The financial and programmatic policies of the national government therefore are supposed to be implemented more faithfully than under the earlier methods of ambiguous DHSS guidelines and general grants of money.[9] But whether the lay managers have power to overrule the consultants has still not been settled.

Enterprising Hospital Managers

Because of nationwide financing and health care cost-containment policies, every individual hospital must follow general rules. To accomplish this, some countries have adopted new methods of selecting or training hospital managers. Although technically employed by and subordinate to the individual hospital's board, the manager becomes attentive to national public policy.

When the newly expanded financing does not include strict controls or nationally standardized methods, the hospital manager remains oriented to his organization and its community. Since both costs and opportunities for revenue steadily grow, the organization encourages its managers to use the payment system to maximize revenue and reputation. The manager is rewarded for exploiting the situation, not for obeying the strictures of distant policy makers.

United States. In a society of independent business firms, the American hospital has gradually come to resemble them. In contrast to their counterparts in Europe, American hospital managers—in both the nonprofit and for-profit sectors—have come to think and work like business managers.

During the nineteenth and early twentieth centuries, as in Europe, American hospital administration involved the routine oversight of buildings, personnel, materials, and financial accounts. The financial functions were simple.[10] Once many doctors managed hospitals; but as medicine became more successful and more glamorous, and as medical education became more technical, fewer doctors were interested in management. By the 1940s American acute hospitals usually were managed by nonclinicians. In the nonconfessional hospitals, the managers were laymen. In the religious hospitals, the executives were still representatives of the religious orders, but now they were closely assisted by lay deputies. At first these lay administrators were accountants promoted from the once lowly business office.[11]

After World War II, the more successful American hospitals became more dynamic, and the tasks of management grew rapidly. The key was the lavish and permissive funding after the mid-1960s under Medicare, Medicaid, Blue Cross, and commercial health insurance. The attending physicians—that is, the outside salesmen—have constantly pressed the hospitals to install the newest methods and additional staff. Costs constantly mounted, and hospitals more than ever needed to please the attendings to bring in revenue. The hospital market has been very competitive, and hospitals have always needed to please the community's office doctors, lest the physicians refer their patients elsewhere and throw the lagging hospital into bankruptcy. Different third parties had different payment rules, and clever calculations could maximize revenue. Some payers—Medicare, Medicaid, and Blue Cross in many states—agreed to reimburse costs, and the hospital had to develop the capacity to identify and document the costs of treating particular patients. Government set standards of safety. To cope with this volume of staff, money, paper, and activity, the once rudimentary hospital business office became a large department, which itself had to be managed.

The increasingly difficult tasks were beyond the capacity of accountants and personnel clerks promoted from within the hospital. The new lay managers required considerable professional education. Growing numbers were graduates of generic curricula in organizational management or special curricula in hospital management. Some obtained joint degrees, with an MPH from a university's School of Public Health and an MBA from its School of Business. The new managements applied to hospitals the trends in American business. The once formless acute hospital—like many other industrial organizations—was treated as if it were a multiproduct multidivisional firm. The executive offices gave considerable autonomy to the operating units in the organization (they had to do so, since the doctors really ran current operations) and monitored the activity of the divisions through records of revenue, expenditure, and materials use. The management's goal was survival in the market and improvement through greater market share. The rules of third parties and the capacities of paying customers were studied, in order to maximize revenue and accumulate extra cash. To attract the most prolific doctors and increase reimbursement, managers bought new equipment, launched new construction, and hired more staff. The capital market—the source for productive new investment—became the key to success of the hospital. Effective executives were skilled in managing debt.[12] Instead of passively conforming to facilities planning and reimbursement rules of governments and of third parties, the new hospital managers try to circumvent them or to maneuver within them, so that they can continue to maximize their own hospital's growth and revenue, regardless of external constraints.[13]

The leading managers must be enterprising not only in marketing but also in reorganizing their own structures. The prospect of tighter reimbursement by payers of hospital costs during the 1980s led to a wave of internal reorganization. Managements with large numbers of salaried senior doctors and residents created medical practice groups that could earn fees outside the hospital financing channels, as I described in the last chapter. Many hospitals introduced internal structural changes in response to payment by DRGs. (Hospital structures often conform to each country's predominant methods of reimbursement.) American hospitals previously were organized by functional department: the leading managers oversaw a comprehensive nursing department, the laboratories, the pharmacy, and other infrastructure services consumed by patient care. The hospital's economic health now depends on its using resources from these functional departments in such a way that the total costs do not exceed the payment from Medicare for each DRG. Some hospitals appointed new "DRG managers" or "product line managers" who monitored clusters of similar patients under the DRG classification (for example, oncology, women and children, and cardiology), who learned resource use and costs for each DRG, and who persuaded doctors and functional managers to economize.[14] Each American hospital can run its affairs differently, and no two responded to DRGs identically.

The role of financial manager has emerged in the top leadership of the American hospital. Previously, financial administrators were accountants and bookkeepers, who counted and recorded past expenditures and ticked off payment of bills. Now they are oriented to the future, participate in all major decisions, and estimate how future plans increase revenue and offset increases in costs. They plan new investments by designing the bond offerings and calculating depreciation. As in American business, the new chief financial officer is a close associate of the chief executive officer.

American chief executive officers once spent much of their day moving about the hospital, conversing with employees and observing clinical care—as they still do in Europe. Now the Americans devote less than 10 percent of their time to visiting the floors and three-quarters of their time to strategic planning, marketing, finance, and responding to government regulations.[15]

If someone's ingenuity enables any American organization to survive, prosper, and grow, he earns a high salary and bonuses. The competition among American hospitals for leadership and the need to keep managers from deserting to other industries have led to high salaries. During the 1970s and 1980s, base salaries of executives (not including bonuses, fringe benefits, and perquisites) rose faster in hospitals than in other American industries. By 1983 the base salaries in hospitals had reached:

	Median	*75th percentile*
All hospitals		
Chief executive officer	$79,700	$95,849
Chief financial officer	$50,800	$58,909
Hospitals with over 450 beds		
Chief executive officer	$97,355	$107,790
Chief financial officer	$60,000	$70,000

The hospitals with the highest revenue—$80 million or more annually—paid the chief executive officers between $100,000 and $200,000 plus perquisites.[16] Because of their growing importance to hospitals and because they can find well-paying jobs in other industries, the chief financial officers have risen in pay faster than all other ranks. Among the larger hospitals, their salaries increased 21.3 percent from 1982 to 1984.[17]

The new generation of managers multiplied and profited as the American hospital sector grew. They were even more essential to the survival and prosperity of their organizations when payers contained utilization and costs during the 1980s. Their salaries and job security continued to improve, while the incomes of other hospital workers stabilized.

Performing simple jobs in hospitals that do not depend on their ingenuity for survival, European hospital managers earn much less. In several countries, such as France and Great Britain, they earn the usual salaries of middle-level government managers; but substantial individual variations occur (as in France) according to size of hospital, the economic level of the community, and the manager's seniority.[18] Germany's heterogeneous hospital ownership and the independence of each hospital make the system somewhat like America's. No surveys of managers' pay have been conducted, but the principal directors of large nonprofit hospitals in Germany around 1983 earned about 120,000 DM a year. Many earned less. (In 1983, 120,000 DM was equal to about $50,000.) Limited to the civil service pay scales, directors of the largest German municipal hospitals earned about two-thirds of the nonprofit hospitals' rates.

While European and Canadian hospitals have stable market shares and predictable utilization levels, many of their managers have marketing strategies— not to grow but to avoid decline. In the face of changes in the population, they try to ensure that utilization does not drop.[19] If it diminishes, regulators and negotiators reduce the prospective budget, the hospital may have to cut its services and personnel, and it may be pressed to close or to convert to extended care. Unless the European and Canadian manager is rewarded for making economies—as in Great Britain and France—he defends the existing organization. The regulators and payers are alert to such marketing when population changes should be bringing about changes in utilization. They also are alert to signs that the hospital managers and chiefs of service are increasing utilization beyond the demand expected by the growth and aging of the local population. Vigorous competition for market share among nonprofit and public hospitals is discouraged everywhere but in the United States.

Bilateral Collaboration. Resourceful managers are willing to desert the model of the independent competitive organization if the results are mounting costs and limited sales. Cooperation to head off bankruptcy is common in other industries and eventually was adopted by American hospital owners and managers.

The problem was that the boom in hospital financing could not escalate forever. Innovations and costs of capital rose cumulatively. More personnel were being added. Medicare, Medicaid, and Blue Cross limited the annual increases in rates. Utilization stabilized. Hospital managers soon realized that not everyone could create expensive and underutilized new services. Throughout the United States, some otherwise independent hospitals started to share services—such as materials purchasing, blood banks, laundries, pharmacies, laboratories, and data processing—in order to save money. Such hospitals remain competitive and self-centered in patient care technology and in marketing.[20]

Outsiders have pressed some hospitals to give up their hopes for complete self-sufficiency and to collaborate in patient care. In a few states with expensive hospital systems, the planning bodies—the Health Systems Agency and the state government's Department of Health—attempt to force regionalization by denying certificates of need for expensive equipment for all hospitals. They hope that two or more applicants will agree among themselves to share CT scanners, cobalt therapy, open-heart surgery, and so on. Hospital managers reluctantly agree to share if they cannot obtain their own CON or if their own utilization makes purchase risky, but they eventually try to purchase their own units if their utilization is sufficient, lest the physicians admit patients in the hospitals where the units are located.[21]

Some pressures to share new services come from lenders. A bond issue will not be underwritten by local government or rated attractively by Moody's or Standard and Poor's if utilization will not be profitable enough to pay it off. As a result, only one hospital in the area might write an offering for a particular new program. A division of labor might be negotiated among the community's hospitals in expensive new services, so that each is assured of sufficient utilization when writing its own proposal. The managers of the hospitals must work out the terms of patient referrals in these specialized sectors while remaining competitive in all others.

The dictates of the capital market lead to some mergers. Older hospitals cannot sell enough bonds or attract enough donations to modernize; their reimbursement rates are too low to generate large enough funds in depreciation and profit. Their management may then be taken over by more modern, higher-priced, and more occupied hospitals that can attract more capital.

Investor-Owned Chains. America has been unique not only in the adoption of businesslike methods in marketing and managing individual nonprofit hospitals but also in the creation of for-profit corporations that own hospitals and other medical care services. The creators and original owners were nonphysicians; their present owners are stockholders.[22]

The United States and other developed countries have long traditions of private clinics owned by individual doctors as their for-profit practice sites, and many remain. When the doctor-owner of one American private clinic had a chance to buy another in 1968, he joined with several laymen to create an appropriate entity, the Hospital Corporation of America. Another principal multiunit company (Humana, Inc.) was created by lawyers and real estate operators who began in the nursing home business. Another (Hospital Affiliates International) began as a partnership of doctors and lay financial experts who managed private clinics owned by doctors; eventually, the firm incorporated, went public, and acquired title to the private clinics in return for stock.[23]

By 1982 forty-one chains owned 668 of the 1,045 for-profit acute, psychiatric, and specialized hospitals in America, with 89,171 of their 120,848 total beds. The chains were highly unequal in size: seventeen owned six or fewer hospitals; three owned over seventy hospitals apiece. Despite considerable publicity designed to market their services and attract capital, the for-profit chains were dwarfed by the nonprofit sector, which had 139 chains, with 967 hospitals, 185,857 beds, and more than twice the revenue. Besides managing their own hospitals, the investor-owned chains' managerial experience enables them to offer services on contract: in 1982 they managed 283 nonprofit and public hospitals, some earmarked for acquisition.[24]

Each for-profit chain has a corporate headquarters that—like any nationwide manufacturing/service corporation—raises capital and monitors its geographically dispersed units. As in other dynamic American companies, the divisions can be diversified, including several of the following: acute hospitals, nursing homes, dialysis centers, addiction treatment centers, psychiatric centers, home care, day care, laboratories, and medical supplies. Competing with each other and with nonprofit hospitals for market share, several chains during the 1980s added ambulatory centers and HMOs with employed doctors, in order to find patients. Humana and others offered to employed groups and to individuals prepaid arrangements guaranteeing full care for an annual capitation fee. These "multi-health care corporations" therefore became vertically integrated systems, a structure common in other American industries.[25]

A multi-health care structure gives the corporation's managers the flexibility much prized by American business management. The manager's strategy is to maximize profits from the chain's entire holdings, not from the hospitals alone. If a payer limits its hospital inpatient payment (such as Medicare DRGs) or if a state government regulator limits all hospital inpatient rates, the company can avoid these limits by treating the patient in an ambulatory site or in home care, with lower costs and more generous prices.

A for-profit chain's strategic planning resembles that of any large business. Careful studies of the local market are made before the chain takes over an existing hospital or builds a new one.[26] The best prospects are regions with growing populations and few nonprofit hospitals, such as the South and West. Taking over an existing hospital is safer than creating a new one. The chain's planners estimate whether the population has enough cash and third-party coverage to ensure profits. The planners prefer an area with at least one public or nonprofit hospital, so that patients without money can be steered there. The chain favors communities under permissive governments, without public facilities planning and without rate regulation. They prefer reimbursement practices whereby third parties pay charges set by the hospital rather than costs; any cost-based reimbursement allows a "return on equity." If the chain acquires an existing hospital, it prefers maximum freedom to modernize it and raise charges.

As in all chain ownership, headquarters performs certain centralized functions for all units. These centralized functions include financial management, raising capital in national markets, personnel recruitment, political lobbying, advertising, materials management, and architectural design. The chains are managed in the decentralized fashion common in nationwide American corporations: unit managers have considerable discretion in details, headquarters monitors the units through financial reports, and the efficiency of the units is judged by their profits.

Medical care in American for-profit hospitals probably is little different from care in the nonprofits. Medical care depends on the attending doctors, technology, and staffing; competition and the expectations of the doctors cause both types of hospitals to provide similar working conditions for the doctors and similar environments for patients. Some differences in operations arise from the types of patients accepted. Few for-profits are set up for tertiary care, and they direct complex and long-stay cases elsewhere—for instance, to the academic medical centers that have nonprofit owners. Because the for-profits get inpatients from office doctors and almost none from walk-in outpatient departments, they have fewer Medicaid patients and hardly any of the poor lacking third-party coverage. Some for-profits may save money by using fewer employees and reassigning them more flexibly.[27]

Their growth in a humanitarian market with many indigents prevents the chains from erecting the financial barrier against nonpayers typical of other commercial markets. During the 1970s and 1980s, the chains bought or leased over 180 public hospitals from financially burdened county governments. After a wave of controversies over loss of access by the poor, the chains and county governments created special funds to cover indigents. The for-profits would no longer turn away the poor, but they still did not invite them.

The for-profits have higher administrative expenses than the nonprofits because—in addition to the offices in individual hospitals—the chain as a whole must be responsible for long-term strategic planning, marketing research, coordination, start-up planning and investment in new hospitals, and the maintenance of headquarters. As in other American business, the headquarters is lavishly housed and generously paid.

The chains acquire new hospitals by purchase—often with little cash because the once publicly owned establishments are decrepit and financially stressed—and by giving former private owners stock in their corporations. The chains cannot raise capital from tax-exempt revenue bonds (such help by local government is limited to nonprofit and public hospitals), but they can borrow in commercial markets, by mortgages and other instruments. Commercial debt is not as restrictive in the use of funds as revenue bonds are. Through growing utilization and profitable charges (particularly on supplies and tests), the chains have been able to repay debt and accumulate additional cash from operating revenue. During this period of growth and financial turnover, the original owners have profited considerably. However, no business sector can grow indefinitely. The investor-owned chains' rapid expansion has left them with one of the highest levels of debt in American business. Managing such debt requires a rate of growth in patient services that cannot be maintained indefinitely for all the firms: eventually they will saturate all markets; third-party payers by the mid-1980s were already limiting prices and utilization.[28]

Controls over Practice

Every hospital must monitor and regulate the quality of its work. Particularly in the present age of vigilance by payers about costs, hospitals' prices and utilization are being observed and limited. For both cost and quality, some control machinery is situated inside the hospital's own management while some is imposed from outside by payers, regulators, and consumers.

Price and Utilization Controls. Payers and governments seek price and utilization controls, but the hospitals' managers and doctors do not. The managers wish more admissions of more profitable patients and—if beds are unprofitably empty—longer stays. If the doctors are paid by fee-for-service, they favor admissions of profitable patients and care little about extended convalescence. Salaried doctors favor filling beds in order to prevent the hospital from reducing and shutting their services.

While hospital managers' efforts are oriented toward increasing revenue, recently the restrictions by payers upon revenue have made managers in all countries aware of the need to prevent operating costs from rising faster than revenue. Payers and regulators no longer allow revenue to drift upward ahead of costs, and their limits now force managers to introduce systems to control costs. Managers in all countries are computerizing financial accounts and supply records. The American investor-owned chains are committed to such methods, in order to minimize costs and maximize profits. The nonprofit and public hospital managers, previously guaranteed full operating costs and never committed to saving society's money, adopt these methods less enthusiastically, only to survive.

At first controls over costs were aimed at price per service. As Chapters Six through Eight said, payers and regulators pressed hospitals to perform their work efficiently, so that prices would not be inflated because of waste. But limiting unit prices is not enough to control costs, since total costs are the product of price times utilization. Therefore, payers and regulators began to limit the provision of medical care that was completely unnecessary or that was done in unduly expensive settings. Effective restraint on excessive utilization requires payers or regulators to intrude into the hospital, monitor the flow of work, distinguish between efficient and wasteful clinical services, and challenge the handling of individual cases.

But such intrusion challenges the organization of medical practice. In every country clinical custom and the wording of health insurance laws delegate utilization decisions to the patient's needs and the doctor's expert judgment. Lay hospital managers are not supposed to become involved: they only provide the means. If a payer or regulator challenges an admission, treatment, or additional days of hospitalization, he is challenging the doctor. But he cannot confront the hospital's doctors, in order to monitor and challenge them, since hospital payers and rate regulators have official relations with the hospital's owners and managers but never with the hospital's doctors.

Controls over Admissions and Stays. Sickness funds in many countries attempt to prevent unnecessary admissions and excessive patient-days. They employ "control doctors" whose professional credentials authorize them to judge medical necessity from the patient's records and whose membership in the medical profession supposedly qualifies them to speak to hospital doctors as equals.[29]

In theory the decision to hospitalize in France, Holland, and several other countries is not supposed to be made by the attending specialist himself; he recommends to the sickness fund's control doctor that a patient be hospitalized, and the control doctor orders the hospitalization. But the system never works this way. The attending specialist and patient always consider admission to be urgent; the control doctor is always busy with his many other administrative duties (particularly performing examinations and certifying patients to receive disability allowances); the patient is admitted before the control doctor sees the papers; the control doctor hesitates to disallow hospitalization and to tell the hospital to bill the patient; therefore, the control doctor's approval is automatic. In practice, control doctors shrink from challenging the judgment of specialists, particularly in teaching hospitals. The control doctor is often a former GP from a smaller community, and specialists bridle if he overrules their clinical judgments; moreover, specialists always give plausible reasons for hospitalization.

The sickness funds have more leverage over length of stay. The hospitals must renew their guarantees in advance. For example, as the twentieth day approaches for a patient in a French hospital, the establishment must notify the sickness fund of any intent to keep the patient longer; and the extension must be supported by the service chief's explanation. During the years when French sickness funds paid all-inclusive daily charges, the fund's control doctor could then recommend continued coverage for a certain number of days at the full rate or at a reduced rate for convalescence. If a reduced rate was recommended, the hospital could bill the patient for the rest, thereby activating his preference for going home; or the hospital could settle for the reduced rate and look for new and more profitable patients.

In every other country, the sickness fund and its control doctor either renew stays of all patients at fixed intervals or review the files of patients from time to time. The German control doctor works more informally. Whenever he visits a hospital, he looks at the records of patients who have been there for a substantial time (as the sickness fund defines it) and asks the chief of service (or his assistant) about the prospects for discharge. In practice, Germany has weaker controls and longer stays than countries with stricter methods have.

If rate regulators notice that a hospital's admissions and length of stay exceed those of similar hospitals, they might complain. But rate regulators have a mandate to guaranteee coverage of a hospital's legitimate costs; and, when per diems and services are the units of payment, they lack instruments to force reduction of admissions and stays. For example, a per diem is awarded as a result of dividing total annual costs by total annual patient-days:

Hospital's total prospective budget: $\qquad \dfrac{\$28,000,000}{140,000} = \$200$
Hospital's total predicted patient-days:

If the regulator (or a negotiator) argues that some of the days are superfluous, and that the hospital will be awarded only the daily rate to cover that effort, the result is a higher rate. Because more hospital costs are fixed than variable, the prospective budget does not decline proportionately to the reduction in utilization. For example:

$$\dfrac{\$25,000,000}{110,000} = \$227.27$$

If the hospital is awarded the new rate for the year and does not reduce utilization as much as requested, the hospital earns a larger profit than before. Nonprofit and public hospitals may add personnel and equipment to use up the cash, and the sickness funds cannot find any profits to recapture during next year's rate setting.

New methods of payment were adopted during the 1980s, in large part because traditional methods were unable to contain costs by motivating lower utilization. For example, France scrapped the daily charge. The DDASS now approves a total prospective budget and can reduce the hospital's application if admissions and stays have appeared excessive. To work within the total, a hospital must reduce utilization. Several Canadian provinces (particularly

Quebec and British Columbia) have demonstrated that global grantors can successfully enforce a freeze or even a reduction in prospective budgets, utilization, and costs.[30]

To discourage overuse, flat-rate methods other than global budgets may be substituted for per diems. For example, American Medicare during the 1980s adopted DRGs instead of cost-based per diems, in order to motivate the more expensive hospitals to reduce stays, tests, pharmaceuticals, and personnel. However, since DRGs generate the perverse incentive of motivating the hospital to increase admissions, Congress created Peer Review Organizations (PROs), independent corporations with mandates to scrutinize the medical necessity of admissions of Medicare cases. The PRO is America's counterpart for the monitoring by the control doctors employed by European sickness funds under per diem payment. Flat-rate payment methods—such as DRGs and global grants—generate another perverse incentive to underservice patients and to pocket the money. Besides scrutinizing excessive admissions, an American PRO also protects the patient and the integrity of the system: it guards against readmissions to earn revenue, and it investigates premature discharges to save operating costs.[31]

Rate regulators must monitor many hospitals, cannot know the internal details of each, and are committed to provide each hospital with enough money. The reforms of payment in France and Holland during the 1980s included a preregulatory step wherein the sickness funds examine the hospital's prospective budget and negotiate with the hospital managers. The reform was instituted because of the sickness funds' insight into specific areas of overutilization in each individual hospital. The sickness funds were expected to negotiate lower utilization levels with the hospital managers. If the hospitals refused, the sickness funds reported their suspicions of waste to the regulators who scrutinized and approved the global budgets.

Controls over Clinical Services. Payers and regulators can reduce costs by discouraging tests and treatments that are excessive in number or in complexity. Restraining them involves challenges to the clinical judgments of the medical chiefs of service in individual cases, not merely questioning the overall policies of the organization. In nearly every country, controlling the chiefs collides with the basic principles of the supremacy and autonomy of the doctor in medical practice. In addition, controlling them often is administratively unfeasible. If the hospital doctors are paid by salary rather than by fee-for-service, their work does not generate individual claims forms that are delivered to sickness funds. Costly medical practices are part of the total cost reports and prospective budgets of the hospital, and specific forms of clinical overutilization cannot be pinpointed. Regulators and sickness funds lack the authority to examine all clinical records, and the chiefs resist investigations where the sickness funds' control doctors would question their clinical practice styles.

When doctors are paid by fee-for-service, lists of individual acts by each doctor for each patient are eventually delivered to the sickness funds. Most bills are for ambulatory services. Included among these bills are claims for care given to inpatients in hospitals: all the nonprofit hospitals and some (or all) public hospitals in several countries (the Netherlands, Switzerland, Canada, the United States, and some *Belegarzt* situations in Germany); and all for-profit hospitals in all countries. The sickness funds now computerize the claims in order to pay the doctors efficiently, and many run special computer programs on the data files to identify the average numbers of each procedure per doctor for all practitioners, for those in particular regions, and for those in particular specialties. The computer programs identify the outliers—that is, individual doctors who submit far more bills than their peers do. The computer programs identify larger volumes rather than higher prices, since all billing under statutory health insurance follows the official fee schedules. (In Germany the work is done not by the sickness funds but by a special association of the doctors in sickness fund practice, the *Kassenärztliche Vereinigung,* or KV.) The German KVs and the sickness funds' control doctors may visit the outliers, ask the reasons for their unusual practice profiles, and urge them to moderate signs of overproduction of bills or frequent use of excessively expensive procedures. Since selection of the clinical procedure depends on each doctor's judgment of the diagnosis and the most effective therapy, the control doctors usually shrink from challenging use of any methods on the official fee schedule. Rather, control usually focuses on volume: the control doctor discourages numbers of bills that unrealistically exceed average frequencies of work.[32]

Utilization control over doctors is administered separately from utilization control over hospitals. Each doctor's practice profile is constructed from all his claims—both extramural and intramural—and is not run separately for each practice site. Each doctor's practice profile is calculated and reviewed individually, and no sickness fund ever aggregates or compares all the doctors practicing in the same hospital. The medical association usually obtains pledges from sickness funds to keep utilization data of doctors confidential, and hospital rate regulators cannot consult them to learn whether medical practice in any hospital is wasteful. Since the computerization of claims is designed primarily to reimburse doctors quickly, the sickness funds invest little in utilization review. Great efforts may result in trouble rather than savings, since the medical association protests step-ups in utilization control, the doctors might go on administrative strike (asking patients to pay them and seek reimbursement from the carriers), and the control doctors cannot prove many of their suspicions about overbilling in individual cases.

The recent trend toward capped methods of paying the hospitals largely resulted from difficulties in imposing utilization controls over doctors by means of regulations. If the hospital is given a global grant for the entire year, it must perform all its work within that limit. Therefore, the chiefs of service themselves must agree on shares, each must limit his methods to his share, and all other chiefs may combine to press overspenders to reduce their shares to average levels. No outsider, such as the sickness fund's control doctor, need intrude and pursue the overspender, thereby triggering the collective resistance of the entire medical staff. The American DRG payment system forces the lay manager to appeal to overspending doctors to become more conscious of their practice styles and try to work within each DRG's price.[33] Fundamental conflicts of interest had to be settled between managers and doctors: during the years when DRGs were being implemented in America, the increasing risk of lawsuits for malpractice was motivating doctors to order more tests than ever before. Therefore, instead of externally imposed controls, hospitals under capped payment systems must create internal management structures whereby the medical chiefs influence each other and (in countries with open staffs, as in America) whereby the lay manager monitors, informs, and persuades the attending physicians.[34] American hospitals have begun to include in their top managements a full-time salaried vice-president for medical affairs, a physician, whose several duties include educating the attendings about more economical practice styles.

Controls over Venal Underservicing. Under cost-based reimbursement, doctors and hospitals are guaranteed full payment for all their work and have incentives to practice more complex techniques in larger number. If capped payments are adopted—such as global budgets, DRGs, or fixed charge lists for hospitals and fee schedules for doctors—the rates are set in light of average costs of care. But some providers might underservice and pocket the profits. Prevention of underservicing involves second-guessing physicians in individual cases. It is stymied by the fact that assuring the quality of care is a fundamental attribute of the medical profession, and doctors and hospitals as matters of principle resist investigations by payers into clinical management of individual cases.

The medical staff structure of the European hospital has been assumed to guarantee high quality. Chiefs of service are selected after a career in full-time hospital service, where they were constantly observed and evaluated by their superiors. Chiefs are picked after a competition which (as in France) is often demanding and calls on testimony from former associates. The chief is responsible for all the work in a specialty, oversees his junior staff, and usually has only one or two other seniors to monitor. Unskilled or unethical junior doctors are dropped from hospital staffs; consequently, the quality-control problem is transferred to the ambulatory sector. The unresolved problem in European quality assurance is how to control the chief of service if his skills or ethics decline before his date of automatic retirement. Usually the chief's principal assistant, the other chiefs, and the hospital management quickly learn about the problems and intervene to steer cases away from the offender.[35].

The United States always has had fundamental problems of quality assurance. Its permissive licensing allows any doctor to perform and collect fees for any specialized procedure, including surgery, regardless of training and experience. In contrast, most European statutory health insurance systems will pay for specialized procedures only when they are performed by specialists fully credentialed in that field. America's hospitals, which give full facilities to nearly every doctor, have had few methods of controlling the many and heterogeneous doctors who constantly enter and leave the buildings.[36] Europeans make hospital medicine more orderly by limiting the number of senior physicians, requiring them to be fully credentialed in their specialties, and making them responsible for the clinical standards. Therefore, no European country has external machinery to review the quality of care within every hospital.[37]

At first each admitting doctor in an American hospital could do what he liked with "his own" patients. The license to practice medicine was qualification enough. After 1910 leading teaching hospitals, which needed to protect their reputations and demonstrate only high standards for students, created "tissue committees" whereby the medical staff guarded against occasional deficiencies and identified individuals who should not operate. Quality controls were also introduced into the education of doctors at the same time. The American College of Surgeons began to accredit hospitals that maintained quality-review machinery, and its efforts evolved in 1951 into the Joint Commission on the Accreditation of Hospitals. A condition for accreditation is a set of medical staff committees to review the necessity of utilization and to audit the quality of work. Among the many thousands of hospitals in the United States, these committees have varied in diligence.[38]

When Medicare and Medicaid were first enacted, hospitals were required to have utilization committees similar to those in the earlier private accreditation programs. Medicare and Medicaid were supposed to protect their patients, but since only medical professionals customarily regulated the quality of care, the new law delegated the task to committees of the hospital's own doctors. Results were disappointing in the many hospitals that had never had vigorous tissue committees. Excessively numerous and excessively expensive treatments were thought to raise costs without benefit to patients. Therefore, the problem was control of costs as well as quality.[39]

The United States Congress in 1972 created 203 Professional Service Review Organizations (PSROs) that would be independent of hospitals and that would perform both quality assurance and cost control for Medicare. The staffs were laymen financed by the national government. Since the PSROs' jurisdiction included the quality of care, their independence from the hospitals was compromised by the medical profession's insistence that only doctors could judge quality and influence the clinical performance of other doctors. Every PSRO was governed by doctors of the local medical society, and nearly all these doctors had hospital affiliations; therefore, clinical performance was still being judged by colleagues. Every PSRO was autonomous in making judgments and administering sanctions; the national government had statutory authority to send them few and only vague guidelines.[40]

Finance officers in Washington hoped that concurrent review of admissions, stays, and utilization by PSROs would reduce admissions and patient-days, but they were disappointed for several reasons:

- Implementation was uneven. State and local medical societies directed the PSROs, and many were opposed to their mere existence. Therefore, some parts of the country never activated them, most operational PSROs were delayed, and many were weak.
- Mandates were contradictory and confusing. The doctors who dominated PSROs often expressed more concern about protecting patients and professional standards by quality assurance than about protecting Medicare from excessive costs. They contended that Medicare was reponsible for covering better care and that quality might be protected by many admissions, adequately long stays, and more tests. Identified as a utilization outlier by the statisticians on a PSRO's staff, a doctor might be absolved by the governing board of doctors as commendably cautious and thorough.[41]
- Monitoring applied only to the hospital records, not to the physicians who actually made the decisions. Office practices were not within the jurisdictions of PSROs. They could not address directives and sanctions to doctors.

Critics of the PSROs argued that the costs of the program exceeded savings.[42] When the Reagan administration came to power, it favored elimination of the PSROs, since they violated its free-market ideology on two grounds: the program was a form of regulation imposed by government; the PSROs themselves were professional cartels restricting competition. But the Reagan administration also enacted a flat-rate payment system (DRGs), which inherently presents incentives to seek profits by underservicing. To guard against these and other abuses, Congress revived the control committees in a stronger form. Each of the state Peer Review Organizations is given specific guidelines from Washington about both minima and maxima in utilization, and each by contract is obligated to enforce program standards on the hospitals. Most Peer Review Organizations are governed by physicians, but the agencies are statewide rather than local, and relations between a hospital medical staff and the PRO board may be less cozy than under the PSROs.

Summary

When revenue came from large donations by the community, owners overshadowed managers in the leadership of the hospital. The internal financial function consisted of paying employees and suppliers in small amounts; few skills and little discretion were required. Within the hospital the managers were subordinated to the doctors and (often) to the principal nurses.

Management in all countries has grown in skill, importance, and numbers of personnel, in response to changes in reimbursement and in the hospitals' internal resource consumption. Revenue depends on skillful billing for patients' services; it also depends on clever maneuvers against payers and regulators. The managers now overshadow the owners' representatives and the leading nurses; the doctors rely on them for the mounting resources for clinical work.

The managers have not only become crucial for the prosperity of the individual hospitals; their cooperation also is essential for the success of public policies to control costs and to implement plans. Precisely how to reach all the hospital managers often eludes governments and sickness funds. Managers cooperate with public policy when the hospitals are owned by governments, when the national Ministries send out clear guidelines, and when managers are rewarded by promotion in the public service. But such coherent structures for communication and rewards are unusual. In most countries the managers are committed to the survival and improvement of their individual hospitals and are committed to pleasing the medical staffs.

Managers are intermediaries between the doctors and (on the other hand) the payers and government regulators. Public policies to control costs and regionalize health services require management structures combining both medical chiefs of service and lay managers, but these arrangements are only now appearing. To commit doctors and managers to the public policies, a country must create national decision-making machinery, so that the national medical association and the national hospital association participate in making the policies.

From such incipient trends, the United States remains an exception. The manager's career depends on competitive success of his individual organization, pitting him against the restraints of payers and governments. The open-staff arrangement prevents creation of a team of full-time chiefs of service committed to organizational stability within a national policy. Rather, the American staff structure makes the hospital the workshop of private doctors oriented toward their practices, and the managers of competing hospitals must please their medical staffs to win their own ceaseless struggles for market share. If managers of independent hospitals try to limit costs and construct a division of labor among themselves, often they do so involuntarily, because of market constraints and stricter payments. Eventually, as in all unstructured markets, some organizations face bankruptcy, disappear, or are taken over by chain managements. Lay multihospital management is nearly unique to America but resembles the rest of the American economy.

Restraints over clinical utilization and over the quality of care cannot easily be implanted inside the management of hospitals. Restraints originate among payers trying to protect their budgets and subscribers. The payers negotiate their complaints irregularly with hospital managers and service chiefs. The doctors resist intrusion of laymen from outside, since they argue that judgments about clinical practice are entirely their responsibility. At present, therefore, no country has a management structure that ties utilization review and quality assurance into a strict national structure led by laymen dedicated to cost containment and consumer protection.

13

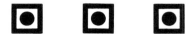

Effects on Costs, Efficiency, and Patient Care

Previous chapters have described a great variety of methods in managing hospitals' internal finances and in paying them. In addition, the chapters show that hospital finance in each country is often changed (whereas, in contrast, methods of paying doctors are simple, few, and durable).

What are the effects of these methods of internal financial management and external payment? What difference do they make? Ideally, a financial arrangement should mobilize the right numbers and types of personnel and resources in each hospital organization. Balances should be struck between waste and underservicing, between excessive clinical intervention and neglect. Appropriate treatments should be provided to patients in need. Do some financial arrangements accomplish these goals better than others? Do some methods have undesirable consequences?

Limitations on Attempting Comparative Analysis

An ideal evaluation of the effects of different payment methods would first create a framework for identifying the most important consequences, and would then obtain comparable data from all countries. Some theoretical frameworks have been proposed.[1] The most significant effects in the comparison of alternative systems are:

- Total costs to the country. Relations to the societal indicators, such as the general price level and the gross national product.
- Efficiency in the relation between total costs and work and between resources and clinical output. Amount of waste.
- Attracting appropriate mixes of employees and resources to where patients live. Ensuring a steady supply matching fluctuations in clinical need.

- Inspiring optimum volume of effective treatments and tests. Not encouraging ineffective or dangerous treatments and tests.
- Incomes of hospital workers and doctors. Incomes of suppliers and surrounding communities.
- Administrative ease and clarity.
- Conflicts.

Pinpointing the effects of payment methods on costs and clinical work in this fashion is nearly impossible at present for several reasons:

☐ Economic statistics about hospitals are generated according to each country's needs and are not comparable. Estimating comparative effects of different national payment systems will be possible only in a special new research project that first redefines and standardizes the hospital data from many countries.

☐ Within many countries important data about hospitals are collected and reported with many mysteries and errors. During abortive attempts to estimate comparative effects, I could not reproduce aggregates for individual countries from the component reports that had supposedly generated them. Different reporting agencies report different totals for the same set of operations. Estimates and errors are corrected subsequently for a few data sets (such as the fundamental GNP and GDP) but not for most. The same statistics (such as proportion of GDP spent on hospitals in a particular year) change when the corrected numbers are announced. The basic data sets become "final" only because the statistical agency must assign its limited manpower to other tasks.

☐ Time series within individual countries—crucial for every analysis of comparative effects—are fallible. Collection or reporting methods change from time to time, often without full explanation of the changes, and the analyst cannot establish whether a statistical fluctuation is due to the payment method or the changes in reports.

☐ Comparisons of payment methods require comparisons of results for comparable organizations. In some countries hospital data now are mixed together—for example, for-profit and nonprofit, acute short-stay and long-stay—and the analyst cannot easily disaggregate them. Specialist physicians' ambulatory services are counted in hospital data in a few countries (such as Britain) but not in most.

☐ Most countries' hospital statistics cover very simple topics, such as total costs, patient-days, length of stay, and principal diagnosis at admission. Few countries collect and report information about hospitals' clinical work and personnel. Until the United States began payment by DRGs, no country combined financial and clinical records.

☐ It is very difficult to isolate the effects of each country's payment system, and then compare it with others'. Many other events affect hospitals' finances and work. A payment system's characteristics should have definite effects after the first few years of phasing in, but recently each country has tinkered with its payment system too often.

☐ Most countries do not distinguish between specialists' intramural and extramural clinical work and earnings. Therefore, the doctors' contributions to the work and costs of hospitals may be underestimated in many countries, particularly in private clinics.

☐ In many federal countries, reimbursement and investment methods vary among provinces. Hospital financial and clinical statistics are usually published by province, and few data are aggregated for the entire country.

These deficiencies can be repaired only in an immensely laborious new research project to collect, verify, standardize, and analyze statistics from many countries, as I explained in Chapter One. As the itinerant researcher discovers at present, apparently sound published hospital statistics are frequently based on incomplete and erroneous sources. Many statisticians are not curious or critical of their own materials, and a cross-national researcher cannot obtain reliable information from them by correspondence. Different sources produce contradictory results. Blindly generalizing from presently available numbers is very risky. Cross-national econometric inferences about effects cannot be performed now; econometric modeling can be done, but only as a theoretical exercise. In the country that appears to have the most copious data and the most brilliant researchers, the United States, attempts to infer the effects of different administrative and financial arrangements are remarkably inconclusive.[2]

In part because of the limited number of topics in the financial statistics and because of their low reliability, the policy debates and academic analyses of hospital payment systems do not penetrate very deeply. Many repetitious publications discuss proportions of GNP going into all of health care. But remarkably little evidence can be found about options in hospital finance.

Even if exhaustive and reliable statistics can be gathered, a fundamental obstacle to simple generalizations always will be that outcomes depend on how a payment method is administered. For example, rate regulation can be administered strictly or generously, with different consequences for services and costs.

The following pages summarize impressions about the effects of different financing arrangements on performance and costs. Many other important effects on the operation of hospitals cannot be identified even impressionistically, since the measures are not widely collected. While the following pages will present some evidence, I cannot make the chapter too prolix—particularly not when the statistics are so uncertain. The text will present many generalizations; supporting details can be found in the publications cited in the notes at the back of this book.

Effects on Costs

In every country recently, the policy debate has revolved around the costs of hospitals. A reimbursement method is sought that will limit hospital spending to a constant or declining proportion of GNP.

Proportions Spent on Hospital Care. The total spent by a country on hospitals is not simply a function of the reimbursement method but depends partly on the country's wealth and partly on the priority given to hospitals. Richer countries often (but not always) spend higher proportions of national resources on health,[3] but this does not automatically produce high hospital spending. As shown in the first column of Table 13-1, three of the richer countries (Sweden, the Netherlands, and the United States) spend high proportions, while

Table 13-1. Effects of Hospital Payment Methods on Nationwide Costs.

System	Proportion of GDP[a] spent on all hospitals in 1980, in %	Expenditure on all hospitals per capita in 1980, converted into U.S. dollars[b]	Average annual increase in total hospital spending, 1970 through 1982, in %	Average annual increase, relative to rise in general consumer price index, 1970 through 1982
Global budgeting:				
United Kingdom	2.77	225.81	19.1	1.6
Canada	4.01	434.30	14.6	1.9
Sweden	6.50	971.57	15.4	1.7
Rate regulation:				
France	3.96	484.10	20.2	2.2
Netherlands	4.87	584.87	12.3	1.8
Negotiations:				
West Germany	3.01	400.46	11.2	2.2
Mixed:				
Switzerland	3.35	497.60	13.9	3.0
United States	4.67	546.77	14.0	2.0

[a]Gross domestic product (GDP) = GNP + (income earned in the domestic market accruing to foreigners abroad) – (income accruing to domestic residents arising from investment abroad).

[b]Exchange rates against the United States dollar (= 1.00 in 1980) were British pound = 0.43, Canadian dollar = 1.17, Swedish krona = 4.23, French franc = 4.23, Dutch guilder = 1.99, Deutsche Mark = 1.82, Swiss franc = 1.68. During subsequent years the American dollar rose and several others dropped, altering the relative values in the second column.

Sources: my calculations from Jean-Pierre Poullier, *Measuring Health Care, 1960–1983* (Paris: Organisation for Economic Co-operation and Development, 1985), Tables A3, A4, H3; from *OECD Economic Outlook*, No. 36 (Dec. 1984), Tables R11, R16; and from several compendia of national hospital statistics (primarily from Switzerland's VESKA and Britain's Office of Health Economics).

two others (West Germany and Switzerland) do not. In Sweden, Holland, and America, technically advanced and expensive work is performed in the inpatient and outpatient departments of hospitals; in Germany and Switzerland, much of it is done in physicians' offices. Except for the academic medical centers, German hospitals until recently were modest in personnel and investment.

Because of the variations among countries in wealth and priorities, a payment system may be associated with very high as well as very low expenditures. For example, although global budgeting and public grants can control costs very strictly, Sweden (as shown in the first column of Table 13-1) devotes the highest proportion of any country to hospitals. After World War II, Sweden adopted a policy of hospital-centered care and built advanced structures that were expensive to operate. Hospital finance has been decentralized to the regional governments (the "county councils"), where politicians win votes and retain office by constantly improving the hospitals. While other countries have fluctuated in their annual expenditures on hospitals, Sweden maintained a steady growth and tightened controls only moderately during the late 1970s.

In Great Britain (as the first and second columns of Table 13-1 show) global budgeting can be associated with low expenditures for hospital investment and operations. Britain entered the National Health Service with a small hospital sector, only about 2.15 acute beds per thousand inhabitants.[4] Government budgeting gave priority to housing over the modernization of hospitals. Public policy finally turned to hospital development during the 1960s but soon foundered over the country's problems of economic stagnation and international trade imbalances. Over 60 percent of the country's health expenditure is devoted to the hospital services[5]—one of the highest shares of any country—and the National Health Service is the largest item in the national government's budget, but the NHS and its hospitals are kept under a lid because of Britain's limited resources and its struggle to reverse the growth in public expenditure.

Sources of Annual Increases in Spending for Hospitals. A reimbursement method might seem more effective in controlling costs if it steadily reduces annual increases in a country's total hospital spending. However, unless it contains a very rigid fixed lid, a payment method has limited leverage over short-run growth. It must concede some increase.

The rise in total spending each year is the product of price increases per unit and increases in units of service:[6]

- Higher prices and wages from one year to the next. Hospitals must pay employees and must buy food, supplies, fuel, and electric power from outside markets.
- Higher prices charged by hospitals and doctors for each service, beyond the rise in general market prices.
- Greater demand due to a larger population. Such annual growth usually is small.
- More admissions and outpatient visits per capita ("utilization").
- More tests and treatments per inpatient admission and outpatient visit ("service intensity").

The strongest determinant of higher expenditure is the general rise in market prices for workers and supplies—particularly wages, since hospitals are labor intensive. The society's general wages and prices are beyond the reach of the decision makers in reimbursement policy and in individual hospitals. As I said in Chapter Ten, the practice in all countries is to pass through prevailing wages. Instead of substituting cheaper labor or cheaper supplies, as in some other industries, hospitals have tended to use more expensive labor and supplies.

Hospital charges beyond the general inflation rate—used to pay higher-than-market wages, to purchase very expensive supplies, or to earn profit—are the only objects that a unit reimbursement method can control directly. Many unit reimbursement systems—such as the fixing of daily charges—have reduced hospitals' ability to pay extra wages or earn extra cash. But restricting unit prices can have only a limited effect on total costs. For example, in America—one of the more permissive countries—increases in unit prices per service in excess of general market prices account for only about 10 percent of the annual increases in total hospital spending.

A hospital reimbursement system cannot control utilization and service intensity by direct orders or by paying (or refusing to pay) individual services, since these result from the decisions of the doctors, based on the steadily improving state of medical science. In the modern era of high-technology medicine, the second strongest determinant of the annual increases in national hospital costs is service intensity, consisting of more tests, more treatments, and more expensive methods of care. A strict reimbursement method can brake the annual growth in utilization and service intensity by motivating or forcing doctors and managers to work in the hospital more economically or to do the same care extramurally. The latter option evades hospital reimbursement controls but transfers the larger cost-containment problem to other sectors.

Annual increases in total hospital spending in every country since World War II have exceeded annual increases in consumer prices and wages for several reasons.[7] The once underpaid and overworked hospital workers have been given extra wage increases to catch up with the general labor force, their hours have been shortened, and more employees have been added. The reimbursement problem has been to find levers that not only limit prices paid to hospitals but also affect the operations, utilization, and service intensity. Criteria must be developed about the "right number" of employees, and the hospital must be prevented from hiring "more than it needs." On the other hand, methods of cost containment must not deprive doctors and patients of "what they need." Criteria must be developed to identify the "appropriate" levels of use.

Variations in Annual Increases. Each payment system can produce different results—when one compares different national versions or the same country's performance at different times—depending on:

☐ The government's policies.
  • Ensuring maximum services to all social classes and communities.
  • Limiting social expenditures and inflation.
☐ The government's capacity to resist:
  • Demands by doctors and hospital employees for higher incomes and shorter hours.
  • Demands by small communities for easily accessible hospitals.
☐ Source of the money for operating and capital costs—that is, the object of the rate regulation.
  • Tax revenue, paid into the government Treasury and sickness funds.
  • Private health insurance, the patients' cash.

The complete time series from 1970 through 1982 (underlying the summary figures in the third column of Table 13-1 but not presented in full) shows that changes in public policy are at least as important as the reimbursement method. Any payment system can be administered generously or thriftily. For example, while German annual increases in total spending were lower than 10 percent after 1974, they averaged about 20 percent during the four previous years, because of great increases in wages and employment (described in Chapter Ten) and the initial effects of the new capital investment law (described in

Chapter Nine). At times Holland has had large annual increases because of "catch-up" wage increases and—on top of these during the late 1970s—the jump in operating costs when new acute-care and extended-care hospitals went into full service. While Great Britain and Canada usually apply global budgeting strictly, at times they allow large general wage increases and, therefore, large spurts in the totals. Examples occurred in Great Britain in 1973 and 1980, and in Canada in 1971 and 1975. Usually the uncontrolled American system yields increases higher than the other countries', but temporary American nationwide price and wage controls in 1973 limited the rise to 11 percent.

Merely comparing countries' annual increases in total hospital spending (the figures summarized in the third column of Table 13-1) is misleading. At least half of every annual increase in the total is a response to prevailing wages and prices; therefore, countries may appear to have exceptionally large increases in hospital spending when they merely have greater inflation. Payment methods can be compared only by their effectiveness in keeping the annual increases close to the society's general inflation rate—that is, the number in the fourth column of Table 13-1.

Throughout the 1970s and early 1980s, global budgeting and public grants restrained hospital spending more strictly than rate regulation, rate negotiations, and the mixed Swiss and American systems. Global budgeting and public grants can force hospital managers to constrain both utilization and service intensity in order to avoid deficits. Global budgeting and public grants coordinate and control both operating costs and investments. In contrast, a unit price-fixing method (such as regulation and negotiation) usually has no instruments to restrain higher-than-predicted admissions and may be legally obligated or pressured to cover more credentialed personnel, more expensive treatments, and some capital costs.

Whenever a country suffers from high inflation, the hospital payment system overshoots its obligation to cover costs, and the general confusion results in considerable extra increases in total hospital spending. For example, Europe suffered from high inflation during the mid- and late 1970s, and annual increases in hospital spending often were 2.5 times the general price index. Since every payment system is an instrument of public policy, it is generous when government and the payers favor modernization and expansion of the hospital sector; in the 1960s and 1970s, for example, some annual increases were 3 to 4.5 times the consumer price index. And each payment system can be strict when government and payers combat inflation and control their taxes; in the early 1980s, for example, most increases were 1.2 to 1.5 times the consumer price index.

Because hospital spending always grows, it can appear to grow much faster than general inflation in the unusual cases when a country controls all its nonmedical prices and wages. For example, Switzerland during the 1970s prospered in the volatile world economy by controlling domestic inflation better than any other country. But its decentralized and unsystematic hospital payment system allowed hospitals to modernize and become more expensive every year. Providing technically advanced and comfortable care was a Swiss public priority. Therefore, as shown in Column 4 of Table 13-1, hospital spending as a multiple of general prices rose faster in Switzerland than in any other country, even though Switzerland's real annual increases were smaller.

Chapter Seven described the variety of political and administrative forms of rate regulation. The range of possible outcomes is evident when one compares France, Holland, and the United States:

☐ France and Holland were once permissive, but they tightened procedures during the late 1970s. Since NHI is part of social security and is supported by government payroll taxes, the two governments invoked rate regulation to protect their own finances. During the 1970s French and Dutch rate regulators were expected to allow hospital budgets to keep pace with the increase in wages and costs in the rest of the economy. They approved prospective budgets with assumptions of high wage and price increases; hospitals then paid their workers and suppliers generously; greater utilization and services increased total costs further; and total costs increased faster than the revenue of the sickness funds. During the 1980s the Ministries writing guidelines gave the regulators much smaller allowances for wage and price inflation, in contrast to the earlier presumption that hospital budgets must keep pace.[8]

☐ American state regulatory programs vary. All of them control rates more strictly than the less constrained market in the unregulated states; a few states (such as Washington) have been permissive; others (such as Maryland and formula-based New York) are stricter.[9] For a variety of reasons—such as conflicting policy priorities, the political leverage of the hospitals and doctors, and the limited legal authority of any state rate regulation[10]—no American state has ever controlled rates as tightly as France and Holland finally did during the early 1980s. The urgency of government fiscal stability—so important under French and Dutch NHI—is absent in the United States. American rate regulation originated in the need of states to limit their own Medicaid payments to hospitals but now is conducted to protect private payers, such as Blue Cross and the privately insured. American national and state governments adopted payment by DRGs—at first for Medicare and later for Medicaid—so that they could protect their own finances and not rely on politically vulnerable state regulators.

A "mixed" system can allow considerable autonomy to each hospital, as in the United States and Switzerland. Each management can constantly modernize its hospital, with expensive consequences for the entire country—as is particularly evident in the United States. As I explained in Chapters Nine and Twelve, hospitals in many American communities compete for market share and must install the newest technology to attract use by attending physicians. Well-paid technicians are added to run the equipment. The more competitive a community, the more expensive its hospitals.[11]

All the foregoing discussion refers to national variations among developed countries in short-term changes in expenditures. Definite patterns in utilization appear in the long-term evolution from less developed to more developed societies. As a society becomes more developed, the utilization profile of hospitals changes: smaller proportions of inpatients are young adults, apparently because they are healthier and the medical care system can treat them extramurally; larger proportions of inpatients are children and the elderly, because populations in developed countries have less infant mortality, longer life expectancies, and a great commitment to treat the vulnerable. Older populations are more expensive medically, since they have more chronic disease, multiple conditions, longer hospital stays, and more readmissions. Such long-range utilization changes correlate roughly but not precisely with expenditure growth, since population-based demand does not automatically dictate forms of hospital service. Provision depends on the actions of churches and governments.[12]

Administrative Devices. Certain administrative features cut across different payment systems and result in higher or lower expenditures. Two of the most important are:

- *Interim rates.* If a payment system allows the hospital to increase its rates during the year—even with screening by a regulator—its annual increase in total costs will be higher. For example, French hospitals until the late 1970s routinely replaced the initial prospective budget with a new one, and the per diems automatically rose. American hospitals have always been able to petition their cost reimbursers for increases during the year or to announce them unilaterally. When France required hospitals to function within the start-of-the-year per diems, the annual increase in total costs moderated. The American DRG system is designed to enforce prospectivity.
- *Carryovers of deficits.* Dutch hospitals for many years could recapture their losses by a surcharge on next year's daily charge, thereby clearing the bank debt; annual increases in costs slowed during the 1980s—partly because the carryovers were eliminated. Under global budgeting and global grants, several Canadian provinces permitted carryovers for many years but eliminated them during the 1970s, to contain costs. Forcing hospitals to work entirely within the start-of-the-year rates was one of the cost-containment reforms in the rate negotiation system of Germany in 1985: the hospital no longer reported last year's profit or loss in its submission to the sickness fund.

Motivating More Efficient Work

Ideally, a payment system should reward efficient care and should not encourage waste. Many theories predict outcomes from methods of payment; for example, per diems are assumed to prolong stays, while fixed amounts per admission reduce them. Per diems and provider-dominated methods of rate setting are thought to keep unnecessary beds full and therefore prevent reduction in hospital establishments and in costs. However, Table 13-2 does not demonstrate any simple connection. If one country uses beds more intensely than another, and if its stays are shorter, several institutional features are at work, and not the reimbursement form alone.

Numbers of Beds. Total hospital costs are the product of numbers of beds, turnover per bed, and costliness per hospital stay. All European countries at present have potentially high costs, since all have more hospital beds than the Anglo-Saxon countries (Britain, Canada, the United States, and Australia). European churches and religious associations for centuries built up hospitals as treatment centers and as long-term housing for the afflicted. Large rooms were filled with beds, operating costs were low, and considerable excess capacity could be kept available in case of epidemics. Very long stays were customary. In contrast, Britain—always partially isolated from European practices—built fewer hospitals[13] and let many people find their own care. Canada and the United States

Table 13-2. Efficiency of Hospital Systems, 1980.

	Numbers of beds in all hospitals per 1,000 inhabitants	Average number of cases treated per nonpsy-chiatric hospi-tal bed	Average length of stay in acute hospitals	Change in length of stay, 1970–1980
Global budgeting:				
England[a]	7.8	25	8.6	−24.9
Canada	6.9	22	12.9	+11.3
Sweden	14.2	16	24.4	−10.3
Rate regulation:				
France	11.1	21	14.0	−26.2
Netherlands	12.3	22	13.3	−24.0
Negotiations:				
West Germany	11.6	19	19.7	−20.9
Mixed:				
Switzerland	12.9	18	14.3	−13.9
United States	6.1	35	10.0	−32.9

[a]British data are from England alone, since average length of stay is not calculated for the entire United Kingdom.

Sources: My calculations from Poullier, *Measuring Health Care, 1960–1983* (see source note, Table 13-1, above), Tables D1(b), D4, E6; from several statistical reports from VESKA, Aarau, Switzerland; from *Compendium of Health Statistics*, 5th ed. (London: Office of Health Economics, 1984); and from several issues of the *Vademecum gezondheidsstatistiek Nederland* (The Hague: Centraal Bureau voor de Statistiek, annual). The number of hospital beds in Sweden is the official inventory but is exaggerated; some are permanently out of service because of nursing shortages, but the statistical reports make no corrections.

had fewer beds per capita than Europe, because they were new and rapidly growing societies. Their population growth constantly outpaced the creation of hospitals. Until recently Canada and the United States lacked the large urban agglomerates where European churches and charities erected huge buildings with many beds.

Only recently have policy makers in all developed countries realized that controlling bed supply is essential for controlling costs. "Hospital beds that are built tend to be used. . . . [T]he more hospital beds are provided in a community, the more days of hospital care will be used."[14] By then, Europe had installed operating-cost payment systems that committed third parties to full coverage of the average daily costs of care and to automatically higher per diems as clinical methods and wages became more expensive. The system for covering operating costs lacked any mechanism for challenging the total number of beds in the country, since it reviewed each hospital individually; and it could not challenge numbers of beds and patient-days in each hospital because (until recently) these were left to the professional judgments of doctors and hospital managers.

Because the method of reimbursing operations lacked techniques for defining and reducing excess beds, the planning and investment systems (originated for expansionist purposes) were finally redirected during the 1960s and 1970s. But, as I said in Chapter Nine, only a few European countries applied planning and investment to overbedding, their reductions were tied to expensive new construction, and they altered the use of beds rather than cut the numbers. For example, when a French hospital was allowed to build a more modern structure, the old building often was preserved for extended care or for an old-age home, often under the same management as the new acute facility. When several old and small Dutch hospitals merged to create a modern new facility, the planners pressed them to reduce the total number of beds; but, at the same time, the country expanded national health insurance to include long-term care, and many new nursing homes were built.

Global budgeting and public grants might be used to set caps on hospital services for the country as a whole and for individual establishments. If a hospital is occupied too little or wastefully, the global grant could be cut to the level of work deemed necessary by the grantor. But, in the few overbedded countries with public grants, this strategy has not been followed. Sweden has always financed hospitals generously, because social policy makes hospitals the focus of ambulatory and inpatient health care and because the politicians in county councils compete to increase hospital services. The officials in Swiss cantonal Ministries of Health examine hospital budgets and supplement sickness fund per diems with cantonal grants, but they always have thought that generous and modern hospital services were leading public assets. The countries with strict global budgeting—Britain and Canada—were already the ones with fewer beds. They have used their grants to prevent expansion (in Canada) and to eliminate underused beds in declining regions (in London under the British NHS).

Fewer beds, more intensive use, and shorter stays have gradually become goals in Europe. The countries that have already been using hospital resources in this style—Britain, Canada, and the United States—have done so from national traditions rather than because of the conscious effects of reimbursement policies. One reason for the spreading interest in global budgeting in France, Holland, and elsewhere is the belief that only such a cap on the hospital can discourage filling unoccupied beds, and the cap might be ratcheted down each year to reduce beds and stays. Rate regulation and rate negotiation based on per diems fail to reduce admissions and stays.

Hospitals can be reduced or completely closed more easily in North America than in continental Europe because of North America's transitory social structure, not because of the payment and planning systems alone. Many European hospitals have been prominent pillars of religious denominations and communities for centuries. Many administrative offices and some clinical services are housed in national monuments. With their shorter histories and frequently changing buildings, American hospitals are viewed more pragmatically, even by their owners and managers. These key people seek a profitable and vibrant organization and are willing to reduce, sell, or close a declining establishment. They readily consider other industries for their investment.[15] In contrast, the owners of a historic European hospital remain loyal to its survival; payers and government try to preserve its market share and revenue.

Turnover and Length of Stay. The countries with few beds have shorter stays and more cases per bed during the year, according to the second and third columns of Table 13-2. All countries (except Canada) have been reducing length of stay regardless of method of payment, according to the fourth column. Although many observers believe that per diems motivate hospitals to lengthen stays and never reduce them, this is not true. Stays diminish because modern medical care is more active than earlier styles, emphasizing rapid interventions and less time for observation and convalescence. (When hospitals are understaffed and the work pace is slower, as in Sweden, stays have been reduced less rapidly.) Another reason for the shortening of stays in nearly all countries is that modern patients more forthrightly insist on going home. With universal coverage, hospitals can maintain occupancy with new admissions.

Despite global budgeting, Canada's stays may have increased slightly. They were already quite short. The increase may be due in part to the aging of the population. (Another possible reason for the unexpected Canadian increase is that there are eccentricities in the data. Historical changes in length of stay for an entire country are difficult to measure in a standardized way.)

The United States has always had the shortest—or nearly the shortest— stays of any country. The principal reason has been organizational rather than pecuniary. American hospitals have had open medical staffs, as I reported in Chapter Eleven. The primary physician did not lose his patient—and the fees— to a hospital specialist but treated the patient before, during, and after hospitalization. He could perform diagnostic workups before hospitalization and could monitor convalescence afterward. Until Blue Cross and other payers during the 1970s protested about excessive admissions, many doctors had two short stays per case—a very short one for testing and a later one for treatment. In contrast, European hospital staffs have always used longer stays to conduct all diagnoses, perform all treatments, and make sure the patient has recovered.

The incentives from American reimbursement methods have made shorter stays acceptable to many American hospital managers. A hospital earns a large share of its revenue from charge lists if the Medicare volume is low, if Blue Cross pays charges rather than per diems, and if commercially insured volume is high. The hospital's earnings from diagnostic and therapeutic charges occur in the first days of each stay, and the residual per diem for nursing and housekeeping is not profitable. The hospital may lose money from longer stays and will gain from admitting a new patient.

Close study of each country's data on length of stay and on other indicators of efficiency shows that no payment system produces a standard reaction. Doctors' practice styles vary widely, even when they are paid by the same method. These practice styles are shared within a community but vary among communities. (The data are summarized in Chapter Eleven; see pp. 314, 316, and the notes accompanying the text.) Length of stay varies as widely within as among countries. For example, in the United States, stays are 50 percent higher in the Northeast than in the West, regardless of diagnosis.[16]

Britain provides the best example of the effects of supply constraint on efficiency. It also demonstrates that capital planning and management must be combined with reimbursement of operating costs in a consistent policy. Data from the Office of Health Economics indicate that, between 1960 and 1980, the total number of beds in England declined 20 percent, while admissions increased. With a declining supply of beds, admissions per bed grew 83.7 percent from 1960 to 1980. To accommodate the demand and avoid excessive waits for beds, stays in acute care halved, from 15.7 days in 1960 to 8.6 days in 1980, so that they became shorter in England than in much of the United States. (Stays in Britain dropped to 8.1 days by 1983.)

Cost per Admission. Total cost is a multiple of unit prices and utilization—that is, cost per admission times number of admissions. Ideally, a payment system should avoid encouraging either excessive cost through wasteful overtreatment or excessive economies through underservicing. Controlling costs per admission results from a combination of controls on length of stay and service intensity. If optimum cost per admission is achieved, total hospital costs might still grow through more admissions, a matter left to the discretion of the doctors and supposedly beyond the power of the regulators and negotiators who examine hospital prospective budgets and set unit prices.

Permissive rate regulation and negotiations can allow costs per admission to rise rapidly, approaching twice or more the general rate of inflation. Strict regulation and negotiations can keep the annual increase in costs per admission about equal to—or, in unusual cases, even below—general inflation. The complete time series for the Netherlands shows both extremes, demonstrating the possible range in administering any payment system. Following are the increases in Dutch costs per admission relative to the annual increase in the general rate of inflation from 1973 through 1983. If the entry is 1.0, costs per admission exactly equaled inflation outside medicine.[17]

1973:	1.9	1979:	1.8
1974:	1.6	1980:	1.1
1975:	1.7	1981:	0.9
1976:	1.3	1982:	1.1
1977:	1.6	1983:	0.8
1978:	1.8		

The changes in Dutch policy and tightening of the regulatory methodology were described in Chapter Seven and in previous pages of this chapter. Even though rate regulation had become stricter, policy makers in Dutch government, the sickness funds, and policy research institutes still considered it vulnerable. Regulating per diems had little leverage over admissions. If occupancy diminished through fewer admissions and shorter stays, hospital managers might protect their cost base by encouraging more tests and billing the sickness funds under the charge list. (Holland was one of the few countries with an itemized charge list supplementing the per diems.) The previous rapid annual increases in costs might resume if changes in the government-of-the-day changed policies, and the reformers wanted a system that could limit and reduce hospitals' entire expenditure. The Dutch regulatory methods that brought down annual increases were very complicated and occasionally contentious. So, after 1983, Holland moved toward global budgeting and assigned the sickness funds a negotiating role—particularly over expected utilization—before the regulating agency (COTG) gave the final approval to the prospective budgets. Because one agency could not perform both oversight tasks, a collaboration and division of labor were created between the local office of the sickness funds (to contain admissions) and COTG (to contain unit costs per admission).

American state rate regulation was first intended to make annual expenditure increases by Medicaid and Blue Cross more predictable and more bearable. Some regulators tried to achieve these goals by persuading hospitals to become more efficient. Ceiling penalty formulas were common: if a hospital was far above its peer groups in unit costs (such as length of stay or some ratio of costs to work), it could not collect its full per diem. A few state rate-setting commissions—particularly in Washington and Maryland—offered advice to hospital managers when they discussed cost reports and prospective budgets. While the state rate-setting programs limited annual increases in total costs—as I said earlier in this chapter—their success in reducing cost per admission was mixed:

- Previous trends to add employees were slowed or stopped, so the hospital could work within the constrained per diems. Forces other than state rate controls may have contributed.[18]
- In some regulated states, stays became longer and not shorter, thereby nullifying savings per admission.[19]
- The most expensive hospitals continued to be most expensive.[20]

The American state rate regulation methods were too weak to make hospitals less inefficient:

☐ The standard of comparison was statewide rather than national: peer groups were selected from other hospitals in that state. The states that were apparently more successful in restraining annual *increases* in both aggregate and unit costs—New York and Massachusetts—had the most expensive hospitals and the longest stays in the country. The apparent successes in annual rates of increases were statistical triumphs, not real financial triumphs, since they were proportions of high cost bases. The totals could not be forced downward to levels of personnel, costs, and stays prevailing in the rest of the country.

☐ The state programs had varying mandates. The national government did not enunciate a policy of controlling costs and improving efficiency, as in other countries. The national government did not distribute guidelines tying costs to national economic indicators.

☐ When state commissions challenged prospective budgets and personnel levels, they were worn down by arguments. The hospitals could appeal to higher officials and to courts.

☐ The regulators lacked full authority over the several elements that governed program costs—namely, prospective budgets and length of stay. They could not investigate whether stays were justified, an essential power in forcing hospitals to become more efficient.

☐ American regulation limited each year's increase over the previous year, instead of rolling back overprovision and costs. In particular, the United States had added so many health personnel during the decades after World War II that its hospitals were inevitably more expensive than Europe's. In 1978 the numbers of personnel per hundred beds were 237.5 in the United States, 179.7 in France, 132.5 in Switzerland, and equally low in other European countries. Many American teaching hospitals had six employees per bed, nearly double their European counterparts.[21] Isolated from Europe, American regulators, payers, and hospital managers did not realize that hospitals could operate with fewer people and did not try to roll back staffing. (In contrast, European visitors to American hospitals are always struck by the larger numbers of employees.[22]) Not until DRGs did Americans have a payment system that motivated reductions.

New York State provided an unintended case study in the vulnerability of a purely formula approach to rate regulation. A formula can be addressed to only one or two cost-containment objects and carries perverse incentives as well as its principal incentives; it leads to unintended cost-raising behavior, whereby hospitals compensate for the losses from the cost-containment effects. Since a group of human regulators is not in place, no one notices and reverses the perverse effects for a considerable time, and a prolonged legislative process must be employed to alter the rules.

☐ New York State had too many hospitals, too many beds, too many admissions, and excessively long stays. The first target of both rate regulation and state hospital planning was the excessive number of hospitals and beds. Throughout the 1970s the formula for calculating the per diem rate raised the denominator of the fraction (that is, expected operating costs divided by expected patient-days) to a minimum. Underoccupied hospitals otherwise would obtain higher per diems. The minima assumed that occupancy should be at least 60 to 85 percent, depending on specialty and size of community. Underoccupied hospitals would receive per diems insufficient to cover their costs; either they reduced their costs or (more likely) they closed. The state's planning agency denied Certificates of Need for improvements in underoccupied hospitals, so they could not revive.

☐ Some hospitals closed because they could not increase admissions to earn more money and avoid the occupancy penalties. Seeing them deteriorate, their attending physicians accelerated the decline by placing their patients elsewhere. On the other hand, many hospitals avoided the fate intended under the occupancy formula by increasing admissions. Every hospital had an incentive to avoid reducing length of stay. (The formulas included penalties against hospitals with extremely above-average stays, but no penalties for failure to reduce stays.) Therefore, compared to the rest of the country, New York continued to have the most expensive hospitals and the longest stays: compared to the average figures for the entire country, New York's costs per admission were one-third higher, its stays were two days longer, and its occupancy rates were nearly eight percentage points higher.[23]

☐ During the early 1980s, the state added more formulas designed to cushion declines in utilization and discourage increases. If a hospital reduced patient-days (through fewer admissions and/or shorter stays), its per diem billings of third parties were increased to enable the hospital to recover the fixed-cost component of the per diem payments that it had lost. The "volume change and adjustment" included a penalty for increasing admissions and stays over the numbers predicted at the start of the year: as patient-days rose, per diem payments were reduced, since the hospital's fixed costs were spread over more billings. Admissions fluctuated down and then up again during the 1980s in New York, and length of stay remained remarkably stationary. Neither followed the declines in the rest of the United States.

Every country regulating payment units seems to move toward capped methods. In Europe the trend is toward global budgeting. American Medicare adopted DRGs, because of the disillusioning struggles in state rate regulation, the Reagan administration's decision to avoid all-payers standardization, the national government's hope to shock the hospital industry into cost consciousness, and the national government's desire to force the high-cost states downward. Instead of substituting a third generation of formulas, the weary officials of New York State planned an all-payers DRG method of their own.

North America provided a demonstration of the effects of contrasting systems on hospital labor costs: the steadily tighter Canadian global budgeting and the essentially uncontrolled American situation. From 1972 to 1980, full-time-equivalent employees per patient-day remained constant in Ontario but rose 20 percent in the United States.[24] Lower costs per admission were due partly to the higher Canadian productivity (fewer hospital workers doing the same work) and partly to lower technological level and service intensity than in American hospitals.[25] As I explained in Chapter Ten, Canadian hospitals had to concede higher wages than American hospitals did, but they could economize by freezing employment.

Effects of DRGs on Cost and Efficiency. American DRGs had two different goals: to limit average costs of admission throughout the country, and to provide incentives for greater efficiency. This flat formula method was designed to pay every hospital the average national cost of admission. It was an incentive reimbursement scheme to penalize the more expensive hospitals and redistribute the payer's cash from the more costly to the less costly establishments. If it had been designed to reduce costs per admission throughout the system, it would have frozen the less costly hospitals instead of giving them more money than ever before.

DRGs are effective in limiting the average costs per admission only if the rules limit the number of expensive outliers, who receive additional payments. DRGs are effective in limiting payers' total expenditures only if the number of admissions is kept within expectations.[26] This is possible only if DRGs are supplemented with extra incentives and regulations: hospitals and doctors could be rewarded for treating patients in ambulatory or home-care programs; a regulatory agency might forbid unnecessary admissions.

DRGs are effective in improving efficiency only if the managers and doctors respond as expected. The more expensive hospitals are assumed to be inefficient and reorganize to do the same work with fewer resources: the number of personnel is reduced; doctors order fewer tests; doctors discharge patients earlier; underused services are closed; separate departments (such as intensive care and coronary care) are consolidated. The less expensive hospitals use the additional cash to acquire more resources and perform more work with the same efficiency as before. Certain types of patients are no longer accepted by the hospitals that cannot treat them efficiently and are referred to the more efficient establishments.

Identifying the actual effects of any payment system always founders because so many other administrative events occur simultaneously and because it can be administered with varying strictness over time. And so it was during the use of DRGs in the United States in the 1980s:

☐ DRGs were applied differently in New Jersey and in Medicare.
- Annual increases were higher in New Jersey, because DRGs began as an experiment necessitating the cooperation of all hospitals; the state government was less punitive than the national government toward high-cost hospitals; and New Jersey hospitals were supposed to earn extra cash to cover the uninsured.
- New Jersey had an all-payers system. Medicare's DRGs were idemulated by a few state Medicaid programs; but in every other state, hospitals billed other payers by other methods and at higher rates. Therefore, hospitals could survive despite strict Medicare payments.
- New Jersey's DRG payment used the statewide average for only half the payment. The rest was calculated from the hospital's own costs. Medicare adopted national rates after a three-year transition.
- Outliers reimbursed separately were 30 percent of all New Jersey cases and about 6 percent of all American Medicare cases.
☐ The effects of Medicare DRGs on the expensive teaching hospitals were cushioned by large extra grants for teaching costs and overhead.
☐ Cost-consciousness became the watchword of the hospital and health insurance industries.
- Hospital managements worried that all other payers would become strict, and some did.
- Hospital managers pursued new standards of excellence in their professional careers, running efficient and lean organizations, reducing operating costs, and adding extramural alternatives to inpatient care.
- To provide health benefits for their employees and families, many companies stopped purchasing group policies from third parties and administered the benefits themselves. They insisted that hospitals treat beneficiaries cheaply, and often they limited referrals to the low bidders. Employers required higher cost sharing by their workers, by cutting benefits and by eliminating coverage of the workers' dependents.[27]
- Even though every DRG yielded as many profits to some hospitals as losses to other establishments, the industry was gripped by a contagious fear of losses and frantically searched for remedies. The structure of the health care market intensified the mania. The many competing suppliers to hospitals encouraged the anxiety by warning that each establishment risked bankruptcy if it did not buy each vendor's management advice, cost-finding computer software, systems for communications and materials management.
☐ Regulatory agencies (Peer Review Organizations) were established to combat the potential increase in admissions to earn more cash payments.

During the year after Medicare's introduction of DRGs—that is during 1984—American hospitals suddenly reversed the earlier trends of growth.[28]

- Total expenses rose 4.6 percent, closer to the rise in general consumer prices than ever before.
- Number of beds dropped 1.1 percent.
- Number of full-time-equivalent personnel dropped 2.3 percent.
- Number of inpatient admissions dropped 4 percent for all patients and 2.9 percent for Medicare patients. Work in an ambulatory mode was substituted: 1.5 million fewer patients were admitted, but 1.1 million more outpatient visits were performed.
- Average length of stay was reduced. From 7 to 6.7 days for all patients, from 9.6 to 7.4 days for Medicare patients.
- Average occupancy rate in community hospitals dropped from 72.2 percent (in 1983) to 66.6 percent (in 1984).
- Expenditures for supplies, services, and related nonlabor expenses had risen 10.2 percent in 1983 but only 3.5 percent in 1984. The once booming hospital supply corporations suffered great drops in earnings.
- All these reductions continued during 1985.

Besides the financial and utilization changes in the entire country, many hospital organizations experienced internal changes. Cost accounting and medical records improved and became computerized. More work was contracted out. Overtime and per diem hiring were reduced. Management learned about the practice of each doctor and identified the most costly. Managers advised the medical staff about possible economies. Services were unbundled in the billing, so payers could be billed separately for professional services of doctors and technicians.

The public debate attributed the sudden reductions in costs and utilization to the introduction of DRGs, but that could be only part of the explanation. Many other incentives and controls were being applied simultaneously by Medicare and other payers. The owners and managers of hospitals seemed to adopt a new philosophy of cost containment and efficiency—and this force might be more important than any other. These additional controls by payers and the hospital management profession therefore counteracted certain cost-increasing incentives of DRGs: admissions diminished and outpatient visits were substituted, even though DRGs implied the reverse; economies were made even by hospitals that were prospering, in order to hedge against a possibly constrained future. As a result, unexpectedly, the entire hospital industry in 1984 earned higher profits than ever before.[29]

A hospital responds to general trends in the total constellation of management and reimbursement, even when every payer follows different rules. Doctors, the clinical staff, and even the administrators cannot make fine distinctions in treating patients of different third parties, but they adopt a general policy toward all. A single payer cannot have conspicuous effects on clinical and management practices in an American hospital unless it dominates the market. (The trend in Europe has been to eliminate distinctions among payers through all-payers arrangements.)

The restraints on American hospital costs per admission would have been even greater during 1984 except for certain cost-raising trends that managers and payers could not control:

☐ *Capital.* After twenty years of accelerated modernization based on debt, hospitals were saddled by a need to repay principal and interest incurred before 1984, and they had to replace equipment from earnings or from new debt. Therefore, while other items in the hospitals' utilization, revenue, and costs rose little or diminished in 1984, depreciation rose 16.8 percent and interest rose 21.9 percent.[30]

☐ *Tests ordered by doctors.* While payers and hospital managers were becoming increasingly cost-conscious, the medical profession believed that it was facing a sudden increase in the number and monetary value of malpractice suits. Forty-three percent of all American doctors said that they had been performing tests and treatments beyond normal clinical requirements for some time, in order to build potential defenses against lawsuits. Twenty percent said that they had increased tests and treatments in 1984 over previous levels.[31] Previously, hospitals had earned more money from the increased testing by their attending physicians, but now the hospitals wanted to reduce costs from tests within each DRG. Therefore, a conflict of interest arose between hospitals and their doctors.

Fixed-limit payment systems are supposed to induce closer cooperation between managers and doctors, so that the hospital can break even under the ceilings. But cooperation requires thorough explanations to medical staffs. Few American hospitals attempted to explain the intricate and unfamiliar DRG payment method to their doctors, and HCFA did not create an instructional program. American doctors bombarded letters-to-the-editor columns of newspapers and television programs with complaints and mistaken analyses, and probably most doctors consistently misinformed their patients. (For example, many described DRGs as a list of maximum days for hospital stays, beyond which their patients must be discharged.) DRGs intensified American doctors' hostility toward Medicare and toward the United States government—a hostility already fueled by Medicare's confusing method of paying their fees. At the same time, throughout France the Division of Hospitals of the Ministry of Social Affairs was conducting workshops with specially prepared teaching modules, explaining to every hospital doctor all details about the new system of global budgeting.

Substituting Cheaper Modes. Ideally, a payment system should inspire hospital managers and health professionals to treat patients in settings that are clinically equivalent to but less expensive than inpatient hospitalization—settings such as outpatient departments, patients' homes, or nursing homes.

Europe did not suddenly shift from intramural to extramural care during its economy wave of the 1970s and 1980s. The financing system and the structure of services discouraged rather than rewarded substitution:

☐ *No gains for the hospital.* Under cost-based reimbursement, the hospital does not obtain additional net revenue from extramural care. The per diems or global grants are calculated from net costs, after earnings are subtracted from the hospital's total costs. Billings by the outpatient department are included in such earnings.

If a hospital management controls extended-care beds in addition to acute-care beds—as in many French public hospitals—the hospital collects a lower per diem for the extended-care beds, since operating costs are lower. If the acute-care beds are not fully occupied, referral results in lower revenues.

☐ *Few facilities.* Many European countries lack extensive home care and nursing home programs. The acute hospital traditionally had many elderly and chronic patients. For this reason several European countries (such as Germany and Holland) had more beds, longer stays, and lower per diem rates than countries with higher turnover and greater service intensity (such as the United States and Great Britain).

☐ *No third-party coverage.* NHI traditionally paid for acute care in doctors' offices and in hospitals. Only recently are programs adding coverage for nursing homes and for home care.

Fee schedules for the payment of doctors under NHI usually cover visits to the hospital OPD. But the office doctors who practice under German NHI have blocked coverage of ambulatory visits to hospital OPDs, thus retaining a monopoly. (Only the hospital *Belegärzte* can bill the official system for their inpatient and outpatient care. The other salaried doctors can collect fees after discharge only from persons covered by private health insurance.) When the national Parliament considered a reform during the late 1970s—wherein hospital doctors would be encouraged to reduce stays and would collect fees for continuing care in an ambulatory mode—the office doctors protested throughout Germany, the office doctors throughout Lower Saxony conducted a strike, and the clause was not enacted in the law.

Certain methods of financing hospitals and organizing delivery promote substitutes for inpatient hospitalization. Great Britain has always performed much care through home visits by general practitioners, district nurses, and community organizations. The United States copied some methods, greatly expanded them during the 1980s, and therefore could reduce hospital admissions and stays. The successful methods are:

☐ *Combining ownership and management.* When Britain's NHS reorganized in 1974, the new DHA was given management of both the hospitals and the home-care services. The District Nursing Officer managed the nurses in both the hospital and the community health services. The DHA was expected to reallocate funds and personnel to the community services if the hospitals seemed overdeveloped and if good work at lower cost could be done at home.

In the United States during the late 1970s and 1980s, nonprofit acute hospitals and for-profit multi-health care corporations developed their own home care programs and nursing homes. At the urging of several state Blue Cross Plans (particularly around New York City) and the National Association of Blue Cross Plans, hospitals developed same-day surgery.[32]

☐ *Limiting hospital beds.* Great Britain tried to reduce beds—and certainly not increase them—in part to discourage hospitalization of patients who could be tested or treated in home care or in neighborhood health centers. General practitioners were given higher practice allowances so that they could modernize their offices. The NHS tried to persuade the GPs to join district nurses and others in well-equipped health centers.

☐ *Coordinating inpatient and outpatient transactions.* New Jersey's numerous outliers include the very short stays within each inpatient DRG. The hospital does not collect the full DRG rates, but only per diems. For these cases the state rate regulators fix DRG rates for outpatient care and same-day surgery that exceed the revenue from the per diems. Inpatient admissions in New Jersey increased—from 154.7 per thousand inhabitants in 1981 to 160.4 per thousand in 1983[33]—since a DRG system apparently carries a powerful incentive to hospitalize. But the countervailing formula for the short-stay outliers may have reduced the increase below its full potential.

☐ *Reducing amount of cost sharing.* By requiring less cost sharing, payers give financial incentives to the patients to prefer ambulatory or home care. The method is used by American Medicare: patients must pay a deductible for inpatient hospitalization but none for home care.

☐ *Creating government grants.* Under global budgeting and public grants, government can create new grants for community providers. The Canadian national and provincial governments were determined to limit hospital spending during the late 1970s. The new financing system enacted in 1977 eliminated the shared-cost method whereby Ottawa automatically paid about half the provinces' global grants to their hospitals. The provinces obtained increased taxing power, transitional block grants, full responsiblity for the hospitals, and stronger incentives to curb the hospitals' spending. One new federal-provincial conditional block grant was added, the Extended Health Care Services Program. Ottawa would pay a certain amount per capita to each province—initially $20, increased annually as GNP grew—to support provincial grants for home care, respite care, community health care, and nursing homes for the aged. As a result, the number of acute-care beds diminished throughout Canada, acute hospitals absorbed a smaller proportion of all Canadian health spending (from 62.4 percent in 1975 to 56.1 percent in 1982), and the community programs grew everywhere.

Guaranteeing Appropriate Care

Ideally, a payment system should "promote good medicine" by minimizing financial barriers for patients who need care, paying for the right amounts and quantities of care, and discouraging excessive treatment or the use of inappropriate therapies.

Access. The methods of covering the population and the methods of paying hospitals have led to nearly universal access to mainstream hospital services in nearly all developed countries. Once hospital care and specialist treatments varied by social classes; the poor got inferior services or nothing.

In countries with universal coverage under general public financing (such as Britain or Canada), no one can experience a financial barrier. Every inhabitant has the right to enter a hospital and receive the standard treatments prescribed by the physicians and available at the establishment. No point-of-service charges are made for intramural or extramural acute hospital services under the official scheme. Patients are expected to pay the bills of private clinics and nursing homes, since these benefits are not provided by general Treasury financing.

In countries with universal coverage under national health insurance (such as France), financial barriers are nearly impossible. Every inhabitant is covered by some sort of insurance scheme that pays standard rates to doctors and hospitals for standard treatments. France has cost sharing by patients for the bills of doctors and hospitals, but this is not a barrier to essential access, since the charges are waived for the seriously ill and for the poor.

In other countries with national health insurance (such as Germany), small proportions of the population may not be covered by the official scheme. Some of those not covered are the more affluent with private insurance, extra cash, and better access than anyone else, since hospital specialists treat them personally. Others are very poor and outside the official schemes—once a common situation and now rare; the municipal welfare office covers their hospital bills. Foreign visitors may be required to post a deposit in advance, as in Switzerland. Since hospitals and their salaried medical staffs have long been accustomed to treating everyone alike, the few uninsured are not identified specially in the clinical charts and are treated in the standard manner. One no longer hears of citizens of developed countries lacking care because of deficient or no third-party coverage.

In all countries with a national health service or national health insurance—except for Canada—persons are free to buy additional private health insurance. This coverage has little effect on basic clinical access, aside from attracting the personal attention of the chief of service. The policies enable the patient to purchase more comfort in the general hospital, such as a private room and more personal attention from the domestic staff. The principal motives for purchase of private coverage are easier access to the for-profit hospitals and the more attractive fees offered to physicians. (As the general NHI schemes have improved benefits in France, Germany, Switzerland, and other countries with many private clinics, the private clinics fill their potentially unoccupied beds with general NHI patients.) Private policies make a difference in posthospital convalescence, often covering spas and nursing homes.

Financial barriers to mainstream medicine still exist in the United States, which has resisted universal equal coverage through either public financing or statutory health insurance. In the total mosaic, many gaps exist.

☐ Access for most Americans depends on insurance provided as a fringe benefit of employment. Coverage of services and amounts of patient cost sharing vary among employers. Some workers and the families of many other workers lost coverage during the 1980s, as employers cut back their labor costs. Because of these cuts and the lack of employment by some, at least 15.2 percent of the American population during late 1983 lacked any third-party coverage.[34]

☐ If someone has neither insurance nor cash, few office doctors will see him. Since office doctors hospitalize patients, such persons can enter no for-profit and few nonprofit hospitals, as either inpatients or outpatients. In a national survey in 1982, 17 percent of the American people said that they had no regular doctor. A determined person can enter a hospital by queuing at the emergency room or outpatient department of a teaching hospital or a public general hospital. Of those without family doctors, nearly two-thirds in the 1982 survey— 10 percent of the entire American population—said that they relied on such hospital services as their principal source of care, as their regular entry point.[35] But the hospitals' outpatient facilities cannot deliver comprehensive primary care, either to single patients or to entire families. Swamped by many indigents and often underfunded because of their many bad debts, such hospitals often cannot deliver mainstream medicine.

☐ During the early 1980s, when insurance coverage declined and hospitals' bad debts rose, about 15 percent of all American hospitals explicitly limited their charity care. "Economic transfers" from private to public hospitals sharply increased.[36]

The intent of planning and investment systems has been to spread facilities to underserved areas and ultimately to equalize services. The intent of insurance and granting systems for the payment of operating costs has been to eliminate financial barriers to access. But payment systems do not guarantee universality and equality in results; they do not guarantee full and appropriate utilization for all clinical needs. Health depends on heredity and life-style, not on hospital services alone. Utilization depends on an understanding of one's own needs, skill in using services, freedom from competing family and work responsibilities, and convenient transportation—all independent of the reimbursement system. Utilization differences are narrower than they were earlier. But they persist, even in the countries with the fewest financial barriers to access.[37]

Offering or Denying New Services. A payment system can convert the patient's need into opportunity but cannot guarantee prompt service if demand exceeds supply. Modern universal financing methods would have to be matched by generous provision and widespread distribution of facilities in all specialties. National health insurance schemes usually guarantee that every subscriber is eligible to receive any recognized nonexperimental therapy if a physician prescribes it. The health care system is expected to provide enough personnel and facilities to satisfy the demand. Since utilization fluctuates, the system must maintain idle capacity, leading to the costs that modern health policy now tries to reduce. To avoid deficits and closures, providers may then find new users to occupy the facility at all times, thereby raising costs further. Very modern facilities are particularly expensive because they are constantly updated.

A common practice in large European nations is to centralize expensive and less frequently used programs, instead of spreading them throughout the country, closer to the users. Often these programs are located in academic centers, and patients must travel there. The national government—with the advice of the leadership of the sickness funds—can control the numbers and sites of such expensive programs, since they require large public grants for construction and equipment. The specifications and expected utilization of the programs often are included in the national hospital plans. If demand presses upon capacity in the few special centers, the larger developed countries eventually install such facilities in many regional hospitals, closer to the patients. Once such treatment ceases to be experimental, it is fully covered under NHI: if a doctor prescribes it, the sickness fund pays according to its normal procedure.

Selective cost sharing to ration particular hospital services is very unusual, except in the United States. Where it exists abroad, it applies to physicians' services or (more often) to extra benefits, such as prescription drugs.[38] Even during the financial crisis of the late 1970s and 1980s, few countries reversed the trend toward full coverage of *hospital* care and added user charges.[39] Where they exist for hospital care, charges are a standard proportion of the bill or a standard copayment per service and do not vary according to the cost of or demand for individual services. The more expensive and unusual services are usually needed by the sicker patients, and (as in France) the more seriously ill patients are exempt from the cost sharing.

Countries differ not only in resource levels but also in clinical styles; the two correspond, and the reimbursement and planning methods fit. The countries with a more interventionist clinical style—most notably, the United States—have more dynamic equipment and drug industries, and they have payment systems that underwrite generous use. The medical profession in the United States—and probably in Germany and other high-technology countries—has long been inclined to perceive correctible pathology and to intervene.[40] Great Britain has had fewer advanced clinical facilities and lower utilization of them than the United States and Germany, not merely because of its stricter method of controlling expenditure but also because its medical profession has always been more cautious. English doctors have been the authors of several influential books listing the popular therapies—often expensive and clinically risky—that were subsequently abandoned as ineffective or unsafe.[41] *The British Medical Journal* and the *Lancet* have become principal outlets for reports about the clinical ineffectiveness and dangers of popular treatments and drugs.[42]

Countries with a cautious clinical style always appear underdeveloped by the standards of high-technology countries, but the discrepancy in instrument/ population ratios is true only for the newest methods.[43] Britain is always catching up, spending its limited resources to correct the once great regional inequalities and eventually modernizing the better-provided places. Eventually, Britain achieves comparable levels of high-technology services in the therapies that are finally vindicated. But even then, British doctors—because of their more cautious prognoses about benefits to patients and their concern for the patients' likely quality of life—will prescribe certain interventions less often. As I said in Chapter Nine, the American reimbursement and investment system enables America to be the testing site—closely watched by interested Britons—for the newest advanced techniques. To many Britons and Europeans, it is not they who are "underprovided"; it is the United States that is "overprovided" and excessively expensive.[44]

Waiting Lists for Accepted Therapies. Small but highly developed countries under national health insurance hesitate to spread expensive programs throughout the country, even after they are fully recognized. NHI is expensive enough for such countries without widespread proliferation and constant modernization of the newest therapies. A few centers for open-heart surgery transplants, cancer therapy, CT scanning, and other such services are created in the principal teaching hospitals. But waiting lists can develop quickly, in violation of the principle of universal and prompt access. Genuine need and physicians' orders cannot be deterred by user charges.

One strategy for affluent small countries in many economic sectors is international trade, and the same method can be applied to hospital care. For example, Holland has generous entitlements in its health insurance, no deterrent fees, and no expectations that patients will contribute large shares of unusual costs. Holland created open-heart surgery centers cautiously; and patients on waiting lists for such surgery often were flown to Switzerland, Great Britain, and the United States. Between 1977 and the early 1980s, over one thousand patients a year—during some years one-quarter of all Dutch heart surgery cases—had care and international transportation paid by the sickness funds.[45] As a permanent policy, this was too expensive, since the sickness funds had to pay for travel and lodging for both the patient and a family member, and since Swiss and American private clinics charged high prices. When Holland could predict regular annual utilization, enough domestic open-heart surgery centers were established, and foreign trips ceased.

Use by many such foreign patients has enabled Switzerland to construct and maintain larger numbers of advanced units than the Swiss population alone can use economically. But such expansion is risky. When the foreign countries develop adequate services of their own, Swiss private clinics—such as the hospital in Genolier used by Dutch heart patients—face bankruptcy. Similarly, Great Britain's for-profit hospitals depend on Arab patients and are threatened by improved capacity in the Middle East.

Countries with national health insurance only now are applying the cutbacks and investment controls that may eventually produce shortages and waiting lists in hospitalization. Great Britain has had to manage the situation for some time, because a national health service must provide both entitlement and facilities. Britain's task has been particularly difficult because its entitlement has been universal and generous, while the country's economic problems require strict limits on facilities. Patients cannot be priced out of the hospital market, since public policy has always insisted on the price of zero. (In contrast, charges in Britain equilibrate supply and demand for spectacles, nursing homes, and some other services.) Hospital admissions have always been managed by waiting lists, and critics have constantly cited the queues and delays as proof of the failure of the NHS.

Are large numbers of Britons denied inpatient care by constrained resources? At first sight a massive problem seems to exist: in 1983 in England alone, inpatient waiting lists totaled 725,600 persons. But an anomaly also exists: the English inpatient occupancy rate in acute care is about 78 percent, one of the lowest in any developed country.[46] While waiting lists attract frequent debate, they are only part—and a very confused part—of the allocation process.

From the start of the NHS, demand and utilization greatly exceeded expectations. To everyone's surprise, private practice virtually disappeared almost at once. Despite a wrangle over pay and conditions of service on the eve of the Appointed Day, nearly every general practitioner joined the NHS at once, nearly every inhabitant enrolled with a GP, and private general practice disappeared. Pay and conditions of service for hospital consultants were so attractive that nearly every specialist signed up as a full-timer or maximum part-timer. Almost every inpatient was treated in an NHS bed by a consultant during his salaried hours, and private specialty practice nearly disappeared.

When services became available, they were used more than expected. The potential untreated demand was greater than predicted. The first evidence was the immediate rush to dentists, who soon had long waiting lists for ambulatory appointments.

The National Health Service took over everything from the voluntary hospitals—including their waiting lists. The hospitals always had them; the pressure to enter was relieved only partially between the World Wars, when the local authority hospitals added consultants in acute care.[47] The NHS has retained the voluntary hospitals' unsystematic method of creating and administering waiting lists. Beds are not pooled in a hospital-wide fashion and are not divided by service. The unit of organization is the "firm" of doctors, and the beds are assigned to a consultant when he is appointed. He controls their use, deciding admissions and discharges. He can treat anyone in those beds; if a GP refers a patient with a problem outside the consultant's specialty, he can hospitalize and treat that patient rather than send him to another consultant. Since every consultant decides admissions to his own beds, he administers his own waiting lists. Some consultants put names on their lists themselves; others let their chief assistants (their "registrars") do it. The admissions office of the hospital has limited administrative work and does not handle waiting lists.

"Numbers of persons on waiting lists" are often reported by consultants to the persons who fill out annual questionnaires sent from DHSS. National aggregates for the entire country are published for such measures as total numbers of persons on waiting lists, ratio of length of list to admissions for each diagnosis, and mean time waiting before admission.[48] But the meaning of each entry varies widely among consultants. Some put many names on the list as contingencies; others add only patients who realistically need and wish to enter the hospital soon. The consultant's outpatient waiting list contains the names of all patients referred by the local GPs; the inpatient waiting list contains the names of patients chosen for admission by the consultant or his registrar.

In practice the waiting list nonsystem is a disorderly way of distinguishing life-threatening from nonthreatening conditions and placing the nonthreatened patients in order based on a mixture of clinical and waiting-time criteria. As in all countries, most inpatient admissions are emergencies or urgent. Nearly all of these patients are admitted without a wait, and probably most consultants do not bother with the formality of adding the names and clearing them from the tops of their waiting lists. Every consultant holds a few of his beds for emergencies. Or, to make space, he discharges a convalescent. Most persons on inpatient waiting lists need nonurgent ("cold") surgery, such as operations for hernias and varicose veins in general surgery; hip replacements in orthopedics; minor operations on the cervix and colporraphy in gynecology; and operations for cataracts and strabismus in ophthalmology. The patients are not forgotten: they continue under the regular care of their GPs; if they deteriorate, their GPs request their immediate admission as urgent. Some are treated by consultants in the OPD or (in many cases of cold surgery) in nearby private hospitals; but their names continue to appear on the inpatient waiting list.

Most inpatient waiting lists are really a grab bag of names that might be phoned when beds become available. They are not rigorously administered. The names appear in rough order of clinical need, as defined by the consultant or registrar. Different consultants seem to keep them in different forms: some make several categories of severity, rank-ordering patients within each category by date; others mix names without any fixed principle of priority. No standard methodology exists for rating the urgency of a case; so the categories vary in meaning. No management office regularly purges the list to learn whether the patients are still interested in treatment, whether any have remitted, whether any have gotten private care. Names are purged from lists only when patients are offered admission and refuse. Occasionally the Department of Health and Social Security, the Regional Hospital Boards, or the Regional Health Authorities check the accuracy of names on waiting lists; such laborious special investigations always find that lists are inflated by the same names: a patient has seen several consultants. Inpatient waiting lists were never intended to be a rigorous measure of need or demand.[49]

Amidst the confusion over the meaning and content of waiting lists, apparently some "urgent" cases wait, scattered unevenly throughout the country and among specialties. "Urgent" cases may steadily increase in the country, while numbers of beds are cut; stays do not shorten, and day surgery does not increase quickly enough to clear these cases off waiting lists.[50]

A barrier to the clearing of urgent cases is the firm system: each consultant controls the set of beds given him on appointment and will not relinquish them. But the composition and severity of patient loads change. Since the consultant in a specialty with increasingly severe patients does not gain more beds from those in other specialties, one consultant has more severe cases on his waiting list than other consultants have. For example, "urgent" urology cases might have to wait longer than "urgent" cases in internal medicine.

One remedy would require a reorganization of medical practice in the hospitals. Admissions offices would supersede the consultants in admitting patients and assigning them to beds. A consultant's work load no longer would be defined by number of beds and number of inpatients. The admissions office would administer a waiting list formula accounting for time and urgency, where urgency is multivariate.[51]

Reorganizing the fundamentals of medical staff structure is always difficult. An easier method of clearing patients in genuine need from inpatient waiting lists without reorganization is to emulate the Dutch, but by using the domestic rather than the international market. The NHS would pay private hospitals to treat such patients. Then the NHS could continue long-term cost containment by reducing its own hospital services.[52] For example, with the encouragement of DHSS, Brighton's District Health Authority in 1984 sent thirty-five patients for hip replacements—a leading cause of waiting lists—to the nonprofit King Edward VII Hospital located in its district, at a total cost of £40,000.

Another possible remedy would override the decentralized structure of the NHS and the local-mindedness of the British people. The GP would refer a patient to any consultant anywhere in the country whose waiting list was shorter than the local ones. Regions already have some "cross-boundary flows," but habit prevents British GPs and patients from using this option regularly. Public preference for local hospitalization—even at the price either of waiting or of paying for expensive underutilized services—is common in many countries.

Reallocating Resources. Before the enactment of an NHI or an NHS, wide inequalities in resources are common. Facilities and health professionals (especially specialist physicians) clustered in richer and more urbanized regions, and particularly in the richer neighborhoods of cities, where the prosperous self-payers lived. Governments and churches tried to install facilities in poor areas, but the shortages were not fully remedied. These hospital outpatient departments and inpatient wards were crowded with the poor, but they were constantly in deficit, since the patients could pay little or nothing. Governments, churches, and charitable associations covered the deficits by gifts or by ceaseless community fund-raising drives.

Once common in Europe and still common in all developing countries, this situation survives today in the one developed country without universal and equal third-party coverage—namely, the United States. American health finance guarantees adequate—and even profitable—financing of the operations of hospitals in most communities. But in poor urban neighborhoods, where patients lack any insurance or have only Medicaid, hospitals have high utilization (particularly in the outpatient department and emergency room), low revenue, and chronic financial difficulties. Modern technology and staffing make the operation of such establishments much more expensive and the deficits much larger than in previous centuries. One-fourth of American hospitals lost money each year during the early 1980s. Of the hospitals with a substantial proportion of poor patients, between one-fourth and one-half ran large and chronic deficits. Without special public grants and without sufficient operating revenue to keep pace with other hospitals in staffing and technology, about one-seventh of nonprofit hospitals in the principal fifty-two cities closed or relocated during the 1970s. Several cities closed their public general hospitals, since the requirements for subsidies burdened their municipal budgets.[53]

Unable to cover deficits by charitable fund raising, the financially stressed hospitals try to stave off bankruptcy by overcharging the commercially insured and the self-payers. But the cost payers (Medicare and Medicaid) have refused to join the cost shifting, and Blue Cross has limited its contribution in its rate negotiations. Faced by many bankruptcies and by a disappearance of hospitals with poor clienteles, several states during the 1980s designed rate regulation to cover the gaps in third-party coverage of the population. New Jersey calculated DRGs to give each hospital extra cash to cover its uninsured. New York State required every hospital to contribute some of its revenue to a state pool covering the bad debts. The New York method did not merely shift revenue within each hospital from one payer to the nonpayers; it shifted revenue from the less stressed to the more stressed hospitals.

National health insurance spreads purchasing power to all social classes in areas with local imbalances, and to regions of the country with few hospitals and doctors. Subscribers are guaranteed services, but the sickness funds are not responsible for providing them. Nonprofit owners of hospitals, doctor-owners of private clinics, and government create facilities—the owners because they are now guaranteed reimbursement, government because of its responsibility to solve unmet needs. As I said in Chapter Nine, government capital grants are a common source for building hospitals in neglected areas, but the private or municipal owner-managers must take the initiative in making the plans. Guaranteed high fees according to the national NHI fee schedules, more young doctors go to previously understaffed areas. Regional deficits slowly moderate.

When a national health service is enacted, the national government at once must guarantee both demand and supply. Every citizen in previously underprovided areas gains full entitlement to the standard benefits, and the national government must supply the facilities.

NHI contributes to improvements in underprovided areas, in both capital and operating cost. Inequalities diminish because operating deficits are reduced. But NHI lacks enough instruments to reduce excessive costs in overprovided areas. The sickness funds can pay less money to hospitals with declining utilization in contracting catchment areas, but the funds and the national government usually cannot force privately and municipally owned hospitals to close, reduce their beds, or merge. At best, the sickness funds and rate regulators can stop the increase in operating costs in the overprovided areas. But if services are still being expanded in the underprovided areas, total costs for the country still rise.

An NHS can attack both underprovision and overprovision simultaneously, since the national government is the owner-manager of facilities everywhere, as well as the source of all operating and investment money. The Ministry of Health can force a reduction and consolidation in the areas losing population; at the same time, it can build new hospitals in previously neglected regions. The result can be modernization in both types of region, without great increases in costs for the country as a whole.

The RAWP method of distributing operating funds and the RAWP-like methods of distributing capital funds—described in Chapters Eight and Nine— have enabled Great Britain to reduce and consolidate hospitals in overprovided areas with declining populations (particularly in London) while also creating more facilities in the chronically neglected areas (such as the northwest, the northeast, and the Midlands). Capital expenditures to create and modernize hospitals have been coordinated with operating expenditures.

In France, the country with the most successful form of traditional facilities planning and investment, public grants and public loans are targeted on areas with low population/bed ratios; redundant new hospitals cannot easily be created in areas with sufficient beds; and new facilities usually must be fitted into a regional division of labor. The agency that manages and finances all the Paris municipal hospitals often consolidates units and reduces beds during modernization, but France elsewhere has few instruments to close beds when populations move out.

Both Britain and France began the postwar period with great regional inequalities. Like other European countries, France had more hospital beds than Britain had. To achieve greater regional equality, France would have to level down substantially as well as level up, while the British would have to reduce overprovision only slightly. But Britain reduced the total numbers of beds drastically—a 24.6 percent net reduction from 1951 to 1982[54]—while building new ones. By 1977 the coefficient of variation among regions in bed/population ratios in England was 0.109. (The coefficient of variation is the ratio for the standard deviation to the mean.) But the coefficient was 0.179 in France and 0.153 in the Netherlands. Regional variations in numbers of doctors are much wider in France and Holland than in England.[55]

RAWP steadily reallocates operating expenditures to the underprovided British regions, by setting targets according to population characteristics and morbidity, not merely by past utilization. Each year's growth money goes entirely or predominantly to the less provided regions. Table 8-1 shows the close distance between target and expenditure achieved by the mid-1980s: the London regions are still 9 percent or less above target; the least provided regions are now only 5 percent below target and come closer each year. In contrast, when the RAWP formulas are applied to the distribution of hospital bed utilization among regions in France, one-third of the regions are 25 percent above or below target.[56]

Few other countries have consolidated management and financing of intramural and extramural services, and therefore few can reallocate. In a few big cities, such as Paris and New York, a municipal agency owns many hospitals and community services and can reallocate.

Paying hospitals by all-inclusive daily rates covering full costs hinders policies to treat patients in day care and in home care. During the 1970s the French government and CNAMTS encouraged these alternatives. The hospital was given special *prix de journée* for programs of day care and home care, based on parts of their prospective budgets and awards by the DDASS. Some hospitals developed such programs, and chiefs of service treated patients extramurally. Home care required special teams. The sickness funds saved money, since they had to pay lower daily rates than the average figures for inpatient hospitalization. The hospital management was willing to transfer patients, since the acute inpatient rate dropped for long stays. But incentives to continue inpatient hospitalization also existed: the hospital lost money if its beds were empty; the medical staffs preferred to observe patients in the hospital rather than make brief house calls and rely on reports by the home-visiting staff. One advantage of strict global budgeting is the incentive to reduce costs; therefore, French hospitals now have a greater incentive to do more work in day care and home care.[57] But more than incentives were needed, the French government and payers decided. A memorandum from the Ministry of Social Affairs recommended that the hospital reduce the number of beds if occupancy dropped below 85 percent; and the government considered supporting the creation of more hospital-based home care programs (*services de soins gradués à domicile*, or SGAD).

Encouraging Professionally Approved Therapies. Ideally, a payment system should motivate the most qualified professional to use the most appropriate tests and treatments to cure patients in need; it should provide the hospital with the cash to obtain the right supplies, equipment, and personnel in sufficient number; it should produce the greatest possible clinical success. However, evidence of the therapeutic outcomes of payment systems is scarce. Hospitals admit sick people, and the very few follow-up studies after discharge show high frequencies of death and relapse. For example, a survey of patients discharged from four hospitals in West Scotland during the early 1950s showed the following outcomes two years after discharge:[58]

Died	26.0%
Alive:	
In worse health	13.5
Still in weak health but not deteriorated	22.4
In better health	29.6
Could not be located	8.5
	100.0%
Total number of patients	(705)

Of the 462 patients who were still alive and could be located, 27.2 percent had been hospitalized again during the intervening two years.

Correlating aggregate health expenditure with nations' health indicators is not a reliable method of evaluating hospital services. Health indicators depend on each population's complaints to survey interviewers and on health providers' uneven reports about their work. Even if the health status of each population could be measured reliably, it is determined by many causes in addition to hospital care—causes such as heredity, life-style, safety at work, and safety on the highway. As a result, health indicators are more favorable in some countries that spend less on hospitals (such as Great Britain) than in countries that spend more (such as the United States).[59] Marginal expenditures on public health services may affect certain indicators of wellness—such as infant mortality—more substantially than marginal expenditures on hospitals do.[60]

Choice of tests and therapies is the responsibility of the medical profession, taught and regulated by professional institutions. Undergraduate and postgraduate education acquaint the student with normal practice in medicine generally and in his specialty. Journals, meetings, and the grapevine keep the practitioner up to date. Hospital doctors are supposed to use the best methods and avoid ineffective and dangerous ones.

Payment units for hospitals are usually aggregate rates—per diems, DRGs, and global budgets—and do not underwrite specific tests and treatments. Negotiators and regulators deal with aggregate budgets and broad rates, rather than investigating clinical practice in detail. Within the aggregate funding, hospital doctors have discretion in using the tests and treatments generally accepted by the specialty plus any new developments. If the hospital has a chief of service, he is responsible for the quality of clinical practice. Payers do not probe unless they hear rumors of substantial error; even the control doctors employed by the sickness funds do not regularly investigate hospitals' clinical performance.

Since tests and treatments are the responsibility of doctors, the reimbursement channel affecting them is the fee schedule for doctors, not the less itemized payment of hospitals. Elsewhere I have reported that the joint committees of doctors from the medical associations and sickness funds often think they are validating or encouraging certain tests and treatments by adding them to the fee schedule for the first time or by increasing their fees.[61] However, many of these tests and treatments are listed in fee schedules in broad language—such as "cholecystectomy," "muscle transfer," or "repair of meningocele"—and the doctors have discretion in choice of procedure. Because so much of medical practice is uncertain, a considerable range of methods is legitimate.[62]

Hospital reimbursement encourages specific therapies only if they require the use of very expensive equipment. These large expenditures require special applications, approvals, and financing, as I explained in Chapter Nine. The hospital medical staff—supported by the country's professional consensus—makes the case for the superiority of the method over inaction and over alternative tests or treatments. The persons who screen the proposal and pay the money expect the new procedure to be used very often, to justify installation. Less expensive methods are not screened and approved by regulators and payers; the hospital buys the equipment, supplies, and staff from its own operating revenue (as in Holland, France, and the United States) or from broad capital grants by government (as in Germany).

Limiting Disapproved Therapies. Professional machinery discourages some therapies, just as it encourages others. Reimbursement systems for hospital care have little direct influence, because they deal with general units and because choice of therapy is left to the doctors. At most, the investment screening system can reject applications for expensive equipment on clinical grounds; but that rarely happens, because the medical staff and the hospital board usually do not request expensive items that are opposed by professional opinion.

Ideally, new methods should not become popular until their clinical effectiveness has been established. Otherwise, investment and operating money could be reserved for more effective methods. The methodology of technology assessment has been developed in America, where many demonstration projects have been performed; and the techniques have attracted attention in Europe. Technology assessment and cost-effectiveness analysis have not yet become integral and widespread parts of investment appraisal in any country.[63] But even if such screening were inserted into every country's investment decisions, technology assessment and cost-effectiveness analysis might not restrain costs very much. Much expenditure on equipment and technicians is devoted to diagnostic testing, which produces reliable and potentially valuable information. Testing has greatly increased in volume and costs for many illnesses without improving clinical outcomes, since treatments have not progressed. The testing capacity is never cut back, because the information may pay off some day.[64]

As in the support of new therapies, other tests and treatments are discouraged by the methods of paying doctors, since the clinical decisions are made by the doctors rather than by hospital organizations. Therapies disapproved by the fee-schedule committees are dropped from the list or are reduced in payments. When a method—such as acupuncture in France—has partisans as well as critics, the compromise is to retain it in the fee schedule and reduce its payment. If a new therapy is gradually superseding a traditional one—such as medical instead of surgical treatment of gastric ulcer—the fee-schedule committee simultaneously increases the value of the new therapy while reducing the value of the traditional procedure.

Volumes of Approved Therapies. An ideal payment system should motivate and underwrite the appropriate frequencies in tests and treatments—

neither too many nor too few. Suddenly extending third-party coverage to groups who had not shared the access available to others can visibly solve the "too few" problem. For example, the enactment of Medicare in the United States gave to nearly all persons over sixty-five years of age general coverage either identical to or even more generous than the benefits available to the younger. The elderly and an activist medical profession took full advantage. Within fifteen years the American elderly utilized hospitals far more frequently than the young. Between 1965 and 1977, surgical operations rose 58 percent for the elderly—from 105 to 166 per thousand persons over sixty-five—and 24 percent for the younger. Rates of surgery on the American elderly—higher than surgery on the elderly in other countries—raised new questions about whether the payment system had swung from the "too few" problem to the "too many" problem, from the perspectives of both costs and clinical appropriateness.[65] (The DRG payment unit—adopted several years later—motivated greater efficiency per admission but further encouraged surgery, since many DRGs had surgical and medical versions, the former paying more.[66])

Attributing precise frequencies of services to hospital payment methods is difficult for several reasons. Tests and treatments are ordered by doctors and not by hospital organizations. The most relevant financial incentives are in the method of paying doctors. (I have summarized briefly the theoretical incentives and actual effects of methods of paying hospital doctors in Chapter Eleven.) But professional norms are the most powerful influence upon practice, particularly among the specialists who work in hospitals, observing and influencing each other. National differences in payment systems do not dictate clear-cut differences in clinical methods, in part because medical techniques have become transnational, and the most successful or fashionable ones spread across boundaries regardless of the methods of paying hospitals and doctors. Payment systems also fail to generate clear-cut differences because of the variations among each country's communities in the practice styles of their doctors, mentioned in earlier chapters.

Certain tests or treatments seem frequent if three dispositions are present in a country: professional approval of their value, paying the doctor by fee-for-service, and heavy reliance by the hospital upon charge lists. An additional disposition is the need of the hospital to amortize debt incurred when it purchased expensive equipment for the doctors' use. Probably few hospital managers explicitly urge frequent use of the equipment, but its installation and staffing are sufficient encouragement. The doctors predicted high use when they petitioned the managers and owners for its acquisition. Amortization is an incentive to high use if the hospital uses charge lists, as many private clinics do. American for-profit hospitals differ most from nonprofit hospitals in their higher frequency of profitable tests.[67] Amortization can be an incentive to high use even under per diem charges: the hospital attracts the patients needing the advanced treatments, instead of letting them go elsewhere. The limited European competition for market share takes this form.

When doctors are paid by salary or capitation and when hospitals are paid by capped rates (global budgets, per diems, or DRGs), an economic determinist might predict very low frequencies of tests and treatments. But doctors practice medicine in order to diagnose and cure. If the international culture of medicine judges that certain diagnoses require a course of investigation and treatments, the doctors will act. If personnel, equipment, and materials are inadequate for tests and treatments that the medical profession deems clearly necessary, government and the payers will be pressed to supply them. American visitors to Great Britain repeatedly point to certain tests and treatments that are given less often than in the United States, but they rarely point out that many other procedures are used just as often or even more often.[68] British consultants—who alone make clinical decisions—believe that many of the less frequent procedures are unproven and subject to offsetting side effects. If certain methods are eventually vindicated, waiting lists may exist for a while, but eventually they will be cleared by wider distribution of facilities within the NHS.

A familiar hypothesis is that an inverse relationship exists between cost containment and quality of care: payment systems that reduce expenditures might have the perverse effects of undertreating and neglecting patients.[69] Obviously, minimum expenditure results in minimum service. But remarkably little is understood—either theoretically or empirically—about the effects of service reduction on the health of patients. For example, as services decline, the effects may be insignificant or even beneficial at first; after a point, deprivation and damage may occur; but no research has ever been done on the shapes of such curves for specific clinical conditions in even simple treatment variables, such as length of stay.[70] Payment systems tend to cover all treatments by the same methods, and cost containment affects them all equally, but discouraging some treatments probably affects health more seriously than cutting others.[71]

Summary

At the start of a research project, it is easy to predict that some payment systems control costs, inspire efficiency, and foster good care better than others. Such predictions actually are based on theoretical incentives rather than reality. After studying each payment system's history and after comparing countries, one has to conclude that all these hypotheses fail. Overriding the potentials of all payment systems is how they are administered by governments, payers, hospital managers, and doctors. Payment systems reputed to allow cost escalation and inefficiency can become strict; others that often keep tight lids can be permissive. Every country changes, often by simply administering the same method differently.

One must also investigate the precise effects of a political or administrative change. Widespread perceptions may be mistaken. For example, it is commonly believed that national-provincial shared-cost programs in federal countries are wasteful: since the province can count on national contributions, it overspends. The national government lacks a voice in screening hospital prospective budgets and suffers a drain on its own finances. A common belief in Canada was that the provincial governments did not control hospital spending under HIDS because it paid only "50-cent dollars" of its own, forcing Ottawa to supply the rest. As I said in Chapter Eight, the payment method was changed in the Fiscal Arrangement Act of 1977: the national government no longer paid half the costs of all provincial grants to hospitals; the national government gave new taxing power and transitional block grants to the provinces; and the provinces were left with full authority to grant their own money to the hospitals. When hospital spending was lower thereafter, a common belief was that the change in the financial methodology caused a sudden tightening. But a study of the full time series shows that the change made little difference. The provinces always paid more than half, always saved more than half when they limited payments, and had been steadily tightening expenditures throughout the 1970s.[72]

Similarly, a sudden drop in American hospital spending in 1984 and widespread restructuring of hospitals were attributed to the adoption of DRGs by Medicare. But, as I said earlier in this chapter, Medicare DRGs could be no more than a contributor. Medicare payments had already been capped earlier. Most American hospital business is not paid by Medicare, and the other third parties and hospital managers introduced their own reforms.

Nevertheless, certain financial and clinical outcomes are associated with some payment methods more often than with others, because of their usual styles of administration. Following are some generalizations based on the evidence in this and previous chapters.

Costs. In all countries the recent debate over hospital finance has been driven by cost containment. Certain administrative devices restrain costs, and others allow spending to increase. In the first column are the administrative determinants that make a difference in controlling costs. The second column shows the characteristics of each determinant resulting in higher costs. The third column shows the characteristics of each determinant associated with lower costs. If the policy goal is cost containment—regardless of any other consequences— payment systems should be organized according to the right-hand column.

Determinant	*Higher Costs*	*Lower Costs*
Unit of payment	Rates related to services rendered: itemized charges, per diems	Global budget, case payments
Pricing and billing	Itemized	Bundled
If global budgeting and public grants	Bottom-up	Top-down
Source of money	Insurance, especially private	Government Treasury
Characteristics of payers.		
—Number	Many	One or few
—Relations among payers	Rivals	United
Nature of the agency that regulates rates or screens budgets	Commission dominated by interest groups	Line agency of government, staffed by civil servants
Procedure of the regulator or grantor:		
—Parent bodies issue guidelines about allowable increases	None. Or few and vague	Yes

Determinant	Higher Costs	Lower Costs
—Can prescribe allowable increases in utilization, not merely rates	No	Yes
—Can authorize any new jobs in hospital	No	Yes
—Has voice in planning of building and programs	No	Yes
Uniform reporting by hospital to regulators and payers	No	Yes
Interim monitoring during the year by the regulator or grantor by means of:		
—Expenditure reports	No	Yes
—Liaison officers	No	Yes
Possible increases in budget or rates during year	Yes	No
Carry-over of deficit into next year	Yes	No
Relations between reviews of last year's expenditure report and next year's prospective budget	Combined	Separate
Annual increases in prospective budgets:		
—Basis	Movements in general prices and wages	Fiscal capacity of the payers
—Inflation allowance	Flexibility at discretion of regulator	Fixed by national guidelines
—Calculation of the inflation allowance	Prediction of next year	Last year plus an increment
Regulator or payer can examine the hospital's books	No	Yes
Scope of hospital budget review by regulator or grantor	Inpatient only	Inpatient and outpatient
Subsidies by government, if any	To sickness funds	To hospitals directly
Planning of hospital services:		
—Does it exist	No. Or indicative planning with voluntary compliance	Yes, with sanctions for noncompliance
—Coordination between planning and reimbursement. If hospital refuses to cooperate.	Payer reimburses patient at high rate	Payer reimburses patient little or nothing
—Source of money for new building and major equipment	Borrowed, with amortization in rates	Granted, with no amortization

Determinant	Higher Costs	Lower Costs
Organization of the hospital:		
—Position of individual establishment	Autonomous	Part of regional or larger system
—Function	Teaching	Nonteaching
—Appointment of managers by	Individual hospital	Public authorities
—Basis of managers' pay	Revenue of each hospital	National salary scales
Physicians:		
—Medical staff structure	Open	Closed
—Relations to hospital	Hospitals compete for doctors	Doctors compete for hospital posts
—Authority of regulators or grantors over pay of senior hospital doctors	No	Yes
—Payment of senior doctors	Fees	Salaries
—Existence of a system to arbitrate pay disputes	Yes	No
Wage determination:		
—Scope of decisions	National or regional	Each unit
—Number covered by agreement	Entire hospital work force together	Separate contracts, each for different period
—Connection with rest of labor force	Linked	Not linked
—Indexed to consumer price movements	Yes	No
—Automatic increments for seniority	Yes	No
—Wage increases are automatically passed through to hospital rates	Yes	No
Standards by law:		
—Quality of personnel	Strong	Weak
—Safety	Strong	Weak
Characteristics of population:		
—Trends	Growing	Stationary
—Age	Older	Younger
—Health	Poor	Good

Some often-discussed proposals by definition reduce costs and utilization, so I have not listed them above.

□ *Very strong controls over utilization.* Some people—classified by such personal characteristics as age or classified by clinical diagnosis—are not admitted. The greater the limits, the lower the operating and capital costs of hospitals.

□ *Very strong controls over supply.* At once, the controls limit capital costs. If supply is much less than demand and if patients must queue, the operating costs of the total hospital system will be lower than otherwise. For-profits may raise their prices and therefore increase their revenue and expenditures, but they are unlikely to clear the entire market.

□ *Great reduction in purchasing power,* such as reduction of insurance coverage and elimination of welfare medicine. By definition, this would reduce spending. Americans in particular have long speculated that finely tuned user charges would lead to lower expenditure and greater efficiency in hospitals and other health services.[73] America already has more cost sharing by patients than any other country, so it alone considers widespread cuts in third-party expenditure a plausible public policy option. Experiments have found that such cost sharing leads to fewer ambulatory visits, but to only a small reduction in hospital admission, reflecting a less elastic demand.[74] The widespread cuts in American third-party coverage during 1983-84, as I reported earlier in this chapter, indeed led to slightly lower utilization of hospitals, a more limited annual increase in hospital revenue, and greater internal economies. (One-tenth of the American people needing care in 1985 did not seek it because they had completely lost insurance coverage or because their coverage did not keep pace with providers' charges.[75]) Events merely demonstrated the truism that less money spent, less money used; they also show that significant reductions in hospital spending through inpatient cost sharing require a reversal of history through a very large reduction in third-party coverage.

Efficiency. No payment system automatically inspires the allocation of resources to the places of need and the most economical use of these resources. Efficiency depends on the skills and dedication of managers, both among hospitals and among payers. Since government is interested in satisfying the population's needs and protecting the payers, government becomes an important monitor.

The trend outside the United States has been to force efficiency by prospective budgeting under caps. Since detailed investigations and regulations become burdensome and contentious—that is, forcing specific efficiencies upon individual hospitals results in an inefficient payment system—the trend has been toward global budgeting. Many countries are moving toward national investment and service planning, to locate and coordinate facilities; but the methodology of such planning has lagged. National coordination is difficult unless all hospital managers and medical staffs cooperate with national decisions. Gradually, a consensus has recently spread in each country about efficient management practice, hospital managers gain credit for applying it, and the payers and government monitor hospital performance more closely.

The United States has followed such trends in disseminating good management practices throughout its hospital industry, through professional training programs of many types, publications, management consulting firms, and management technologies marketed nationally. Medicare and Blue Cross have spread throughout the country payment systems aiming at economical care everywhere. But otherwise, America avoids the pattern of nationwide standardization found in other countries, either to create a more efficient hospital industry or to do anything else. One advantage is America's greater scope for innovation in organizational features that improve efficiency. America can test out in some hospitals and then disseminate new methods—such as same-day surgery and hospital-based home care—that contain costs.[76]

Clinical Effectiveness. Adopting therapies is the responsibility of doctors rather than hospital managers. Some financial encouragement and discouragement of treatments are possible in the construction of fee schedules for doctors and in the utilization review of doctors' work. In contrast, methods of paying hospitals are too broad to target the use of specific therapies at particular hospitals.

Investment finance methods for hospitals affect the adoption of new expensive therapies. More restrictive methods of proposing, evaluating, and approving these therapies can slow their introduction throughout a country. Those methods can limit installation to a few sites where they can be used most often and can be evaluated. In countries where hospitals can self-finance capital— as in the United States and Holland—expensive new equipment and new therapies can spread more widely. If they bring the hospital revenue—as under American charge lists—the new therapies can spread before their clinical effectiveness is established. Then they can be replaced by improvements, with little financial loss to the hospital and much gain to the doctors. As a result, the United States is the principal testing site for new equipment and new therapies, and its instrument companies are the world's largest. Clinical effectiveness is ultimately established through professional consensus and widespread adoption. The flow of new methods can stop suddenly if self-financing of capital, charge lists, and cost shifting among payers end.

It is not possible to fine-tune payment systems to promote "efficiency" and "clinical effectiveness," because the operational meaning of these worthy goals is not clear. Resource use is supposed to be "efficient" when substitution of methods reduces costs in money and time, with no or small reductions in health outcomes. Therapies are supposed to be "effective" when they improve health. But there is still little consensus about defining the health outcomes affected by hospital work, measuring variations, and attributing them to particular causes. One reason for the trend toward global budgeting is that payers and government regulators became weary after their prolonged and contentious attempts to ratify particular resources and therapies and to fix their volumes. Global budgeting hands the perplexing decisions about resources and therapies completely to hospital managers and doctors.

Conflicts. A payment system can be expensive not only in money but in contention. Weary policy makers and administrators can testify that harmony is just as valuable as economy, and often they are tempted to be generous with the payers' money, just to buy peace. Contention increases expenses for government, hospitals, and payers. Following are some system attributes that result in high and low conflict in hospital regulation:

Determinant	Higher Conflict	Lower Conflict
Type of government	Federal	Unitary
Life of the statute	Must be renewed frequently and is amended often	Permanent; amended rarely

Determinant	Higher Conflict	Lower Conflict
Power of legislature	High	Low
Role of courts	Active; overrule regulators and legislators	Passive; accept executive discretion
Security of the civil service	Low	High
Method of regulation	Automatic formulas	Personal administration
Complexity of the system in rules and in administration	High	Low
Stability in the rules	Changes are frequent and numerous	Changes are rare and few
Coverage of litigation costs	Included in budget for care of patients	Cannot be passed on to third parties
Structure of hospital system	Most hospitals are autonomous; heterogeneous; many private clinics	Most are in a few multi-hospital systems; uniform; few private clinics
Role of medical profession in hospital finance	Strong	Limited

Whether a system is "generous" or "stingy" has no effect on contention. The biggest spenders include a country that placidly accepts government decisions (Sweden) and one that constantly fights and evades them (the United States).

Strengths and Weaknesses. Every payment system has administrative advantages as well as disadvantages, in addition to financial and clinical consequences. One might list strong and weak points of every device mentioned in this book. Any policy maker considering a new device that has already been practiced abroad should be aware of the complete mix. As an illustration, following are the strengths and weaknesses of the principal units of payment used today in developed countries. (I omit payment by the case, since it is just beginning in only one country.)

☐ All-inclusive daily charges.
- Strengths.
  — Administrative simplicity.
  — Economy in billing. Lists of patients and their days are sent to sickness funds.
  — Usually all payers are on the same footing. Rivalry among them in the coverage of basic hospital services is reduced, and they can form common negotiating fronts. Their competition moves to other subjects.
  — The work and income of the doctors are controlled more closely by the hospital organization.
- Weaknesses.
  — Not enough data about treatments.
  — If the daily charge is uniform, costing by type of patient is hindered. Some payers subsidize others.
  — Incentive to avoid shortening stays.

    — Because the hospital management and sickness funds do not get prompt information about services, utilization control over individual doctors' work is weak.

    — If the daily charge includes amortization of debt, new equipment and programs can proliferate.

☐ Itemized billings, more or less. The minimum itemization is highly debundled.

  • Strengths.

    — More statistical information about the work of the hospital and of the doctors.

    — Cost-center accounting within the hospital is feasible under the more itemized methods.

    — More accurate costing of types of patients. Accurate individual billing is possible.

    — Costing of individual procedures conduces to the efficient assignment of personnel, space, and equipment. The costs and benefits of individual procedures can be compared.

    — Since individual procedures are recorded, utilization control is possible.

    — Incomes of some doctors can be higher—a strong point for them. Doctors' incomes are more differentiated, determined more by their own efforts.

  • Weaknesses.

    — Incentive to proliferation of tests and treatments in inpatient and particularly in outpatient departments.

    — More administrative work for hospitals and payers.

☐ Global budget.

  • Strengths.

    — Spending for all hospital services in the region or country can be controlled and predicted.

    — Fits planning of facilities and investments.

    — Administrative simplicity.

    — Hospital spending can be tied into larger expenditure planning, such as maintaining a constant proportion of GNP.

    — Payers can plan their premiums and taxes with greater certainty.

    — Health managers and doctors must work more closely with officials in other economic sectors; they must become involved in public priority setting more generally.

  • Weaknesses.

    — Provides insufficient data about treatments and costs of procedures.

    — Utilization control over work of individual doctors is handicapped by lack of data.

    — Incentive to save money by underserving.

    — Usually no cost-center accounting within the hospital.

    — Hospital managers complain that global budgeting is often used to squeeze the hospitals unduly. (As in many aspects of hospital finance, this is not inevitable: it depends on how global budgeting is administered, whether payers cover deficits.)

— Can become involved in politics, and hospital spending might experience stop-and-go fluctuations.
— In practice, hospital managers are not given all the discretion they expect. They might have received a fixed budget and expected to keep all existing services open. The grantors who constrain the money and services do not always think through how to deal with excess demand.

14

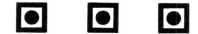

Conclusion: Improving Hospital Finance Systems

The central question in any economic transaction is "Who should pay how much money to whom for what output to achieve which goals?" The question can be phrased and answered simply in most economic transactions, because their buyers, sellers, products, and customer goals are clear-cut. But health markets in general and hospital finance in particular are quite different: means and outcomes are full of uncertainties, alternative services can be substituted, and different actors have competing goals. Health care and hospitals have changed in recent decades, so the phrasing and answers to the foregoing questions vary by time and place.

After comparing the systems of developed countries, the traveler is always asked a second question, "Which one is the best?" But in a complex and varied field like hospital finance, the analyst must ask the questioner to specify "best" for whom, according to what criteria, with what tradeoffs? The one "optimal" and "rational" hospital financing arrangement—the goal of much health financing literature—is a mirage.

Several parts of this book—particularly Chapters Six, Seven, and Eight— conclude with comprehensive lists of advantages and disadvantages of particular payment arrangements for different participants. Many chapters conclude with overviews of trends. This concluding chapter will highlight some principal generalizations about trends, countries' difficulties under certain payment arrangements, the consensus about remedies, and still unsolved disadvantages. It will not prophesy the future; many writers about health care financing eagerly impress their audiences with confident scenarios about the future, but they merely project a few current events (usually in the chronically unsettled American situation), and these prophecies are always wrong in retrospect. This chapter will not present a simple cookbook of recommendations, since the important task is to design a complete political and economic system in hospital and health care together. Every arrangement must be adapted to each country and must be capable of change. Judging from the complaints one hears from at least one important source in each country, the popular and perfect hospital payment system cannot be found at present. Even if it existed, events will strain any frozen model.

Who Should Pay? In developed countries the payers of hospital operating costs once were diverse and their limited resources curbed the hospitals' modernization. However, third-party coverage of the entire population has become virtually universal, to eliminate political protests over patients' access and over the adequacy of the hospitals' funding. Benefits are leveled upward in all developed countries, so the several third parties have nearly identical minimum coverage in the hospital.

Countries vary in the structure of third parties, in the carriers' interrelations, and in the carriers' benefits outside basic hospital care. The differences will probably persist because of the configurations among funds that evolved historically and because of the vested interests of current organizations.

If the third-party insurance mechanism never becomes universal (as in Canada) or if it becomes strained (as in Italy and Spain), government may nationalize the financing of hospital operating expenditures. But the tendency now is to try to keep the statutory insurance system solvent, because the sickness funds wish to survive and because government officials now fear the burdens of full public financing of such an insatiable sector.

Therefore, public policy is now directed at setting the payment of the third-party payers. Sickness funds and hospitals must become stabilized, while the social security taxes and general taxes must not be increased. Therefore, hospital cost containment becomes an essential part of general fiscal stabilization in health and social security, managed in each country by frequent communications among government, sickness funds, and hospital associations.[1]

National health insurance statutes create universal all-payers systems that universalize access and standardize hospital finance. Such systems can tolerate gaps in coverage only if the exempt are the richer persons, who cover themselves voluntarily and more generously. Such a substantial gap in an otherwise universal statutory system exists only in Holland, and the richer buy equivalent private coverage.

The only developed country without universal basic coverage is the United States, which attempts the same result with a mosaic of employer-financed fringe benefits, statutory insurance for the aged, public welfare for some of the poor, heterogeneous private insurance for many others, and patient cost sharing. This precarious edifice crumbled during the 1980s, and the periodic American debate over enacting typical European statutory health insurance then revived. As in all countries, an important advocate doubtless will be the hospitals, who need reliable and affluent third-party payers.

Who pays operating costs is not identical with who pays for capital. Over the last century, there has been a trend in many countries toward governmental financing of investment. Government could raise the large sums and could impose plans to help underserved regions. But the widespread crisis in public finance during the 1970s stopped the trend. Government finance officers are happy to let the hospitals borrow investment money from private markets and amortize the debt in operating costs charged to the sickness funds. If cost containment ceases to dominate hospital finance policy, the trend toward government payment of capital may resume. Health care policy makers (as distinct from the finance officers) prefer it as the essential instrument to implement plans. The hospital managers are happy to accept investment money from all sources.

How Much Money for What? The hospital payment systems described in this book fix amounts. Usually the decision has been to set the size of the per diem, although occasionally a country has adopted another unit. As the documentation and logic for fixing the rate became more elaborate, the regulators, negotiators, and payers investigated the hospital's inputs more thoroughly. The debate revolved around the hospital's prospective budget. Therefore, reimbursement analysis shifted from a unit of service to the hospital's entire budget, laying the basis for a trend toward the setting of global expenditure caps.

Rate setting has been administered to achieve several different goals: provide enough resources for appropriate hospital care, prevent waste of resources, and limit the growth of costs and strains upon the payers. These goals are quite different: the first implies substantial increases in spending; the third can result in cutbacks. But no criteria exist to fix adequate levels of resources or tolerable costs for the insurance system. When cost containment became a high priority, rate setters took the hospital's historical costs and trended them by inflation or by some other simple criterion. This merely perpetuated the status quo, even though a country might have benefited from a different distribution of resources.

More recently, many economists and some policy makers have urged that prospective budgets and unit rates be set to encourage greater "efficiency" in the hospital's use of resources and greater "effectiveness" in its clinical achievements. But the hospital's achievements are not clearly defined and calibrated, the output cannot be clearly traced to particular inputs, and the quantities of inputs and outputs cannot yet be correlated. So the regulators, negotiators, and payers use simple methods of calculating payment and utilization. They increasingly prefer global budgets and expenditure caps, enabling them to avoid detailed discussions about resources and transferring the responsibility for priorities and resource allocation to the hospital's doctors and managers.

But this is only a temporary political solution for the payers, and it provides no guidance to the providers about purposes, their relative merits, and the outcomes of different techniques. During the intellectual confusion at the time when the policy of resource growth was superseded by the opposing policy of cost containment, it became fashionable to debunk hospital care. Many health economists and government finance officers generalized that medical interventions were more wasteful than efficient, more dangerous than effective. Therefore, the population's health would improve if hospital capacity and costs were reduced. This brief vogue is now being replaced by serious research to identify the therapies and the forms of service delivery that are effective clinically, moderate in costs, and feasible for patients and doctors.[2]

The new approach enables the clinicians to reassert leadership in health care policy, to reaffirm that the chief health policy priority is improvement of health. Research in technology assessment is spreading among developed countries,[3] can provide a common meeting ground for the clinicians and finance officers, and will probably be integrated into hospital financial planning in the future. Estimating the clinical effectiveness of therapies will never become simple and actually is becoming increasingly difficult, as more of every country's hospital population are the chronically disabled elderly.

Pay to Whom? Hospital management and hospital reimbursement are locked into the traditional image of an autonomous organization. The unit is calculated for each hospital and is paid to its managers.

Every country now realizes more or less that the fragmentation among health care organizations is mistaken, particularly with the increase in chronically disabled and elderly persons. Hospitals should be connected with other organizations in a total system, so that patients can be referred back and forth wherever appropriate. The payment system should be designed for the entire network and should neither overencourage nor underencourage referrals in and out of the hospital. The payment system should provide adequate resources for the health care system within the society's priorities, but the specific treatment and referral decisions should be made by doctors and managers on professional and not pecuniary grounds.

Creating a clinically neutral payment method for an integrated health care system will reduce the problem of skewed utilization of the acute hospital. At present in every country, a very small proportion of all patients incurs at least half of all spending, particularly in hospitals. These patients, such as elderly persons with cancer, have poor prognoses.[4] Only one course of action—maximum testing and treatment—is legitimate in an acute hospital; but this may be inhumane in many cases, as well as cost-ineffective.[5] Organizing and financing a complete health care system would permit assignment of patients to the most appropriate levels.

Signs of such a reform can be seen in a few countries. The National Health Service of Great Britain manages and finances several programs in each district. Many municipal hospitals in France have acute-care, extended-care, and residential divisions, and a few are now adding home care. Government can most easily combine investment, management, and the financing of several operations, but integrated systems can be created in the private sector. Several American multi–health care corporations operate coordinated programs in the same community and offer prepaid subscriptions. In all countries government, private installations, and managers will need to plan together. And, above all, the physicians must understand and cooperate.

How to manage and finance comprehensive networks of health services (including the hospitals) is now being explored in countries with fragmented systems of organization and reimbursement.[6] The subject will doubtless be studied much more during the coming years.

Which Goals? For many years hospital reimbursement begged this part of the question. Third-party reimbursement by sickness funds or by government simply perpetuated the status quo. It was left to the hospital's clinicians and managers to define the work. The third parties automatically renewed their payments, unless patients and doctors stopped using the hospital.

But by the 1980s countries began to seek definitions of the outcomes of health care and to debate whether other sites were better than the acute-care hospital for certain results. The literature of business previously had preached "strategic planning" and "management by objectives," and these ideas entered hospital administration in several countries. During reforms of reimbursement, several countries decided that the prospective budget should no longer be screened in the light of traditional statistical guidelines but according to clinical objectives. In France and Holland, the new hospital finance laws have created a preliminary negotiation step, wherein the local sickness fund and the hospital managers discuss the clinical objectives that the prospective budget is supposed to accomplish. The new law in Germany set a new negotiating agenda between the local sickness fund and the hospital. Instead of merely arguing over the prospective budget in the light of previous spending, the negotiators are supposed to discuss the hospital's clinical objectives. The German hospital's budget is supposed to explain the reasonable costs of the required effort.

Policy makers in many countries now seek to characterize each hospital by its total objectives and to price each hospital's distinctive mix of objectives. To perform the analysis, Europeans recently have become interested in DRGs. The case mix and its costs would be used to plan the prospective budget. At present DRG methods estimate only the historical costs of treating different cases. The problem now is to recommend the most appropriate treatments of various single-diagnosis and multiple-diagnosis conditions, calculate the costs of each type of case, and then calculate the expected caseloads and budgets for each organization in a constellation.

Creating and Managing a Payment System

Paying hospitals involves conflicts of interest among organizations (hospitals, sickness funds, government agencies) and among individuals (doctors, hospital workers, insurance subscribers, taxpayers). Every payment system in a public sector in a democracy must be enacted by the legislature. To get a majority vote, to prevent any party from making enemies, and to adopt a system that can be implemented satisfactorily, every interest group must participate in the creation of the arrangement. Harmonious management of the system in practice requires periodic consultations among the interest groups. Officials of government cannot dictate any important arrangements unilaterally; if they try, the costs in trouble ultimately weaken both the government-of-the-day and the health sector.

Every developed country has learned this except the United States. American health economists and many officials imagine that if perfect formulas can be devised, they can be enacted, and all will go well. As a result, large numbers of econometric research projects are commissioned, extremely complicated procedures are enacted for the government's own programs (particularly Medicare and Medicaid), and providers (particularly the doctors) refuse to cooperate. Hospitals accept the new procedures under protest, since they must have Medicare and Medicaid business for survival, but implementation is conflict ridden and contentious. Except in the payment of hospitals in a few states, no basis is created for any harmonious all-payers system.

The voluminous American publications and policy reports about hospital finance are full of advanced calculating procedures for cost accounts, DRGs, and so on. Every country needs such instructions to guide the accountants for hospitals and payers. Outside the United States, these methods are used by hospitals and payers in developing their rival positions, and they are used by regulators in calculating rates. But these formulas are only guidelines; the final results involve adjustment among the rivals. The American literature implies that the calculating procedures automatically dictate outcomes, and it does not explain the methodologies of bilateral negotiation and of rate regulation. Trapped by this style of thinking, the United States Congress during the 1980s tried to solve its problems over Medicare by commissioning many research projects to discover the best formulas for hospital operating payment rates, hospital investment, physicians' relative values scales, and so on. Hardly any thought—and no research grants—was given to the central issues of how to construct arrangements acceptable to the hospital industry and to the medical profession, how to involve them in the operation of the payment system, how to settle disputes, and so on.

How to design and manage reimbursement is the principal European lesson for the United States. Americans have yet to grasp that paying for health care is both politics and economics. Even if the Americans still wish to avoid creating an all-payers system, they will still need to understand how a decentralized market operates in actual practice, but their health research studies theoretically "perfect" markets more often than real-life markets.

Understanding real-life interactions remains as important as ever in the more structured decision-making systems of Europe. Several now try to combine different decision-making forms in subtle new ways. For example, hospital rate regulation once was a bilateral confrontation over the prospective budget between the hospital's manager and the government's regulator. But the regulator was at a disadvantage in his understanding of each hospital. France and Holland recently have introduced an initial stage of negotiation, wherein the local sickness fund and the hospital's managers and service chiefs discuss the hospital's objectives, past performance, and future utilization. In some Canadian provinces, local consumer councils might cushion the frequently tense relations between Ministries of Health and hospitals forced to operate under strict caps. In order to avoid pressures for more subsidies, some governments encourage hospitals to revive their forgotten skills in private fund raising. Spreading the techniques of all these negotiating relationships is at least as important as teaching rules of finance.

The Limited Effects of Payment Systems

A hospital is a complex organization, with many participants, motivations, and external influences. It is fashionable to ignore this complexity and to speculate about the straightforward consequences of one or another reimbursement arrangement. But a payment system is too crude to dictate precise results.

A payment system is simply a method of delivering money to a hospital to cover the costs of its personnel and resources, with some limits to avoid waste and to protect payers.

Since payment systems can deliver money only according to general principles, they cannot be calibrated to bring about the many specific organizational and clinical goals. It is the doctors, managers, and other staff members—motivated by their professional aims—who accomplish goals. Motivating and supervising them involve more than paying them and supplying them with resources. Effective and economical work requires conscientious management, with the full participation of the medical staff. An additional trend is to involve the sickness funds in dialogues about clinical performance as well as about money alone.

Therefore, it is a delusion to try to regulate all of health care providers' behavior in great detail by finely tuned pecuniary incentives. The positive incentives that count most are professional conscience and prestige. The danger of running a loss can induce hospital managers to avoid waste. For that reason, many payers of hospitals and other health services are adopting global budgets and expenditure caps. But, on the other hand, the pursuit of cash profits cannot improve efficiency and other desirable behaviors on a large scale throughout a country's hospital industry. The medical staff will not reduce its own clinical work levels and personal incomes to provide extra cash for the hospital; statutory sickness funds and governments will not allow hospitals to earn profits over many years; managers will try to break even if savings will tempt payers and regulators to reduce their cost base.

The Challenges of Hospital Financial Management

After reading his college textbooks, the manager might look forward to a life of rational calculation, applying formulas to data. Instead, he must mediate among conflicting interests; whenever his current life is calm, he must head off future disputes. He must make judgments about resources when the alternatives are uncertain, when some choices might ultimately prove mistaken.

Conflicting demands from society have always beset hospital managers. They have always been expected to serve the needs of the unfortunate but not cost too much. For example, the managers of today can empathize with their predecessors of 1563, threatened by the Council of Trent with demotion and fines either for underservicing the public or for maintaining expensive excessive capacity.[7]

Under pressure to avoid waste during the centuries of little money, lay managers often limited clinical services. A few may have won their arguments with doctors, but were ultimately shown to have misjudged the progress of medicine.[8] As statutory health insurance and government grants pumped more money into hospitals, lay managers could avoid disputes with the increasingly prestigious doctors by satisfying their demands and passing the costs to the third parties. Then they had to cultivate skills in persuading regulators and payers. But as cost containment has again been imposed on management and as global budgeting has transferred detailed allocation decisions to the hospital staff itself, managers again have had to work out priorities with doctors. A common trend now is to organize the hospital's medical staff as an integral part of management and to make it a responsible participant in all financial decisions about programs, equipment, and operating costs. The doctors as well as the lay managers must learn new skills.

The Role of Government

Hospitals have always been part of the public sector. For many centuries they were financed and managed by private alternatives to the central government: churches, charitable associations, and philanthropists. In many countries municipal governments managed and financed many hospitals. During the twentieth century, national governments everywhere have rapidly become central actors in hospital finance. This fact is irreversible, as demonstrated by the failure of recent efforts to reprivatize hospital finance in Great Britain and the United States.

National governments became drawn into hospital finance by enacting health insurance laws to expand access, when they guaranteed generous third-party payments to hospitals, when they subsidized operating costs and investments, and when they rescued some underfinanced systems by full-scale takeovers. Since statutory health insurance is financed from social security payroll taxes and (in many countries) by additional government subsidies, every national government in recent decades has directed the containment of hospital payments by instructing regulators, negotiators, sickness funds, and hospital managers or by limiting its own grants. National and provincial governments have become more active in providing or guiding hospital investment, and they may impose more planning of facilities and services in the coming years. Events have moved quickly, the arrangements have been controversial, hospitals and doctors have complained about their losses in money and in power, and adjustments have been made. Eventually, government-hospital relations may settle down in their procedures. If developed countries become more affluent again, hospital managers and doctors will be appeased by more money. But government-hospital-doctor teamwork will have to cope with the difficult tasks of reorganizing the health services system, integrating separate organizations, and reallocating resources among regions and sectors. Government, hospital directors, and doctors will have to plan and manage together.

This trend and future requirements are no surprise to public officials, hospital managers, and medical associations in most countries. The only exception is the United States. Its national government has not enacted any mechanism for regular consultations and negotiations with the hospital industry and medical associations in deciding the ground rules and reimbursement for its own programs of Medicare and Medicaid, let alone for the entire health sector. The Americans try to set pay rates for hospitals and doctors by means of elegant calculations by civil servants and advisory commissions. One result is that most members of the American medical profession refuse to accept assignment of Medicare claims, and almost all of them refuse to practice under Medicaid. A showdown with the hospitals is postponed by their ability to survive under DRGs during the first years, but low annual "update factors" will eventually produce a crisis. Settling each year's Medicare pay rates during the 1980s is constantly chaotic: the executive branch fails to take all the advice of the study commissions, the hospitals and doctors refuse to accept the recommendations of either the officials or the commissions, the hospitals and doctors press Congress for more favorable rates in the annual government budget and in Social Security amendments, and a complicated result emerges from political logrolling. Amidst all this turmoil, the hospital planning laws have lapsed as national policy and as a program in most states.

Weary of this enervating and expensive situation, the Americans may eventually look for stable negotiation and coordination mechanisms that can avoid the waste of energy as well as the waste of money. But that will require recognition of what every other developed country has long understood: government, hospitals, and organized medicine must learn how to work together. Free markets can continue to flourish in America, but health needs its own special form of collaborative management.

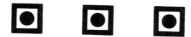

Appendix A:
Principal Countries
in this Research

This book has been written analytically and avoids country-by-country descriptions. The following pages provide a brief overview of the countries where I focused my field research, in order to orient the reader. As I said at the beginning of Chapter Thirteen, each country collects and reports even the simplest data by different formats. Therefore, the following tables are only approximations, and countries cannot be compared precisely.

I have tried to present numbers from nearly the same year. Because of lags in publication in a few countries, most statistics date from the late 1970s. Slowly the statistical reports of each country move the dates forward, but they always lag behind the current date. The patterns described in the following text remain true long after the dates of the statistics.

Basic Facts About Hospitals

Tables A-1 and A-2 give the characteristics of each country's hospitals and personnel.* While the United States is very large, several of the others are substantial too—namely, France, Germany, and England. The United States has a large number of hospitals, but so do the European countries. Their bed density exceeds America's.

Continental Europe has longer stays and higher occupancy than the United States. The Americans have greater service intensity—that is, for each

*Tables A-1 through A-6 are found on pages 401–406.

bed, shorter stays, more admissions, and higher turnover. When a country has more admissions and longer stays—as in Germany and France—it has more patient-days relative to its population. The three Anglo-Saxon countries have fewer patient-days relative to their populations because of their shorter stays.

In all countries except England, hospitals are owned by voluntary associations and local governments. Proprietary hospitals are large in number in France, Germany, and the United States, but they are small in size and handle only a fraction of the patient load.

Germany and Switzerland have more doctors than Britain and the United States. This has been the most volatile of the basic national counts: medical schools were expanded in all countries during the 1960s and 1970s, and the numbers of doctors rapidly increased during the late 1970s and 1980s. Throughout Europe the doctor/population ratios rose between 50 percent and 100 percent (varying among countries) from 1961 to 1983. In the United States, the increase was 40 percent.[1]

According to Table A-2, every country has a considerable number of nurses. But they are not fully employed. Unknown numbers are part-timers or have dropped from practice. In some countries many hospital employees do nursing work without the title.

Because hospitals are labor intensive, different levels of staffing should be the principal determinants of cross-national differences in costs. Table A-3 rank-orders the countries by employee/bed ratios and by costs per day, and the variables are highly related. (Spearman's rank correlation coefficient $r_s = 0.80$.) The spread is not as wide as one might expect, since, as I said in Chapter Ten, America's more lavish staffing is partially offset by lower wages. Compared to Europe, Canada also employs more workers and pays lower wages, but lately it has tried to reduce hospital employment.

Total Spending

Table A-4 attempts to show total expenditure in each country. (One might think such estimates are firm, but researchers disagree. For example, some think the totals for Germany and Holland are higher.[2])

While hospital spending makes important contributions to the totals in Table A-4, the two types of spending do not perfectly correlate. Distribution by service appears in Table A-5. France and Germany have high totals in large part because they spend so much on ambulatory acute care. France also spends much on extended care for the elderly. The Netherlands has a high total because of programs in caring for the elderly as well as the recent growth in acute-care hospital investment.

Countries participated unequally in the health care cost explosion that began during the 1960s and peaked during the late 1970s. Some estimates appear in Table A-6. Germany and Holland started from a low initial base and grew rapidly. Sweden and the United States were more expensive than other countries at first and continued to grow. Britain has always operated thriftily.

Overview of Organizations and Payment Systems

Following are a summary and comparison of the methods of organizing and paying hospitals in six countries studied in depth during this research.

The United States can be included in aggregate statistical counts, as in Tables A-1 through A-6, but not in simple cross-national institutional descriptions, such as the following. It cannot be included because of a central theme in this research. Every other developed country has certain general patterns in the management and finance of hospitals. But the United States has none: every payer follows different practices; every state has somewhat different ground rules.

Abbreviations in the following array:

DNA = Does not apply, since the payment system operates on different
    principles
NHI = National health insurance, rather than private insurance
NHS = National health service run by government
FTE = Full-time equivalent, when counting numbers of employees

	France	Holland	West Germany	Switzerland	Canada	Great Britain NHS
Program characteristics:						
Coverage of population	Complete under NHI Extensive for cost sharing	70% under NHI About 30% under commercial	90% under NHI About 9% under commercial	94% under various programs	Complete	Complete
Benefit coverage standard for all	Yes	Yes to those covered by NHI	Yes to those covered by NHI	Yes for basic; supplemental coverage varies	Yes	Yes
Number of payers	Very few, one principal	One or few in each area	Several in each area	In most cantons, several	One per province	One
Principal revenue source for insurance or benefits program	Payroll taxes	Payroll taxes	Subscriber and employer premiums	Subscriber premiums	General revenue in most provinces	General revenue
General Treasury payments to each hospital	No	No	No	Yes, in part	Yes, almost in full	Yes, in full
General Treasury payments to sickness funds	Begins recently	Yes	No	Yes	DNA	DNA
Out-of-pocket payments for benefits in basic package	Few	No for NHI Yes for some commercial	No for NHI Yes for commercial	Some	No	Few
Decision-making methods:						
System used	Public: budget regulation Private: negotiation with sickness funds	Rate regulation preceded by negotiation with sickness funds	Negotiation with sickness funds	Mixture in each canton	Government grants	Legislation and administration
Where regulation is used:						
Source of guidelines	National government	National government; commissions	Provincial government	Cantonal government	DNA	DNA
Rates fixed by	Local civil servants representing national government	Autonomous commission	Arbitration panel, if negotiations fail	Cantonal Ministry of Health	DNA	DNA
Control over regulatory system	Elected government	Elected government and interest groups	DNA	Elected government	DNA	DNA
Some hospitals exempt in practice	No	No	DNA	Very few	DNA	DNA
Hospital association represented in approval of guidelines	No	Yes	Yes	No in most cantons Yes in a few	DNA	DNA

	Col 1	Col 2	Col 3	Col 4	Col 5	Col 6
Public authority discusses rates or grants with hospital before final award	Yes	Yes	DNA	Yes	Yes in most provinces No in Ontario	DNA
Where government grants hospital part or all its budget:						
Level of government	DNA	DNA	DNA	Province	Province	Regional subdivision of national government
Source of money	DNA	DNA	DNA	General revenue	General revenue; a few premium systems	General revenue
Appeals procedure	External	External	None	None	Internal	None
Form of review by public authority:						
Prospective review of budget	Line-by-line	Line-by-line	DNA	Line-by-line	Once line-by-line; trend toward general categories or global	Global, general categories
Retrospective monitoring	Line-by-line	Line-by-line	DNA	Line-by-line	Mixed	Line-by-line
Payers coordinate with investment planners	CRAM, a little	No	No	Yes, where cantonal government	Yes, identical	Yes, identical
Regulators coordinate with investment planners	DDASS, a little	No	No	Yes, where cantonal government	Yes, identical	Yes, identical
Wage rates decided by	Public: national civil service	Nationwide collective bargaining	Public: national civil service Nonpublic: nationwide collective bargaining	Cantonal civil service governs many	Individual bargaining in some provinces; province-wide elsewhere	Nationwide collective bargaining for workers; government commission for nurses
Public authority (regulators or grantors) approve new hiring by hospital	Only general ceilings	Bed/FTE guideline	DNA	Specific approvals in some cantons	Bed/FTE guideline in some provinces	Only general ceilings
Payment method:						
Basic unit	Public: budget Private: daily rate, some items	Daily rate that generates a budget	Daily rate	Daily rate plus budget	Budget	Budget
Differentiated by:						
Type of service	No	No	A few	No	No	No
Type of patient	No	No	No	No	No	No
Orientation	Prospective	Prospective	Prospective	Prospective	Prospective	Prospective

	France	Holland	West Germany	Switzerland	Canada	Great Britain NHS
Base of payment	Public: cost / Private: charge	Cost	Cost	Cost	Cost, limited by government's financial ability	Hospital's programmatic needs, limited by government's financial ability
Additional charges for items	Public: No / Private: Yes	Some hospitals	No	Yes for a few private hospitals	No	No
Hospital can choose among alternative formulas or rates	No	No	No	No	No	No
Annual increase:						
Automatic across-board, in %	No	Yes	No	No	Some provinces	No
Individualized, according to budget	Yes	Special applications	Yes	All	Some provinces	Yes, according to government's judgment of hospital's programmatic needs
Regulation extends to private room rates	Yes	Yes	No	No	Yes	Yes
Uniformity or variations:						
Price discrimination among insured persons	Not in same hospital	Not in same hospital	Not in same hospital	No	DNA	DNA
Different hospital systems with different payment methods	Yes, public-private	No	No, but diverse owners	No, but diverse owners	No	No
Self-payer same as insured	Yes	Yes	Yes	Yes	No	No
Regional variations in the system	None	None	Provincial	Treasury share varies by province	Provincial	Regional and local administrative units
Allowable costs vary by program	No	NHI: no / Private: some	No	No	DNA	DNA
Difference between acute and chronic	Yes	Not in same hospitals / Yes in different hospitals	No	Yes	Yes	Yes
Out-of-jurisdiction patients pay more	No	No	No	Yes	No	No
Cross-subsidization among services	Public: DNA, global budget / Private: yes	DNA, one hospital-wide rate	Yes	DNA, one hospital-wide rate	DNA, global budget	DNA, global budget

Hospitals free to charge private patients without limit	Public: no / Private: yes	Yes	Yes, in theory	Yes, in theory	No	No
Costs allowable in payment to hospital:						
Purchase and financing of building	Yes	Yes	No	No	No	No
Purchase of equipment	Yes	Yes	Only minor	Varies by canton	Only minor	Only minor
Depreciation	Yes	Yes	No	Usually no	No	No
Interest charges	Yes	Yes	Yes	Usually no	No	No
Last year's deficit	Public: yes / Private: rarely	No	No	No	No	No
Doctors' earnings	Public: yes / Private: no	No	Yes, salaries	Some yes, some no	No	No
Educational costs for:						
Doctors	Yes	Mixed	No	Only some	Yes	Yes
Nurses	Yes	Yes	Yes	Only some	Yes	Yes
Wage pass-through	Public: yes / Private: no	Yes	Yes	Yes	Usually yes	Yes
Bad debts	No	No	No	No	Yes	No
Outpatient costs	Public: some / Private: no	No	Yes	Yes, under subsidy by canton	Yes	Yes
Constraint on utilization as part of the award	Public: yes, but not systematic / Private: no	No	No	No	Some provinces yes, some no	Yes, because of cash limits
Cost sharing by patient	Public: yes, part of charge / Private: yes, in addition to official charge	NHI: no / Privately insured: yes	NHI: no / Privately insured: yes	Yes	No	No
Reporting and accounting:						
Uniform internal hospital accounts	Yes	No	Yes	Yes	Yes	Yes
Uniform report to regulators or grantors	Yes	Yes	Yes	Yes	Yes	Yes
Are the foregoing two the same	Yes	No	No	Yes	No	Yes

	France	Holland	West Germany	Switzerland	Canada	Great Britain NHS
Nationwide uniformity in:						
Internal hospital accounts	Yes	No	Yes	Yes	Yes	Yes
Report to regulators or grantors	Yes	Yes	Yes	No	No	Yes
External expenditures audit is reviewed by regulator or grantor	Yes	No	Yes	Yes	Yes	Yes
Regulator or grantor prescribes and examines carefully reports on:						
Interim expenditures	No	No	No	Yes, in many cantons	Yes, in many provinces	Yes
End-of-year expenditures	No	No	No	Yes	Yes	Yes
Reporting by clinical department	Yes	Yes	No	Yes	No	No
Cash flow:						
Handling of patient cost sharing	Separate billing by hospital	NHI: DNA Private: cash benefits system in theory	NHI: DNA Private: cash benefits system in theory	Collected by sickness fund	DNA	NHS: DNA Private: separate billing by hospital
Administrative costs of billing:						
For sickness fund	Low	Some	Some	Some	Almost none	NHS: some
For hospital	Low	Low	Low	Some	Almost none	Almost none
Speed of payment	Automatic installments	Quick	Quick	Quick	Automatic installments	Automatic installments
Medical staffs organized to participate in financial decision in each hospital	Yes	No	Yes	Some	No	No
A "profit" can be retained by	Public: no Private: yes	Occasionally	Yes	No	No	No

Table A-1. Characteristics of Countries.

	France	Holland	West Germany	Switzerland	Canada	England	United States
Population (est.)	52,920,000	13,853,000	61,396,000	6,327,000	23,316,000	46,350,000	216,383,000
Year of data	1976	1976	1977	1976	1976	1977	1977
General (acute hospitals)							
Total number	3,030	238	2,185	214	894	922	6,322
Owned by government	524	27	897	113	888	797	2,212
Private nonprofit	337	211	877	82		125	3,335
Private for-profit	1,305	0	411	19	6		775
Beds per 10,000 pop.	57.1	51.1	79.5	57.6	54.4	37.5	49.5
Admissions per 10,000 pop.	1,677.4	1,071.1	1,511.0	1,119.8	1,577.5	1,041.0	1,672.4
Admissions per bed	20.7	21.0	19.0	19.5	29.0	27.8	33.8
Morbidity (patient-days per 10,000 pop.)	2.35	1.52	2.14	1.61	1.50	1.15	1.34
Occupancy, in %	79.6	84.4	82.6	76.2	76.2	72.0	73.7
Average length of stay in days	14.0	15.3	15.7	14.3	9.6	9.5	8.0
All hospitals							
Total number	3,566	772	3,416	474	1,389	2,250	7,234
Owned by government	1,035		1,258	199	1,299	2,125	2,641
Private nonprofit	772		1,141	207		1,228	3,618
Private for-profit	1,722	0	1,017	68	90		975
Beds per 10,000 pop.							
Owned by government	68.3	123.6	61.9	71.4	84.6	82.7	25.9
Private nonprofit	13.4		41.5	34.7			32.8
Private for-profit	20.2	0	14.3	8.5	17.9	7.2	1.9
Admissions per 10,000 pop.							
Owned by government	1,125.9	1,135.0	922.9	856.5	1,659.2	1,153.0	268.2
Private nonprofit	163.2		631.8	416.2			1,135.8
Private for-profit	516.3	0	155.9	119.8	96.3		143.5

Notes: Blank spaces mean that the data were not separately run for those categories. Some categories are combined in the data files in some countries. For example, Holland has so few governmentally owned hospitals that the data are always merged with the voluntary hospitals'; England has so few private hospitals that the nonprofits and for-profits are always combined.

Data in Canada always combine hospitals, regardless of ownership. After a search in directories, I identified 338 general hospitals with 30,406 beds owned by municipal, provincial, and national governments; 510 general hospitals with 94,389 beds were owned by religious groups and voluntary associations.

Data are for England alone and do not include Scotland, Wales, or Northern Ireland.

Sources: My calculations from statistical publications in each country. Many of them are cited and the information reproduced in *World Health Statistics Annual* (Geneva: World Health Organization, 1980, 1983).

Table A-2. Number of Doctors and Nurses.

	France	Holland	West Germany	Switzerland	Canada	England and Wales	United States
Population	52,890,000	13,853,000	61,396,000	6,327,000	23,316,000	49,119,000	215,118,000
Year of data	1976	1977	1977	1977	1977	1977	1976
Doctors							
Total number	83,306	23,769	125,174	12,715	41,398	74,500	361,443
Population per doctor	613	583	490	498	563	659	595
Doctors per 10,000 people	16.3	17.2	20.4	20.1	17.8	15.2	16.8
Nurses and midwives							
Total numbers							
Qualified	221,955	33,826	196,833	25,600	140,000	145,393	961,000
Assistant, practical	90,720	18,150	45,079	4,400	41,000	59,380	489,000
Population per nurse	165	267	254	211	125	240	148
Nurses per 10,000 people	55.1	37.5	39.4	47.4	77.6	41.7	67.4

Note: The nurses in Britain are only those employed by the National Health Service.
Source: World Health Statistics Annual (Geneva: World Health Organization, 1980, 1983).

Table A-3. Comparisons in Staffing and Costs.

| Country | Hospital employees per 100 beds | Cost per patient-day | | Year of data |
		In original currency	Converted to U.S. $	
U.S.A.	237.5	$194.34	$194.34	1978
Canada	206.6	$147.92	$131.60	1978
Switzerland	184.5	Fr 266.85	$144.24	1978
Netherlands	155.2	312.01 fl	$139.91	1978
France	between 116.5 and 187.1	between 378.2 F and 620.1 F	between $84.04 and $137.80	1978
West Germany	73.1	168.52 DM	$81.41	1978

Notes: All data are for acute general hospitals. Because of their open-staff structures, American and Canadian personnel figures do not include the many attending physicians.

French acute hospitals manage extended care facilities and homes for the elderly, and many data are combined. It is not possible to isolate personnel data and total patient care costs for the entire country for the acute hospitals alone. The employees per 100 beds are 116.5 if all beds are counted in the denominator of the fraction, and 187.1 if only the acute and long-stay beds are counted. The cost per patient-day is 378.2 F if all patient-days are counted (including the homes for the elderly) in the denominator of the fraction, and 620.1 F if they are not included.

Except for the medical, nursing, and technical employees, personnel data cannot be isolated for acute hospitals in England. The many ancillary workers are assigned to all the services in the District Health Authority.

Sources: My calculations from the following:

United States: *Hospital Statistics: 1979 Edition* (Chicago: American Hospital Association, 1979).

Canada: Unpublished data from the Institutional Statistics Section, Health Division, Statistics Canada. All public general and allied special hospitals. To estimate number of FTEs, I have counted all the full-timers and have counted each part-timer as if he were half-time.

Switzerland: *Jahresbericht 1979* (Aarau: Vereinigung Schweitzerischer Kranken-häuser, 1980).

Netherlands: *Statistiek personeelssterkte 1978* and *Financiële statistiek 1978* (Utrecht: Nationaal Ziekenhuisinstituut, 1979).

France: Danielle Douxami, "Statistique annuelle des hôpitaux généraux publics de France métropolitaine," *Santé, Sécurité Sociale: Statistiques et commentaires,* No. 5 (Sept.–Oct. 1979), esp. pp. 137–142; and M. Duriez, *La consommation médicale finale 1979: Evaluations provisoires* (Paris: Centre de Recherche pour l'Etude et l'Observation des Conditions de Vie, 1980), esp. pp. 5 and 12.

West Germany: Bundesminister für Jugend, Familie und Gesundheit, *Daten des Gesundheitswesens* (Stuttgart: W. Kohlhammer, 1980), pp. 233, 249, 272.

Conversion into U.S. dollars at the free-market exchange rates prevailing at the end of June 1978. $1 (US) = $1.24 (Canadian) = 1.85 Fr S = 2.23 fl = 4.50 F = 2.07 DM. Source: *Pick's Currency Yearbook 1977–1979* (New York: Pick Publishing Company, 1981).

Table A-4. Total Expenditures for Health in 1982.

Country	US $ per head	Percentage of GDP
United States	1,388	10.6
Sweden	1,239	9.7
France	996	9.3
Netherlands	851	8.7
West Germany	883	8.2
Canada	1,058	8.2
Switzerland	990	7.8
United Kingdom	539	5.9

Source: Jean-Pierre Poullier, *Measuring Health Care, 1960–1983* (Paris: Organisation for Economic Co-operation and Development, 1985), Tables 1 and 2.

Table A-5. Total Health Care Spending by Service.

Country	Sweden	West Germany	United States	Switzerland	Netherlands	Canada	France	United Kingdom
Year	1975	1975	FY 1974–75	1975	1974	1975	1975	FY 1974–75
Hospitals	71.5%	35.0%	50.4%	44.9%	52.6%	59.0%	38.0%	62.8%
Primary and specialist care	24.6	30.2	40.0	41.0	41.9	27.6	44.5	21.3
Self-medication	3.5	4.5		5.0	?	4.5	3.8	3.2
Other (public health, research, education, etc.)	0.4	24.3	4.9	9.1	1.1	7.2	4.4	11.8
Administration	0.4	6.0	4.7	?	4.4	1.7	9.3	0.9
Total	100.0%	100.0%	100.0%	100.0%	100.0%	100.0%	100.0%	100.0%

Source: Robert J. Maxwell, *Health and Wealth* (Lexington, Mass.: Lexington Books, 1981), p. 83.

Table A-6. Average Annual Increases in Total Health Spending, 1960–1976.

Country	Actual	CPI	Relative
Sweden	14.42	6.21	2.32
West Germany	14.45	3.81	3.80
United States	10.80	4.21	2.57
Netherlands	17.35	5.80	2.99
Canada	12.18	4.46	2.73
France	14.84	5.89	2.52
United Kingdom	13.00	7.63	1.70

Source: Average annual increases in actual expenditures and in consumer prices from Joseph G. Simanis and John R. Coleman, "Health Care Expenditures in Nine Industrialized Countries, 1960–76," *Social Security Bulletin,* Vol. 43, No. 1 (Jan. 1980), p. 6. I calculated the "relative price effect" by dividing CPI into actual expenditures. The statistic shows the increase in health spending beyond the country's general inflation rate.

Publications

Following are the books that present basic descriptions of each country's health services in general and hospitals in particular:

All Countries

Report on the World Health Situation (Geneva: World Health Organization, quadrennial).

Each European Country

Alan Maynard, *Health Care in the European Community* (London: Croom Helm, 1975; a second edition is in preparation).

Brian Abel-Smith (ed.), *Eurocare* (Basel: Health Service Consultants, 1984).

Gordon McLachlan and Alan Maynard (eds.), *The Public/Private Mix for Health* (London: Nuffield Provincial Hospitals Trust, 1962).

Jan Blanpain and others, *National Health Insurance and Health Resources* (Cambridge, Mass.: Harvard University Press, 1978).

Norbert Paquel and others, *Le coût de l'hospitalisation: Comparaisons internationales* (Paris: Documents du Centre d'Etude des Revenus et des Coûts, 1979).

France

Economic Models Ltd., *The French Health Care System* (Chicago: American Medical Association, 1976).

Ministère des Affaires Sociales et de la Solidarité Nationale, *La santé en France* (Paris: La Documentation Française, 1985).

Jean-Marie Clément, *L'hôpital* (Paris: Berger-Levrault, 1983).

West Germany

Romuald Schicke, *Soziale Sicherung und Gesundheitswesen* (Stuttgart: W. Kohlhammer Verlag, 1978).

Statistisches Bundesamt, *Die Struktur der Ausgaben im Gesundsheitsbereich und ihre Entwicklung seit 1970* (Bonn: Bundesminister für Arbeit und Sozialordnung, 1978).

Donald W. Light and Alexander Schuller (eds.), *Political Values and Health Care: The German Experience* (Cambridge, Mass.: MIT Press, 1986).

Netherlands

J. M. Boot and M. H. J. M. Knapen, *De Nederlandse gezondheids* (Utrecht: Uitgeverij Het Spectrum, 1983).

A. Th. L. M. Mertens, *In goede handen: De Nederlandse gezondheidszorg* (Leiden: Spruyt, Van Mantgem & Does, 1981).

Switzerland

Pierre Gygi and Heiner Henny, *Das schweizerische Gesundheitswesen,* 2nd ed. (Bern: Verlag Hans Huber, 1977). The tables are updated periodically.

United Kingdom

Ruth Levitt and Andrew Wall, *The Reorganised National Health Service,* 3rd ed. (London: Croom Helm, 1984).

Royal Commission on the National Health Service, *Report* (London: Her Majesty's Stationery Office, 1979).

Department of Health and Social Security, *Health Care and Its Costs* (London: Her Majesty's Stationery Office, 1983).

Canada

Lee Soderstrom, *The Canadian Health System* (London: Croom Helm, 1978).

Robert G. Evans, *Strained Mercy: The Economics of Canadian Health Care* (Toronto: Butterworths, 1984).

United States

Steven Jonas (ed.), *Health Care Delivery in the United States,* 3rd ed. (New York: Springer, 1986).

Florence A. Wilson and Duncan Neuhauser, *Health Services in the United States* (Cambridge, Mass.: Ballinger, 1982).

Appendix B:
Principal Informants

I am deeply indebted to the following persons, who granted at least one hour in interviews. In addition, there were many others who provided invaluable information in shorter discussions.

Fieldwork about hospitals alone was concentrated into two or three consecutive months for each country. Additional interviews for this project were spread over several years, during my visits for other research, as well as this one.

France

Paris, Government of France. Claude Ameline, Mme Bellegarde, Mme Chaix, Mr. Choisselet, Mme Conrad-Bruat, Danielle Douxami, Daniel Gautier, Claude Girbon, Patrick Hermange, Jean de Kervasdoué, Gérard Moine, Ph. Grenier de Monner, O. Rateau, Claude Renou, Jean-Marie Rodrigues, Mme Tatout, Patrick Terroir, Jean-Claud Veysseix.

Paris, Assistance Publique. Mme Angelin, J. C. Gorra, Alain Grenon, Jean Hue, Marc Kerebel, Jean-François Lacronique, Marc Lorey, Béatrice Majnoni d'Intignano, Jean Rougemont, Jean-Marc Simon.

Paris and Vicinity, Other. M. Bouak, Robert F. Bridgman, R. Cappe, Antoinette Catrice-Lorey, Patrice Legrand, François Meillier, Arié Mizrahi, Michel Moujart, A. Rauch, Simone Sandier.

Lyons, Dijon, and Beaune. Pierre Barbier, André Bellis, Georges Camus, Marcel Chovet, Henriette Deslorieux, Marc Dubulle, Mr. Geffroy, Frédéric Guilloux, M. R. Lengagne, Mr. Mano, Jacques Menard, Odette Mingoutaud, Maurice Rochaix.

West Germany

Bonn. Ulrich Geissler, Gunnar Griesewell, Herbert Harsdorf, Gerhard Konow, Thea Krämer, Hans-Jürgen Maass, Wolfgang Nüsche, Hans Stein, Eberhard Thiel, Walter Thürk, Rudolf Vollmer, Axel Weber, Eckhardt Westphal.

Düsseldorf. Jürgen Abshoff, Siegfried Eichhorn, Maria Gehrt, Wolfgang Holz, Heinz Hübner, Rolf Klingenhagen, Karl Jeute, Hans-Dietmar Laas, Hubertus Müller, Udo Müller, Willi Quadt, Mr. Schiffers, H. G. Schmidt-Jensen, Paul Swertz.

Cologne. Günther Aumüller, Gerhard Brenner, Schwester Claresia of the Genossenschaft der Armen Dienstmägde Jesu Christi, Wally Esch, Hans-Günther Krautwald, Wilhelm Lempken, Mr. Müller, Thea Münsch, F. W. Schwartz, Hans Trawinski.

Hanover. Ernst Bruckenberger, Joachim Gäde, Heinz Glünder, Klaus-Dirk Henke, Herwig Matthes, Romuald Schicke, Martin Zeymer.

Elsewhere. Christa Altenstetter, Joachim Baumgarten, Fritz Beske, Wilfried Bolles, Christian von Ferber, Hartmut Krukemeyer, Heinz Laufer, Nikolaus Lobkowicz, Alex Mennicken, Heinz Naegler, Fritz Schnabel, Theo Thiemeyer, Hans-Werner Wachtel.

Netherlands

Utrecht. Josef H. van Aert, Jan van Amstel, D. Blanken, A. Brouwer, E. H. Brouwer, G. J. de Cock, R. A. M. Dorresteijn, C. Elich, H. J. Hannessen, Luuk Huiskes, C. Kleemans, E. J. van Kooten Niekerk, H. J. Lammers, J. A. Machielsen, D. van der Meer, A. P. W. P. van Montfort, Jan J. Onnes, W. G. van der Putten, A. T. T. Rosendaal, A. Sliedrecht, W. Slobbe, P. M. W. Starmans, S. Verbeek, H. van Vondel, I. Th. van der Vos, J. de Waard, Th. J. Weterman, H. H. M. Willems.

The Hague. J. J. Baaij, Roger H. Bakker, J. van Dijk, Chiel Huffmeijer, Frank Mauta, J. Steuer, Dane Wagenaar, F. V. J. M. Werner, E. Wiebenga.

Amsterdam and Amstelveen. J. J. de Bruijn, C. Dalmeyer-Henneke, C. W. A. van den Dool, H. A. Faas, R. H. M. Hendriks, Th. R. Himlopen, A. J. Klip, S. Koopal, E. Lammerts van Bueren, H. Ris, W. A. Roschar, Carel Jan Royer, Adolf H. Wiebenga.

Elsewhere. G. W. J. Bol, L. M. J. Groot, Andries Querido, J. Wolf.

Switzerland

Bern. Danielle Bridel, Werner Frischknecht, Alfred J. Gebert, Martin Gienel, Rudolf Gilli, Carlo Graf, J. H. Häfliger, Heiner Henny, Dr. Hoffman of Schweiz Rotes Kreuz, Roger Kübler, Jürg Lehmann, Roland Löffel, Ulrich Naef, Rudolf Oester, Hans Ott, Erhard Ramseier, Pierre-M. Vallon, Max Zürcher.

Aarau. Hermann Engler, Peter Hess, A. Küster, Hans-Christoph Reinhard, Erhard Trommsdorf.

Zürich. Markus Bächi, György J. Csihák, Gerhard Kocher, H. Langmack, Ernest Menzi, M. Peter, Hermann Plüss, Hans Rathgeb, Hansruedi Schudel, Paul Stiefel, Wilhelm Wohlgemuth.

Elsewhere. Elie Benmoussa, Ervin Gregor, Ulrich Raeber, Jean-Paul Robert, Daniel Schmutz, Josef Schurtenberger, Edwin von Büren.

Great Britain

London, Department of Health and Social Security. Patricia W. Annesley, Anthony J. Anstey, George Brechin, Joan Firth, V. J. Green, Douglas Harris, Gordon Harris, Malcolm A. Harris, John James, Edwin Ko, J. F. Mann, John Middleton, Jill Moore, C. J. Nickless, Michael A. Parsonage, Stephen Thorpe-Tracy, John Vaughan, Robert Weeden, Michael L. Whippman, Don White.

London, H. M. Treasury. John Caff, Anthony J. Goldman, Michael Prescott, Michael Spackman.

London, National Health Service. Glyn Barnes, Michael Bellamy, Anthony Foster, D. Joines, Dennis Jones, Edwin Linehan, Don Russell, Alvin Stockmarr.

London, Other. Brian Abel-Smith, R. Gwyn Bevan, W. F. Eales, Susan Ellen, Robert L. Jones, Michael Lee, Robert Maxwell, Gordon McLachlan, Simon N. G. Patterson, Hugh Sanderson, George Teeling-Smith, Peter West, Iden Wickings.

Elsewhere. Frank Burns, T. E. Chester, George Cree, Stuart Dimmock, John Dodd, James S. Fishwick, Katharine Fussell, Sidney Hampshire, Colin Hayton, Anne Ludbrook, K. S. Morris, Robin Pearson, John W. Stewart, David Wooff.

Canada

Ottawa. Robert Armstrong, Paul Brown, Louis de G. Fournier, A. Thurlow Frazier, Cyril M. MacKay, Donald C. MacNaught, Jean-Claude Martin, William Mennie, David Stewart.

Quebec. Pierre Bergeron, Marc Boucher, Thomas J. Boudreau, Maurice Crépin, Robert Dallaire, Roland Dubois, Craig Gauthier, Charles E. Germain, Fernand Hould, Victorin B. Laurin, Sidney Lee, Pierre P. Mercier, Fernand Picard, Anton Torunian, Alain Tremblay.

Ontario. F. W. Carvel, William Lindsay Clark, Jack Cooper, Stephen Dreezer, Herbert F. Eichler, Douglas Enright, Robert E. Foster, George Hamilton, Lawrence Kaplan, James A. Kendree, Ron Leneveu, Frank Markel, Anne Murray, J. B. S. Rose, Glen Siegel, Malcolm Taylor, Jack Timpson, Erwin Waschnig.

British Columbia. D. A. Belton, John J. Benham, J. Duncan Bradford, James Burslem, Walter Dietiker, Gerry Fisher, R. W. Foreman, Al C. Laugharne, William John Lyle, Eric O'Dell, L. E. Ranta, W. E. Selwood, Earl Snook, Bryan Stoodley, Eugene Tomasky, G. O. Hughes Waitt, Fred Worthington.

Elsewhere. Robert W. M. Boyd, Gary Cox, G. H. Loewen, A. H. McLean, Charles D. Porter, Lorne E. Rozofsky.

United States

Washington, D.C. Gerard Anderson, Thomas Antone, Katharine G. Bauer, Sheila Burke, Gerald Connor, Jay Constantine, Robert Froehlke, Paul

Ginsburg, Warren Greenberg, Robert Hoyer, David C. Main, Glenn Markus, Paul Rettig, James Vertrees.

New York. Anthony Heckel, Lou Imhoff, Henry Karpe, John Lovett, Norman Metzger, Stanley Peck, Paul Selbst, Steven Sieverts, Joseph Terenzio, Jerry Trask.

New Jersey. Joanne Finley, Donald Heil, James Hub, John Reiss, Bruce Vladeck.

Elsewhere. Mark Albertz, Allen Antisdel, Francis Baker, Mary Bensen, David Bertke, Paul Bliss, Warren Falberg, Thomas Johnson, James Kelly, Alexander McMahon, Walter McNerney, Eugene Ott, James Sammons, Carl J. Schramm.

Other Countries, International Organizations

Per Carlsson, Luc Delesie, Miles Hardie, Goran Hedsund, Emile P. Mach, P. Owe Petersson, Jean-Pierre Poullier.

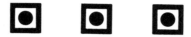

Notes

Chapter One

1. Data about hospital spending in many countries earlier during the 1970s appear in Robert J. Maxwell, *Health and Wealth* (Lexington, Mass.: Lexington Books, 1981), pp. 82–86; and Norbert Paquel and others, *Le coût de l'hospitalisation: Comparaisons internationales* (Paris: Documents du Centre d'Etude des Revenus et des Coûts, 1979).

2. Hospital costs are the biggest component in the rise of health care costs in every country, according to G. Janssen, *Report of Cost Evolution, Financing of Health Insurance and Measures with a View to Curbing Costs* (Geneva: Association Internationale de la Mutualité, 1981), pp. 6–7. For time series of hospital and other health data back to the early 1960s, see John R. Coleman and Joseph G. Simanis, "Rising Health Care Costs: A World Problem," *Appalachian Business Review*, No. 3 (1979), p. 8; Jean-Pierre Poullier, *Public Expenditure on Health Under Economic Constraints* (Paris: Organisation for Economic Co-operation and Development, 1984), Part 2; and unpublished data from the Health Industries Department, SRI International, Menlo Park, Calif.

3. *Paying the Doctor* (Baltimore and London: Johns Hopkins University Press, 1970) and *Health Insurance Bargaining* (New York: Gardner Press and Wiley, 1978).

4. For discussions of current statistical practices, along with recommendations for standardized formats, see Alain Foulon, *Les dépenses de santé dans les comptes nationaux du S.E.C.* (Paris: Centre de Recherche pour l'Etude et l'Observation des Conditions de Vie, 1979); and Francis H. Roger, *The Minimum Basic Data Set for Hospital Statistics in the EEC* (Luxembourg: Commission of the European Communities, 1981).

5. Some of the difficulties are mentioned in John Deering's review of Robert Maxwell's book on comparative health statistics, *Health Affairs*

(published by Project HOPE), Vol. 1, No. 1 (Winter 1981), pp. 107–111. In countries that have developed advanced and expensive statistical systems, imperfections underlie the most basic facts. For a comparison of the varying reliability of methods for collecting American utilization data, see James Lubitz, "Different Data Systems, Different Conclusions? Comparing Hospital Use Data for the Aged from Four Data Systems," *Health Care Financing Review,* Vol. 2, No. 4 (Spring 1981), pp. 41–60. Economists analyzing the same data set may get conflicting results, as in Ellen Pryga, "Hospice Care Under Medicare" (Chicago: Office of Public Policy Analysis, American Hospital Association, 1983), pp. 14–15 and p. 10 of the Appendix; and J. R. Ashford, "Is There Still a Place for Independent Research into Public Policy in England and Wales in the 1980's? A Case Study from the Field of Health Care: Modelling Hospital Costs," *Journal of Operational Research,* Vol. 32 (1981), pp. 851–864. Any cross-national comparisons of utilization must be corrected for subtle variations in recording, such as those discovered in Lola Jean Kozak and others, "The Status of Hospital Discharge Data in Six Countries," in *Vital and Health Statistics,* Series 2, No. 80 (Washington, D.C.: National Center for Health Statistics, 1980).

6. The CERC report (cited in note 1, above) repeatedly discusses whether statistical differences among countries reflect reality or are artifacts of statistical methods. For example, page 66 contains two different estimates of proportions of GNP spent on health among OECD countries, resulting from the statistical methods of the reporting agencies. The two most laborious comparative analyses of health financial data often made different estimates of the same facts; contrast Maxwell (note 1, above) and Poullier (note 2, above).

7. William Glaser, *Paying the Hospital: Foreign Lessons for the United States* (New York: Center for the Social Sciences, Columbia University, 1982; a report for the Health Care Financing Administration, U.S. Department of Health and Human Services, available from the National Technical Information Service, Springfield, Va.). Summarized in Glaser, "Paying the Hospital: Foreign Lessons for the United States," *Health Care Financing Review,* Vol. 4, No. 4 (Summer 1983), pp. 99–110; and in Glaser, "American Health Care Problems and Foreign Solutions," in *International Perspective on Health Care: Learning from Other Nations—Hearing Before the Select Committee on Aging, House of Representatives, 98th Congress, 2d Session* (Washington, D.C.: U.S. Government Printing Office, 1984), pp. 7–16. In *Health Insurance Bargaining: Foreign Lessons for Americans* (New York: Gardner Press and Wiley, 1978), Appendix A, I have described how to derive policy lessons from cross-national research. Lessons from other countries have startled Americans and Europeans in other fields where competition has serious effects; note the attention attracted by Ezra Vogel's *Japan as No. 1: Lessons for America* (Cambridge, Mass.: Harvard University Press, 1979).

8. Such field research about the organization and work of government agencies and high-level public organizations has become common. See, for example, Robert Bendiner, *Obstacle Course on Capitol Hill* (New York: McGraw-Hill, 1964); Eugene Eidenberg and Roy D. Morey, *An Act of Congress: The Legislative Process and the Making of Education Policy* (New York: Norton, 1969); Hugh Heclo and Aaron Wildavsky, *The Private Government of Public Money: Community and Policy Inside British Political Administration* (Berkeley:

University of California Press, 1974). Only one textbook has been written about the methodology: Lewis Anthony Dexter, *Elite and Specialized Interviewing* (Evanston, Ill.: Northwestern University Press, 1970).

9. My previous work about hospitals has been published in various books and journals. See esp. *Social Settings and Medical Organization: A Cross-National Study of the Hospital* (New York: Lieber-Atherton, 1970) and "American and Foreign Hospitals: Some Sociological Comparisons," in Eliot Freidson (ed.), *The Hospital in Modern Society* (New York: Free Press, 1963), Chap. 2.

10. William Glaser, "Internship Appointments of Medical Students," *Administrative Science Quarterly*, Vol. 4, No. 3 (Dec. 1959), pp. 337–356; William Glaser and Frances A. McVey, "Effects of Public Health Field Practice upon Career Preferences and Career Plans," *Nursing Research*, Vol. 14 (Winter 1965), pp. 61–66; and other articles and books.

11. See, for example, *Paying the Doctor* (note 3, above), *Health Insurance Bargaining* (note 7, above), and *Federalism in Canada and West Germany* (New York: Center for the Social Sciences, Columbia University, 1979; distributed by the National Technical Information Service, Springfield, Va.).

Chapter Two

1. See, for example, the attempted typologies in Robert F. Bridgman and Milton I. Roemer, *Hospital Legislation and Hospital Systems* (Geneva: World Health Organization, 1973).

2. Henri Anrys and others, *Les hôpitaux dans le Marché Commun* (Brussels: Maison Larcier, 1977); the comparative manual of terminology by the Hospital Committee of the European Economic Community, *Hospitals in the EEC* (Lochem, Netherlands: Uitgeversmaatschappij de Tijdstroom, 1978); and unpublished papers from the Workshop on Hospital Finance Systems, conducted by the Regional Office for Europe, World Health Organization, 1984.

3. See, for example, Paul Quaethoven, *Het statuut van de ziekenhuisge-neesheer in de lid-staten van de Europese Economische Gemeenschap* (Leuven, Belgium: School voor Maatschappelijke Gezondheidszorg, Katholieke Universiteit Leuven, 1969).

4. The history of the British hospital system is described in Brian Abel-Smith, *The Hospitals, 1800–1948* (London: Heinemann, 1964).

5. The history of the French hospital system is described in Jean Imbert and others, *Histoire des hôpitaux en France* (Toulouse: Editions Privat, 1982).

6. The rise and decline of private hospitals owned by doctors are summarized in William Glaser, "For-Profit Hospitals: American and Foreign Comparisons," *Health Care Management Review*, Vol. 9, No. 4 (Fall 1984), pp. 27–34.

7. Ekaterini Siafaca, *Investor-Owned Hospitals and Their Role in the Changing U.S. Health Care Systems* (New York: F & S Press, 1981).

8. Montague Brown and Howard L. Lewis, *Hospital Management Systems* (Rockville, Md.: Aspen Publishers, 1976); Montague Brown and Barbara P. McCool (eds.), *Multihospital Systems* (Rockville, Md.: Aspen Publishers, 1980).

9. "Corporate Reorganization," *Topics in Health Care Financing,* Vol. 11, No. 1 (Fall 1984); Samuel J. Tibbitts, "Future Belongs to New Multihealth Corporations—Hospitals Should Join Now," *Modern Healthcare,* Vol. 14, No. 12 (Sept. 1984), pp. 203, 206, 208, 211.

10. See, for example, Simone Sandier, *Comparison of Health Expenditures in France and the United States, 1950–1978* (Washington, D.C.: National Center for Health Statistics, 1983).

11. Howard M. Leichter, *A Comparative Approach to Policy Analysis: Health Care Policy in Four Nations* (New York: Cambridge University Press, 1979), pp. 95–99; Joseph P. Newhouse, "Medical-Care Expenditure: A Cross-National Survey," *Journal of Human Resources,* Vol. 12, No. 1 (Winter 1977), pp. 115–125.

Chapter Three

1. The complete wage scale appears in Alfred Wendehorst, *Das Juliusspital in Würzburg* (Würzburg, West Germany: Stiftung Juliusspital, 1976), Vol. 1, pp. 109–111.

2. Ernest Coyecque found such annual accounts in the principal hospital of Paris, beginning in 1363. *L'Hôtel-Dieu de Paris au moyen âge: Histoire et documents* (Paris: Chez H. Champion, 1891), Vol. 1, pp. 7–13. Each fiscal year began at Christmas.

3. For examples of such lists in Paris's principal hospital, see Coyecque (note 2, above), pp. 146–148. The widespread adoption of "estate accounting" in Western Europe is described in Derek T. Bailey, "European Accounting History," in H. Peter Holzer and others, *International Accounting* (New York: Harper & Row, 1984), pp. 20–22.

4. For example, experiences of French hospitals during the fourteenth and fifteenth centuries are described in Jean Imbert and others, *Histoire des hôpitaux en France* (Toulouse: Editions Privat, 1982), pp. 87, 90.

5. For the history of French accounting and the structure of recent schemes, in both private and public sectors, see André Reydal, *Le nouveau plan comptable français* (Paris: Editions Sirey, 1981); Kenneth S. Most, "Accounting in France," in H. Peter Holzer and others, *International Accounting* (New York: Harper & Row, 1984), Chap. 12. Accounting methods for hospitals during the nineteenth century are described in Eugène Durieu and Germain Roche, *Répertoire de l'administration et de la comptabilité des établissements de bienfaisance* (Paris: Au Bureau du Mémorial des Percepteurs, 1842), Vol. 2; and Gabriel Cros-Mayrevieille, *Traité de l'assistance hospitalière* (Paris: Berger-Levrault, 1912), Vol. 3, Part 5. Recent accounting and reporting by government agencies are described in André Sonrier, *La comptabilité publique* (Paris: Berger-Levrault, 1978).

6. "Instruction M21 sur la comptabilité des hôpitaux et hospices publics" (Paris: issued jointly by the Direction Général de la Santé Publique, Ministère de la Santé Publique et de la Population, and by the Direction de la Comptabilité Publique, Ministère des Finances et des Affaires Economiques, in effect from Jan. 1, 1961). A revised nomenclature took effect on Jan. 1, 1979. For an interpretation of the rules and an explanation of the forms used during those decades, see André

Sonrier, *Comptabilité hospitalière*, 9th ed. (Paris: Berger-Levrault, 1979). Hospital accounting methods were changed after 1984.

7. Information from Theodor Kogge, *Hundert Jahre Evangelisches Krankenhaus Düsseldorf* (Düsseldorf: privately printed, 1949), p. 36.

8. Kogge, pp. 36–49, showing the evolution of the hospital in Table 3-1. For a French example, see Maurice Garden, *Le budget des Hospices Civils de Lyon, 1800–1976* (Lyon: Presses Universitaires de Lyon, 1980), Chap. 4. Many German nonprofit hospitals are combined in Hagen Kühn, *Politisch-ökonomische Entwicklungsbedingungen des Gesundheitswesens* (Königstein/Ts., West Germany: Verlag Anton Hain, 1980), p. 300. Many English nonprofit hospitals are combined in Robert Pinker, *English Hospital Statistics, 1851–1938* (London: Heinemann, 1966), pp. 155–158.

9. The *Krankenhaus-Buchführungsverordnung* (KHBV), published in Karl Jung and Marianne Preuss, *Rechnungs- und Buchführung im Krankenhaus* (Stuttgart: Verlag W. Kohlhammer, 1978).

10. William O. Cleverley (ed.), *Handbook of Health Care Accounting and Finance* (Rockville, Md.: Aspen Publishers, 1982), Chap. 3; Albert A. Cardone (ed.), "Uniform Reporting," *Topics in Health Care Financing*, Vol. 6, No. 2 (Winter 1979). American state governments trying to regulate rates and control costs have had a constant struggle to mandate and collect uniform reports from all hospitals, according to James Vertrees and Julian Pettengill, *Report on Hospital Prospective Payment Systems Mandated by Section 2173 of Public Law 97-35* (Washington, D.C.: Health Care Financing Administration, U.S. Department of Health and Human Services, 1982), pp. 84–85.

11. The decentralized multidivisional structure developed first in the United States. See Alfred D. Chandler, Jr., *Strategy and Structure* (Cambridge, Mass.: MIT Press, 1962).

12. The first stage of Swiss financial reporting is described in Martin Wipf, "Der VESKA Kontenrahmen 1971—Schweizerische Einheitskontenrahmen für Krankenanstalten," *ÖKZ: Österreichische Krankenhaus-Zeitung*, Jan. 1975. Recent cost-center accounting is described in György Csihak, "Kostenstellenrechnungen in einem Grossspital in der Schweiz," *Krankenhaus-Umschau*, No. 4 (1980), pp. 259–261; and Arthur Kuster, "Elargissement de la comptabilité analytique de la VESKA," *Schweizer Spital*, Vol. 48, No. 4 (1984), pp. 23–25.

13. Jean-Marie Clément, *Les réformes hospitalières, 1981–1984* (Paris: Berger-Levrault, 1985); Claude Renou and others, *Rapport . . . relatif à l'évaluation de l'experimentation de nouveaux modes de financements et de gestion des établissements hospitaliers* (Paris: Ministère de la Santé, 1982); Chantal Cuer and others, "D'une expérience tarifaire à une mutation d'hôpital: Le budget global," *Gestions hospitalières*, No. 215 (April 1982), pp. 331–340.

14. For detailed guides with many illustrations, see André Sonrier, *Gestion et finances hospitalières*, 9th ed. (Paris: Berger-Levrault, 1978), Chap. 6; André Sonrier, *Comptabilité hospitalière* (see note 6, above), Chap. 8. A convenient overview is provided in Suzy Chalavet, *Le prix de revient hospitalier* (Paris: Editions Médicales et Universitaires, 1976), pp. 75–81, 92–174.

15. American "stepdown" calculations are explained in L. Vann Seawell, *Introduction to Hospital Accounting* (Chicago: Hospital Financial Management

Association, 1977), Chap. 23, esp. pp. 437–440; and Cleverley, *Handbook of Health Care Accounting and Finance* (see note 10, above), Chap. 11.

16. Explained in Donald F. Beck, *Principles of Reimbursement in Health Care* (Rockville, Md.: Aspen Publishers, 1984), Chaps. 6–7.

17. Arthur L. Brien, "Effective Reporting for Reimbursement Under Medicare," *CPA Journal,* Vol. 42, No. 4 (April 1972), pp. 289–295.

18. John L. Ashby, "An Analysis of Hospital Costs by Cost Center, 1971 Through 1978," *Health Care Financing Review,* Vol. 4, No. 1 (Sept. 1982), pp. 37–53.

19. David Burik, "Cost Accounting's Useful, but Don't Expect Too Much from It," *Modern Healthcare,* Vol. 14, No. 9 (July 1984), pp. 168–174.

20. Recording unit data, aggregating them, and using diagnosis-related groups in general are summarized in Robert Fetter and others, "Case Mix Definition by Diagnosis-Related Groups," *Medical Care,* Vol. 18, No. 2 (Feb. 1980), Supp.; J. Joel May (ed.), "Diagnosis Related Groups," *Topics in Health Care Financing,* Vol. 8, No. 4 (Summer 1982); and Paul L. Grimaldi and Julie A. Micheletti, *Diagnosis Related Groups: A Practitioner's Guide* and *DRG Update: Medicare's Prospective Payment Plan* (Chicago: Pluribus Press, 1983). The enactment of Medicare reimbursement by DRGs caused sudden changes in American hospital accounting and an acceleration in computerization, evident in many articles about current events in American hospital journals. See, for example, "Strategies for Change," *Hospitals,* Vol. 57, No. 13 (July 1, 1983), pp. 58–63; "Financial Modeling," *Topics in Health Care Financing,* Vol. 10, No. 1 (Fall 1983); Task Force on Federal Health Care Legislation, Health Care Subcommittee, American Institute of Certified Public Accountants, "Medicare Changes Create Accounting, Reporting, and Auditing Problems," *Healthcare Financial Management,* Vol. 14, No. 11 (Nov. 1984), pp. 28–38. Similar cost accounting is attempted experimentally in other national hospital systems. See, for example, Pieter F. P. M. Nederstigt, *Diagnosis Related Groups: Een patiënt-georiënteerd kosteninformatiesysteem* (Utrecht: Nationaal Ziekenhuisinstituut, 1985).

21. See, for example, Joan Trofino, "A Reality Based System for Pricing Nursing Service"; and Patricia A. Prescott, "DRG Prospective Reimbursement: The Nursing Intensity Factor," *Nursing Management,* Vol. 17, No. 1 (Jan. 1986), pp. 19–24, 43–48.

22. Illustrated in Werner Siepermann, "Gewinn- und Verlustausgleich," *Die Ortskrankenkasse,* Vol. 57, No. 7 (April 1, 1975), pp. 237–245.

23. Explained in William O. Cleverley, "Return on Equity in the Hospital Industry: Requirement or Windfall?" *Inquiry,* Vol. 19 (Summer 1982), pp. 150–159.

24. J. H. van Aert and A. P. S. P. van Montfort, *Training Functions and Their Cost Consequences for General Hospitals* (Utrecht: Nationaal Ziekenhui-sinstituut, 1978); *Aufwand für Lehre und Forschung an den Universitätsspitäl-ern: Bericht der Arbeitsgruppe* (Aarau: Schweizerisches Krankenhausinstitut, 1975); Roger Grégoire and others, *Rapport de la Commission chargée d'étudier les charges supportées par les régimes de protection sociale et par l'Etat* (Paris: submitted to the Ministry of Labor and thence to Parliament, Dec. 1975), pp. 54–58 and Annex 3. The issue was examined in Great Britain, since the question was

possible division of costs between two Ministries: see A. J. Culyer and others, *Joint Costs and Budgeting for English Teaching Hospitals* (York: Institute of Social and Economic Research, University of York, 1976), published in part in A. J. Culyer and others, "What Accounts for the Higher Costs of Teaching Hospitals?" *Social and Economic Administration,* Vol. 12, No. 1 (Spring 1978), pp. 20–30. For an attempt to estimate the additional costs in the many American hospitals that have some teaching, see Frank A. Sloan and others, "Effects of Teaching on Hospital Costs," *Journal of Health Economics,* Vol. 2 (1983), pp. 1–28.

25. Harold A. Cohen and Jack C. Keane, *Approaches to Setting the Level of Payment for Hospital Capital Costs Under a Prospective Payment System* (Washington, D.C.: Assistant Secretary for Planning and Evaluation, U.S. Department of Health and Human Services, 1984), pp. 9–11; Michael J. Kalison and Richard Averill, "The Response to PPS: Inside, Outside, over Time," *Healthcare Financial Management,* Vol. 38, No. 1 (Jan. 1984), p. 80.

26. The American experience is summarized in Cohen and Keane (see note 25, above), pp. 14–17, 42, 54, 56.

27. William O. Cleverley, *Essentials of Health Care Finance,* 2nd ed. (Rockville, Md.: Aspen Publishers, 1986), esp. Chaps. 7, 13; John Byron Silvers and C. K. Prahalad, *Financial Management of Health Institutions* (Jamaica, N.Y.: SP Medical & Scientific Books, 1974).

Chapter Four

1. The characteristics and payment of for-profit hospitals are summarized in William Glaser, "For-Profit Hospitals: American and Foreign Comparisons," *Health Care Management Review,* Vol. 9, No. 4 (Fall 1984), pp. 27–34.

2. A glossary of hospital terms in the principal languages appears in Hospital Committee of the European Economic Community, *Hospitals in the EEC* (Lochem, Netherlands: Uitgeversmaatschappij de Tijdstroom, 1978). The various words for "daily charge" are listed on p. 404.

3. Maurice Rochaix, *Essai sur l'évolution des questions hospitalières de la fin de l'ancien régime à nos jours* (Paris: Fédération Hospitalière de France, 1959), pp. 43–44, 91; Paul Coudurier, *Les prix de journée,* 4th ed. (Paris: Berger-Levrault, 1978), pp. 19–21.

4. The evolution of fee schedules is evident in the examples in J. M. Schulenburg, *Systeme der Honorierung frei praktizierender Ärzte und ihre Allokationswirkungen* (Tübingen, West Germany: Mohr-Siebeck, 1981). Bills by apothecaries and fees of physicians in seventeenth-century Britain are described in C. J. S. Thompson, *The Mystery and Art of the Apothecary* (London: Bodley Head Ltd., 1929), Chap. 16.

5. Gabriel Cros-Mayrevieille, *Traité de l'administration hospitalière* (Paris: Paul Dupont, 1886), pp. 458–483.

6. Rochaix, *Essai sur l'évolution . . .* (see note 3, above), pp. 255–264.

7. Gabriel Cros-Mayrevieille, *Traité de l'assistance hospitalière* (Paris: Berger-Levrault, 1912), Vol. 2, pp. 14–16, 45–54, 547–559, 569–575.

8. Henry C. Burdett, *Pay Hospitals and Paying Wards Throughout the World* (London: J. & A. Churchill, 1879).

9. French methods for calculating the daily charge are described in Coudurier, *Les prix de journée* (see note 3, above).

10. The payment system and its drawbacks are described in *Bericht über die finanzielle Lage der Krankenanstalten* (Bonn: Bundestag, Drucksache V/4230, May 19, 1969); and Siegfried Eichhorn, *Krankenhaus Betriebslehre*, 2nd ed. (Stuttgart: Verlag W. Kohlhammer, 1971), Vol. 2, esp. pp. 247-252.

11. See, for example, Konrad Elsholz, *Krankenhäuser Stiefkinder der Wohlstandsgesellschaft* (Baden-Baden: Nomos Verlagsgesellschaft, 1969), pp. 44-46; *Modellversuch "Alternative Pflegesatzmodelle"—Theoretische Vorstudie* (Cologne: Gesellschaft für Betriebschaftliche Beratung and Deutsches Krankenhausinstitut, 1983), pp. 14, 39-42. Econometric hypotheses about the consequences of different designs appear in Bertram Schwemin and Heinz Hermann Stollenwerk, "Die wirtschaftlichen Auswirkungen des linearen Pflegesätzes," *Die Ortskrankenkasse*, Vol. 57, No. 18 (1975), pp. 678-686.

12. Roger Grégoire, "Pour une réforme hospitalière: Rapport presenté au Ministre de la Santé Publique et de la Sécurité Sociale," in *Pour une politique de la santé* (Paris: Ministère de la Santé Publique et de la Sécurité Sociale, 1971), p. 178.

13. For example, the Inspector General of French hospital affairs has proposed that physicians' procedures—whether billed by the hospital or by the physician personally—be paid for at the full tariff when performed during the first five days of hospitalization, at 50 percent between the sixth and fifteenth days of hospitalization, and at 20 percent during all subsequent days. *L'hospitalisation: Rapport annuel, 1971* (Paris: Inspection Générale des Affaires Sociales, 1972), pp. 57-58.

14. John Diffenbach and Katharine G. Bauer, *The Philadelphia Blue Cross 1971 Contract Negotiations* (Boston: Intercollegiate Case Clearing House, 1972), p. 11.

15. The problems confronting the committee and its instructions are summarized in D. J. Wagner, "Efficiency en effectiviteit in de gezondheidszorg," in Stichting Studiecentrum voor Ziekenhuiswetenschappen, *Het kostenvraagstuk van de gezondheidszorg* (Lochem, Netherlands: Uitgeversmaatschappij de Tijdstroom, 1973), pp. 112-113. The committee's report is *Interim verslag van de Commissie Minimumbezettingsgraad* (Utrecht: Centraal Orgaan Zickenhuistarieven, 1973).

16. Some writers have suggested, therefore, that the French all-inclusive daily charge be replaced with itemized prices for all services. See Maryse Gadreau, *La tarification hospitalière* (Paris: Editions Médicales et Universitaires, 1976), passim, esp. pp. 344-369; Béatrice Majnoni d'Intignano, "Maîtriser les dépenses d'hospitalisation," in *Une meilleure santé à un moindre prix?* (Paris: Les Editions Ouvrières, 1978), pp. 31-60.

17. Beratergruppe Wannagat, *Gutachten zur Neuordnung der Krankenhausfinanzierung* (Bonn: Bundesministerium für Arbeit und Sozialordnung, 1983), esp. the Appendix.

18. See, for example, the paucity of information about utilization and finances available in Pierre Gilliand, *L'hospitalisation en Suisse: Statistiques, 1936-1978* (Aarau: Schweizerisches Krankenhausinstitut, 1980).

19. Attempts to disentangle the effects of charges by econometric comparisons of all-out and all-in hospitals proved inconclusive. See J. H. van Aert and A. P. W. P. van Montfort, *Basisonderzoek kostenstructuur ziekenhuizen* (Utrecht: Nationaal Ziekenhuisinstituut, 1977), pp. 12, 26.

20. Periodic surveys on rates have been conducted by the American Hospital Association since the end of World War II. A particularly detailed summary of charging practices appears in *Hospital Rates, 1959* (Chicago: American Hospital Association, 1960).

21. Some estimates are given in Louis F. Rossiter and Gail R. Wilensky, *Out-of-Pocket Expenses for Personal Health Services,* and Amy K. Taylor, *Inpatient Hospital Services: Use, Expenditures, and Sources of Payment* (Washington, D.C.: National Center for Health Services Research, U.S. Department of Health and Human Services, 1982 and 1983).

22. David E. Rosenbaum, "Audits Catching More Errors in Hospital Bills," *New York Times,* July 8, 1984, pp. 1, 22.

23. For an early proposal that case-mix reimbursement of hospitals is the best method for voluntarily inspiring efficiency, see Judith R. Lave and others, "A Proposal for Incentive Reimbursement for Hospitals," *Medical Care,* Vol. 11, No. 2 (March–April 1973), pp. 79–90.

24. The early thinking and evolving methods for classifying hospitals by case mix are summarized in J. Joel May (ed.), "Diagnosis Related Groups," *Topics in Health Care Financing,* Vol. 8, No. 4 (Summer 1982). Payment by the case was made possible by earlier American research about the costs of treating each illness, beginning with Dorothy P. Rice, *Estimating the Cost of Illness* (Washington, D.C.: Division of Medical Care Administration, U.S. Public Health Service, 1966); and Anne A. Scitovsky, "Changes in the Costs of Treatment of Selected Illnesses, 1961–1965," *American Economic Review,* Vol. 57 (Dec. 1967), pp. 1182–1195.

25. This research project, the Yale DRG project, is described in Robert B. Fetter and others, "Case Mix Definition by Diagnosis-Related Groups," *Medical Care,* Vol. 18, No. 2 (Feb. 1980), Supp.

26. The New Jersey system, its calculations, and possible alternatives are described clearly and thoroughly in Paul L. Grimaldi and Julie A. Micheletti, *Diagnosis Related Groups: A Practitioner's Guide,* 2nd ed. (Chicago: Pluribus Press, 1983). How it has worked out in practice is described in Jeffrey Wasserman and others, *DRG Evaluation* (Princeton: Health Research and Educational Trust of New Jersey, 1982–1984), 4 vols.; and *Diagnosis-Related Groups: The Effect in New Jersey, the Potential for the Nation—Conference Proceedings* (Washington, D.C.: Health Care Financing Administration, U.S. Department of Health and Human Services, 1984). The unusual calculations giving each hospital extra cash to cover bad debts from nonpaying patients are described in "The All-Payers DRG System: Has New Jersey Found an Efficient and Ethical Way to Provide Indigent Care?" special issue of *Bulletin of the New York Academy of Medicine,* Vol. 62, No. 6 (July–Aug. 1986).

27. Such as the methods used in all other developed countries, as presented in William A. Glaser, *Paying the Hospital: Foreign Lessons for the United States* (New York: Center for the Social Sciences, Columbia University, 1982; a report to the Health Care Financing Administration, U.S. Department of Health and

Human Services; available from the National Technical Information Service, Springfield, Va.). Government officials' motives for preferring DRGs over other methods are summarized in Alfonso D. Esposito, "Medicare's Prospective Payment Demonstration Program," in *Diagnosis-Related Groups . . . Conference Proceedings* (see note 26, above), pp. 22–23.

28. Richard S. Schweiker and others, *Report to Congress: Hospital Prospective Payment for Medicare* (Washington, D.C.: U.S. Department of Health and Human Services, 1982).

29. Jean-Marie Rodrigues and others, "Le projet de médicalisation du système d'information: Méthode, définition, organisation," and "Définition de l'éventail des malades hospitalisés par des Groupes de Diagnostic Homogènes," *Gestions hospitalières*, No. 224 (March 1983), pp. 205–220. See also *Note explicative sur le budget global pour l'exercice 1985* (Paris: Direction des Hôpitaux, Ministère des Affaires Sociales et de la Solidarité Nationale, 1983), p. 8.

30. Much more sophisticated peer grouping in the investigation of global budgets has been proposed for the Ministry of Social Affairs in Quebec in Jean-Marie R. Lance and André-Pierre Contandriopoulos, "Le régroupement des hôpitaux selon leur production: Base d'évaluation de leur performance," *L'actualité économique*, April–June 1980, pp. 308–338.

31. The European studies are summarized in papers submitted to a conference on "The Management and Financing of Hospital Services," London, Dec. 1986; and in Mahesh Patel and others, "DRG version européenne," *Schweizer Spital*, Vol. 50, No. 6 (1986), pp. 27–28.

32. The idea was not unique to Britain. It had been proposed in Europe even earlier but never implemented to a significant extent. For example, Jean Imbert and others, *Histoire des hôpitaux en France* (Toulouse: Editions Privat, 1982), pp. 228–229.

33. For a history of the British Contributory Schemes, see Veronica Dawkins, *A Study of the Development of Hospital Contributory Schemes in England and Wales* (Bristol: British Hospitals Contributory Schemes Association, 1982); and Joseph E. Stone, *Hospital Organisation and Management*, 4th ed. (London: Faber & Faber, 1952), Appendix M.

34. James Tull Richardson, *The Origin and Development of Group Hospitalization in the United States, 1890–1940* (Columbia: University of Missouri, 1945), pp. 14–17. Their conversion into county-wide systems became the transition to Blue Cross (pp. 17–18).

35. Robert M. Sigmond, "Capitation as a Method of Reimbursement to Hospitals in a Multihospital Area," in *Medical Care* (Washington, D.C.: Office of Research and Statistics, Social Security Administration, 1968), pp. 49–59; Walter J. Unger and Robert M. Sigmond, "Can New Capitation Experiment Cut Hospital Costs?" *Healthcare Financial Management*, Vol. 10, No. 12 (Dec. 1980), pp. 22–26.

36. William B. Elliott and others, "The Hospital Capitation Payment Project: New Incentives and Tools for Cost Containment," *Inquiry*, Vol. 20, No. 2 (Summer 1983), pp. 114–120; William B. Elliott, *The Hospital Capitation Experiment: A Progress Report* (Chicago: Blue Cross and Blue Shield Association, 1983). A few hospitals economized on costs and prospered, such as the one described in Richard M. Mangion, "Capitation Reimbursement: A

Progress Report," *Hospital and Health Services Administration,* Vol. 31, No. 1 (Jan.-Feb. 1986), pp. 99–110.

Chapter Five

1. Jean Imbert, *Les hôpitaux en droit canonique* (Paris: Librairie Philosophique J. Vrin, 1947), pp. 287–301.

2. Charging methods in British, European, and American hospitals during the nineteenth century are summarized in Henry C. Burdett, *Pay Hospitals and Paying Wards Throughout the World* (London: J. & A. Churchill, 1879).

3. The American controversies are summarized in David Rosner, *A Once Charitable Enterprise: Hospitals and Health Care in Brooklyn and New York 1885–1915* (New York: Cambridge University Press, 1982), Chaps. 2, 3; and Morris J. Vogel, *The Invention of the Modern Hospital: Boston 1870–1930* (Chicago: University of Chicago Press, 1980), Chap. 5. Since paying patients were brought into hospitals by office doctors, the medical staffs came to dominate the American hospital.

4. British methods are described in Joseph E. Stone, *Appeals for Funds and Hospital Publicity* (Birmingham: Birbeck & Sons, 1934).

5. American hospital income during the first half of the twentieth century is described in Edward H. L. Corwin, *The American Hospital* (New York: Commonwealth Fund, 1946), pp. 57–73; and Commission on Hospital Care, *Hospital Care in the United States* (New York: Commonwealth Fund, 1947), Chap. 34.

6. Descriptions of the social services of the guilds appear in Jean Bennet, *La Mutualité Française des origines à la Révolution de 1789* (Paris: Coopérative d'Information et d'Edition Mutualiste, 1981); and George Clune, *The Medieval Gild System* (Dublin: Browne & Nolem, 1943), passim.

7. Edgcumbe Staley, *The Guilds of Florence* (London: Methuen, 1906), Chap. 19; Bennet, *La Mutualité Française* (see note 6, above), pp. 507–523.

8. No history of health insurance exists in general, but it is included in two histories of social security: Peter A. Köhler and Hans F. Zacher (eds.), *The Evolution of Social Insurance, 1881–1981* (London: Frances Pinter, 1982); and Gaston V. Rimlinger, *Welfare Policy and Industrialization in Europe, America and Russia* (New York: Wiley, 1971). Among the very few histories of health insurance in any country are Horst Peters, *Die Geschichte der sozialen Versicherung,* 3rd ed. (Sankt Augustin, West Germany: Asgard-Verlag, 1978); and Paul Biedermann, *Die Entwicklung der Krankenversicherung in der Schweiz* (Davos-Platz, Switzerland: Buchdruckerei Davos, 1955). For a good history of health insurance and health financing in the United States, see Odin W. Anderson, *The Uneasy Equilibrium* (New Haven, Conn: Yale University Press, 1968). Some very revealing comparisons of the Anglo-Saxon and continental European (especially German) philosophies and methods were made when Britain enacted its NHI law. The differences in philosophies and methods are summarized in R. W. Harris, *National Health Insurance in Great Britain, 1911–1946* (London: Allen & Unwin, 1946), Chaps. 2–3. The contrasting traditions in workmen's compensation are described briefly in George Rohrlich, "Compara-

tive Approaches to Work Injury Compensation in International Perspective," in *Compendium on Workmen's Compensation* (Washington, D.C.: National Commission on State Workmen's Compensation Laws, 1973), Chap. 6. For details on health insurance in every European country at the beginning of the twentieth century, see *Twenty-Fourth Annual Report of the Commissioner of Labor, 1909: Workmen's Insurance and Compensation Systems in Europe* (Washington, D.C.: U.S. Government Printing Office, 1911), 2 vols.

9. The evolution of welfare bargaining in American labor relations and health finance is described in Raymond Munts, *Bargaining for Health: Labor Unions, Health Insurance, and Medical Care* (Madison: University of Wisconsin Press, 1962). The large share of American health insurance connected with employment is reported in Deborah J. Chollet, *Employer-Provided Health Benefits* (Washington, D.C.: Employee Benefits Research Institute, 1984). The resulting coverage of the American population is summarized in Pamela J. Farley, *Private Health Insurance in the United States* (Washington, D.C.: National Center for Health Services Research, U.S. Department of Health and Human Services, 1986).

10. For descriptions of statutory health insurance generally and in individual countries, see the bibliography at the end of Appendix A in this volume.

11. The 1890 data are taken from Philipp Herder-Dorneich, *Honarreform und Krankenhaussanierung* (Berlin: Erich Schmidt Verlag, 1970), p. 76. I have calculated 1981 data from Bundesministerium für Jugend, Familie, und Gesundheit, *Daten des Gesundheitswesen—Ausgabe 1983* (Stuttgart: Verlag W. Kohlhammer, 1983), p. 199.

12. Described in *Private Health Insurance in Europe* (Paris: Comité Européen des Assurances, 1983).

13. The national health services of Britain, Sweden, the Soviet Union, and China are described in Victor W. Sidel and Ruth Sidel, *A Healthy State*, 2nd ed. (New York: Pantheon Books, 1983). Great Britain's National Health Service is described in Ruth Levitt and Andrew Wall, *The Reorganised National Health Service*, 3rd ed. (London: Croom Helm, 1984).

14. William Laing, *Private Health Care* (London: Office of Health Economics, 1985).

15. Canada's health system is described in Lee Soderstrom, *The Canadian Health System* (London: Croom Helm, 1978). How it came about is summarized in Malcolm G. Taylor, *Health Insurance and Canadian Public Policy* (Montreal: McGill–Queen's University Press, 1978).

16. Described in Steven Jonas and others, *Health Care Delivery in the United States*, 2nd ed. (New York: Springer, 1981); Marshall W. Raffel, *The U.S. Health System* (New York: Wiley, 1980); and Florence Wilson and Duncan Neuhauser, *Health Services in the United States*, 2nd ed. (Cambridge, Mass.: Ballinger, 1982).

17. Paul Starr, *The Social Transformation of American Medicine* (New York: Basic Books, 1982), Book 2.

18. David Stockman, "The Social Pork Barrel," *The Public Interest*, No. 39 (Spring 1975), pp. 3–30.

19. For a comparison between the United States and another country with a once identical health financing system, see Sidney S. Lee, "Health Policy, A Social Contract: A Comparison of the United States and Canada," *Journal of Public Health Policy*, Vol. 3, No. 3 (Sept. 1982), pp. 293–301.

20. Jack Hadley and others, *Care for the Poor and Hospitals' Financial Status: Results of a 1980 Survey of Hospitals in Large Cities* (Washington, D.C.: Urban Institute, 1983); Jack Hadley and others, "The Financially Distressed Hospital," *New England Journal of Medicine*, Vol. 307 (Nov. 11, 1982), pp. 1283–1287.

21. The characteristics of large donations and methods of obtaining them are summarized in Jerold Pana, *Megagifts: Who Gives Them, Who Gets Them* (Chicago: Pluribus Press, 1984).

22. Some financial comparisons between the *Ersatzkassen* and the other German statutory sickness funds appear in Paul-Helmut Huppertz and others, *Beitragssatzdifferenzen und adäquate Finanzausgleichsverfahren in der gesetzlichen Krankenversicherung* (Bonn: Bundesministerium für Arbeit und Sozialordnung, 1981). Rivalries between *Ersatzkassen* and other statutory sickness funds, and the consequences for benefits and cost containment, are discussed in Renate Mayntz and others, *Analyse von Planungs- und Steuerungsfunktionen der gesetzlichen Krankenversicherung in Versorgungsschwerpunkten des Gesundheitswesens* (Bonn: Bundesministerium für Arbeit und Sozialordnung, 1982); and Heinz Lampert, "Strukturfragen aus ordnungspolitischer Sicht: Gesundheitswesen und gesetzliche Krankenversicherung in der Sozialordung der Bundesrepublik Deutschland," in *Strukturfragen im Gesundheitswesen in der Bundesrepublik Deutschland* (Bonn: Wissenschaftliches Institut der Ortskrankenkassen, 1983), pp. 85–91, 95–96.

23. F. J. Werner and others, report of an interdepartmental work group on the financial consequences of *volksverzekering* (universal health insurance) (Leidschendam, Netherlands: Ministerie van Volksgezondheid en Milieuhygiëne, 1977).

24. Alain Foulon, *Comparaison des régimes de Sécurité Sociale: Cotisations et prestations* (Paris: Documents du Centre d'Etude des Revenus et des Coûts, 1983).

25. Clark C. Havighurst, "Antitrust Enforcement in the Medical Services Industry: What Does It All Mean?" *Health and Society*, Vol. 58, No. 1 (1980), pp. 112–113; Clark C. Havighurst, "The Role of Competition in Cost Containment," in Warren Greenberg (ed.), *Competition in the Health Care Sector* (Washington, D.C.: Bureau of Economics, Federal Trade Commission, 1978); Jules M. Fried and Michael J. Rabinowitz, "Antitrust May Pose New Legal Issues for Hospitals," *Hospitals*, Vol. 56, No. 11 (June 1, 1982), pp. 66–69.

26. For example, the complications introduced into the supposedly straightforward New Jersey DRGs, as described in Paul L. Grimaldi and Julie A. Micheletti, *Diagnosis Related Groups: A Practitioner's Guide*, 2nd ed. (Chicago: Pluribus Press, 1983), pp. 137–144.

27. Data in Frank A. Sloan and Edmund R. Becker, "Cross-Subsidies and Payment for Hospital Care," *Journal of Health Politics, Policy and Law*, Vol. 8, No. 4 (Winter 1984), pp. 660–685. For an extensive comparison of European standard rates and American multiple rates, see William Glaser, "Juggling

Multiple Payers: American Problems and Foreign Solutions," *Inquiry*, Vol. 21, No. 2 (Summer 1984), pp. 178–188.

Chapter Six

1. See, for example, David Burik, "The Changing Role of Hospital Prices: A Framework for Pricing in a Competitive Environment," *Health Care Management Review*, Vol. 8, No. 2 (Spring 1983), pp. 65–71.

2. The only interview survey of how hospital managers make these decisions was conducted in a few Massachusetts hospitals during the 1960s, before the great expansion of paid-in-full cost reimbursement changed the system there, making the charge lists a supplement rather than the principal revenue source. See Edward M. Kaitz, *Pricing Policy and Cost Behavior in the Hospital Industry* (New York: Praeger, 1968), Chaps. 3–4. The spread of econometric research in health has eclipsed arduous legwork like Kaitz's, but his is the only method that enables one to learn how hospital managers make decisions.

3. Some relative-value scales have been proposed for the charge lists within the more industrialized parts of the hospital, such as radiology and the laboratory. The weights are derived from research about labor time and resource use in those departments. For examples see Howard J. Berman and Lewis E. Weeks, *The Financial Management of Hospitals*, 5th ed. (Ann Arbor, Mich.: Health Administration Press, 1982), Chap. 8. In actual practice these are precisely the departments where American hospitals add large markups to cover revenue shortfalls in other services and in order to earn overall profits. If the markups are constant proportions, the relative values are preserved, but all the charges greatly exceed costs.

4. Such a pricing strategy is summarized in William O. Cleverley (ed.), *Handbook of Health Care Accounting and Finance* (Rockville, Md.: Aspen Publishers, 1982), Chap. 9. Such a computer program is described in Jeffrey G. Long, "Electronic Spreadsheets Help Hospitals Pinpoint Crucial Costs," *Modern Healthcare*, Vol. 14, No. 10 (Aug. 1984), pp. 102–104.

5. The methods are explained in Cleverley, *Handbook of Health Care Accounting and Finance* (see note 4, above), Chap. 15; and Donald F. Beck, *Principles of Reimbursement in Health Care* (Rockville, Md.: Aspen Publishers, 1984).

6. At one time some doctors with multiple affiliations referred self-paying middle-class patients to cheaper hospitals if clinical conveniences were equal. But hospitals did not manipulate their entire charge lists for all their business to attract this small number of extra referrals: Kaitz, *Pricing Policy and Cost Behavior in the Hospital Industry* (see note 2, above), Chap. 4.

7. Linda Punch, "Publicity on Prices Has Little Impact," *Modern Healthcare*, Vol. 13, No. 12 (Dec. 1983), pp. 46, 48.

8. See, for example, the Canadian and British experiences described in William A. Glaser, *Health Insurance Bargaining* (New York: Gardner Press and Wiley, 1978), Chaps. 2, 9.

9. The history of the sickness funds before and after the law of 1883 appears in William Harbutt Dawson, *Social Insurance in Germany, 1883–1911* (London: T. Fisher Unwin, 1912). The resistance to the centralizing tendencies

of the German national government and the resulting structure of health insurance are summarized in Herbert Jacob, *German Administration Since Bismarck* (New Haven, Conn.: Yale University Press, 1963), pp. 37–43.

10. For the history of relations between sickness funds and doctors, see Frieder Naschold, *Kassenärzte und Krankenversicherungsreform* (Freiburg im Breisgau, West Germany: Verlag Rombach, 1967); and Julius Hadrich, *Die Arztfrage in der deutschen Sozialversicherung* (Berlin: Duncker & Humblot, 1955).

11. The organizational and financial history of Germany hospitals appears in Marie-Theres Starke, *Die Finanzierung der Krankenhausleistungen als sozial- und ordnungspolitisches Problem* (Münster, West Germany: Aschendorffsche Verlagsbuchhandlung, 1962), pp. 17–59; Johannes Kessels and others, *Die Gestalt des katholischen Krankenhauses* (Freiburg im Breisgau, West Germany: Katholischer Krankenhausverband Deutschlands, 1981), pp. 132–282 and sources cited; and *10 Jahre P.E.G.* (Munich: Privatklinik- Einkaufs- und Betriebsgenossenschaft, 1980), pp. 22–28. For a history of hospital financing laws, see Beratergruppe Wannagat, *Gutachten zur Neuordnung der Krankenhausfinanzierung* (Bonn: Bundesminister für Arbeit und Sozialordnung, 1983), pp. 7–60.

12. Bundesministerium für Gesundheitswesen, *Gesundheitsstatischer Bericht der Bundesrepublik Deutschland, 1960* (Stuttgart: Verlag W. Kohlhammer, 1962), p. 143.

13. Lee K. Frankel and Miles M. Dawson, *Workingmen's Insurance in Europe* (New York: Charities Publication Committee, 1910), p. 243.

14. Robert J. Maxwell, *Health and Wealth* (Lexington, Mass.: Lexington Books, 1981), pp. 82–83.

15. The current methods are described in Glaser, *Health Insurance Bargaining* (see note 8, above), Chap. 6.

16. Decision making in the German federal system in general is described in Fritz W. Scharpf and others, *Politikverflechtung: Theorie und Empirie des kooperativen Föderalismus in der Bundesrepublik* (Kronberg/Ts., West Germany: Scriptor Verlag, 1976). Hospital finance is summarized on pp. 205–217. For an explanation of how major health decisions are made in the German federal system, see William Glaser, *Federalism in Canada and West Germany* (New York: Center for the Social Sciences, Columbia University, 1979; distributed by the National Technical Information Service), Chaps. 9–15 passim.

17. The provisions of KHG and of its accounting regulations are described in many places. See, for example, Heinz Hübner, *Kostenrechnung im Krankenhaus,* 2nd ed. (Stuttgart: Verlag W. Kohlhammer, 1980); Maria Gehrt and Heiko Jüngerkes, *Selbstkostenrechnung nach der Bundespflegesatzverordung: Ein Ratgeber für die Praxis,* 2nd ed. (Stuttgart: Verlag W. Kohlhammer, 1974); Behrend Behrends, "Das Pflegesatzrecht," *Die Ortskrankenkasse,* Vol. 63, No. 19 (Oct. 1, 1981), pp. 761–776.

18. *Bericht über die finanzielle Lage der Krankenanstalten* (Bonn: Bundestag, Drucksache V/4230, May 19, 1969). The payment system at that time is described in Maria Gehrt and Heinz Schöne, *Bundespflegesatzverordnung* (Stuttgart: Verlag W. Kohlhammer, 1955).

19. An example of such a proposal is *Zwischenbericht der Kommission Krankenhausfinanzierung der Robert Bosch Stiftung* (Stuttgart: Robert Bosch Stiftung, 1983).

20. The original design and early work of the KA are described in Henry Landsberger, *The Control of Cost in the Federal Republic of Germany: Lessons for America?* (Washington, D.C.: Bureau of Health Planning, U.S. Department of Health and Human Services, 1981), Chap. 4. Later experiences of the KA and the consequences of the omission of hospital finance from the KA's recommendations are summarized in *Bericht der Bundesregierung nach Artikel 2 § 6 des Krankenversicherungs-Kostendämpfungsgesetzes* (Bonn: Bundestag, Drucksache 9/1300, Feb. 2, 1982).

21. The history and structure of *verzuiling* are described in J. P. Kruijt and Walter Goddijn, "Verzuiling en outzuiling als sociologisch proces," in A. N. J. van Hollander and others (eds.), *Drift en koers: Een halve eeuw sociale verandering in Nederland* (Assen, Netherlands: Van Gorcum, 1961), pp. 227–263.

22. John Windmuller, *Labor Relations in the Netherlands* (Ithaca, N.Y.: Cornell University Press, 1969).

23. Glaser, *Health Insurance Bargaining* (see note 8, above), Chap. 5.

24. The *Ziekenfondsraad* and INAMI are described in L. V. Ledeboer, *Heden en verleden—van de ziekenfondsverzekering en de verzekering van bijzondere ziektekosten* (Leidschendam, Netherlands: Ministerie van Volksgezondheid en Milieuhygiëne, 1973); M. Delhuvenne and others, *Aperçu du régime belge d'assurance obligatoire contre la maladie et l'invalidité* (Brussels: Institut National d'Assurance Maladie-Invalidité, frequently updated); and Glaser, *Health Insurance Bargaining* (see note 8, above), pp. 61–64, 82–85.

25. For an extensive summary of the characteristics, history, achievements, and weaknesses of COZ, see L. J. de Wolff (ed.), *De prijs voor gezondheid: Het Centraal Orgaan Ziekenhuistarieven, 1965–1982* (Baarn, Netherlands: Uitgeverij Ambo, 1984).

26. The guidelines were published in *COZ-Vademecum: Richtlijnen van de Stichting Centraal Orgaan Ziekenhuistarieven* (Alphen aan den Rijn, Netherlands: Samson Uitgeverij, a loose-leaf book constantly updated).

27. *Financieel overzicht van de Gezondheidszorg: Waarin opgenomen een raming van de kosten* (Leidschendam, Netherlands: Ministerie van Volksgezondheid en Milieuhygiëne, 1977 et seq.).

28. Jean-Pierre Poullier, *Public Expenditure on Health Under Economic Constraints* (Paris: Organisation for Economic Co-operation and Development, 1984), Part 2, Table B-1.

29. Glaser, *Health Insurance Bargaining* (see note 8, above), Chap. 3.

30. The methods of paying private clinics during the 1960s and early 1970s, and their financial consequences, are described in *Les établissements sanitaires et sociaux: Rapport annuel, 1977–1978* (Paris: Inspection Générale des Affaires Sociales, 1979), Part 2. Recent methods and results are described in Norbert Paquel and Pierre Giraud, *Le coût de l'hospitalisation—Les établissements de soins privés—Description et analyse d'ensemble* (Paris: Documents du Centre d'Etude des Revenus et des Coûts, 1980), Chap. 3.

31. Investigators from the Ministries of Labor and Health discovered, for example, that the CRAM in Brittany had given all private clinics a surgical daily

charge comparable to the one in the academic medical center of Rennes. *L'hospitalisation: Rapport annuel, 1971* (Paris: Inspection Générale des Affaires Sociales, 1972), p. 50.

32. For the history of Blue Cross, see Odin Anderson, *Blue Cross Since 1929* (Cambridge, Mass: Ballinger, 1975).

33. The philosophy appears in Robert M. Sigmond and Thomas Kinser, *The Hospital-Blue Cross Plan Relationship* (Chicago: Blue Cross Association, 1976), pp. 40-42.

34. John Diffenbach and Katharine G. Bauer, *The Philadelphia Blue Cross 1971 Contract Negotiations* (Boston: Intercollegiate Case Clearing House, 1972), Case No. 9-373-126.

35. One of the more organized arrangements is described in Katharine G. Bauer and Arva Rosenfeld Clark, *The Indiana Controlled Charges System* (Boston: Harvard Center for Community Health and Medical Care, 1974).

36. Several Blue Cross offices are described in William L. Dowling, "Prospective Rate Setting: Concept and Practice," *Topics in Health Care Financing*, Vol. 3, No. 2 (Winter 1976); Katharine G. Bauer, "Hospital Rate Setting—This Way to Salvation?" *Health and Society*, Vol. 55 (Winter 1977), pp. 117-158; and the studies by Arthur D. Little and Katharine Bauer cited in her article. One arrangement is described extensively in Michael Sumner and Gary Gaumer, *Case Study of Prospective Reimbursement in Western Pennsylvania* (Washington, D.C.: Health Care Financing Administration, U.S. Department of Health and Human Services, 1980).

37. Armand Leco, "Prospective Rate Setting in Rhode Island," *Topics in Health Care Financing*, Vol. 3, No. 2 (Winter 1976), pp. 39-56; James A. Block and others, "Experimental Payments Program: It's Working for Rochester-Area Hospitals," *Hospital Financial Management*, Vol. 11, No. 9 (Sept. 1981), pp. 10-20. Organized American programs—whether negotiations or regulation—often yield uncertain outcomes because they are frequently altered, as is evident in Harvey Zimmerman and others, "Prospective Reimbursement in Rhode Island," *Inquiry*, Vol. 14, No. 1 (March 1977), pp. 3-16.

38. Mary O'Tousa, *Hospital-Blue Cross Contract Provisions: July 1, 1981* (Chicago: American Hospital Association, 1982).

39. Discussed and documented in many issues of HIAA's *Report on Consumer and Professional Relations: Hospital Relations*, esp. No. 7-82, Aug. 6, 1982.

40. America's strong advocates of competitive solutions to health care finance oppose common negotiating teams as monopsonistic and conspiratorial. See, for example, Lawrence G. Goldberg and Warren Greenberg, "An Antitrust Exemption for Commercial Insurers? Answer: No," *Federation of American Hospitals Review*, Vol. 17, No. 1 (Jan.-Feb. 1984); Clark C. Havighurst, "Role of Competition in Cost Containment," in Warren Greenberg (ed.), *Competition in the Health Care Sector* (Washington, D.C.: Federal Trade Commission, 1978), pp. 391-393.

41. *Travelers Insurance Co.* v. *Blue Cross of Western Pennsylvania*, 361 F. Supp. 774 (1972); *Frankford Hospital* v. *Blue Cross of Greater Philadelphia*, 417 F. Supp. 1104 (1976).

42. "Hospital Cost Control—the State Option" and "Hospital Cost Control—The State Option Revisited," *Viewpoint* (of the Health Insurance Association of America), March 1978 and Jan. 1980.

43. William A. Guy, "California Charts a New Competitive Course," *Healthcare Financial Management,* Vol. 36, No. 12 (Dec. 1982), pp. 60–74; Linda Bergthold, "Crabs in a Bucket: The Politics of Health Care Reform in California," *Journal of Health Politics, Policy and Law,* Vol. 9, No. 2 (Summer 1984), pp. 203–222.

44. *Report to the Legislature on the Operations of the California Medical Assistance Commission* (Sacramento: California Medical Assistance Commission, several times annually); Lucy Johns and others, *Selective Contracting for Health Services in California* (Washington, D.C.: Lewin and Associates and National Governors Association, 1985); E. Richard Brown and others, "Competing for Medi-Cal Business: Why Hospitals Did, and Did Not, Get Contracts," *Inquiry,* Vol. 22, No. 3 (Fall 1985), pp. 237–250. As in other American efforts to reduce Medicaid costs, the largest savings in California resulted from a simultaneous reduction in the number of beneficiaries.

45. The original theory and actual experiences of the Arizona system appear in Jon B. Christianson and Diane G. Hillman, *Health Care for the Indigent and Competitive Contracts* (Ann Arbor, Mich.: Health Administration Press, 1986); and Bradford L. Kirkman-Liff and others, "Medicaid and Capitated Competitive Contracting: The Arizona Experiment," *New England Journal of Human Services,* Vol. 5, No. 3 (Summer 1985), pp. 30–36. The scandals were described in Arizona newspapers during late 1983 and 1984 and (with considerable restraint) in *Medicaid Issues: Hearings Before the Subcommittee on Health and the Environment of the Committee on Energy and Commerce, House of Representatives, 98th Congress, 2d Session* (Washington, D.C.: U.S. Government Printing Office, 1984), Serial No. 98–140, pp. 157–352.

46. Michael A. Morrissey and others, "Hospitals and Health Maintenance Organizations: An Analysis of the Minneapolis–St. Paul Experience," *Health Care Financing Review,* Vol. 4, No. 3 (March 1983), pp. 59–69; John E. Kralewski, Dennis Countryman, and Laura Pitt, "Hospital and Health Maintenance Organization Financial Agreements for Inpatient Services," *Health Care Financing Review,* Vol. 4, No. 4 (Summer 1983), pp. 79–84.

47. John E. Kralewski and others, "HMO–Hospital Relationships: An Exploratory Study," *Health Care Management Review,* Vol. 8, No. 2 (Spring 1983), pp. 27–36.

48. Samuel J. Tibbitts and Allen J. Manzano, *PPO's: Preferred Provider Organizations: An Executive's Guide* (Chicago: Pluribus Press, 1984); Dale H. Cowan, *Preferred Provider Organizations: Planning Structure and Operation* (Rockville, Md.: Aspen Publishers, 1984). Most PPOs are lower-fee arrangements with office doctors for ambulatory care. Arrangements with hospitals are included in S. Brian Barger and others, *The PPO Handbook* (Rockville, Md.: Aspen Publishers, 1984).

Chapter Seven

1. The organization of the *département* before 1982 and the work of the prefect are described in Brian Chapman, *The Prefects and Provincial France*

(London: Allen & Unwin, 1955); Marcel Piquemal, "L'administration territoriale: Le département," *Notes et études documentaires* (La Documentation Française), Nos. 4249–4250 (Dec. 29, 1975); and Hervé Detton, *L'administration régionale et locale de la France,* 7th ed. (Paris: Presses Universitaires de France, 1975). Arrangements since 1982 are summarized in Jean-François Auby, *Le commissaire de la république* (Paris: Presses Universitaries de France, 1983). The political dynamics in the *département* and region are analyzed in Pierre Grémion, *Le pouvoir périphérique* (Paris: Editions du Seuil, 1976). The organization and work of the DDASS are described in Pierre Lachèze-Pasquet, *L'administration de l'hôpital,* 5th ed. (Paris: Berger-Levrault, 1979), pp. 95–98; and Dominique Ceccaldi and Michel Lucas, "Santé et Sécurité Sociale: Un ministère en mouvement," *Revue française des affaires sociales,* Vol. 34, No. 4 (Oct.–Dec. 1980), pp. 31–52. The work of the *trésorier-payeur général* is described in Piquemal (in the article cited above), pp. 23–28.

2. The development of the daily charge is summarized in Maurice Rochaix, *Essai sur l'évolution des questions hospitalières de la fin de l'ancien regime à nos jours* (Paris: Fédération Hospitalière de France, 1959), pp. 255–264.

3. A guide to filling out the form for the operating budget in past years, when the goal was to derive a daily charge, appears in André Sonrier, *Comptabilité hospitalière,* 9th ed. (Paris: Berger-Levrault, 1979), Chap. 3. New treatises are being written during the 1980s to explain the forms used for global budgeting. For a convenient short overview of hospital budgeting during modern times, see M. Cl. Beaughon and G. Vincent, "Les finances de l'hôpital," *Gestions hospitalières,* Nos. 177–178 (June–July and Aug.–Sept. 1978), pp. 521–525 and 643–648. The law and calculating procedures for the daily charges during the recent past can be found in Paul Coudurier, *Les prix de journée,* 4th ed. (Paris: Berger-Levrault, 1978).

4. The annual budget is written primarily by the National Institute of Statistics and Economic Studies (INSEE). It is submitted every year to Parliament by the forecasting section of the Ministry of Finance. It bears a title such as *Rapport économique et financier: Comptes prévisionnels de la nation pour 1984 et principes économiques pour 1985.*

5. The involved political maneuvers among the diverse actors occur sporadically at all stages of rate determination. Described in Gérard de Pouvourville and Marc Renaud, "Hospital System Management in France and Canada," *Social Science and Medicine,* Vol. 20, No. 2 (1985), pp. 156–160.

6. Few publications summarize Dutch hospital rate setting in general. An exception is B. H. Weustink, "Ziekenhuizen en ziekenfondsen—Plaatselijk overleg," in *In het kader van de gezondheidszorg* (Lochem, Netherlands: Uitgeversmaatschappij de Tijdstroom, 1978), pp. 255–265. The work of COZ is summarized in L. J. de Wolff (ed.), *De prijs voor gezondheid: Het Centraal Orgaan Ziekenhuistarieven* (Baarn, Netherlands: Uitgeverij Ambo, 1984). For a good analysis of the internal financial management of Dutch hospitals, see A. Mulder, *De economie en het ziekenhuis* (Lochem, Netherlands: Uitgeversmaatschappij de Tijdstroom, 1978).

7. These and other index numbers were collected and printed in *Macro economische verkenning* (The Hague: Centraal Planbureau, annual).

8. H. J. Hannessen, "COZ en beroep," in L. J. de Wolff (ed.), *De prijs voor gezondheid* (see note 6, above), pp. 259–277.

9. *Financieel overzicht van de gezondheidszorg: Waarin opgenomen een raming van de kosten tot 1984* (Leidschendam, Netherlands: Ministerie van Volksgezondheid en Milieuhygiëne, 1982), Tweede Kamer, zitting 1982–83, 17,600 hoofdstuk XVII, No. 10, p. 29.

10. For overviews of Swiss health insurance and hospitals, see Pierre Gygi and Heiner Henny, *Das schweizerische Gesundheitswesen*, 2nd ed. (Bern: Verlag Hans Huber, 1977, updated by periodic supplements); Pierre Gilliand, *L'hospitalisation en Suisse: Statistiques 1936–1978* (Aarau: Schweizerisches Krankenhausinstitut, 1980); Heiner Henny, *La structure des coûts des hôpitaux* (Aarau: Schweizerisches Krankenhausinstitut, 1974).

11. For example, John K. Galbraith, *American Capitalism: The Concept of Countervailing Power* (Boston: Houghton Mifflin, 1952).

12. For a good overview, see Barry M. Mitnick, *The Political Economy of Regulation: Creating, Designing, and Removing Regulatory Forms* (New York: Columbia University Press, 1980).

13. For the history of state insurance regulation, see John G. Day, *Economic Regulation of Insurance in the United States* (Washington, D.C.: U.S. Department of Transportation, 1970), pp. 3–51; Spencer L. Kimball, *Insurance and Public Policy* (Madison: University of Wisconsin Press, 1960). The work of state insurance regulators today is described in Robert H. Miles and Arvind Ghambri, *The Regulatory Executives* (Beverly Hills, Calif.: Sage, 1983).

14. For the legislative history of Medicaid, see Robert Stevens and Rosemary Stevens, *Welfare Medicine in America* (New York: Free Press, 1974). The fiscal burdens on the states are reported in *Report of the Task Force on Medicaid Reform* (Washington, D.C.: National Governors Association, 1977). The cuts in eligibility and benefits in states not opting for rate control are summarized in Allen D. Spiegel and Simon Podair (eds.), *Medicaid: Lessons for National Health Insurance* (Rockville, Md.: Aspen Publishers, 1975), pp. 109–128, 351–356.

15. Andrew B. Dunham and James A. Morone, *The Politics of Innovation: The Evolution of DRG Rate Regulation in New Jersey* (Princeton: Health Research and Educational Trust of New Jersey, 1983), Vol. IV-A of the "DRG Evaluation," pp. 1–26.

16. Descriptions of the American state programs can be found in Abt Associates, *First Annual Report of the National Hospital Rate-Setting Study* (Washington, D.C.: Health Care Financing Administration, U.S. Department of Health and Human Services, 1980), 10 vols.; James Vertrees and others, *Report on Hospital Prospective Payment Systems Mandated by Section 2173 of Public Law 97-35* (Washington, D.C.: Health Care Financing Administration, U.S. Department of Health and Human Services, 1982); and Paul L. Joskow, *Controlling Hospital Costs: The Role of Government Regulation* (Cambridge, Mass.: MIT Press, 1981), pp. 113–128. A handy summary of the Abt investigation appears in Diane Hamilton (ed.), "Rate Regulation," *Topics in Health Care Financing*, Vol. 6, No. 1 (Fall 1979).

17. The defeat of national hospital rate regulation during the Carter administration is described in David S. Abernethy and David A. Pearson,

Regulating Hospital Costs (Ann Arbor, Mich.: Health Administration Press, 1979). The method of national policy implemented by state governments—used in hospital facilities planning but not in hospital rate regulation—is described in David B. Walter and others, *Regulatory Federalism* (Washington, D.C.: Advisory Commission on Intergovernmental Relations, 1984).

18. See reports by Abt Associates and by Vertrees and others (cited in note 16, above).

19. The content of guidelines is summarized in Abt Associates, *First Annual Report of the National Hospital Rate-Setting Study* (see note 16, above), vol. 1, pp. 83–103.

20. William Glaser, "Hospital Rate Regulation: American and Foreign Comparisons," *Journal of Health Politics, Policy and Law,* Vol. 8, No. 4 (Winter 1984), pp. 702–731. Political and procedural differences between American and European regulation in another sector are described in Ronald Brickman and others, *Controlling Chemicals: The Politics of Regulation in Europe and the United States* (Ithaca, N.Y.: Cornell University Press, 1985).

21. The weak design and short life of the Colorado Hospital Commission are reported in Gail H. Klapper and Rebecca L. Harrington, "Viewpoint: The Rise and Fall of Cost Containment in Colorado," *Health Care Management Review,* Vol. 6, No. 2 (Spring 1981), pp. 79–83; and Donald Rice, "Government Regulation of the Hospital Industry in Colorado," *Journal of Public Health Policy,* Vol. 2, No. 1 (March 1981), pp. 58–69.

22. American conservatives' push to eliminate many national and state regulatory programs during the late 1970s and the 1980s is summarized in Martin Tolchin and Susan J. Tolchin, *Dismantling America: The Rush to Deregulate* (Boston: Houghton Mifflin, 1983). Opposition to hospital rate regulation and health facilities planning became a vogue among American health economists. See, for instance, Robert B. Helms, "The Health Cost Problem: Is Regulation Our Only Hope?" *Bulletin of the New York Academy of Medicine,* Vol. 56, No. 1 (Jan.–Feb. 1980), pp. 26–37; John C. Goodman, *The Regulation of Medical Care: Is the Price Too High?* (San Francisco: Cato Institute, 1980); Clark Havighurst, *Deregulating the Health Care Industry* (Cambridge, Mass.: Ballinger, 1982).

23. For an example of cost shifting under state rate regulations, see Michael D. Rosko, "The Impact of Prospective Payment: A Multi-Dimensional Analysis of New Jersey's SHARE Program," *Journal of Health Politics, Policy and Law,* Vol. 9, No. 1 (Spring 1984), pp. 96–98.

24. Allen S. Meyerhoff and David A. Crozier, "Health Care Coalitions: The Evolution of a Movement," *Health Affairs,* Vol. 3, No. 1 (Spring 1984), pp. 120–128.

25. The frequent challenges to government programs in American courts are described in Jethro K. Lieberman, *The Litigious Society* (New York: Basic Books, 1981).

26. Harold A. Cohen and Carl J. Schramm, "A Design for Resolving the Conflicts Resulting from Separate Regulation of Hospital Rates and Hospital Capacity," in Mancur Olson (ed.), *A New Approach to the Economics of Health Care* (Washington, D.C.: American Enterprise Institute, 1981), pp. 258–273.

27. Alexander Hamilton, John Jay, and James Madison, *The Federalist,* esp. Nos. 9, 10, 51.

28. Mitnick, *The Political Economy of Regulation* (see note 12, above), pp. 45–72, 206–237; Daniel J. Fiorino and Daniel S. Metlay, "Theories of Agency Failure" (paper presented at annual meeting of the American Political Science Association, Washington, D.C., 1977).

29. Jack A. Meyer (ed.), *Market Reforms in Health Care* (Washington, D.C.: American Enterprise Institute, 1983); see also the publications by Helms, Goodman, and Havighurst, cited in note 22, above.

30. The American preference for formula methods over negotiation is expressed in Richard S. Schweiker and others, *Report to Congress: Hospital Prospective Payment for Medicare* (Washington, D.C.: U.S. Department of Health and Human Services, 1982), pp. 39–40. During the years just before this decision about paying American hospitals under Medicare, I had supplied the policy makers with national monographs describing methods of negotiation and regulation in Europe. They interpreted the information as negative lessons from abroad: such methods were unfeasible and undesirable in America.

31. Formula methods of projecting new cost bases and rates from past costs are compared with review of prospective budgets by regulatory staffs in *Recommendations for Financing Hospital Inpatient Care* (Albany: Council on Health Care Financing, State of New York, 1980), pp. 99–102. The council reaffirmed a preference for New York's formula methods over the budget screening used in other states.

32. The Economic Stabilization Program is described in Paul B. Ginsburg, "Inflation and the Economic Stabilization Program," in Michael Zubkoff (ed.), *Health: A Victim or Cause of Inflation?* (New York: Neale Watson Academic Publications, 1976), pp. 31–51. The several formulas for a national hospital cost-restraint policy during 1977 and 1978 are described in Abernethy and Pearson, *Regulating Hospital Costs* (see note 17, above), passim.

33. The New York and Massachusetts methods are described in two monographs by Abt Associates, *Case Study of Prospective Reimbursement in New York* and *Case Study of Prospective Reimbursement in Massachusetts* (Washington, D.C.: Health Care Financing Administration, U.S. Department of Health and Human Services, 1980).

34. Michael A. Morrissey and others, "State Rate Setting," *Health Affairs*, Vol. 2, No. 2 (Summer 1983), pp. 16–47; Brian Biles and others, "Hospital Cost Inflation Under State Rate-Setting Programs," *New England Journal of Medicine*, Vol. 303 (Sept. 18, 1980), pp. 664–668; Joskow, *Controlling Hospital Costs* (see note 16, above), Chap. 7 passim.

35. Some examples appear in Paul L. Grimaldi and Julie A. Micheletti, *Diagnosis Related Groups: A Practitioner's Guide,* 2nd ed. (Chicago: Pluribus Press, 1983), p. 93. Changing any decision rules in any sort of rate regulation is inherently full of uncertainties and conflicts of interest, as described in Stephen Breyer, *Regulation and Its Reform* (Cambridge, Mass.: Harvard University Press, 1982), esp. Chaps. 2–5.

36. Hirsch S. Ruchlin and Harry M. Rosen, "The Process of Hospital Rate Regulation: The New York Experience," *Inquiry*, Vol. 18 (Spring 1981), pp. 70–78. The bottlenecks in the New York appeals machinery—particularly during the early years—are described in Katharine G. Bauer and Arva Rosenfeld Clark, *New*

York: The Formula Approach to Prospective Reimbursement (Boston: Harvard Center for Community Health and Medical Care, 1974).

Chapter Eight

1. For a convenient summary of budgeting during the first decade of the National Health Service, see Claude Guillebaud and others, *Report of the Committee of Enquiry into the Cost of the National Health Service* (London: Her Majesty's Stationery Office, 1956), pp. 99-103. Financial management and problems during the first decades are summarized in Gwyn Bevan and others, *Health Care Priorities and Management* (London: Croom Helm, 1980), Chap. 2.

2. The earlier problems and the reforms of the 1960s are described in Richard Clarke, *Public Expenditure, Management and Control: The Development of the Public Expenditure Survey Committee (PESC)* (London: Macmillan, 1978); and Samuel Brittan, *Steering the Economy: The Role of the Treasury,* 2nd ed. (Harmondsworth, England: Penguin Books, 1971), esp. Chap. 3. For a convenient short description of the appropriations procedure in the past and present, see Eric Taylor, *The House of Commons at Work,* 9th ed. (London: Macmillan, 1979), Chap. 6. The history of PES during its first years appears in Clarke, cited above. Systematic descriptions of the procedure after it had settled down can be found in Samuel Goldman, *The Developing System of Public Expenditure Management and Control* (London: Her Majesty's Stationery Office, 1973); and Her Majesty's Treasury, *Public Expenditure White Papers: Handbook on Methodology* (London: Her Majesty's Stationery Office, 1972).

3. How decisions are actually made in practice within Treasury and between Treasury and the spending departments is described masterfully in Hugh Heclo and Aaron Wildavsky, *The Private Government of Public Money* (Berkeley: University of California Press, 1974). The application of PES to DHSS is summarized in Bevan, *Health Care Priorities and Management* (see note 1, above), pp. 69-80, 124-131.

4. The evidence is summarized in Nick Bosanquet and Alan Maynard, *Public Expenditures on the NHS* (London: Institute of Health Services Management, 1985-1986), 2 vols.

5. The extreme regional inequalities before the war are documented in "Political and Economic Planning, Medical Care for Citizens," *Planning,* No. 222, June 30, 1944.

6. Figures are taken from M. H. Cooper and A. J. Culyer, "Equality in the National Health Service," in M. M. Hauser (ed.), *The Economics of Medical Care* (London: Allen & Unwin, 1972), pp. 55-57. Trends in regional differentials during the 1950s and 1960s—how some regions moved toward the national average and others away from it—are summarized in D. A. T. Griffiths, "Inequalities and Management in the NHS," *Hospital,* Vol. 67, No. 7 (July 1971), pp. 229-230.

7. The difficulties faced by one Hospital Board are described in Christopher Ham, *Policy-Making in the National Health Service: A Case Study of the Leeds Regional Hospital Board* (London: Macmillan, 1981), Chap. 6.

8. Peter A. West, "Allocation and Equity in the Public Sector: The

Hospital Revenue Allocation Formula," *Applied Economics*, Vol. 5 (1973), pp. 153–166.

9. This new structure is described in Ruth Levitt and Andrew Wall, *The Reorganised National Health Service*, 3rd ed. (London: Croom Helm, 1984). Financing is discussed in Chap. 6. The leading work on resource allocation and financial management since the reorganization is Bevan, *Health Care Priorities and Management* (see note 1, above).

10. *Priorities for Health and Personal Social Services in England: A Consultative Document* (London: Her Majesty's Stationery Office, 1976); and *Care in Action: A Handbook of Policies and Priorities for the Health and Personal Social Services in England* (London: Her Majesty's Stationery Office, 1981).

11. The RAWP recommendations appear in two Department of Health and Social Security publications: *Sharing Resources for Health in England: Report of the Resource Allocation Working Party* (London: Her Majesty's Stationery Office, 1976) and *Advisory Group on Resource Allocation* (London: Her Majesty's Stationery Office, 1980). The administration of RAWP is described in R. G. Bevan and A. H. Spencer, "Models of Resource Policy of Regional Health Authorities," in M. Clarke (ed.), *Planning and Analysis in Health Care Systems* (London: PION, 1983), pp. 90–118; and Martin J. Buxton and Rudolf E. Klein, *Allocating Health Resources: A Commentary on the Report of the Resource Allocation Working Party* (London: Her Majesty's Stationery Office, 1978).

12. Department of Health and Social Security, *Health Care and Its Costs* (London: Her Majesty's Stationery Office, 1983), pp. 25–26; and Department of Health and Social Security, *The Health Service in England: Annual Report, 1985* (London: Her Majesty's Stationery Office, 1985), p. 3.

13. Martin J. Buxton and Rudolf E. Klein, "Distribution of Hospital Provision: Policy Themes and Resource Variations," *British Medical Journal*, Feb. 8, 1975, pp. 345–349; and D. R. Jones and S. Masterman, "NHS Resources: Scales of Variation," *British Journal of Preventive and Social Medicine*, Vol. 30 (1976), pp. 244–250.

14. S. J. Senn and H. Shaw, "Resource Allocation," *Journal of Epidemiology and Community Health*, Vol. 32, No. 1 (March 1978), pp. 22–27.

15. Davis J. Hunter, "Coping with Uncertainty," *Sociology of Health and Illness*, Vol. 1, No. 1 (1979), pp. 40–68; Howard Elcock and Stuart Haywood, *The Buck Stops Where?* (Hull: Institute for Health Studies, University of Hull, 1980), pp. 36–50; and *The Sub-Regional Application of R.A.W.P. by Regional Health Authorities* (Birmingham: National Association of Health Authorities in England and Wales, 1983).

16. Grass-roots resistance to the shift from the acute to the Cinderella services is described in Stuart C. Haywood, "The Politics of Management in Health Care," *Journal of Health Politics, Policy and Law*, Vol. 8, No. 3 (Fall 1983), pp. 424–443.

17. British newspapers are full of the controversies aroused within districts as services are cut and redesigned. See also the news columns of the weekly magazine *Health and Social Service Journal*. For a thorough case study, see J.

S. Yudkin, "Changing Patterns of Resource Allocation in a London Teaching District," *British Medical Journal*, Oct. 28, 1978, pp. 1212-1215.

18. My calculations from Jean-Pierre Poullier, *Public Expenditure on Health Under Economic Constraints* (Paris: Organisation for Economic Co-operation and Development, 1984), Part 1, p. 37, Table 4.

19. Robert Maxwell, *Health and Wealth* (Lexington, Mass.: Lexington Books, 1981), pp. 51-57.

20. Alain C. Enthoven, *Reflections on the Management of the National Health Service* (London: Nuffield Provincial Hospitals Trust, 1985), pp. 34-42.

21. Bevan, *Health Care Priorities and Management* (see note 1, above), pp. 139-141, 149-162.

22. For a history of Canadian hospital finance, see G. Harvey Agnew, *Canadian Hospitals, 1920-1970* (Toronto: University of Toronto Press, 1974), Chap. 5; and *The Hospitals of Ontario—A Short History* (Toronto: King's Printer, 1934). The governmentalization of hospital finance throughout the country is described in Malcolm Taylor, *Health Insurance and Canadian Public Policy: The Seven Decisions That Created the Canadian Health Insurance System* (Montreal: McGill-Queen's University Press, 1978), Chaps. 1-4.

23. Provincial budgeting from the 1950s to the present is described in Ronald M. Burns, "Budgeting and Finance," in David J. Bellamy and others (eds.), *The Provincial Political Systems* (Toronto: Methuen, 1976), pp. 330-336; and in several books about individual provincial governments, such as Fred F. Schindeler, *Responsible Government in Ontario* (Toronto: University of Toronto Press, 1969), pp. 55-61. Budgeting methods in the national government are discussed in J. C. Strick, *Canadian Public Finance*, 2nd ed. (Toronto: Holt, Rinehart and Winston of Canada, 1978), esp. Chap. 3.

24. The changes are described in Richard van Loon, "From Shared Cost to Block Funding and Beyond," *Journal of Health Politics, Policy and Law*, Vol. 2, No. 4 (Winter 1978), pp. 454-478; William A. Glaser, *Federalism in Canada and West Germany: Lessons for the United States* (New York: Center for the Social Sciences, Columbia University, 1979; distributed by the National Technical Information Service), Chaps. 13-14 and sources cited; and Thomas J. Courchene, *Refinancing the Canadian Federation: The 1977 Fiscal Arrangements* (Montreal: Canadian Economic Policy Committee, C. D. Howe Research Institute, 1979).

25. Ontario's experiences with global budgeting of hospitals are described in Robin G. Milne, *Hospital Budgeting in Ontario* (Glasgow: Department of Political Economy, University of Glasgow, 1977), Chap. 2; and *Government Controls on the Health Care System: The Canadian Experience—Hospital Responses to Budgetary Constraints in Ontario* (Washington, D.C.: Lewin and Associates, 1976; distributed by the National Technical Information Service).

26. The *Québecois* leadership's critique of the earmarked shared-cost programs for hospitals and other sectors and their desire to reallocate the health money according to provincial priorities are discussed in Claude Castonguay and others, *Rapport: Commission d'enquête sur la santé et le bien-être social* (Quebec: Official Publisher, 1967 and 1970); and Claude Morin, *Quebec Versus Ottawa* (Toronto: University of Toronto Press, 1976), esp. Chaps. 4, 10.

27. Methods of payment to Quebec hospitals in recent years are described in Gilles DesRochers, "Le financement des établissements de santé et de services sociaux," *Canadian Public Administration,* Vol. 22, No. 3 (Autumn 1979), pp. 366–379; Agathe Légaré and Monique Langlois, "Le budget global: Formule adoptée qu'il reste à adapter," *65 à l'heure,* Vol. 4, No. 3 (May 1977), pp. 123–125; and André-Pierre Contandriopoulos and others, *A Method for Reviewing Hospital Budgetary Bases* (Montreal: Département d'Administration de la Santé, Université de Montréal, 1977).

28. The merits of the complaints are analyzed in Robert G. Evans, "Health Care in Canada: Patterns of Funding and Regulation," *Journal of Health Politics, Policy and Law,* Vol. 8, No. 1 (Spring 1983), pp. 16–21.

29. Allan S. Detsky and others, "The Effectiveness of a Regulatory Strategy in Containing Hospital Costs," *New England Journal of Medicine,* Vol. 309 (July 21, 1983), pp. 151–159.

30. The evolution of Quebec health policy and the difficulties in implementing it are described in Marc Renaud, "Réforme ou illusion? Une analyse des interventions de l'état québécois dans le domaine de la santé," *Sociologie et sociétés,* Vol. 9, No. 1, pp. 127–152.

31. The methods are summarized in the works cited in note 27 above; in *Le guide budgétaire* (Quebec: Ministère des Affaires Sociales, annual); and in the many working papers of the Etudes Financières, Direction de la Recherche et Statistique, Direction Générale Planification et Evaluation, Ministère des Affaires Sociales.

32. The design and results of the experiment appear in Claude Renou and others, *Rapport à Monsieur le Ministre de la Santé relatif à l'évaluation de l'experimentation de nouveaux modes de financements et de gestion des établissements hospitaliers* (Paris: Ministère de la Santé, 1982); R. Cappe and others, "L'expérience du budget global au Centre Hospitalier de Saint-Germain-en-Laye ou essai pour une direction par objectifs," *Gestions Hospitalières,* No. 191 (Dec. 1979), pp. 1031–1039; and Serge Fontarensky, "L'expérience du budget global au C.H.R. d'Amiens," *La révue hospitalière de France,* No. 367 (Jan. 1984), pp. 32–48.

33. The general reform of the hospital system during the 1980s is summarized in Jean-Marie Clément, *Les réformes hospitalières, 1981–1984* (Paris: Berger-Levrault, 1985). Global budget calculations appear in *Note explicative sur le budget global pour l'exercice 1985* (Paris: Direction des Hôpitaux, Ministère des Affaires Sociales et de la Solidarité Nationale, 1983). A new accounting system is used for retrospective cost reports and prospective budgets, replacing the traditional one described in Chapter Three of this book. It is the "Guide méthodologique de comptabilité hospitalière," 1984 et seq.

34. Dutch hospital and health insurance journals during the 1980s were full of discussions about the need for global budgeting and about the philosophy behind the new approach. Typical essays appear in *Symposium budgettering intramurale gezondheidszorg* (Utrecht: Nationaal Ziekenhuisinstituut, 1983).

35. The canton of Vaud recently enacted some features of global budgeting resembling the methods of France. All sickness funds and the cantonal government negotiate a prospective budget with each hospital; the payers send monthly payments; shares depend on volumes of use by subscribers. The

arrangements are managed by the cantonal government and not by a *centrale*. See Charles Kleiber and Luc Schenker, *Le budget global dans le canton de Vaud, Suisse* (Lausanne: Service de la Santé Publique et de la Planification Sanitaire, 1985).

36. Payment of hospitals by Medicare before DRGs is described in Herman R. Somers and Anne R. Somers, *Medicare and the Hospitals* (Washington, D.C.: Brookings Institution, 1967); Judith M. Feder, *Medicare: The Politics of Federal Hospital Insurance* (Lexington, Mass.: Lexington Books, 1977); and *Medicare After 15 years: Has It Become a Broken Promise to the Elderly?* Report by the Select Committee on Aging, U.S. House of Representatives, 96th Congress, 2d Session (Washington, D.C.: U.S. Government Printing Office, 1980). The formal payment rules are described in Mary Elizabeth Rieder and James M. Kaple, "An Overview of Medicare and Medicaid Reimbursement," in William O. Cleverley (ed.), *Handbook of Health Care Accounting and Finance* (Rockville, Md.: Aspen Publishers, 1982), pp. 670–679, 684, 686.

37. Explained in Richard F. Averill and David A. Sparrow, "TEFRA's Two-Part Strategy Will Reduce Medicare's Financial Liability to Hospitals," *Healthcare Financial Management,* Vol. 37, No. 4 (April 1983), pp. 72–84; and John K. Iglehart, "The New Era of Prospective Payment for Hospitals," *New England Journal of Medicine,* Vol. 307, No. 20 (Nov. 11, 1982), pp. 1288–1292.

38. John E. Wennberg and others, "Will Payment Based on Diagnosis-Related Groups Control Hospital Costs?" *New England Journal of Medicine,* Vol. 311, No. 5 (Aug. 2, 1984), pp. 295–300.

39. Donald W. Simborg, "DRG Creep: A New Hospital-Acquired Disease," *New England Journal of Medicine,* Vol. 304, No. 26 (June 25, 1981) pp. 1602–1604; and Grace M. Carter and Paul B. Ginsburg, *The Medicare Case Mix Index Increases* (Santa Monica, Calif: Rand Corporation, 1985).

40. Discovered by HCFA's Region II under the New Jersey DRG system, since a "Medicare waiver" allowed New Jersey to include all the Medicare cases. Reported to Congress in William Toby, "Memorandum: Region II Experiences with the Diagnostic Related Groups Program in New Jersey," reprinted in *Quality Assurance Under Prospective Reimbursement Programs: Hearing Before the Special Committee on Aging, United States Senate, 98th Congress, First Session* (Washington, D.C.: U.S. Government Printing Office, 1983), pp. 71–82. This report motivated the Congress to retain the Professional Service Review Organizations (renamed PROs).

41. Irwin Cohen, "The Provider Reimbursement Appeals Process: Past, Present and Future," *Healthcare Financial Management,* Vol. 38, No. 6 (June 1984), pp. 80, 82, 84.

Chapter Nine

1. See, for example, the many eighteenth- and nineteenth-century hospital buildings, still used during the 1940s, in *Cent ans d'Assistance Publique à Paris, 1849–1949* (Paris: Administration Générale de l'Assistance Publique à Paris, 1949); and Axel Hinrich Murken, *Das Bild des deutschen Krankenhauses im 19. Jahrhundert* (Münster, West Germany: Verlag Murken-Altrogge, 1978).

2. Examples of such sales are described in Maurice Garden, *Le budget des Hospices Civils de Lyon, 1800–1976* (Lyon: Presses Universitaires de Lyon, 1980), pp. 58–61.

3. No comprehensive history of European capital financing has been written, but information about individual hospitals can be found in the specialized volumes about each. Capital financing in Britain and America are covered in Brian Abel-Smith, *The Hospitals, 1800-1948* (London: Heinemann, 1964), passim; and Edward H. L. Corwin, *The American Hospital* (New York: Commonwealth Fund, 1946), Chap. 3.

4. The evolution of this approach to the planning and organization of hospital services is discussed in Robert Bridgman, "Hospital Regionalization in Europe," in Christa Altenstetter (ed.), *Changing National-Subnational Relations in Health: Opportunities and Constraints* (Washington, D.C.: National Institutes of Health, Public Health Service, U.S. Department of Health and Human Services, 1978), pp. 321–331. Early examples of regionalization are described in Arthur Engel, *Perspectives in Health Planning* (London: Athlone Press, 1968); Malcolm Tottie and B. Janzon (eds.), *Regional Hospital Planning* (Stockholm: Nordiska Bokhandeln, 1967); Hugh Leavell, *Regionalization of Health Services: An Examination of the Regionalization Concept and of WHO's Possible Role in Relation to This Concept* (Geneva: World Health Organization, 1969); and many reports by consultants sent by the World Health Organization to member countries.

5. An overview of the conception and implementation of regionalization appears in Robert F. Bridgman and Milton I. Roemer, *Hospital Legislation and Hospital Systems* (Geneva: World Health Organization, 1973), esp. pp. 175–181. The mixture of achievements and disappointments is summarized in Bridgman, "Hospital Regionalization in Europe" (see note 4, above).

6. An overview of estimating methods in several countries is given in Daniel Le Touzé, "Hospital Bed Planning in Canada," *International Journal of Health Services,* Vol. 14, No. 1 (1984), pp. 113–119.

7. Evident throughout *The Implications of Cost-Effectiveness Analysis of Medical Technology. Background Paper No. 4: The Management of Health Care Technology in Ten Countries* (Washington, D.C.: Office of Technology Assessment, U.S. Congress, 1980).

8. See, for example, *Procedures for Areawide Health Facility Planning* (Washington, D.C.: U.S. Public Health Service, 1963); and Walter J. McNerney and Donald C. Riedel, *Regionalization and Rural Health Care* (Ann Arbor: University of Michigan, 1962).

9. For political history of RMP, see Thomas S. Bodenheimer, "Regional Medical Programs: No Road to Regionalization," *Medical Care Review,* Vol. 26, No. 11 (Dec. 1969), pp. 1125–1166; and Frank D. Campion, *The AMA and U.S. Health Policy Since 1940* (Chicago: Chicago Review Press, 1984), pp. 279–280. The political origins of the Medicare program for physicians are discussed in Theodore R. Marmor, *The Politics of Medicare* (Hawthorne, N.Y.: Aldine, 1973). The political origins of the Medicare program for hospitals are discussed in Herman M. Somers and Anne R. Somers, *Medicare and the Hospitals* (Washington, D.C.: Brookings Institution, 1967); and Judith M. Feder, *Medicare:*

The Politics of Federal Hospital Insurance (Lexington, Mass.: Lexington Books, 1977).

10. Albert W. Snoke, "What Good Is Legislation—Or Planning—If We Can't Make It Work?" *American Journal of Public Health*, Vol. 72, No. 9 (Sept. 1982), pp. 1028-1033. For an analysis of the structural defects in the most recent law, see Bonnie Lefkowitz, *Health Planning* (Rockville, Md.: Aspen Publishers, 1983).

11. For examples see Drew Altman and others, *Health Planning and Regulation* (Ann Arbor, Mich.: Health Administration Press, 1981).

12. Less than 4 percent of patient-care revenue could be used for depreciation and interest, according to the special survey reported in Bundesminister für Gesundheitswesen, *Bericht über die finanzielle Lage der Krankenanstalten* (Bonn: Deutscher Bundestag, 5. Wahlperiode, Drucksache V/4230, May 19, 1969).

13. *The Cost of Medical Care* (Geneva: International Labour Office, 1959), pp. 191, 208; Fritz Kastner, *Monograph on the Organisation of Medical Care Within the Framework of Social Security: Federal Republic of Germany* (Geneva: International Labour Office, 1968), p. 71; and Statistisches Bundesamt Wiesbaden, *Ausgaben für Gesundheit, 1970 bis 1978* (Stuttgart: Verlag W. Kohlhammer, 1980), p. 16.

14. The financial collaborations between the *Bund* and the *Länder* during the 1970s are described in Fritz Scharpf and others, *Politikverflechtung* (Kronberg/Ts., West Germany: Scriptor Verlag, 1976-1977), 2 vols.

15. Described in Fritz Schnabel, "Politischer und administrativer Vollzug des Krankenhausfinanzierungsgesetzes" (unpublished doctoral dissertation, University of Konstanz, 1980), pp. 68-110, 157-172.

16. For a convenient short summary of each province's plan, see A. Schön and others, "Analyse und Bewertung der Krankenhausbedarfspläne der deutschen Bundesländer," *Das Krankenhaus,* Vol. 70, No. 5 (May 1978), pp. 159-166. The limited legal authority of such plans is explained in Udo Steiner, "Die staatliche Krankenhausbedarfsplanung als Gegenstand der verwaltungsgerichtlichen Rechtmässigkeitskontrolle," *Deutsches Verwaltungsblatt,* Vol. 94, No. 23 (Dec. 1, 1979), pp. 865-872.

17. Summaries of the planning and grant system appear in Christa Altenstetter, *Krankenhausbedarfsplanung* (Munich: R. Oldenbourg Verlag, 1985); and Siegfried Eichhorn, *System der Krankenhausplanung in der Bundesrepublik Deutschland* (Düsseldorf: Deutsches Krankenhausinstitut, 1984). The early years of the planning system are summarized in Bundesminister für Jugend, Familie, und Gesundheit, *Bericht der Bundesregierung über die Auswirkungen des Gesetzes zur wirtschaftlichen Sicherung der Krankenhäuser und zur Regelung der Krankenhauspflegesätze (KHG)* (Bonn: Deutscher Bundestag, 7. Wahlperiode, Drucksache 7/4530, Dec. 30, 1975); and Bundesregierung, *Entwurf eines Gesetzes zur Änderung des Krankenhausfinanzierungsgesetzes* (Bonn: Deutscher Bundestag, 8. Wahlperiode, Drucksache 8/2067, Aug. 29, 1978).

18. My calculations from Bundesministerium für Jugend, Familie, and Gesundheit, *Daten des Gesundheitswesens: Ausgabe 1983* (Stuttgart: Verlag W.

Kohlhammer, 1983), pp. 253–266; and from other data supplied by the Bundesministerium für Arbeit und Sozialordnung.

19. The original drafting of §10KHG, subsequent administration, and the hospitals' use of the money are described in Theo Thiemeyer and others, *Einordnung von Krankenhäusern in ein abgestuftes Versorgungssystem* (Bonn: Bundesminister für Arbeit und Sozialordnung, 1982). The accounting rules for assigning equipment to different classes are listed in Karl Jung and Marianne Preuss, *Rechnungs- und Buchführung im Krankenhaus* (Stuttgart: Verlag W. Kohlhammer, 1978). The rules guide the hospital managers in their purchasing plans; in requesting investment funds for particular equipment, either from the *Land* government (under §10KHG) or from the sickness funds (under the *Pflegesatz*); and in answering queries from the payers.

20. How hospitals actually use the maintenance and depreciation money collected under the daily charge from the sickness funds pursuant to §18BPflV is summarized in Theo Thiemeyer and others, *Analyse und Neugestaltung der Pauschalen für Instandhaltung und Instandsetzung nach der Bundespflegesatz-verordnung* (Bonn: Bundesminister für Arbeit und Sozialordnung, 1979).

21. My calculations from *Daten des Gesundheitswesens* (see note 18, above), pp. 253–266; and from other data supplied by the Bundesministerium für Arbeit und Sozialordnung.

22. The most thorough study of the financial shortfalls is *Finanzbedarf im Bereich der Krankenhausinvestionen* (Düsseldorf: Deutsches Krankenhausinstitut, 1984).

23. Günther Orth, "10 Jahre Krankenhausfinanzierungsgesetz—Ziel und Wirklichkeit—aus der Sicht der Krankenhäuser," *Krankenhaus-Umschau,* Vol. 51, No. 12 (Dec. 1982), pp. 816–821; and many others. The German Hospital Association endorsed amortization of all equipment costs as part of the daily charge but continued reliance on public grants for extensive construction: "Thesen zur Neuordnung des Krankenhaus-Finanzierungsystems," resolution adopted by the Vorstand of the Deutsche Krankenhausgesellschaft, Dec. 8, 1982.

24. The proposals of all the central players are summarized in Ernst Bruckenberger, "Vorstellungen und Ziele des Bundes und der Länder zur Novellierung des Krankenhausfinanzierungsgesetzes," *Krankenhaus-Umschau,* Vol. 53, No. 10 (Oct. 1984), pp. 754–762. Bruckenberger examines at length the competing proposals by the national government and the Christian-Democratic-led provinces that went before Parliament and were compromised in the final legislation in December 1984. During the debates of the 1980s, some papers by study commissions also attracted attention, particularly *Zwischenbericht der Kommission Krankenhausfinanzierung der Robert Bosch Stiftung* (Stuttgart: Robert Bosch Stiftung, 1983).

25. The arguments for extending planning to the doctors' offices appear in Ernst Bruckenberger, "Zur Problematik der abgestimmten Nutzung medizinischtechnischer Grossgeräte," in Hans Rüdiger Vogel (ed.), *Bedarf und Bedarfsplanung im Gesundheitswesen* (Stuttgart: Gustav Fischer Verlag, 1983), pp. 49-57. Data about location of equipment in 1984 appear in *Deutsches Ärzteblatt,* Vol. 81, No. 17 (April 24, 1984), p. 1341.

26. For codification of all the cantons' hospital plans, see Gisela Lauber, *Gesundheits- und Krankenhausplanung der Kantone* (Aarau: Schweizerisches

Krankenhausinstitut, 1979). A summary of the goals and techniques of hospital planning, with special reference to Switzerland, appears in Peter Bürki and others, *Probleme der wirtschaftlichen Spitalführung* (Bern: Betriebswirtschaftliches Institut der Universität Bern, 1977), pp. 86-139. For a good discussion of Swiss health planning in general, including the hospital component, see Pierre Gilliand, *Planification de santé publique: Quelques bases et tendances plausible* (Aarau: Schweizerisches Krankenhausinstitut, 1977).

27. The history of French hospital construction policy and the stages in building styles are summarized in Suzanne Gourguechon, "La politique hospitalière et son adaptation à une conjoncture novelle," *Revue française des affaires sociales*, Vol. 34, No. 4 (Oct.-Dec. 1980), pp. 173-187.

28. The debates over planning methods and their applications to individual decisions are summarized in Béatrice Majnoni d'Intignano, *Les investissements hospitaliers* (Paris: Editions Médicales et Universitaires, 1976), pp. 149-173.

29. "La coordination des établissements de soins publics et privés" (Paris: Ministère de la Santé Publique et de la Sécurité Sociale, Note d'information No. 71, Feb. 29, 1972).

30. Planning is described in Gérard Moreau, "La planification dans le domaine de la santé: Les hommes et les équipements," *Revue française des affaires sociales*, Vol. 34, No. 4 (Oct.-Dec. 1980), pp. 135-150; C. Brumter, "La planification sanitaire" (unpublished doctoral dissertation, Université de Sciences Juridiques, Politiques, Sociales et de Technologie, Strasbourg, 1979); and C. Dutreil, "La carte sanitaire," *Revue trimestrielle de droit sanitaire et social*, Nos. 37-38 (Jan.-June 1974), pp. 391-441. The law and methodology are described in *Carte sanitaire: Organisation, indices des besoins, régions et secteurs* (Paris: Berger-Levrault, 1979).

31. Emile Lévy and others, *Introduction à la gestion hospitalière* (Paris: Dunod, 1977), Chap. 12.

32. Several examples are given in Sauveur Berterretche and François Vedelago, *Les décisions d'investissement en matériel endoscopique dans les unités hospitalières* (Talence, France: Département Sociologie de la Santé, Université de Bordeaux II, 1983).

33. Its organization and important role in French public investment are described in "La Caisse des Dépôts et Consignations," *Notes et études documentaires* (La Documentation Française), Nos. 3996-3998, June 20, 1973.

34. Data from Majnoni, *Les investissements hospitaliers* (see note 28, above), p. 184; and from *Les finances du secteur public local: Statistiques des comptes pour l'exercice 1979 des hôpitaux publics . . .* (Paris: Direction de la Comptabilité Publique, Ministère du Budget, 1982), p. 23. Majnoni shows variations in sources of finance by type of hospital.

35. The rules are listed in Paul Coudurier, *Les prix de journée,* 4th ed. (Paris: Berger-Levrault, 1978), pp. 88-97, 137, 195-196.

36. Maryse Gadreau, *La tarification hospitalière* (Paris: Editions Médicales et Universitaires, 1975), pp. 275-282, 355-356, 363-364.

37. *Assurance maladie et hospitalisation* (Paris: Caisse Nationale de l'Assurance Maladie des Travailleurs Salariés, 1972), pp. 16-19.

38. For the history of capital financing, see Donald R. Cohodes and Brian M. Kinkead, *Hospital Capital Formation in the 1980s* (Baltimore: Johns Hopkins University Press, 1984), pp. 17–25; and Brian M. Kinkead, *Historical Trends in Hospital Capital Investment* (Washington, D.C.: Assistant Secretary for Planning and Evaluation, U.S. Department of Health and Human Services, 1984).

39. Besides grants by many state and local governments, the national and state governments collaborated in a shared-cost program, described in Judith R. Lave and Lester B. Lave, *The Hospital Construction Act—An Evaluation of the Hill-Burton Program, 1948–1973* (Washington, D.C.: American Enterprise Institute, 1974).

40. Maureen Metz, *Trends in Sources of Capital in the Hospital Industry* (Chicago: Office of Public Policy Analysis, American Hospital Association, March 1983). Distribution among types of bond and types of philanthropy appears in the articles by Michael Endres and Robert J. Miller, in William O. Cleverley (ed.), *Handbook of Health Care Accounting and Finance* (Rockville, Md.: Aspen Publishers, 1982), Chaps. 53, 57.

41. Steps in the crucial decisions to include capital costs in Medicare operating payments appear in Herman M. Somers and Anne R. Somers, *Medicare and the Hospitals* (Washington, D.C.: Brookings Institution, 1967), Chap. 8; and Judith M. Feder, *Medicare: The Politics of Federal Hospital Insurance* (Lexington, Mass.: Lexington Books, 1977), Chap. 4.

42. The intricacies of this and other recent borrowing methods are summarized in Geoffrey B. Shields (ed.), *Debt Financing and Capital Formation in Health Care Institutions* (Rockville, Md.: Aspen Publishers, 1983); and in Cohodes and Kinkead, *Hospital Capital Formation in the 1980's* (see note 38, above), Chaps. 5–6.

43. *Capital Equipment Spending by Hospitals* (New York: CIT Corporation, annual).

44. Evident in the new American textbooks in institutional financial management. Capital budgeting, the choice of investment, and the financing of debt become the central tasks. See, for example, John Byron Silvers and C. K. Prahalad, *Financial Management of Health Institutions* (Oak Brook, Ill.: Healthcare Financial Management Association, 1974). Such books—taken for granted in the American environment—could not be written in any other country.

45. A declining physical plant results in loss of medical staff and then in lower occupancy. Inferred from closure of two hundred hospitals between 1975 and 1977, in Emily Friedman, "The End of the Line: When a Hospital Closes," *Hospitals*, Vol. 52 (Dec. 1, 1978), pp. 69–75.

46. Because of the entrepreneurial and competitive features throughout, the American system *as a whole* adopts and diffuses new technology more rapidly and more extensively than any other nation's system does. In her very able study of new methods in the United States, Louise Russell attempted to determine whether initial adoption is quicker and diffusion faster in the local hospital markets with more competition and more third-party coverage. Defects in the data, confounding variables, and the restricted perspective of macrostatistical analysis interfered with the results, but some evidence was found that competition and third-party coverage led to such regional variations in adoption and diffusion

within America. See Louise B. Russell, *Technology in Hospitals* (Washington, D.C.: Brookings Institution, 1979). Several other intensive studies of particular markets uncovered many examples of how competitive market situations and third-party cost-based reimbursement (paying both for utilization and debt service) encourage early adoption and widespread diffusion of advanced technology. Summarized in Judith L. Wagner (ed.), *Medical Technology* (Washington, D.C.: National Center for Health Services Research, U.S. Department of Health and Human Services, 1979), pp. 92–104.

47. The methodology of financial feasibility studies is described in Joel M. Ziff and John W. Hlywak, "Financial Feasibility Studies," in Cleverley, *Handbook of Health Care Accounting and Finance* (see note 40, above), Chap. 54; and Harvey J. Gitel, "The Financial Feasibility Study," in Shields, *Debt Financing and Capital Formation in Health Care Institutions* (see note 42, above), Chap. 4.

48. The methodology of rating hospital bonds in the credit market is described in Craig W. Atwater, "Rating Hospital Revenue Bonds," in Cleverley, *Handbook of Health Care Accounting and Finance* (see note 40, above), Chap. 55; William J. Gray, "Debt Capacity, Credit Analysis, and the Rating Agencies," in Shields, *Debt Financing and Capital Formation in Health Care Institutions* (see note 42, above), Chap. 3; and Booz, Allen, & Hamilton, "Historical Linkage Between Selected Hospital Characteristics and Bond Ratings," in *Report of the Special Committee on Equity of Payment for Not-for-Profit and Investor-Owned Hospitals* (Chicago: American Hospital Association, May 1983), Appendix E. If the catchment area and the medical staff are not certain to maintain at least an 80 percent occupancy rate, hospitals will be pressed by creditors to pay higher interest rates, according to William J. Laffey and Stan Lappen, "Tax-Exempt Hospital Financing: Revenue Bonds," *Health Care Management Review*, Vol. 1, No. 4 (Fall 1976), pp. 24–30.

49. The structure, financing, and sales of the medical equipment industry are described in Jane E. Sisk and others, *Federal Policies and the Medical Devices Industry* (Washington, D.C.: Office of Technology Assessment, U.S. Congress, 1984).

50. The great increase in testing—beyond the capacity of therapy to use the information—is described in Stuart H. Altman and Robert Blendon (eds.), *Medical Technology: The Culprit Behind Health Care Costs?* (Washington, D.C.: National Center for Health Services Research, U.S. Department of Health and Human Services, 1979), pp. 39-56, 144-165, 178-212; Thomas W. Moloney and David E. Rogers, "Medical Technology: A Different View of the Contentious Debate over Costs," *New England Journal of Medicine*, Vol. 301, No. 26 (Dec. 27, 1979), pp. 1413-1419; and David Reuben, "Learning Diagnostic Restraint," *New England Journal of Medicine*, Vol. 310, No. 9 (March 1, 1984), pp. 591-593.

51. The absence of price competition in the industries that produce devices used in clinical treatment is reported in Arthur Young and Company, *A Profile of the Medical Technology Industry and Governmental Policies* (Washington, D.C.: National Center for Health Services Research, U.S. Department of Health and Human Services, 1981), 3 vols.

52. For an exposé of competitive sales methods in the lucrative industry for implantable medical devices, see Special Committee on Aging, U.S. Senate,

Fraud, Waste and Abuse in the Medicare Pacemaker Industry (Washington, D.C.: U.S. Government Printing Office, 1982).

53. Jean-Georges Moreau and Patrice Bimont, "L'industrie du matériel biomédical," *Revue française des affaires sociales*, Vol. 34, No. 4 (Oct.-Dec. 1980), pp. 191–204 passim.

54. Mark S. Freeland and Carol E. Schendler, "Health Spending in the 1980's: Integration of Clinical Practice Patterns with Management," *Health Care Financing Review*, Vol. 5, No. 3 (Spring 1984), pp. 14-16; and Sisk and others, *Federal Policies and the Medical Devices Industry* (see note 49, above), pp. 35-37.

55. *Medicare Payments of Return on Equity Capital to Proprietary Providers* (Washington, D.C.: Office of Inspector General, U.S. Department of Health and Human Services, 1983).

56. Institute of Medicine, *For-Profit Enterprise in Health Care* (Washington, D.C.: National Academy Press, 1986), pp. 80-84, 328, and sources cited therein. The chains' methods of raising capital are summarized in Chap. 3.

57. *1983 Directory: Investor-Owned Hospitals and Hospital Management Companies* (Washington, D.C.: Federation of American Hospitals, 1983), pp. 6–9.

58. An example of how a chain makes and finances a takeover decision is described in detail in Ernest G. Barnes (opinion of the Administrative Law Judge), "Initial Decision in the Matter of American Medical International et al." (Washington, D.C.: Federal Trade Commission, Docket No. 9158, July 27, 1983).

59. On the strengths of the chains generally, see Ekaterini Siafaca, *Investor-Owned Hospitals and Their Role in the Changing U.S. Health Care System* (New York: F & S Press, 1981). On the savings in construction, see Lawrence S. Lewin, Robert A. Derzon, and Rhea Margulies, "Investor-Owneds and Nonprofits Differ in Economic Performance," *Hospitals*, Vol. 55, No. 13 (July 1, 1981), p. 58.

60. Denis T. Raihall and J. William Gotcher, "How to Rank Requests for Capital Expenditures in Your Hospital," *Hospital Financial Management*, Vol. 25, No. 12 (Dec. 1971).

61. I will not present the full details of American health planning under Public Law 93-641, since this intricate subject has been covered in other publications. Herbert H. Hyman, *Health Planning: A Systematic Approach*, 2nd ed. (Rockville, Md.: Aspen Publishers, 1982); Lefkowitz, *Health Planning* (see note 10, above); see also the many sources cited in these two books. For a history of American facilities planning, see Symond R. Gottlieb, "A Brief History of Health Planning in the United States," in Clark C. Havighurst (ed.), *Regulatory Health Facilities Construction* (Washington, D.C.: American Enterprise Institute, 1974), pp. 7–26.

62. CT scanners happened to spring onto the American scene during the first years of the planning procedures under Public Law 93-641. They were expensive at first and fell above the CON thresholds. They also appeared at a time when many American health economists were impressed by iconoclastic writings about the clinical ineffectiveness of once popular but expensive technologies, led by Archie L. Cochrane, *Effectiveness and Efficiency* (London: Nuffield Provincial Hospitals Trust, 1972). How the American health-planning system restrained the proliferation and profitability of CT scanners is summarized in Altman and

others, *Health Planning and Regulation* (see note 11, above), pp. 112-128. The uneven implementation of CONs among states and the erratic implementation over time are depicted in Lawrence D. Brown, "Common Sense Meets Implementation: Certificate-of-Need Regulation in the States," *Journal of Health Politics, Policy and Law*, Vol. 8, No. 3 (Fall 1983), pp. 480–494.

63. Donald R. Cohodes, "Interstate Variation in Certificate of Need Programs," in Institute of Medicine, *Health Planning in the United States* (Washington, D.C.: National Academy Press, 1981), vol. 2, pp. 54–88.

64. David S. Salkever and Thomas W. Bice, *Hospital Certificate-of-Need Controls: Impact on Investment, Costs and Use* (Washington, D.C.: American Enterprise Institute, 1979), Chaps. 4–5.

65. An example is given in Ann Lawther-Higgins and others, "The Impact of Certificate of Need on CT Scanning in Massachusetts," *Health Care Management Review*, Vol. 9, No. 2 (Summer 1984), pp. 71-79. The reduction in scale of very expensive capital proposals in Massachusetts in general is described in Julianne R. Howell, *Regulatory Hospital Capital Investment: The Experience in Massachusetts* (Washington, D.C.: National Center for Health Services Research, U.S. Department of Health and Human Services, 1981).

66. *Policy Implications of the Computed Tomography (CT) Scanner: An Update* (Washington, D.C.: Office of Technology Assessment, U.S. Congress, 1981), p. 15. The much stricter controls over the diffusion of new equipment in countries where acquisition depends on public capital grants are evident in *The Implications of Cost-Effectiveness Analysis of Medical Technology. Background Paper No. 4: The Management of Health Care Technology in Ten Countries* (Washington, D.C.: Office of Technology Assessment, U.S. Congress, 1980), esp. Chaps. 2, 3, 6, 10.

67. David Banta, "Computed Tomography: Cost Containment Misdirected," *American Journal of Public Health*, Vol. 70, No. 3 (March 1980), pp. 215–216 and sources cited.

68. Rosanna M. Coffey, "Patients in Public General Hospitals," in *National Health Statistics, 1983* (Washington, D.C.: U.S. Government Printing Office, 1983), pp. 61–65.

69. Anne Bagamery, "Health Care," *Forbes*, Vol. 133, No. 1 (Jan. 2, 1984), pp. 213–214. The only other sector with a higher debt-to-equity ratio was the troubled airline industry (discussed on p. 142 of *Forbes*).

70. *National Gerimedical Hospital and Gerontology Center* v. *Blue Cross of Kansas et al.*, 452 U.S. 378 (1981).

71. Stillborn proposals for more coherent government decisions about lending are summarized in Cohodes and Kinkead, *Hospital Capital Formation in the 1980's* (see note 38, above), pp. 111–116.

72. Designating the provincial authorities as the authors of regional hospital plans anticipated a future reorganization of Dutch health services regionally. All these planning efforts—both under the law and in the work of research institutes—are described in L. M. J. Groot, "Hospital Planning and Regionalization in the Netherlands," in Altenstetter, *Changing National-Subnational Relations in Health* (see note 4, above), pp. 281–296.

73. Jean-Pierre Poullier, *Public Expenditure on Health Under Economic*

Constraints (Paris: Organisation for Economic Co-operation and Development, 1984), Part 1, p. 37.

74. E. Riegen, "Circuitvorming en regionale planning van algemene ziekenhuizen," in Interacademiale Werkgroep Ziekenhuiswetenschappen, *Besturen in de gezondheidszorg: Concerns en circuits* (Lochem, Netherlands: Uitgeversmaatschappij de Tijdstroom, 1984), pp. 104-121. Such regional caps on capital spending were proposed for the United States by the Carter administration in 1977. Opposition by many interest groups led to defeat in Congress. The legislative history is given in David S. Abernethy and David A. Pearson, *Regulating Hospital Costs: The Development of Public Policy* (Ann Arbor, Mich: Health Administration Press, 1979), pp. 41-42, 90-93, 105, 124, 143-144, 157, and passim. In contrast to the lack of regulation in the United States, Holland's COTG can enforce the caps by not allowing amortization and operating costs in prospective budgets.

75. Such persistent difficulties are described in Christopher Ham, *Policy-Making in the National Health Service: A Case Study of the Leeds Regional Hospital Board* (London: Macmillan, 1981), Chap. 3.

76. The planning system from 1974 through 1981 is spelled out in the manual *The NHS Planning System* (London: Department of Health and Social Security, 1976); and in Gwyn Bevan and others, *Health Care Priorities and Management* (London: Croom Helm, 1980), Chaps. 5, 9. A case study of the planning cycle in one region at that time appears in Maurice Kogan and others, *The Working of the National Health Service* (London: Her Majesty's Stationery Office, 1978), pp. 103-125. Since then an intermediate planning and management unit—the Area Health Authority—has been eliminated. Planning is now done by the RHA and DHA alone, and the DHA alone manages facilities.

77. Brian Abel-Smith and Richard M. Titmuss, *The Cost of the National Health Service in England and Wales* (Cambridge, England: Cambridge University Press, 1956), p. 52.

78. On the difficulties of conducting hospital investment through annual government budgets, and on the attempted solutions, see Economic Models Ltd., *The British Health Care System* (Chicago: American Medical Association, 1976), pp. 61-64.

79. *CAPRICODE: Procedure for the Planning and Processing of Individual Building Projects* (London: Department of Health and Social Security, Jan. 1974), 6 vols. The rules for calculating RCCS and the CAPRICODE forms appear in *CAPRICODE: Cost Control* (London: Department of Health and Social Security, 1974), vol. 6 of the work just cited.

80. Report of the Comptroller and Auditor General, *Appropriation Accounts (Volume 3: Classes X-XV and XVII), 1979-1980* (London: Her Majesty's Stationery Office, 1981), pp. xxviii-xxx.

81. The poor condition of the hospitals was documented in a survey conducted by the Ministry of Health in preparation for World War II, later published as *The Hospital Surveys: The Domesday Book of the Hospital Services* (London: Nuffield Provincial Hospitals Trust, 1946).

82. Department of Health and Social Security, *Sharing Resources for Health in England: Report of the Resource Allocation Working Party* (London: Her Majesty's Stationery Office, 1976), Chap. 5 and Annexes D and E.

83. The growing investment in underprovided regions is described in a series "Where the Need Is Greatest" in occasional issues of *Nursing Times* during 1979.

84. Bevan and others, *Health Care Priorities and Management* (see note 76, above), pp. 148-149.

85. Alan Maynard and Arthur Walker, "A Critical Survey of Medical Manpower Planning in Britain," *Social and Economic Administration*, Vol. 11, No. 1 (Spring 1977), pp. 52-75.

86. Social Services Committee, House of Commons, *The Government's White Papers on Public Expenditure: The Social Services* (London: Her Majesty's Stationery Office, 1980), Vol. 2, p. 58.

87. For example, *Draft Regional Strategy* (London: North West Thames Regional Health Authority, 1985).

88. See, for example, the lists in *Avon Leagues of Hospital Friends: A Record of Achievements, 1948-1981* (Bristol: Avon County Association of Leagues of Hospital Friends, 1981).

89. Some examples appear in Roberta G. Simmons and Susan Klein Marine, "The Regulation of High Cost Technology Medicine: The Case of Dialysis and Transplantation in the United Kingdom," *Journal of Health and Social Behavior*, Vol. 25, No. 3 (Sept. 1984), pp. 326-327.

Chapter Ten

1. For a description of employment and remuneration in the past, see William Glaser, *Social Systems and Medical Organization* (New York: Lieber-Atherton, 1970), Chaps. 2-3. The work and lives of hospital employees in successive periods in France are summarized in Jean Imbert and others, *Histoire des hôpitaux en France* (Toulouse: Editions Privat, 1982), pp. 47-55, 110-116, 208-211, 316-319, 360-364. The history and philosophy of a typical religious nursing community are described in Rodolphe von Tavel, *La puissance et la gloire* (Bern: Diakonissenhaus, 1935). A philosophy of nursing conveyed to secular nurses in Europe's confessional hospitals appears in Marcelle Dalloni, *Sous les armes de la charité* (Fribourg, Switzerland: St.-Paul, Imprimerie et Librairie, 1950).

2. A few histories of individual hospitals reproduce lists of employees by rank and by remuneration. See, for example, a list for 1801 in Alfred Wendehorst, *Das Juliusspital in Würzburg* (Würzburg, West Germany: Stiftung Juliusspital, 1976), Vol. 1, pp. 109-112.

3. Maurice Garden, *Le budget des Hospices Civils de Lyon, 1800-1976* (Lyon: Presses Universitaires de Lyon, 1980), pp. 110-112.

4. My calculations from Christian Saint Guilhem and others, *Le coût de l'hospitalisation: Les moyens du système hospitalier public* (Paris: Documents du Centre d'Etude des Revenus et des Coûts, 1978), pp. 102-103. The rapid and intercorrelated increases in personnel-per-bed and cost-per-bed in Switzerland are evident in Ulrich Gessner and Bruno Horisberger, *Gesundheitsversorgungs-Indikatoren* (St. Gallen, Switzerland: Interdisziplinäres Forschungszentrum für die Gesundheit, 1982), Chaps. 4-5; and Ulrich Gessner and Bernhard Güntert, *Ein*

EDV-gestütztes Indikatorensystem für das Spitalmanagement (Saint Gallen, Switzerland: Interdisziplinäres Forschungszentrum für die Gesundheit, 1985).

5. My calculations from data in Jean-Pierre Poullier, *Public Expenditure on Health Under Economic Constraints* (Paris: Organisation for Economic Co-operation and Development, 1984), Part 2, Table D-5. The growth of the health sector in the United States is analyzed extensively in Edward S. Sekscenski, "The Health Services Industry: A Decade of Expansion," *Monthly Labor Review*, Vol. 104, No. 5 (May 1981), pp. 9–16.

6. See, for example, Bui Dang Ha Doan, *Les hôpitaux généraux publics et leurs personnels durant les années 70* (Paris: Centre de Sociologie et de Démographie Médicales, 1983), pp. 62, 74–92.

7. The trend is evident throughout the national reports in Albert A. Blum (ed.), *International Handbook of Industrial Relations* (Westport, Conn.: Greenwood Press, 1981). Unfortunately, no such comprehensive book has been published about public-sector labor relations.

8. Brief histories and current descriptions of the unions in health appear in Hugh A. Clegg and Theodore E. Chester, *Wage Policy and the Health Service* (Oxford: Blackwell, 1957), Chap. 1 passim; and Amarjit Singh Sethi and Stuart J. Dimmock (eds.), *Industrial Relations and Health Services* (London: Croom Helm, 1982), Chap. 5.

9. Nick Bosanquet (ed.), *Industrial Relations in the NHS: The Search for a System* (London: King Edward's Hospital Fund, 1979), Chap. 1.

10. An overview of the hospitals' hostility toward unions and their success in limiting unionization appears in Thomas A. Barocci, *Non-Profit Hospitals* (Boston: Auburn House, 1981). See the remarkable tone of the remarks at a special meeting of the American Society for Nursing Service Administrators, "Improving Communication with Nurses Seen as Key Way to Deter Unionization," *Hospitals*, Vol. 55, No. 3 (Feb. 1, 1981), pp. 21, 23; and the viewpoint throughout William J. Emanuel, "Nurse Unionization Is Dominant Theme," *Hospitals*, Vol. 55, No. 7 (April 1, 1981), pp. 121–128. A typical manual about how to defeat unions is Warren H. Chaney and Thomas R. Beech, *The Union Epidemic: A Prescription for Supervisors* (Rockville, Md.: Aspen Publishers, 1976).

11. Alan M. Sear and Howard T. Bunge, "Trends in Hospital Unionization Since the 1974 Amendments to the National Labor Relations Act," *Hospital and Health Services Administration*, Jan.–Feb. 1982, pp. 26–38.

12. Nick Bosanquet, "Unions and Hospitals: The American Case," *British Medical Journal*, March 15, 1980, pp. 806–807.

13. For a short history of organized labor relations in American hospitals, see Richard U. Miller and others, *The Impact of Collective Bargaining on Hospitals* (New York: Praeger, 1979), Chaps. 2–5. Overviews of the present situation appear in Roger Feldman and others, *Hospital Employees' Wages and Labor Union Organization* (Washington, D.C.: National Center for Health Services Research, U.S. Department of Health and Human Services, 1980), Chap. 1; *Impact of the 1974 Health Care Amendments to the NLRA on Collective Bargaining in the Health Care Industry* (Washington, D.C.: U.S. Department of Labor and Federal Mediation and Conciliation Service, 1979), Chaps. 3, 4, 8; and Sethi and Dimmock, *Industrial Relations and Health Services* (see note 8, above), Chap. 4.

14. Victor Silvera, *La fonction publique et ses problèmes actuels* (Paris: Editions de l'Actualité Juridique, 1969), pp. 431–453.

15. The index numbers for all hospital jobs in France in 1975 are listed in Henri Anrys and others, *Les hôpitaux dans le Marché Commun* (Brussels: Maison Larcier, 1977), pp. 173–183. The wages cited by Anrys are those for private clinics and not public hospitals. Since the same unions bargain with both the government and the national association of private clinics (FIEHP), the unions induce both to adopt the same basic logic of a scale and index numbers for each occupation. Some differences exist, of course.

16. For a good short introduction to French hospital personnel rules, see Emile Lévy and others, *Introduction à la gestion hospitalière* (Paris: Dunod, 1977), Chap. 4. For detailed guides through the many laws and special statutes, see Albert Faure, *Statut général du personnel hospitalier* (Paris: Berger-Levrault, 1977); and Pierre Lachèze-Pasquet, *L'administration de l'hôpital*, 5th ed. (Paris: Berger-Levrault, 1979), Part 2. Faure describes the basic pay rates and fringe benefits on pp. 83–107.

17. Many additional details about European hospital wage determination appear in Donald White, *Pay Negotiations in Six Overseas Health Services* (London: Personnel Division, Department of Health and Social Security, 1980); and in *Employment and Conditions of Work in Health and Medical Services* (Geneva: International Labour Office, 1985), Chaps. 2, 4.

18. The formation and the first seven years' experience of the Whitley Councils are described in Clegg and Chester, *Wage Policy and the Health Service* (see note 8, above).

19. Earl of Halsbury and others, *Report of the Committee of Inquiry into the Pay and Related Conditions of Service of Nurses and Midwives and . . . of the Professions Supplementary to Medicine and Speech Therapists* (London: Her Majesty's Stationery Office, 1974 and 1975); and Standing Commission on Pay Comparability (H. A. Clegg and others), *Reports* (London: Her Majesty's Stationery Office, 1979–1980).

20. Lord McCarthy, *Making Whitley Work* (London: Department of Health and Social Security, 1976); Bosanquet, *Industrial Relations in the NHS* (see note 9, above); Royal Commission on the National Health Service, *Report* (London: Her Majesty's Stationery Office, 1979), pp. 162–167, 457–469; and Daniel Vulliamy and Roger Moore, *Whitleyism and Health* (London: Workers' Education Association, 1979).

21. Emulating the longer contracts of other countries is recommended by White, *Pay Negotiations in Six Overseas Health Services* (see note 17, above).

22. Manuel L. English, "British Hospitals and Incentive Bonus Schemes," *World Hospitals,* Vol. 8 (1974), pp. 87–91.

23. Systematic studies of the wage system in practice within British hospitals do not exist. Some exposés have appeared in newspapers. See, for example, "Why It Pays Public Service Managements to Collaborate in Their Workers' Fiddles," *The Guardian,* Aug. 4, 1979; and "One Disease Hospitals Cannot Wipe Out Easily," *Daily Telegraph,* Dec 10, 1979.

24. Evidence submitted by DHSS to the Nurses and Midwives and Professions Allied to Medicine Pay Review Body, early 1984.

25. For the unions' case for automatic linking and the arguments against it, see Standing Commission on Pay Comparability (H. A. Clegg and others), *Report No. 1: Local Authority and University Manual Workers; NHS Ancillary Staffs; and Ambulancemen* (London: Her Majesty's Stationery Office, 1979), pp. 13–15. The several reports of the Clegg Commission compare the wages in the various occupations; they also compare NHS wages with the wages paid in private occupations. One cannot quote a simple across-the-board percentage differential, since each NHS occupation is slightly different from its private counterparts and because the ratio frequently changes. A principal objection to linking is the disputed nature of comparability, particularly in the case for a monopsony employer like NHS.

26. *Compendium of Health Statistics*, 3rd ed. (London: Office of Health Economics, 1979), Figure 1.4, based on data from DHSS.

27. Clément Michel, *The Cost of Hospitalization* (Brussels: Commission of the European Communities, 1978), p. 54.

28. The most complete description of Canadian hospital labor relations can be found in Sethi and Dimmock, *Industrial Relations and Health Services* (see note 8, above), Chaps. 3, 6, 9–11, 13, 16.

29. The system made the hospital managers weak bargainers; wages rose quickly during the 1960s and early 1970s, and hospital costs exploded, according to Robert G. Evans, "Beyond the Medical Marketplace," in Richard N. Rosett (ed.), *The Role of Health Insurance in the Health Services Sector* (New York: Neale Watson Academic Publications and National Bureau of Economic Research, 1976), pp. 447–462. Ontario's attempts to lid hospital costs after 1969 were foiled by the militance of the unions, according to John J. Deutsch and others, *Report of the Minister of Health's Committee to Examine the Effect of Fiscal Constraints on Hospital Employees* (Toronto: Ministry of Health, Province of Ontario, 1974).

30. The creation and operation of the anti-inflation policy are described in Allan M. Maslove and Gene Swimmer, *Wage Controls in Canada, 1975–1978* (Montreal: Institute for Research on Public Policy, 1980); and Sethi and Dimmock, *Industrial Relations and Health Services*, (see note 8, above), Chap. 16.

31. For example, in Ontario, where hospital wages exceeded private industrial wages by the 1980s. Allan S. Detsky and others, "The Effectiveness of a Regulatory Strategy in Containing Hospital Costs," *New England Journal of Medicine*, Vol. 309 (July 21, 1983), p. 156.

32. Turnover is higher among American hospital nurses than among any other service workers, in some years nearly 50 percent higher. James L. Price, *The Study of Turnover* (Ames: Iowa State University Press, 1977), pp. 58–64; James L. Price and Charles W. Mueller, *Professional Turnover: The Case of Nurses* (Jamaica, N.Y.: SP Medical & Scientific Books, 1981).

33. Whether the wages of American hospital workers are "lower," "higher," or "equal to" other workers' wages therefore depends on time, area, and comparison groups. See the contradictory results in Victor R. Fuchs, "The Earnings of Allied Health Personnel," *Explorations in Economic Research*, Vol. 3, No. 3 (Summer 1976), pp. 408–432; and Frank Sloan and Bruce Steinwald, *Hospital Labor Markets* (Lexington, Mass.: Lexington Books, 1980), pp. 76–78.

34. Sloan and Steinwald, *Hospital Labor Markets* (see note 33, above), passim.

35. As in the midwestern hospitals studied by Miller and his colleagues in *The Impact of Collective Bargaining on Hospitals* (see note 13, above), Chaps. 7-10.

36. Richard Miller and others, "Union Effects on Hospital Administration," *Labor Law Journal*, Vol. 28, No. 8 (Aug. 1977), pp. 512-519.

37. Barocci, *Non-Profit Hospitals* (see note 10, above), pp. 123-130. Comparative earnings data for recent years are published frequently in HCFA's periodical, *Health Care Financing Trends*.

38. My calculations from *Hospital Statistics: 1983 Edition* (Chicago: American Hospital Association, 1983), Table 1. The unusual American trend was noticed in Martin Feldstein and Amy Taylor, *The Rapid Rise of Hospital Costs* (Washington, D.C.: Council on Wage and Price Stability, 1977), pp. 13-19.

39. Paul Coudurier, *Les prix de journée*, 4th ed. (Paris: Berger-Levrault, 1978), pp. 68-77.

40. The elaborate minuet in New York State is described in Lucretia Dewey Tanner and others, *Impact of the 1974 Health Care Amendments to the NLRA on Collective Bargaining in the Health Care Industry* (Washington, D.C.: Office of Research, Federal Mediation and Conciliation Service, U.S. Department of Labor, 1979), Chap. 9.

41. For example, the Maryland Health Services Cost Review Commission, described in Carl J. Schramm, "Containing Hospital Labor Costs—A Separate-Industries Approach," *Employee Relations Law Journal*, Vol. 4, No. 1 (Summer 1978), pp. 89-91.

42. David Kidder and Daniel Sullivan, "Hospital Payroll Costs, Productivity, and Employment Under Prospective Reimbursement," *Health Care Financing Review*, Vol. 4, No. 2 (Dec. 1982), pp. 96-99.

43. William Glaser, *Health Insurance Bargaining* (New York: Gardner Press and Wiley, 1978), Chap. 9.

44. The problems of unit and district managers are described in Brian Edwards, "Managers and Industrial Relations," in Bosanquet, *Industrial Relations in the NHS* (see note 9, above), Chap. 6.

45. As in *Draft Regional Strategy* (London: North West Thames Regional Health Authority, 1985), pp. 67-70.

46. Morris L. Barer and others, "Manpower Planning, Fiscal Restraint, and the 'Demand' for Health Care Personnel," *Inquiry*, Vol. 21, No. 3 (Fall 1984), pp. 262-264.

Chapter Eleven

1. For a history of office practice paid by fee-for-service in Europe, England, and the United States, see Fielding H. Garrison, *An Introduction to the History of Medicine*, 4th ed. (Philadelphia: Saunders, 1929), pp. 90-91, 135, 170-171, 236, 292-294, 391-392, 751-752, and the sources cited on p. 912.

2. Jean Imbert and others, *Histoire des hôpitaux en France* (Toulouse: Editions Privat, 1982), pp. 130-133; and George Rosen, "The Hospital: Historical

Sociology of a Community Institution," in Eliot Freidson (ed.), *The Hospital in Modern Society* (New York: Free Press, 1963), pp. 17–18.

3. Imbert and others, *Histoire des hôpitaux en France* (see note 2, above), pp. 212–213, 254–262, 319–328.

4. Erwin Ackerknecht, *Medicine at the Paris Hospital, 1794–1848* (Baltimore: Johns Hopkins University Press, 1967), esp. Chap. 4; and Pierre Vallery-Radot, *Deux siècles d'histoire hospitalière* and *Nos hôpitaux parisiens* (Paris: Paul Dupont, 1947 and 1948), passim.

5. I encountered it in the early 1960s, during the fieldwork for *Paying the Doctor* (Baltimore: Johns Hopkins University Press, 1970); and "American and Foreign Hospitals," in Freidson, *The Hospital in Modern Society* (see note 2, above), Chap. 2.

6. The early arrangements whereby patients paid charitable hospitals for private rooms and paid fees to the chiefs of service are described in Henry C. Burdett, *Pay Hospitals and Paying Wards Throughout the World* (London: J. & A. Churchill, 1879).

7. Details about the work rules and staff structures during the 1960s in hospitals in Belgium, France, Germany, Italy, Luxembourg, and Holland appear in Paul Quaethoven, *Het statuut van de ziekenhuisgeneesheer in de lid-staten van de Europese Economische Gemeenschap* (Leuven, Belgium: School voor Mattschappelijke Gezondheidszorg, Katholieke Universiteit Leuven, 1969).

8. France best illustrates the rapid change from the old to the new medical staffs. The new arrangements are described in Jean-Marie Clément, *L'hôpital: Environnement, organisation, gestion* (Paris: Berger-Levrault, 1983), pp. 274–296; and *Les médecins hospitaliers—Rapport sur les professions sanitaires et sociales* (Paris: Inspection Générale des Affaires Sociales, 1979). The laws and regulations are explained in Raymond Piganiol and others, *Le médecin hospitalier* (Paris: Berger-Levrault, 1976 and supplements).

9. My calculations from data in Bui Dang Ha Doan, *Les hôpitaux généraux publics et leurs personnels durant les années 70* (Paris: Centre de Sociologie et de Démographie Médicales, 1983), p. 73.

10. The history of British specialty practice before and under the NHS appears in Rosemary Stevens, *Medical Practice in Modern England* (New Haven, Conn.: Yale University Press, 1966). The exclusion of GPs from most NHS hospitals is described in Frank Honigsbaum, *The Division in British Medicine* (London: St. Martin's Press, 1980).

11. Brian Abel-Smith and Kathleen Gales, *British Doctors at Home and Abroad* (Welwyn, England: Cadicote Press, 1964).

12. Stevens, *Medical Practice in Modern England* (see note 10, above), pp. 197-199.

13. Review Body on Doctors' and Dentists' Remuneration, *Eighth Report, 1978* (London: Her Majesty's Stationery Office, 1978), p. 80.

14. "Physician-Hospital Relations," *SMS Report* (American Medical Association), Vol. 1, No. 11 (Dec. 1982); John C. Gaffney and Gerald L. Glandon, "The Physician's Use of the Hospital," *Health Care Management Review*, Vol. 7, No. 3 (Summer 1982), p. 55.

15. Michael A. Morrisey and others, "A Survey of Hospital Medical Staffs," *Hospitals*, Vol. 57, No. 24 (Dec. 1, 1983), p. 91.

16. Morrisey and others, pp. 92–93.

17. Michael A. Morrisey, "The Composition of Hospital Medical Staffs," *Health Care Management Review,* Vol. 9, No. 2 (Summer 1984), p. 13.

18. Two guides for managers in recruiting and keeping productive office doctors are I. Donald Snook, *Building a Winning Medical Staff* and Harry Olson, *Physician Recruitment and the Hospital* (Chicago: American Hospital Association, 1984).

19. Enactment of reforms of the teaching hospitals is described in Haroun Jamous and others, *Contribution à une sociologie de la décision: La réforme des études médicales et des structures hospitalières* (Paris: Centre d'Etudes Sociologiques, Centre National de la Recherche Scientifique, 1967).

20. British hospital doctors' salaries are described in Glaser, *Paying the Doctor* (see note 5, above), pp. 61–65, 215–222. The method of deciding them is described in Glaser, *Health Insurance Bargaining* (New York: Gardner Press and Wiley 1978), Chap. 9.

21. Functional budgeting and the difficulties in implementing it within the NHS are described in Irvine Lapsley and Malcolm Prowle, *The Effectiveness of Functional Budgetary Control in the National Health Service* (Coventry, England: Centre for Industrial Economic and Business Research, University of Warwick, 1978). The consultants' complaints about their committee work led to the survey of all consultants' work schedules, reported in the Review Body's *Eighth Report, 1978* (see note 13, above), Appendix D.

22. All rules concerning hospital doctors are summarized in Marburger Bund, *Ärztliche Versorgungswerke der Bundesrepublik Deutschland* (Stuttgart: A. W. Gentner Verlag, constantly updated).

23. Explained in Guido Braun, *Zum Tarifrecht des Arztes: Arbeitszeit und Bereitschaftsdienst,* rev. ed. (Erlangen, West Germany: Perimed Fachbuch-Verlagsgesellschaft, 1983).

24. The tangle of private practice rights of chiefs is explored by Wolfgang Gitter, *Zum Privatliquidationsrecht der leitenden Krankenhausärzte* (Cologne: Verband der privaten Krankenversicherung, 1975).

25. Bui, *Les hôpitaux généraux publics* (see note 9, above), p. 23.

26. The private clinics then argue that they are cheaper and more efficient than the nonprofit and public hospitals; the latter reply that the patient and sickness fund pay more in the clinics. See the rival brochures: *Hospitalisation privée: Un facteur d'économies pour la Sécurité Sociale* (Paris: Fédération Intersyndicale des Etablissements d'Hospitalisation Privée, 1979); and *Non: L'hôpital public ne coûte pas toujours plus cher . . . c'est autre chose* (Paris: Fédération Hospitalière de France, 1980).

27. Glaser, *Paying the Doctor* (see note 5, above), Chap. 3; and Glaser, *Health Insurance Bargaining* (see note 20, above), Chaps. 2–7.

28. For example, the report of the Commissie Van Mansvelt to Holland's Ministry of Health, 1980.

29. This unique American invention intends to keep the doctors completely free under organized financing programs, an unlikely combination never attempted abroad. Jonathan A. Showstack and others, "Fee-for-Service Physician Payment: Analysis of Current Methods and Their Development," *Inquiry,* Vol. 16 (Fall 1979), pp. 230–246; Thomas L. Delbanco, "Paying the

Physician's Fee: Blue Shield and the Reasonable Charge," *New England Journal of Medicine*, Vol. 301 (1979), pp. 1314–1320.

30. Janet B. Mitchell and others, *Alternative Methods for Describing Physician Services Performed and Billed* and *Creating DRG-Based Physician Reimbursement Schemes: A Conceptual and Empirical Analysis* (Chestnut Hill, Mass.: Center for Health Economics Research, 1983 and 1984).

31. Summarized in the special issue of *Health Affairs*, Vol. 3, No. 2 (Summer 1984).

32. David T. Pieroni (ed.), "Physician Compensation," *Topics in Health Care Financing*, Vol. 4, No. 3 (Spring 1978). The history of the organization and payment of doctors based entirely in hospitals rather than primarily in offices is summarized in Bruce Steinwald, "Hospital-Based Physicians: Current Issues and Descriptive Evidence," *Health Care Financing Review*, Vol. 2, No. 1 (Summer 1980), pp. 63–75.

33. For a defense of carefully designed arrangements without perverse incentives, see Frank Matthews, "The Case for Percentage Contracts with Hospitals," *Medical Economics*, June 25, 1973, pp. 98–108.

34. Cour des Comptes, *Rapport au Président de la République suivi des réponses des administrations* (Paris: Journaux Officiels, 1980), pp. 35–49, 168–173; and Comité de Liaison d'Etude et d'Action Républicaines (CLEAR), *L'hôpital en question: Dossier pour la réforme hospitalière* (Paris: Editions Emile Paul, 1970), pp. 188–189.

35. Giving operational responsibility to the senior doctors was considered one of the most promising results of the experimental trials in global budgeting: Claude Renou and others, *Rapport à Monsieur le Ministre de la Santé rélatif à l'évaluation de l'experimentation de nouveaux modes de financements et de gestion des établissements hospitaliers* (Paris: Ministère de la Santé, 1982), pp. 42–43.

36. Mark Pauly, "The Effect of Medical Staff Characteristics on Hospital Costs," in Jon R. Gabel and others (eds.), *Physicians and Financial Incentives* (Washington, D.C.: Health Care Financing Administration, U.S. Department of Health and Human Services, 1980), pp. 75–85; Michael Redisch, "Physician Involvement in Hospital Decision-Making," in Michael Zubkoff and others (eds.), *Hospital Cost Containment* (New York: Neale Watson Academic Publications, 1978), pp. 217–243; Milton Roemer and Jay W. Friedman, *Doctors in Hospitals: Medical Staff Organization and Hospital Performance* (Baltimore: Johns Hopkins University Press, 1971), pp. 288–290.

37. The great variation in practice style by American doctors with comparable cases is documented in research by John Wennberg, summarized in his "Dealing with Medical Practice Variations," *Health Affairs*, Vol. 3, No. 2 (Summer 1984), pp. 6–32; in research by Steven A. Schroeder, summarized in his "Variations in Physician Practice Patterns: A Review of Medical Cost Implications," in Edward J. Carels and others (eds.), *The Physician and Cost Control* (Cambridge, Mass.: Oelgeschlager, Gunn and Hain, 1980), pp. 23–50; and in many other studies summarized in Avedis Donabedian, "The Epidemiology of Quality," *Inquiry*, Vol. 22 (Fall 1985), pp. 283–284.

38. These cost-awareness efforts are described and evaluated in John M. Eisenberg and others, "Cost Containment and Changing Physicians' Practice

Behavior," *Journal of the American Medical Association*, Vol. 246, No. 19 (Nov. 13, 1981), pp. 2195–2201; and Lois P. Myers and Steven A. Schroeder, "Physician Use of Services for the Hospitalized Patient: A Review, with Implications for Cost Containment," *Milbank Memorial Fund Quarterly: Health and Society*, Vol. 59, No. 4 (Summer 1981), pp. 481–507.

39. Richard B. Saltman and David W. Young, "The Hospital Power Equilibrium: An Alternative View of the Cost Containment Dilemma," *Journal of Health Politics, Policy and Law*, Vol. 6, No. 3 (Fall 1981), pp. 391–418; David W. Young and Richard B. Saltman, "Preventive Medicine for Hospital Costs," *Harvard Business Review*, Jan.–Feb. 1983, pp. 126–133; Jeffrey E. Harris, "The Internal Organization of Hospitals: Some Economic Implications," *Bell Journal of Economics*, Vol. 8, No. 2 (Autumn 1977), pp. 467–482.

40. The collapse of America's most publicized community hospital with a closed staff is described in Lloyd B. Wescott, "Hunterdon: The Rise and Fall of a Medical Camelot," *New England Journal of Medicine*, Vol. 300 (April 26, 1979), pp. 952–956, 977–979.

41. Robert Rubright (ed.), *Persuading Physicians: A Guide for Hospital Executives* (Rockville, Md.: Aspen Publishers, 1983); Everett A. Johnson and Richard L. Johnson, *Hospitals in Transition* (Rockville, Md.: Aspen Publishers, 1983); Paul M. Ellwood, "When MDs Meet DRGs," *Hospitals*, Vol. 57, No. 24 (Dec. 16, 1983), pp. 62–66; and many others.

42. Lee Soderstrom, "Federal-Provincial Cost-Sharing: Can Ottawa Influence Provincial Health Policies Using Financial Carrots?" (paper presented at the Conference of Canadian Health Economists, Regina, Sask., 1983), footnote 14.

43. Some hospitals published hortatory guides for their doctors, such as *Santé: Ses coûts* (Quebec: L'Hôtel-Dieu de Québec, 1977).

44. Robert G. Evans, "Health Care in Canada: Patterns of Funding and Regulation," *Journal of Health Politics, Policy and Law*, Vol. 8, No. 1 (Spring 1983), pp. 10–16 passim.

45. National Council of Welfare, *Medicare: The Public and Private Insurance* (Ottawa: Health and Welfare Canada, 1982); *Preserving Universal Medicare: A Government of Canada Position Paper* (Ottawa: Health and Welfare Canada, 1983), pp. 19–21.

46. See, for example, J. S. A. Ashley and others, "How Much Clinical Investigation?" *Lancet*, April 22, 1972, pp. 890–892; G. Ferster and M. Butts, "Estimation of Notional Savings in Revenue Expenditure by Specialty at District Level," *Hospital and Health Services Review*, March 1978, pp. 87–90; and others cited in Michael H. Cooper, *Rationing Health Care* (London: Croom Helm, 1975), pp. 55–57.

47. Björn Smedby and C. Sundelin, "Admission Rate and Length of Stay for Nonspecific Enteritis in Pediatric Departments in Sweden," *International Journal of Health Services*, Vol. 2, No. 4 (1972), pp. 541–550.

48. Department of Health and Social Security, *Reports on the Organisation of Medical Work in Hospitals* (London: Her Majesty's Stationery Office, 1967, 1972, 1974). These were the "Cogwheel Reports."

49. Iden Wickings and others, "Review of Clinical Budgeting and Costing Experiments," *British Medical Journal*, Vol. 286 (Feb 12, 1983), pp. 575–578.

50. Theo de Vries, *Het klinisch-chemisch laboratorium in economisch perspectief* (Leiden: H. E. Stenfert Kroese, 1974), Chaps. 3–4.

51. Lawrence Lewin and others, "Investor-Owneds and Nonprofits Differ in Economic Performance," *Hospitals*, Vol. 55, No. 13 (July 1, 1981), pp. 52–58; Thomas W. Moloney and David E. Rogers, "Medical Technology: A Different View of the Contentious Debate over Costs," *New England Journal of Medicine*, Vol. 301, No. 26 (Dec 27, 1979), pp. 1413–1419.

52. Johanna Sonnenfeld, "The Blue Cross and Blue Shield Association's Medical Necessity Program," *Voluntary Effort Quarterly*, Vol. 3, No. 2 (June 1981), pp. 5–8.

53. John P. Bunker, "Surgical Manpower: A Comparison of Operations and Surgeons in the United States and in England and Wales," *New England Journal of Medicine*, Vol. 282, No. 3 (Jan. 15, 1970), pp. 135–144; John C. Pearson and others, "Hospital Caseloads in Liverpool, New England, and Uppsala," *Lancet*, Sept. 7, 1968, pp. 559–566; Egon Jonsson and Duncan Neuhauser, "Hospital Staffing Ratios in the United States and Sweden," *Inquiry*, Vol. 12, No. 2, Supp. (June 1975), pp. 128–137; Eugene Vayda, "A Comparison of Surgical Rates in Canada and in England and Wales," *New England Journal of Medicine*, Vol. 289 (Dec. 6, 1973), pp. 1224–1229.

54. Klim McPherson and others, "Small-Area Variations in the Use of Common Surgical Procedures: An International Comparison of New England, England, and Norway," *New England Journal of Medicine*, Vol. 307 (Nov. 18, 1982), pp. 1310–1314; Klim McPherson and others, "Regional Variations in the Use of Common Surgical Procedures Within and Between England and Wales, Canada, and the United States," *Social Science and Medicine*, Vol. 15A (1981), pp. 273–288; Noralou P. Roos and Leslie L. Roos, "High and Low Surgical Rates: Risk Factors for Area Residents," *American Journal of Public Health*, Vol. 71, No. 6 (June 1981), pp. 591–600.

55. Victor R. Fuchs, "The Supply of Surgeons and the Demand for Operations," *Journal of Human Resources*, Vol. 13, Supp. (1978), pp. 35–56.

56. Sigrid Lichtner and Manfred Pflanz, "Appendectomy in the Federal Republic of Germany," *Medical Care*, Vol. 9, No. 4 (July–Aug. 1971), pp. 311–330.

57. American and Canadian doctors earn higher income per hour from hospital care than from office care. Therefore, the incentive is toward more work in the hospital than in the office. Mark S. Blomberg, "Physician Fees as Incentives," in *Changing the Behavior of the Physician: A Management Perspective* (Chicago: Center for Health Administration Studies, University of Chicago, 1980), pp. 28–30.

58. Denis J. Rich, Robert G. Evans, and David W. Pascoe, *Manitoba and Medicare: 1971 to the Present* (Winnipeg: Manitoba Health, 1985).

59. C. E. B. Frost, "How Permanent Are NHS Waiting Lists?" *Social Science and Medicine*, Vol. 14C, No. 1 (March 1980), pp. 1–11; *Parliamentary Debates (Hansard), House of Commons*, Vol. 592, No. 153 (July 30, 1958), Columns 1476, 1483–1484.

Chapter Twelve

1. Governance and management of the French public hospital—when it was still oriented toward the community and was monitored only sketchily by the national government—are described in Henri Thoillier, *L'hôpital français* (Paris: Max Brézol Editeur, 1943).

2. Governance and management of the French public hospital today are described in Pierre Lachèze-Pasquet, *L'administration de l'hôpital*, 5th ed. (Paris: Berger-Levrault, 1979); and Jean-Marie Clément, *L'hôpital: Environment, organisation, gestion* (Paris: Berger-Levrault, 1983). Clément describes the present careers of managers at pp. 204–212.

3. H. H. Kreuter and H. J. Schlauss, *Konzertierte Aktion im Gesundheitswesen: Aufgaben, Leistungen, Analysen* (Cologne: Deutscher Ärzte-Verlag, 1981).

4. Robert J. Maxwell, *Health and Wealth* (Lexington, Mass.: Lexington Books, 1981), p. 68.

5. Ministry of Health and Department of Health for Scotland, *A National Health Service* (London: His Majesty's Stationery Office, 1944).

6. The management of the NHS hospital from 1948 to 1974 is described in Joseph E. Stone, *Hospital Organisation and Management,* 4th ed. (London: Faber & Faber, 1952); and T. E. Chester and S. N. Joy, *Hospitals and the State* (London: Acton Society Trust, 1955–1959), 6 vols. Events in the hospital services during those years are chronicled in Almont Lindsey, *Socialized Medicine In England and Wales* (Chapel Hill: University of North Carolina Press, 1962), Chaps. 10–11 and passim. For an excellent concise history, see Brian Abel-Smith, *National Health Service: The First Thirty Years* (London: Her Majesty's Stationery Office, 1978). Reduction in the authority of the nurses is traced by Stuart Dimmock, "What Role for Nurses?" *Nursing Times,* Feb. 20, 1985, pp. 30–31.

7. The NHS after 1974 is described thoroughly in Ruth Levitt and Andrew Wall, *The Reorganised Health Service,* 3rd ed. (London: Croom Helm, 1984). The style of management—in which higher managers review financial indicators of the performance of the next lower tier—is summarized in Department of Health and Social Security, *Management Arrangements for the Reorganised National Health Service* (London: Her Majesty's Stationery Office, 1972). Implementation of the new arrangements during the first years is summarized in R. G. S. Brown, *Reorganising the National Health Service* (Oxford: Blackwell, 1979). For studies of the grass roots of the NHS in practice, see Rosemary Stewart and others, *The District Administrator in the National Health Service* (London: Pitman Medical, 1980); Howard Elcock and Stuart Haywood, *The Buck Stops Where?* (Hull: Institute for Health Studies, University of Hull, 1980).

8. The new "team management" was proposed in the "Gray Book"—that is, *Management Arrangements for the Reorganised National Health Service* (see note 7, above). Difficulties in implementation are summarized in Gwyn Bevan and others, *Health Care Priorities and Management* (London: Croom Helm, 1980), Chap. 12. A survey of how teams worked is summarized in David J. Hunter, "Cometh the NHS Chief Executive?" *Hospital and Health Services Review,* Nov. 1983, pp. 273–280.

9. The new management was recommended in Roy Griffiths and others, *NHS Management Inquiry* (London: Department of Health and Social Security, Oct. 1983). It was carried out according to the circular *Health Services Management: Implementation of the NHS Management Inquiry Report* (London: Department of Health and Social Security, June 1984). Possible changes in the structure of budgets are described in Philip Davies and Malcolm Prowle, "Management Budgets in the NHS," *British Medical Journal,* Vol. 289 (Dec. 1, 1984), pp. 1552–1554.

10. John Allen Hornsby and Richard E. Schmid, *The Modern Hospital* (Philadelphia: Saunders, 1913).

11. The structure and management of American hospitals just before the great financial growth and transformation of the 1960s are described in James A. Hamilton, *Patterns of Hospital Ownership and Control* (Minneapolis: University of Minnesota Press, 1961); and in the leading textbook of that period, Malcolm T. MacEachern, *Hospital Organization and Management,* 3rd ed. (Chicago: Physicians' Record Company, 1957).

12. The new philosophy and methods of management are discussed in John Byron Silvers and C. K. Prahalad, *Financial Management of Health Institutions* (New York: SP Medical & Scientific Books, 1974); Everett A. Johnson and Richard L. Johnson, *Hospitals in Transition* (Rockville, Md.: Aspen Publishers, 1982); and many articles throughout *Modern Healthcare* and *Healthcare Financial Management.* For a protest, see Philip R. Alper, "The New Language of Hospital Management," *New England Journal of Medicine,* Vol. 311, No. 19 (Nov. 8, 1984), pp. 1249–1251.

13. There is much informal folklore about how to beat the rules. Some is published, as in Donald F. Beck, *Principles of Reimbursement in Health Care* (Rockville, Md.: Aspen Publishers, 1984); and in *Prospective Payment Guide,* a monthly magazine that tells financial managers how to maximize revenue under DRGs. The American practices are described and contrasted with the simpler and standardized European methods in William A. Glaser, "Juggling Multiple Payers," *Inquiry,* Vol. 21, No. 2 (Summer 1984), pp. 178–188.

14. An organizational theory by the inventors of DRGs is presented in Laurence F. McMahon and others, "Hospital Matrix Management and DRG-Based Prospective Payment," *Hospital and Health Services Administration,* Vol. 31, No. 1 (Jan.–Feb. 1986), pp. 62–74. A specific example of reorganization of a hospital appears in Ralph G. Goodrich and G. Richard Hastings, "St. Luke's Hospital Reaps Benefits by Using Product Line Management," *Modern Healthcare,* Vol. 15, No. 4 (Feb. 15, 1985), pp. 157–158. Several books guided the managers in methods of reorganizing hospital structure and operations, in order to increase income and reduce costs under DRGs. See, for example, Howard L. Smith and Myron D. Fottler, *Prospective Payment: Managing for Operational Effectiveness* (Rockville, Md.: Aspen Publishers, 1985), esp. Chap. 8.

15. Bill Jackson and Joyce Jensen, "Strategic Planning and Marketing Will Be Administrators' Top Concerns," *Modern Healthcare,* Vol. 15, No. 1 (Jan. 4, 1985), pp. 68-70.

16. Linda I. Collins, "A Survey of Hospital Salaries," *Hospitals,* Vol. 57, No. 24 (Dec. 16, 1983), pp. 73–82 passim. The survey also identified their

educational preparation: nearly all the CEOs came from programs in hospital administration; nearly all the CFOs came from schools of business.

17. "Cole Compensation Survey," *Modern Healthcare*, Vol. 14, No. 4 (Nov. 1, 1984), p. 138. As a result, the basic salaries of chief financial officers in American hospitals keep pace with those in banking and other industries: "Cole Compensation Survey," *Modern Healthcare*, Vol. 15, No. 23 (Nov. 8, 1985), p. 118. Many bankers ultimately earned more, because many received cash incentive bonuses from the banks' profits; but by the mid-1980s, even bonuses were being offered to chief financial officers in the supposedly nonprofit hospitals.

18. The involved rules about the basic salary, supplements, and fringe benefits of French hospital managers are explained in Albert Faure, *Statut général du personnel* (Paris: Berger-Levrault, 1977), pp. 9–13, 83–107.

19. Hansjürgen Meyer and others, "Instrumente der Wirtschaftsführung im Krankenhaus unter besonderer Berücksichtigung der Kosten- und Leistungs-rechnung," *Krankenhaus-Umschau*, Vol. 54, No. 2 (Feb. 1985), pp. 85–86.

20. Many examples of sharing and mergers are described in Montague Brown and Howard L. Lewis, *Hospital Management Systems* (Rockville, Md.: Aspen Publishers, 1976); Montague Brown and Barbara P. McCool (eds.), *Multihospital Systems* (Rockville, Md.: Aspen Publishers, 1980); and "Shared Services: Group Purchasing Spurs Growth of Shared Service Organizations," *Modern Healthcare*, Vol. 16, No. 18 (Aug. 29, 1986), pp. 65–80 passim.

21. Sharing in response to planners' restraints is described in Diana Barrett, *Multihospital Systems* (Cambridge, Mass.: Oelgeschlager, Gunn & Hain, 1980), pp. 27–31.

22. These investor-owned for-profit chains are outnumbered by commonly owned and centrally directed nonprofit chains, described in Barrett (see note 21, above); and in B. Jon Jaeger (ed.), *A Decade of Implementation: The Multiple Hospital Management Concept Revisited* (Durham, N.C.: Department of Health Administration, Duke University, 1975).

23. Management of the investor-owned chains is described in Institute of Medicine, *For-Profit Enterprise in Health Care* (Washington, D.C.: National Academy Press, 1986), and sources cited therein. A case example appears in Gwen Kinkead, "Humana's Hard-Sell Hospitals," *Fortune*, Vol. 102, No. 10 (Nov. 19, 1980), pp. 68–70, 76, 81.

24. My calculations from *1983 Directory* (Washington, D.C.: Federation of American Hospitals, 1983); from Dan Ermann and Jon Gabel, *Multihospital Systems: Issues and Empirical Findings* (Washingon, D.C.: National Center for Health Services Research, U.S. Department of Health and Human Services, 1983); and from unpublished information supplied by the Hospital Data Center, American Hospital Association.

25. Samuel J. Tibbitts, "Future Belongs to New Multihealth Corporations," *Modern Healthcare*, Vol. 14, No. 12 (Sept. 1984), pp. 203, 206, 208, 210; and "Hospitals Restructure for New Markets in Move to Establish Health Systems," *Federation of American Hospitals Review*, Vol. 17, No. 6 (Nov.–Dec. 1984), pp. 16–47.

26. An example is described in Ernest G. Barnes (Administrative Law

Judge), "Initial Decision in the Matter of American Medical International et al." (Washington, D.C.: Federal Trade Commission, Docket No. 9158, July 27, 1983).

27. Steven C. Renn, "The Effects of Ownership and System Affiliation on the Economic Performance of Hospitals," *Inquiry,* Vol. 22, No. 3 (Fall 1985), pp. 219–236; Robert V. Pattison and Hallie M. Katz, "Investor-Owned and Not-for-Profit Hospitals," *New England Journal of Medicine,* Vol. 309 (Aug. 11, 1983), pp. 347–353; and J. Michael Watt and others, "The Comparative Economic Performance of Investor-Owned Chains and Not-for-Profit Hospitals," *New England Journal of Medicine,* Vol. 314 (Jan. 9, 1986), pp. 89–96. Considerable statistical information about the chains appears in Montague Brown and others, "Trends in Multihospital Systems: A Multiyear Comparison," *Health Care Management Review,* Vol. 5, No. 4 (Fall 1980), pp. 9–22.

28. The change from euphoria to caution can be traced in the sections on "Health Care" in the "Annual Report on American Industry," *Forbes,* every January throughout the 1970s and 1980s.

29. A Dutch control doctor's work schedule is described in Arnold M. F. B. Crousen, *Analyse van het werk van een controlerend geneeskundige voor de ziektewet* (Assen, Netherlands: Van Gorcum, 1968). A textbook about the control doctor's duties in Holland is Jan A. van der Hoeven, *De controlerend geneesheer* (Leiden: Uitgeverij L. Stafleu, 1960). The work of the control doctor in Germany is described in Erich-Michel Simon, *Le contrôle médical de l'assurance-maladie dans la République Fédérale Allemande* (Strasbourg: Université Louis Pasteur, Faculté de Médecine de Strasbourg, 1971). The work in France is discussed in Claude Fournier and Claude Rousseau, *Le médecin-conseil d'assurances: Déontologie, méthodologie* (Paris: L'Argus, 1984).

30. Described in Gordon H. Hatcher, *Universal Free Health Care in Canada, 1947–77* (Washington, D.C.: Fogarty International Center, National Institutes of Health, U.S. Department of Health and Human Services, 1981), pp. 101–108, 131–133.

31. *Implementation of Peer Review Organization (PRO) Program: Hearing Before the Subcommittee on Health of the Committee on Finance, United States Senate, 98th Congress, 2d Session* (Washington, D.C.: U.S. Government Printing Office, 1984); Kathleen N. Lohr, *Peer Review Organizations (PROs): Quality Assurance in Medicare* (Washington, D.C.: Office of Technology Assessment, U.S. Congress, 1985).

32. Described in William Glaser, "Controlling Costs Through Methods of Paying Doctors: Experiences from Abroad," in Stuart O. Schweitzer (ed.), *Policies for the Containment of Health Care Costs and Expenditures* (Washington, D.C.: Fogarty International Center, National Institutes of Health, U.S. Department of Health and Human Services, 1978), pp. 225–230; and Hatcher, *Universal Free Health Care in Canada* (see note 30, above), pp. 46–50, 88–91, 114–118, 138–139, 231–255.

33. American doctors show wide variations in practice styles and costliness when treating patients within the same DRG. See John E. Wennberg and others, "Will Payment Based on Diagnosis-Related Groups Control Hospital Costs?" *New England Journal of Medicine,* Vol. 311, No. 5 (Aug. 2, 1984). Therefore, hospital managers must persuade their attendings on two scores: the more

expensive doctors should work more economically; the less expensive doctors should admit more patients.

34. New arrangements in manager-physician relations triggered by DRG payment methods are described in Paul L. Grimaldi and Julie Micheletti, *Prospective Payment* (Chicago: Pluribus Press, 1985); and Keith H. McLaughlin, "Medicare's Changes Should Prompt Execs to Try New Ideas for Managing," *Modern Healthcare*, Vol. 14, No. 16 (Dec. 1984), pp. 134, 136.

35. They may find it difficult to intervene, though, if the chief has been very famous and is strong willed. The most famous case of the system's inability to control a deteriorating chief before the date of his automatic retirement is described in Jürgen Thorwald, *The Dismissal: The Last Days of Ferdinand Sauerbruch* (New York: Pantheon Books, 1962). During field research in the early 1980s, I encountered another example in another country.

36. The hospitals that are most permissive in granting surgical privileges have more operations, greater risks, and higher mortality, according to Osler Peterson, "Why Do High Surgery Rates Raise Case Fatality Rates?" *American Journal of Public Health*, Vol. 71, No. 6 (June 1981), pp. 574–576.

37. *Health Services in Europe*, 3rd ed. (Copenhagen: World Health Organization, Regional Office for Europe, 1981), Vol. 1, Chap. 8; and Schweitzer, *Policies for the Containment of Health Care Costs and Expenditures* (see note 32, above), Chaps. 21, 23.

38. The history and performance of quality-assurance committees are discussed in Milton Roemer and Jay Friedman, *Doctors in Hospitals* (Baltimore: Johns Hopkins University Press, 1971), passim, esp. pp. 223–227. The history and work of the Joint Commission are summarized in Jesus J. Peña and others, *Hospital Quality Assurance* (Rockville, Md.: Aspen Publishers, 1984), Chap. 3.

39. Judith M. Feder, *Medicare: The Politics of Federal Hospital Insurance* (Lexington, Mass.: Lexington Books, 1977), Chap. 3.

40. The work of PSROs is described in John W. Bussman and Sharon V. Davidson (eds.), *P.S.R.O.: The Promise, Perspective, and Potential* (Reading, Mass.: Addison-Wesley, 1981); and Michael J. Goran and others, "The PSRO Hospital Review System," *Medical Care*, Vol. 13, No. 4, Suppl. (April 1975).

41. The contradictory demands on the PSRO from cost containment and quality improvement, and the contradictory implications for costs, are discussed in Harry M. Rosen, "Conflict in Regulatory Goals" (paper prepared for annual convention of the American Political Science Association, 1977).

42. *The Effect of PSROs on Health Care Costs* (Washington, D.C.: Congressional Budget Office, 1979) and *Wasted Health Dollars: Evaluation of Professional Standards Review Organizations—Hearing Before the Subcommittee on Oversight and Investigations of the Committee on Interstate and Foreign Commerce, House of Representatives* (Washington, D.C.: U.S. Government Printing Office, 1980).

Chapter Thirteen

1. William O. Cleverley, "Evaluation of Alternative Payment Strategies for Hospitals: A Conceptual Approach," *Inquiry*, Vol. 16, No. 2 (Summer 1979), pp. 108–118; *Study of British Columbia Hospital Funding Program* (Vancouver:

Ernst & Whinney, 1979), Vol. 2; David Abernethy, "A Tentative Checklist of Questions to Ask When Analyzing a Government Program," *Policy Studies Journal*, Vol. 6, No. 4 (Summer 1978), pp. 552-554.

2. The American literature is reviewed in W. Richard Scott and Ann Barry Flood, "Costs and Quality of Hospital Care," *Medical Care Review*, Vol. 41, No. 4 (Winter 1984), pp. 213-261. For evidence that the current American "research" produces more theoretical models than empirical generalizations, see T. G. Cowing and others, "Hospital Cost Analysis: A Survey and Evaluation of Recent Studies," in Richard M. Scheffler and Louis F. Rossiter (eds.), *Advances in Health Economics and Health Services Research* (Greenwich, Conn.: JAI Press, 1983), Vol. 4, pp. 257-303.

3. Robert J. Maxwell, *Health and Wealth* (Lexington, Mass.: Lexington Books, 1981), pp. 37-47; Joseph P. Newhouse, "Medical-Care Expenditure: A Cross-National Survey," *Journal of Human Resources*, Vol. 12, No. 1 (Winter 1977), pp. 115-125.

4. Robert Pinker, *English Hospital Statistics, 1861-1938* (London: Heinemann, 1966), p. 84.

5. *Compendium of Health Statistics*, 5th ed. (London: Office of Health Economics, 1984), Table 2.6.

6. Explained in Mark S. Freeland and Carol Ellen Schendler, "National Health Expenditures: Short-Term Outlook and Long-Term Projections," *Health Care Financing Review*, Vol. 2, No. 3 (Winter 1981), pp. 100-104. The reasoning is applied to American time series by Freeland and Schendler and (with slightly different results about relative weight of the variables) by Jack A. Meyer and others, *Passing the Health Care Buck* (Washington, D.C.: American Enterprise Institute, 1983); to Swiss data by Pierre Gilliand, "Les coûts d'exploitation hospitalière," *Hospitalis*, Nos. 11-12, 1980, and Nos. 1-2, 1981; and to Dutch data by A. P. W. P. van Montfort, *Analyse van de kostenstijging in prijs- en volumecomponenten* (Utrecht: Nationaal Ziekenhuisinstituut, 1978).

7. A typical time series comparing general consumer prices and total hospital spending appears in Simone Sandier, "Les dépenses de soins médicaux en France depuis 1950," *Revue française de finances publiques*, No. 2 (1983), p. 25.

8. The development of the French fiscal crisis and the mixture of remedies are described in Louis Roche and others, *L'économie de la santé* (Paris: Presses Universitaires de France, 1982), pp. 112-124.

9. Charles L. Eby and Donald R. Cohodes, "What Do We Know about Rate-Setting?" *Journal of Health Politics, Policy and Law*, Vol. 10, No. 2 (Summer 1985), pp. 299-327 and the sources cited therein.

10. Explanations and data are presented in William A. Glaser, "Hospital Rate Regulation: American and Foreign Comparisons," *Journal of Health Politics, Policy and Law*, Vol. 8, No. 4 (Winter 1984), pp. 702-731.

11. Dean E. Farley, *Competition Among Hospitals: Market Structure and Its Relation to Utilization, Costs and Financial Position* (Washington, D.C.: Hospital Studies Program, National Center for Health Services Research, U.S. Department of Health and Human Services, 1985); James C. Robinson and Harold S. Luft, *Does Competition Reduce the Cost of Hospital Care?* (San

Francisco: Institute for Health Policy Studies, School of Medicine, University of California, 1985).

12. Robert F. Bridgman, *Hospital Utilization: An International Study* (Oxford: Oxford University Press, 1979), pp. 217–218, 232, and passim.

13. Evident in Pinker, *English Hospital Statistics, 1861–1938* (see note 4, above).

14. Max Shain and Milton Roemer, "Hospital Costs Relate to the Supply of Beds," *Modern Hospital*, Vol. 92, No. 4 (April 1959), p. 71. See also Milton I. Roemer, "Bed Supply and Hospital Utilization: A Natural Experiment," *Hospitals*, Vol. 35, No. 21 (Nov. 1, 1961), pp. 36–42. The principal cross-national comparison of health services utilization found that bed/population ratios were the principal correlate of admission rates: Robert Kohn and Kerr L. White (eds.), *Health Care: An International Study* (Oxford: Oxford University Press, 1976), Chap. 8.

15. See, for example, the unsentimental negotiations described in Eugenia S. Carpenter and Pamela Paul-Shaheen, "Implementing Regulatory Reform: The Saga of Michigan's Debedding Experiment," *Journal of Health Politics, Policy and Law*, Vol. 9, No. 3 (Fall 1984), pp. 453–473.

16. Mark R. Chassin, *Variations in Hospital Length of Stay: Their Relationship to Health Outcomes* (Washington, D.C.: Office of Technology Assessment, U.S. Congress, 1983), Chap. 2. Likewise, wide variations in length of stay among British districts are reported in G. Ferster and M. Butts, "Estimation of Notional Savings in Revenue Expenditure by Specialty at District Level," *Hospital and Health Services Review*, March 1978, p. 88.

17. My calculations from *Kosten en financiering van de gezondheidszorg* (The Hague: Centraal Bureau voor de Statistiek, biennial); *Vademecum gezondheidsstatistiek Nederland* (The Hague: Centraal Bureau voor de Statistiek, annual); and *Statisch zakboek* (The Hague: Centraal Bureau voor de Statistiek, annual).

18. David Kidder and Daniel Sullivan, "Hospital Payroll Costs, Productivity, and Employment Under Prospective Reimbursement," *Health Care Financing Review*, Vol. 4, No. 2 (Dec. 1982), pp. 89–99.

19. Nancy L. Worthington and Paula A. Piro, "The Effects of Hospital Rate-Setting Programs on Volumes of Hospital Services: A Preliminary Analysis," *Health Care Financing Review*, Vol. 4, No. 2 (Dec. 1982), pp. 47–66.

20. Gerard Anderson and Judith R. Lave, "State Rate-Setting Programs: Do They Reward Efficiency in Hospitals?" *Medical Care*, Vol. 22, No. 5 (May 1984), pp. 494–498.

21. My calculations from my own field research and from statistics supplied by the American Hospital Association, the French Ministry of Health, and the Swiss VESKA. Comparisons of French and American staffing for different types of hospitals at various times are presented in Simone Sandier, *Comparisons of Health Expenditures in France and the United States, 1950-78* (Washington, D.C.: National Center for Health Statistics, 1983), p. 28. Comparisons of European and American teaching hospitals appear in R. Gwyn Bevan and Frans Rutten, "Comparisons of the Costs, Organisation and Finance of University Hospitals of Different Countries" (paper prepared for the Workshop on the Cost and Financing of University Hospitals, Regional Office for Europe, World

Health Organization, Copenhagen, 1983); and Steven A. Schroeder, "A Comparison of Western European and US University Hospitals," *Journal of the American Medical Association*, Vol. 252, No. 2 (July 13, 1984), pp. 242–244.

22. For example, Heinz-J. Glumski, "Krankenhauswesen in den USA," *Krankenhaus-Umschau*, Vol. 53, No. 11 (Nov. 1984), p. 839.

23. My calculations from *Hospital Statistics* (Chicago: American Hospital Association, annual).

24. Allan S. Detsky and others, "The Effectiveness of a Regulatory Strategy in Containing Hospital Costs: The Ontario Experience, 1967–1981," *New England Journal of Medicine*, Vol. 309 (July 21, 1983), pp. 155–156.

25. Robert G. Evans, *Strained Mercy: The Economics of Canadian Health Care* (Toronto: Butterworths, 1984) pp. 163–164.

26. Communities varied in admission rates for conditions later clustered in DRGs. After adoption of payment by DRGs, doctors in low-admission communities could send more patients to hospitals, on the grounds that they were bringing medical practice up to national norms. The hospitals' revenue would benefit as least as well as the patients' health. John E. Wennberg, "Will Payment Based on Diagnosis-Related Groups Control Hospital Costs?" *New England Journal of Medicine*, Vol. 311, No. 5 (Aug. 2, 1984), pp. 295–300; John R. Griffith and others, "Clinical Profiles of Hospital Discharge Rates in Local Communities," *Health Services Research*, Vol. 20, No. 2 (June 1985), pp. 131–151.

27. Ross H. Arnett and Gordon R. Trapnell, "Private Health Insurance: New Measures of a Complex and Changing Industry," *Health Care Financing Review*, Vol. 6, No. 2 (Winter 1984), pp. 31–42. Management consultants advised firms how to control personnel costs by "take-backs" of their once generous health benefits. See, for instance, Gerard Tavernier, "Companies Prescribe Major Revisions in Medical Benefits Programs to Cut Soaring Healthcare Costs," *Management Review*, Vol. 72, No. 8 (Aug. 1983), p. 9 ff.

28. "1984 Hospital Cost and Utilization Trends," *Economic Trends* (American Hospital Association), Vol. 1, No. 1 (Spring 1985). Changes in hospital practices and expenditures during this period are summarized in Helen Darling, "Charting the Progress of Cost Containment," *Business and Health*, Vol. 2, No. 2 (Nov. 1984), pp. 30–33; and Linda E. Demkovich, "Public and Private Pressures to Control Health Care Costs May Be Paying Off," *National Journal*, Vol. 16, Nos. 50–1 (Dec. 15, 1984), pp. 2390–2393.

29. For an outstanding summary of the hypotheses and early evidence about the effects of Medicare DRGs, see Office of Technology Assessment, U.S. Congress, *Medicare's Prospective Payment System: Strategies for Evaluating Cost, Quality, and Medical Technology* (Washington, D.C.: U.S. Government Printing Office, 1985). The unexpected increase in net profits was discovered in *Financial Impact of the Prospective Payment System on Medicare Participating Hospitals* (Washington, D.C.: Office of Inspector General, Office of Audit, Department of Health and Human Services, 1986) and in other data reported in Prospective Payment Assessment Commission, *Technical Appendixes to the Report and Recommendations to the Secretary, U.S. Department of Health and Human Services—April 1, 1986* (Washington, D.C.: U.S. Government Printing Office, 1986), p. 23.

30. "1984 Hospital Cost and Utilization Trends" (see note 28, above).

31. "Recent Trends in Medical Professional Liability," *SMS Report* (American Medical Association), Vol. 4, No. 2 (March 1985). During another period of anxiety about malpractice liability a decade earlier, doctors had also increased their testing. Patricia Danzon, *Medical Malpractice* (Cambridge, Mass.: Harvard University Press, 1985), p. 149. But before DRGs the hospitals profited from additional testing.

32. Joyce Jensen and William Frock, "Early Discharge of Medicare Patients Pushes Hospitals into Long-Term Care," *Modern Healthcare,* Vol. 15, No. 23 (Nov. 8, 1985), pp. 56–57; Don E. Detmer, "Ambulatory Surgery," *New England Journal of Medicine,* Vol. 305 (Dec. 3, 1981), pp. 1406–1409; Monroe Lerner and others, *The Blue Cross Plan Utilization Differential* (Chicago: Health Services Foundation, 1983); Laurel L. Olson and others, "Providers Preparing for Major Battle over Market for Outpatient Surgery," *Modern Healthcare,* Vol. 14, No. 2 (Sept. 1984), pp. 82–98.

33. Unpublished data from the Health Research and Educational Trust of New Jersey.

34. U.S. Bureau of the Census, *Economic Characteristics of Households in the United States: Fourth Quarter 1983* (Washington, D.C.: U.S. Government Printing Office, 1985), p. 5.

35. Lu Ann Aday and others, *Access to Medical Care in the U.S.: Who Has It, Who Doesn't* (Chicago: Pluribus Press, 1984), Chaps. 2–4; Charlotte Muller, "Review of Twenty Years of Research on Medical Care Utilization," *Health Services Research,* Vol. 21, No. 2 (Part 1) (June 1986), pp. 131–135.

36. Suzanne Mulstein, "The Uninsured and the Financing of Uncompensated Care," *Inquiry,* Vol. 21, No. 3 (Fall 1984), pp. 214–222.

37. The complicated and contradictory evidence concerning differences in utilization is summarized in Pranlal Manga and Geoffery R. Weller, "The Failure of the Equity Objective in Health: A Comparative Analysis of Canada, Britain and the United States," *Comparative Social Research,* Vol. 3 (1980), pp. 229–267; and Alastair M. Gray, "Inequalities of Health: The Black Report, A Summary and Comment," *International Journal of Health Services,* Vol. 12, No. 3 (1982), pp. 349–380.

38. Robin F. Badgley and R. David Smith, *User Charges for Health Services* (Toronto: Ontario Council of Health, 1979), Part 3.

39. Brian Abel-Smith, *Cost Containment in Health Care* (London: Bedford Square Press, 1984), pp. 23–24 and passim.

40. John P. Bunker, "When Doctors Disagree," *New York Review of Books,* Vol. 32, No. 7 (April 25, 1985), pp. 7–12 and sources cited.

41. A. L. Cochrane, *Effectiveness and Efficiency* (London: Nuffield Provincial Hospitals Trust, 1972). For an American catalogue of discarded treatments, see John P. Bunker and others, *Costs, Risks, and Benefits of Surgery* (New York: Oxford University Press, 1977), esp. Chaps. 7, 8, 12, 13, 17.

42. See, for example, J. D. Hill and others, "A Randomised Trial of Home-Versus-Hospital Management for Patients with Suspected Myocardial Infarction," *Lancet,* Vol. 1 (1978), pp. 837–841 and sources cited therein.

43. As in the many comparisons of Britain and the United States in Henry J. Aaron and William B. Schwartz, *The Painful Prescription: Rationing Hospital Care* (Washington, D.C.: Brookings Institution, 1984).

44. This attitude is evident in the British reaction to Aaron and Schwartz's book (cited in note 43). See Rudolf Klein, "Rationing Health Care," *British Medical Journal,* Vol. 289, No. 6438 (July 21, 1984), pp. 143–144; and letters to *New England Journal of Medicine,* Vol. 310, No. 25 (June 21, 1984), pp. 1672–1673. Despite the apparent organizational similarity between Canadian and American hospitals, a Canadian analyst finds the American establishments far more lavish in technology, thereby accounting for the Americans' higher operating costs: Robert G. Evans, "Illusions of Necessity," *Journal of Health Politics, Policy and Law,* Vol. 10, No. 3 (Fall 1985), pp. 450–459.

45. L. M. J. Groot, "Medical Technology in the Health Care System of the Netherlands," in *The Implications of Cost-Effectiveness Analysis of Medical Technology. Background Paper No. 4: The Management of Health Care Technology in Ten Countries* (Washington, D.C.: Office of Technology Assessment, U.S. Congress, 1980), p. 151; and *Verslag van de Ziekenfondsraad over het jaar 1984 met de financiële gegevens over 1983* (Amstelveen, Netherlands: Ziekenfondsraad, 1984), p. 42.

46. *Compendium of Health Statistics,* 5th ed. (London: Office of Health Economics, 1984), Tables 3.15, 3.19.

47. Joseph E. Stone, *Hospital Organisation and Management,* 3rd ed. (London: Faber & Faber, 1939), p. 30.

48. Department of Health and Social Security and Office of Population Censuses and Surveys, *Hospital In-Patient Enquiry* (London: Her Majesty's Stationery Office, annual). The lengths of waiting lists vary widely among districts and specialties, according to *Guide to Hospital Waiting Lists* (London: College of Health, 1985).

49. Since long waiting lists are a persistent political embarrassment, DHSS has commissioned many special investigations of their management and content. Summarized in D. Hicks, *Waiting Lists—A Review* (London: Operational Research Branch, Department of Health and Social Security, 1972); *Reduction of Waiting Times for In-Patients Admission* (London: Department of Health and Social Security, 1975); Harrogate Seminar, *Waiting for Hospital Treatment* (London: Department of Health and Social Security, 1980), esp. pp. 5–13, 51–53.

50. That waiting lists are a real problem despite their inflation is argued in Harrogate Seminar (cited in note 49), pp. 5–13.

51. This is the remedy proposed by Anthony J. Culyer and John G. Cullis, "Some Economics of Hospital Waiting Lists in the NHS," *Journal of Social Policy,* Vol. 5, Part 3 (July 1976), pp. 255–263. A general critique of the firm systems' inefficiency in the management of the modern hospital appears in R. L. Himsworth, "What Price the Old Firm? or The Future of Hospital Practice," in Gordon McLachlan (ed.), *Specialized Futures* (Oxford: Oxford University Press, 1975), pp. 63–82.

52. John G. Cullis and Philip R. Jones, "Inpatient Waiting: A Discussion and Policy Proposal," *British Medical Journal,* Vol. 287 (Nov. 12, 1983), pp. 1483–1486.

53. Judith Feder and others, "Poor People and Poor Hospitals: Implications for Public Policy," *Journal of Health Politics, Policy and Law,* Vol. 9, No. 2

(Summer 1984), pp. 237–250; Alan Sager, "Why Urban Voluntary Hospitals Close," *Health Services Research*, Vol. 18, No. 3 (Fall 1983), pp. 451–481.

54. My calculations from *Compendium of Health Statistics* (see note 5, above), Table 3.11.

55. Alan Maynard and Anne Ludbrook, "Thirty Years of Fruitless Endeavor? An Analysis of Government in the Health Care Market," in Jacques van der Haag and Mark Perlman (eds.), *Health, Economics, and Health Economics* (Amsterdam: North-Holland Publishing Company, 1981), pp. 60–65.

56. Alan Maynard and Anne Ludbrook, "The Regional Allocation of Health Care Resources in the U.K. and France," *Social Policy and Administration*, Vol. 17, No. 3 (1983), pp. 232–248.

57. René Caquet, *Les alternatives à l'hospitalisation* (Paris: La Documentation Française, 1983).

58. Thomas Ferguson and A. N. MacPhail, *Hospital and Community* (Oxford: Oxford University Press, 1954), pp. 81–86.

59. Maxwell, *Health and Wealth* (see note 3, above), pp. 51–57.

60. R. D. Fraser, "An International Study of Health and General Systems of Financing Health Care," *International Journal of Health Services*, Vol. 3, No. 3 (1973), pp. 369–397.

61. Glaser, *Paying the Doctor* (Baltimore: Johns Hopkins University Press, 1970), Chaps. 3, 4, 7 passim; and Glaser, *Health Insurance Bargaining* (New York: Gardner Press and Wiley, 1978), Chaps. 2–7 passim.

62. David M. Eddy, "Variations in Physician Practice: The Role of Uncertainty," *Health Affairs*, Vol. 3, No. 2 (Summer 1984), pp. 74–89.

63. American methods and case studies are summarized in Kenneth E. Warner and Bryan R. Luce, *Cost-Benefit and Cost-Effectiveness Analysis in Health Care* (Ann Arbor, Mich.: Health Administration Press, 1982); and in *The Implications of Cost-Effectiveness Analysis of Medical Technology* (Washington, D.C.: Office of Technology Assessment, U.S. Congress, 1980–1982), several vols. British methods are described and case studies presented in Michael F. Drummond, *Principles of Economic Appraisal in Health Care* (Oxford: Oxford University Press, 1980). European contributions appear in the *International Journal of Technology Assessment in Health Care*.

64. See, for example, S. P. Martin and others, "Inputs into Coronary Care During 30 Years—A Cost-Effectiveness Study," *Annals of Internal Medicine*, Vol. 81 (1974), pp. 289–293.

65. James Lubitz and Ronald Deacon, "The Rise in the Incidence of Hospitalizations for the Aged, 1967 to 1979," *Health Care Financing Review*, Vol. 3, No. 3 (March 1982), pp. 21–40; Joseph Valvona and Frank Sloan, "Rising Rates of Surgery Among the Elderly," *Health Affairs*, Vol. 4, No. 3 (Fall 1985), pp. 108–119; and *Unnecessary Surgery: Double Jeopardy for Older Americans— Hearing Before the Special Committee on Aging, United States Senate, 99th Congress, First Session* (Washington, D.C.: U.S. Government Printing Office, 1985), pp. 71–97. American rates of surgery quoted in my text are taken from Lubitz and Deacon, p. 31.

66. An experimental method of paying for each patient by stage of disease rather than DRG would discourage surgery, since the hospital would be paid the same for medical treatment of the case: Rosanna M. Coffey and Marsha G.

Goldfarb, *DRG's and Disease Staging for Reimbursing Medicare Patients* (Washington, D.C.: National Center for Health Services Research, U.S. Department of Health and Human Services, 1983). But the surgeons would resist, since they would lose fees to the internists.

67. Lawrence S. Lewin and others, "Investor-Owneds and Nonprofits Differ in Economic Performance," *Hospital,* Vol. 55, No. 13 (July 1, 1981), pp. 52-58; Robert V. Pattison and Hallie M. Katz, "Investor-Owned and Not-for-Profit Hospitals: A Comparison Based on California Data," *New England Journal of Medicine,* Vol. 309 (Aug. 11, 1983), pp. 347-353; Hospital Cost Containment Board, State of Florida, *Annual Reports* (Tallahassee: Florida Hospital Cost Containment Board, 1981-82 and 1982-83).

68. See the numerous—but still incomplete—comparisons in Aaron and Schwartz, *The Painful Prescription* (note 43, above).

69. National survey of American hospital administrators, summarized in Bill Jackson and Joyce Jensen, "Most Administrators Fear Care Quality Will Be Hurt by Prospective Payment," *Modern Healthcare,* Vol. 14, No. 15 (Nov. 15, 1984), pp. 108, 110; field visits to hospitals during the first months of American Medicare's DRG payments, summarized in *Information Requirements for Evaluating the Impacts of Medicare Prospective Payment on Post-Hospital Long-Term-Care Services* (Washington, D.C.: U.S. General Accounting Office, 1985), and in Special Committee on Aging, U.S. Senate, *Impact of Medicare's Prospective Payment System on the Quality of Care Received by Medicare Beneficiaries* (Washington, D.C.: U.S. Government Printing Office, 1985).

70. Chassin, *Variations in Hospital Length of Stay: Their Relationship to Health Outcomes* (see note 16, above).

71. Bunker, "When Doctors Disagree" (see note 40, above).

72. Lee Soderstrom, "Federal-Provincial Cost-Sharing" (paper presented at the Conference of Canadian Health Economists, Regina, Sask., 1983). While total spending did not diminish, the new fiscal arrangements gave provinces more flexibility, and some shifted spending from hospitals to extramural programs: *Financing Confederation* (Ottawa: Economic Council of Canada, 1982), pp. 56-58.

73. The proposals for extensive cost sharing are summarized and criticized in Morris L. Barer and others, *Controlling Health Care Costs by Direct Charges to Patients: Snare or Delusion?* (Toronto: Ontario Economic Council, 1979).

74. Joseph P. Newhouse and others, *Some Interim Results from a Controlled Trial of Cost Sharing in Health Insurance* (Santa Monica, Calif.: Rand Corporation, 1982).

75. Joyce Jensen and Ned Miklovic, "High Medical Costs Forcing Patients to Postpone Seeking Medical Care," *Modern Healthcare,* Vol. 15, No. 14 (July 5, 1985), pp. 209-210.

76. Michael Nathanson, "Cost-Saving Technology Still a New Idea," *Modern Healthcare,* Vol. 14, No. 10 (Oct. 1984), p. 151.

Chapter Fourteen

1. I will describe the structure and financial decisions of European health insurance in a book now in preparation.

2. Barbara Starfield and others, *The Effectiveness of Medical Care: Validating Clinical Wisdom* (Baltimore: Johns Hopkins University Press, 1985); Jack Hadley, *More Medical Care, Better Health?* (Washington, D.C.: Urban Institute Press, 1982).

3. A forum for this work is the *International Journal of Technology Assessment in Health Care*. A principal source of information—read in many countries—is the "Health Technology Assessment Reports" commissioned by the National Center for Health Services Research and Health Care Technology Assessment, U.S. Department of Health and Human Services.

4. Thérèse Lecomte, "La concentration des dépenses de santé: Les 10% plus forts consommateurs," *Consommation,* No. 3 (July–Sept. 1978), pp. 65-101; *Qui consomme quoi?* (Paris: Caisse Nationale de l'Assurance Maladie, 1982); Steven T. Fleming and others, "A Multi-Dimensional Analysis of the Impact of High-Cost Hospitalization," *Inquiry,* Vol. 22, No. 2 (Summer 1985), pp. 178-187; James Lubitz, "The Use and Costs of Medicare Services in the Last Two Years of Life," *Health Care Financing Review,* Vol. 5, No. 3 (Spring 1984), pp. 117-131; and *Jahresbericht* (Bern: Krankenkasse KKB, 1984), pp. 7-8.

5. Anne Scitovsky and A. M. Capron, "Medical Care at the End of Life," *American Review of Public Health,* Vol. 7 (1986), pp. 59-75.

6. For example, Interacademiale werkgroep ziekenhuiswetenschappen, *Besturen in de gezondheidszorg: Concerns en circuits* (Lochem, Netherlands: Uitgeversmaatschappij de Tijdstroom, 1984); and *Discussienota inzake een samenhangende zorgstructuur* and *Advies inzake een samenhangende zorgstructuur* (Amstelveen, Netherlands: Ziekenfondsraad, 1983 and 1985).

7. H. J. Schroeder (ed.), *Canons and Decrees of the Council of Trent* (St. Louis: B. Herder, 1941), pp. 240-241.

8. For example, one of America's leading hospital managers, and head of a teaching hospital, reported to the annual conference of the American Hospital Association of his successes in reducing the use of rubber gloves in the operating theater and in selling off the hospital's library: George P. Ludlum, floor discussions in *Transactions of the Association of Hospital Superintendents: Seventh Annual Conference,* Vol. 7 (1905), pp. 186-187; and *Transactions of the American Hospital Association: Ninth Annual Conference,* Vol. 9 (1907), pp. 188-190.

Appendix A

1. My calculations from Jean-Pierre Poullier, *Measuring Health Care, 1960-1983* (Paris: Organisation for Economic Co-operation and Development, 1985), Tables D-6, H-1.

2. As in Robert J. Maxwell, *Health and Wealth* (Lexington, Mass.: Lexington Books, 1981), pp. 35, 38, 41.

Glossary of Abbreviations

Abbreviation	Name	Meaning
GENERAL		
CPI	consumer price index	Measure of annual change in a nation's cost of living.
FTE	full-time equivalent	A count of workers whereby total work hours are divided by the normal workweek.
GDP	gross domestic product	GNP minus net-factor payments (interest, profits, and salary remittances) from nonresidents.
GNP	gross national product	The total value of all goods and services produced each year in a nation.
NHI	national health insurance	Statute requiring persons to join a sickness fund and requiring employers and workers to pay premiums.
OPD	outpatient department	The service of the hospital for treating ambulatory patients.
GREAT BRITAIN		
COHSE	Confederation of Health Service Employees	Union representing nurses and domestics.
DHA	District Health Authority	The basic tier for policy making and management.
DHSS	Department of Health and Social Security	Ministry of the national government.
DMT	District Management Team	Executive at the district tier.
GP	general practitioner	
NALGO	National Association of Local Government Officers	Union representing administrators and clerks in NHS.

473

Abbreviation	*Name*	*Meaning*

NHS	National Health Service	Hierarchy of committees and their employees who plan and manage health services.
NUPE	National Union of Public Employees	Union representing blue-collar workers in NHS.
PES	Public Expenditure Survey	The national government's expenditure-planning system.
RAWP	Resource Allocation Working Party	The formula for distributing funds among regions.
RCCS	Revenue Consequences of Capital Schemes	Operating money added for new programs.
RCN	Royal College of Nursing	Professional association of the diplomaed nurses.
RHA	Regional Health Authority	Regional tier for policy making.
SIFT	Service Increment for Teaching	Additional operating money to RHSs and DHAs to cover their costs of teaching undergraduate medical students.
SMR	Standardised Mortality Ratio	Proxy for morbidity used in RAWP formula.

UNITED STATES

AMA	American Medical Association	National professional association of physicians.
CON	Certificate of Need	A license issued by a state government, authorizing operation of a building or program.
DHHS	Department of Health and Human Services	A Ministry of the national government.
DRG	diagnosis-related group	A classification of patients.
HCFA	Health Care Financing Administration	Agency within DHHS that administers Medicare and Medicaid.
HIAA	Health Insurance Association of America	Trade association of commercial insurers.
HMO	Health Maintenance Organization	A prepaid multispecialty group of physicians, usually with extensive facilities.
NLRA	National Labor Relations Act	Law of the United States government regulating collective bargaining between trade unions and employers.
PPO	Preferred Provider Organization	Any group or organization that offers health care at a lower price.
PRO (formerly PSRO)	Peer Review Organization	A commission created by national law to monitor utilization of hospitals under Medicare.

CANADA

HIDS	Hospital Insurance and Diagnostic Services	National government's program of conditional grants to provinces.

Abbreviation	Name	Literal translation into English	Meaning
FRANCE			
CHR	Centre Hospitalier Régional	Regional Hospital Center	Group of public hospitals that accepts referrals from a region.
CHU	Centre Hospitalier Universitaire	University Hospital Center	A CHR that is affiliated with a university for teaching and research.
CH	Centre Hospitalier	Hospital Center	A public hospital or group that provides clinical specialties other than the most technical.
CNAMTS	Caisse Nationale de l'Assurance Maladie des Travailleurs Salariés	National Fund for the Health Insurance of Wage Earners	Official sickness fund for the large majority of French workers.
CCSMA	Caisse Centrale de Secours Mutuels Agricoles	Central Fund for Cooperative Agricultural Assistance	Official sickness fund for farmers.
CANAM	Caisse Nationale d'Assurance Maladie et Maternité des Travailleurs Non Salariés des Professions Non Agricoles	National Fund for the Health Insurance and Maternity Benefits of Nonwage and Nonagricultural Workers	Official sickness fund for businessmen, professionals, artisans.
CRAM	Caisse Régionale de l'Assurance Maladie	Regional Health Insurance	Regional office of CNAMTS.
CSMF	Confédération des Syndicats Médicaux Français	Confederation of French Medical Syndicates	Principal association of French doctors concerned with economic interests.
DDASS	Direction Départementale des Affaires Sanitaires et Sociales	Departmental Office for Health and Social Affairs	Field staff of the Ministry of Social Affairs.
DRASS	Direction Régionale des Affaires Sanitaires et Sociales	Regional Office for Health and Social Affairs	Field staff of the Ministry of Social Affairs in the region.
FHF	Fédération Hospitalière de France	Hospital Federation of France	National association of all public hospitals.
FIEHP	Fédération Intersyndicale des Etablissements d'Hospitalisation Privée	Federation of Syndicates of Private Hospitals	Principal national association of the for-profit private hospitals.
H	Hôpital	Hospital	An acute hospital with the basic specialties.
WEST GERMANY			
KHG	Krankenhausfinanzierungsgesetz	Hospital Finance Law	Principal law about capital grants and operating costs.
BPflVO	Bundespflegesatzverordnung	Federal Decree on Daily Charges	Regulations specifying allowable costs for the prospective budget.
SKB	Selbstkostenblätter	Sheets with Total Operating Costs	The form for last year's operating costs and next year's prospective budget.
RVO	Reichsversicherungsordnung	Imperial Insurance Decree	Statute that created national health insurance.

Abbreviation	Name	Literal translation into English	Meaning
WEST GERMANY (continued)			
RVO-Kassen	Gesetzliche Krankenkassen	Statutory Sickness Funds	Funds that administer national health insurance.
BOK	Bundesverband der Ortskrankenkassen	Federal Union of Local Sickness Funds	National leadership of the largest association of sickness funds.
KA	Konzertierte Aktion im Gesundheitswesens	Coordinating Body in Health Affairs	Forum of several groups that recommends policy targets.
BAT	Bundes-Angestelltentarif-vertrag	Federal Administrators Wage Contract	Framework contract for administrators and professionals employed by government.
DAG	Deutsche Angestellten-Gewerkschaft	German Union of Administrators	Federation representing salaried and professional workers.
KV	Kassenärztliche Vereinigung	Association of Fund Doctors	Society of doctors in health insurance practice in each province.
NETHERLANDS			
COZ	Stichting Centraal Orgaan Ziekenhuistarieven	Central Agency for Hospital Charges	Commission that fixed hospital rates 1965–1982.
COTG	Centraal Orgaan Tarieven Gesondheidszorg	Central Agency for Health Care Charges	Commission that fixes the rates of hospitals and of other providers, 1982 et seq.
NZI	Nationaal Ziekenhuisinstituut	National Hospital Institute	Research and educational agency for hospital industry.
NZR	Nationaal Ziekenhuis Raad	National Hospital Council	Association of all private and public hospitals.
SWITZERLAND			
VESKA	Vereinigung Schweizerische Krankenhäuser	Association of Swiss Hospitals	National association of all public and private hospitals.

Index